GW00393290

THE VETERINARY FORMULARY
Handbook of Medicines Used in Veterinary Practice

THE VETERINARY FORMULARY

Handbook of Medicines Used in Veterinary Practice

First Edition

Edited by
Yolande M Debuf

Prepared in the Department of Pharmaceutical Sciences of the
Royal Pharmaceutical Society of Great Britain

London
THE PHARMACEUTICAL PRESS
1991

Copyright © 1991 by the Royal Pharmaceutical Society of Great Britain

All rights reserved. No part of this publication may be reproduced, stored in a retrieval system, or transmitted in any form or by any means – electronic, mechanical, photocopying, recording or otherwise – without the prior written permission of the copyright holder.

Copies of this book may be obtained through any good bookseller or, in any case of difficulty, direct from the publisher or the publisher's agents:

The Pharmaceutical Press
1 Lambeth High Street, London SE1 7JN, England

Australia
The Australian Pharmaceutical Publishing Co. Ltd
40 Burwood Road, Hawthorn, Victoria 3122
and
The Pharmaceutical Society of Australia
Pharmacy House, PO Box 21, Curtin, ACT 2605

Germany, Austria, Switzerland
Deutscher Apotheker Verlag
Postfach 10 10 61, Birkenwaldstrasse 44, D-7000 Stuttgart 10

India
Arnold Publishers (India) Pte Ltd
AB/9 Safdarjung Enclave, New Delhi 110029

Japan
Maruzen Co. Ltd
3-10 Nihonbashi 2-chome, Chuo-ku, Tokyo 103
or
PO Box 5050, Tokyo International, 100-31

New Zealand
The Pharmaceutical Society of New Zealand, Pharmacy House,
124 Dixon Street, PO Box 11640, Wellington 1

USA
Rittenhouse Book Distributors, Inc.
511 Feheley Drive, King of Prussia, PA 19406

British Library Cataloguing-in-Publication Data

The veterinary formulary.
  I. Debuf, Yolande
  636.089

ISBN 0 85369 245 9

Typeset, printed, and bound in Great Britain by Page Bros, Norwich, Norfolk
NR6 6SA

THE VETERINARY FORMULARY
Advisory Committee 1987-1991

Chairman
Professor A Steele-Bodger, CBE, MA, BSc, FRCVS

Committee Members

E N Boden, MRPharmS
M Braithwaite, BPharm, MRPharmS
J L Crooks, MRCVS
E G Hartley, MRCVS

Professor P M Keen, BVSc, PhD, MRCVS
B Lazonby, MRPharmS
Professor P Lees, BPharm, PhD, CBiol, FIBiol, Hon Assoc RCVS

W T Turner, BVetMed, MRCVS

Department of Pharmaceutical Sciences

Director
W G Thomas, MSc, PhD, FRPharmS

General Editor of Scientific Publications
A Wade, BPharm, MPhil, FRPharmS

The Veterinary Formulary
Editorial Staff

Editor
Y M Debuf, BSc, BVMS, MRCVS

K B K Davis, MRPharmS
P Gotecha, BSc, MRPharmS
J Martin, BPharm, PhD, MRPharmS

Contents

GUIDANCE ON PRESCRIBING

CLASSIFIED NOTES ON DRUGS AND PREPARATIONS

APPENDIXES AND INDEXES

Preface

Between 1950 and 1970 the Pharmaceutical Society, with the assistance of the veterinary profession, published the British Veterinary Codex (BVetC) 1953 and 1965 and two supplements 1959 and 1970. The BVetC aimed to provide standards for the drugs and medicines in veterinary use together with authoritative statements on their actions and usage, dosage in various species, and methods of preparation. This was a development of the information given for human medicines by the British Pharmaceutical Codex (BPC). In 1972 the Medicines Commission decided that all standards for medicines should be collected in one source, the British Pharmacopoeia, and editions of the British Pharmacopoeia (Veterinary) 1977 and 1985 were subsequently produced. The other information in the BVetC was discontinued.

The success of the revised form of the British National Formulary from 1981 suggested there was a place for a book on animal medicines organised on similar lines. In 1986 the Pharmaceutical Society agreed to start work on a book that would describe veterinary drugs and medicines in a pharmacological and therapeutic classification and present the information in a manner that would be easy to use. Due to the increasing cost of licensing and legislation fewer drugs are becoming available with veterinary licences. It was therefore decided to include information on a selection of medicines licensed only for use in humans, but known to be used in veterinary medicine. The responsibility for the use of such human medicines rests with the veterinarian.

This is the first edition of The Veterinary Formulary. It is intended as a text for rapid reference primarily for veterinarians but will also be valuable for pharmacists and others involved with animal health-care. The Veterinary Formulary does not aim to contain all information necessary for prescribing. Specialised publications and manufacturers' data sheets for veterinary medicines and human preparations should be consulted as necessary and taken into account according to the clinical condition. The book aims to promote rational and effective treatment by grouping together the similar preparations of each drug. Information is classified under a body system, disease or condition. Drug information included in the text comprises mechanism of action, therapeutic indications, side-effects, and dosages considered suitable for use in the domestic species including horses, cattle, sheep, pigs, dogs, cats, and poultry.

Information on fish, rabbits and rodents, and non-domestic species such as exotic birds and reptiles is also provided and includes extensive tables of antimicrobial, parasiticide, and anaesthetic dosages together with notes on diseases and conditions commonly treated in these species and methods of drug administration. The Appendixes include comprehensive lists of drug interactions and drug incompatibilities.

The majority of the text for The Veterinary Formulary was written by expert authors and reviewed by the Advisory Committee. The Royal Pharmaceutical Society would like to thank the following contributors for their valuable assistance.

W M Allen, DVSc, PhD, MSc, MRCVS

Professor J D Baggot, BSc, MVM, PhD, DSc, FAVCPT, MRCVS

K C Barnett, MA, PhD, BSc, DVOphthal, MRCVS

L A Brown, BVSc, PhD, MRCVS

B H Coles, BVSc, MRCVS

M J Cooper, BVM&S, PhD, MRCVS

B M Corcoran, MVB, MRCVS

M J Corke, MA, BVetMed, MRCVS

J L Crooks, MRCVS

R Curtis, PhD, MSc, BVSc, DTVM, DVOphthal, FRCVS

R J Curtis, BSc, MIBiol, PhD

M Davies, BVetMed, CertVR, CertSAO, MRCVS

J M Dobson, DVetMed, MRCVS

P A Flecknell, MA, VetMB, PhD, DLAS, MRCVS

R M Gaskell, BVSc, PhD, MRCVS

G Grant, BVMS, MRCVS

M W Gregory, PhD, BVSc, DipIEMVT, CBiol, MIBiol, MRCVS

L W Hall, MA, BSc, PhD, DVA, MRCVS

M E Herrtage, MA, BVSc, DVR, DVD, MRCVS

Professor D E Jacobs, BVMS, PhD, MRCVS

A M Johnston, BVM&S, MRCVS

Professor R S Jones, MVSc, DrMedVet, DVA, FRCVS

Professor P M Keen, BVSc, PhD, MRCVS

J K Kirkwood, BVSc, PhD, MRCVS

A Knifton, BVSc, BSc, PhD, MRCVS

M P C Lawton, BVetMed, CertVOphthal, GIBiol, FRCVS

Professor P Lees, BPharm, PhD, CBiol, FIBiol, Hon Assoc RCVS

A Livingston, PhD, BSc, BVetMed, MRCVS

D H Lloyd, BVetMed, PhD, MRCVS

W B Martin, PhD, DVSM, FRSE, CBiol, FIBiol, MRCVS

S E Matic, BVSc, MA, DVR, DVC, MRCVS

A R Michell, BVetMed, BSc, PhD, MRCVS

D J Middleton, MVSc, PhD, MRCVS

A R Peters, DVetMed, BA, PhD, FRCVS

R C Pilsworth, MA, VetMB, BSc, CertVR, MRCVS

S W Ricketts, BSc, BVSc, DESM, FRCVS

P D Rossdale, MA, PhD, FACVSc, DESM, FRCVS

G C Skerritt, BVSc, FRCVS

L R Thomsett, DVD, FRCVS

W T Turner, BVetMed, MRCVS

R B Williams, BVSc, MPhil, MRCVS

C D Wilson, MRCVS

J Wingfield, LLM, MPhil, BPharm, DipAgVetPharm, MRPharmS

S S Young, MA, VetMB, PhD, DVA, MRCVS .

We would also like to acknowledge the work of the late James C Stuart who provided text for the sections dealing with poultry. The assistance of his colleague is greatly appreciated.

Many organisations have been extremely helpful and have provided useful information. The assistance of veterinary product manufacturers in providing details of their products is gratefully appreciated as is the help given by the Veterinary Medicines Directorate in checking certain details. The Royal Pharmaceutical Society would also like to acknowledge the assistance of Eric Greenfield who started the work by organising the preparations into a classification and the late Jeffrey Greenfield who continued the work as Editor until 1989. The Committee has also been assisted by Joy Wingfield and Bruce Rhodes. The secretarial assistance provided by Thelma Roberts and the assistance given by Pamela North, BPharm, MRPharmS, MIInfSc and all the staff of the library and information department are greatly appreciated.

The RSPGB is anxious to ensure that The Veterinary Formulary is suited to the needs of its readers. Recognising that amendments and updating will be necessary in future editions, the editor welcomes any comments and constructive criticism that can be considered when the text is revised. These should be sent to the Editor, The Veterinary Formulary, 1 Lambeth High Street, London SE1 7JN.

Arrangement of information

Guidance on prescribing
In this section, different aspects of prescribing in veterinary practice are discussed. General guidance provides information on the safe and appropriate use of medicines; Legal aspects of prescribing covers the control of medicines, prescription writing, labelling requirements, and medicated feeding stuffs including the veterinary written direction. Prescribing for animals used in competitions is considered with reference to the sporting authorities, and their rules and regulations. There are notes on prescribing for the domestic species including specific sections on prescribing for neonates, pregnant animals, hepatic impairment, renal impairment, and lactating animals. The sections on exotic species such as reptiles and exotic birds or less frequently encountered companion animals such as fish, rabbits, and rodents include common clinical conditions, methods of drug administration, and extensive tabular data on drug dosage including antimicrobial drugs, parasiticides, and anaesthetics. Information on the initial management of acute poisoning in animals, symptomatic therapy, and specific antidotes for more frequently encountered poisons are discussed in the section Emergency treatment of poisoning.

Classified notes on drugs and preparations
The main text consists of 18 chapters each covering a particular body system, condition, or drug category. The information provided in the chapters concerns the use and administration of medicines and drugs to the domestic species including horses, cattle, sheep, goats, pigs, dogs, cats, and poultry. Each chapter is divided into numbered sections such that similar drugs are grouped together. Text on the use of these drugs in veterinary practice, mechanism of action, and adverse effects is given, which is followed by drug monographs and relevant medicines, whether generic or proprietary. Preparations that are licensed in the UK for use in animals and, where these are unavailable, products that are licensed for use in humans and commonly used in veterinary medicine are included. The latter are printed in small typeface for easy recognition and occur predominantly in the chapters dealing with the Cardiovascular System, Endocrine System, and Malignant Disease. Occasionally, information on the use of a veterinary preparation for an unlicensed indication is given and denoted by ♦. The responsibility for their use lies with the veterinarian who has the 'animal under his care' (see General guidance, page 5).

Appendixes and indexes
The appendixes include Drug Interactions and Drug Incompatibilities. Information is arranged under drug name, drug group name, or therapeutic category and listed alphabetically. Appendix 3 provides useful conversions of mass, volume, and temperature from imperial to metric units, and an explanation of terms such as tonicity.
The Index of Manufacturers and Organisations lists addresses of manufacturers whose preparations appear in The Veterinary Formulary and also organisations associated with veterinary practice.
The general Index should be used to locate information on drugs, medicines, and diseases. The main information on drugs is given on the page numbers identified in **bold** type.

Symbols used in The Veterinary Formulary

Internationally recognised units and symbols are used in The Veterinary Formulary wherever possible.

≡ — equivalent to
°C — degrees Celsius (centigrade). Unless otherwise stated in the text, temperatures are expressed in this thermometric scale
⧫ — veterinary preparation or veterinary drug used for an unlicensed indication
CD — controlled drug, see Legal aspects of prescribing, page 8
GSL — general sale list, see Legal aspects of prescribing, page 8
P — pharmacy-only medicine, see Legal aspects of prescribing, page 8
PML — pharmacy merchants list, see Legal aspects of prescribing, page 8
PoM — prescription-only medicine, see Legal aspects of prescribing, page 8
™ — trade mark

Abbreviations used in The Veterinary Formulary

For abbreviations of names of manufacturers and organisations associated with veterinary practice *see also* Index of Manufacturers and Organisations, pages 411-422.

ATC — animal test certificate
BEVA — British Equine Veterinary Association
BP — British Pharmacopoeia 1988 and Addenda 1989, 1990, and 1991
BP(Vet) — British Pharmacopoeia (Veterinary) 1985 and Addendum 1988
BSAVA — British Small Animal Veterinary Association
BUN — blood-urea-nitrogen
BVA — British Veterinary Association
BVetC — British Veterinary Codex and Supplement 1970
cm — centimetre(s)
DANI — Department of Agriculture, Northern Ireland
DNA — deoxyribonucleic acid
DVO — District Veterinary Officer
e/c — enteric coated
ECF — extracellular fluid
ECG — electrocardiogram
g — gram(s)
HSE — Health and Safety Executive
i.m. — intramuscular
i.v. — intravenous
kg — kilogram(s)
L — litre(s)
M — molar
m² — square metres
mg — milligram(s)
MIC — minimum inhibitory concentration
mL — millilitre(s)
MMB — Milk Marketing Board
mmHg — millimetre(s) of mercury
NPIS — National Poisons Information Service
pH — the negative logarithm of the hydrogen ion concentration
PL — product licence
p.o. — by mouth
RCVS — Royal College of Veterinary Surgeons
RPSGB — Royal Pharmaceutical Society of Great Britain
RSPCA — Royal Society for the Prevention of Cruelty to Animals
s.c. — subcutaneous
soln. — solution
s/r — sustained release
UK — United Kingdom
units — standard international units, unless otherwise stated in the text. *See also* Appendix 3, page 408
USA — United States of America
VMD — Veterinary Medicines Directorate
VWD — veterinary written direction

Late changes to veterinary preparations

The Review of Veterinary Medicines by the Veterinary Medicines Directorate continues and many changes to details of preparations licensed for use in animals are constantly being received from manufacturers. The following are changes to preparations that could not be incorporated into the main body of text.

New veterinary preparations

GSL **Aerosol Ringworm Remedy** (Alfa-Laval)
Spray, dichlorophen 3%, undecenoic acid 3%; 168 g

PoM **Amoxinsol 50**™ (Univet)
Oral powder, for addition to drinking water, amoxycillin trihydrate 500 mg/g, for *broiler chickens, layer hens*; 150 g
Withdrawal Periods. *Poultry*: slaughter 7 days, eggs from treated birds should not be used for human consumption

PoM **Aquacil**™ (Hand/PH)
Powder, for addition to feed, amoxycillin trihydrate 500 g/kg, for *salmon*; 1 kg, 2 kg
Withdrawal Periods. *Fish*: slaughter 500° days

PoM **Bimoxyl**™ **LA** (Bimeda)
Depot injection (oily), amoxycillin (as trihydrate) 150 mg/mL, for *cattle*; 100 mL
Withdrawal Periods. *Cattle*: slaughter 21 days, milk 72 hours

PoM **Dazole**™ **40%** (Hand/PH)
Oral powder, for addition to drinking water, dimetridazole 400 g/kg, for *pigs* (see section 1.1.8), *chickens, turkeys, game birds*; 120 g, 2 kg
Withdrawal Periods. *Pigs, poultry, game birds*: slaughter 6 days

PML **Dextrose 40%** (Bimeda)
Intravenous infusion, glucose 40%, for *cattle, sheep*; 400 mL

GSL **Footrot Aerosol** (Alfa-Laval)
Spray, cetrimide 6%, diethyl phthalate 2%, for *sheep*; 168 g, 400 g

PoM **Insuvet**™ **Lente** (Fisons)
Injection, insulin zinc suspension (bovine, highly purified) 100 units/mL, for *dogs, cats*; 10 mL

PoM **Insuvet**™ **Neutral** (Fisons)
Injection, soluble insulin (bovine, highly purified) 100 units/mL, for *dogs, cats*; 10 mL

PoM **Insuvet**™ **Protamine Zinc** (Fisons)
Injection, protamine zinc insulin (bovine, highly purified) 100 units/mL, for *dogs, cats*; 10 mL

PoM **Katavac**™ **CHP** (Duphar)
Injection, powder for reconstitution, combined feline calicivirus, FPL, and FVR vaccine, living, prepared from viruses grown on an established feline cell line, for *cats*; 1-dose vial
Dose. *Cats*: *by subcutaneous or intramuscular injection*, 1 dose, see manufacturer details for vaccination programmes

PoM **Navilox**™ (Univet)
Oral powder, isoxsuprine hydrochloride 30 mg/g, for *horses*; 300 g
Withdrawal Periods. Should not be used in *horses* intended for human consumption
Dose. *Horses*: 600 micrograms/kg of isoxsuprine twice daily for 6 weeks, then once daily for 3 weeks, then every other day for 3 weeks

PoM **Omnisol 200**™ (Hand/PH)
Oral powder, for addition to milk, milk replacer, or to prepare an oral solution, chlortetracycline hydrochloride 200 g/kg, for *calves*; 120 g, 2 kg
Withdrawal Periods. *Calves*: slaughter 7 days

PoM **Oralject Sedazine-ACP**™ (Vetsearch; distributed by Millpledge)
Oral paste, acepromazine (as maleate) 8.9 mg/mL, for *horses*; 30-mL metered dose applicator

Withdrawal Periods. Should not be used in *horses* intended for human consumption

PoM **Parvovac**™ (RMB)
Injection, porcine parvovirus vaccine, inactivated, prepared from virus, containing a suitable oil as adjuvant, for *pigs*; 10 mL
Dose. *Pigs: by intramuscular injection*, 2 mL

GSL **Piperazine Citrate BP(Vet)** (Distributed by Millpledge)
Tablets, piperazine citrate 500 mg, for *dogs, cats*; 500

GSL **Prevender**™ **Insecticidal Collar for the Dog** (Virbac)
Diazinon 15%, for *dogs*

GSL **Prevender**™ **Insecticidal Collar for the Large Dog** (Virbac)
Diazinon 15%, for *dogs*

GSL **Ruby Adult Dog Wormer** (Spencer)
Tablets, dichlorophen 500 mg, for *dogs, cats*; 8

GSL **Stardine**™ **3:1** (Lever)
Teat dip, spray, or udderwash, available iodine 1.5%, glycerol, for *cattle*; 5 litres, 25 litres
Teat dip or spray. Dilute 1 volume with 3 volumes water
Udderwash. Dilute 1.67 mL in 1 litre water

GSL **Stardine**™ **RTU** (Lever)
Teat dip or spray, available iodine 0.6%, glycerol, for *cattle*; 25 litres

GSL **Startex**™ **7:1** (Lever)
Teat dip or spray, chlorhexidine 2.55%, glycerol, for *cattle*; 3.125 litres, 25 litres
Dilute 1 volume with 7 volumes water

GSL **Startex**™ **RTU** (Lever)
Teat dip or spray, chlorhexidine gluconate 0.5%, glycerol, for *cattle*; 25 litres

PoM **Synutrim**™ **30% Soluble** (Hand/PH)
Oral powder, for addition to milk, milk replacer, or to prepare an oral solution, co-trimazine 50/250 [trimethoprim 50 g, sulphadiazine 250 g]/kg, for *calves*; 150 g, 2 kg
Withdrawal Periods. *Calves*: slaughter 10 days

PoM **Ventipulmin**™ (Boehringer Ingelheim)
Syrup, clenbuterol 25 micrograms/mL, for *horses*; 355-dose applicator
Withdrawal Periods. Should not be used in *horses* intended for human consumption

PML **Vermisole**™ **Forte** (Bimeda)
Oral solution, levamisole hydrochloride 75 mg/mL, for *cattle, sheep*; 500 mL
Withdrawal Periods. *Cattle*: slaughter 21 days, milk 48 hours. *Sheep*: slaughter 21 days, milk from treated animals should not be used for human consumption

Discontinued veterinary preparations

Abidec™ (Parke-Davis)
Alugan™ (Hoechst)
Corneocaine™ (Bimeda)
Defungit™ (Hoechst)
Furasol™ (SmithKline Beecham)
Head-to-Tail™ **PB Dressing** (Coopers Pitman-Moore)
Head-to-Tail™ **Demodectic Mange Dressing** (Coopers Pitman-Moore)

Hostacain™ **2%** (Hoechst)
Monensin-100 Ruminant (Hand/PH)
Orbisan™ **Forte** (SmithKline Beecham)
Parentrovite™ (SmithKline Beecham)
Powacide™ (SmithKline Beecham)
Vitamin AD₃E (Animalcare)

Changes to Withdrawal Periods statement

PoM **Penbritin**™ **Veterinary** (SmithKline Beecham)
Withdrawal Periods. Should not be used in *horses* intended for human consumption

GUIDANCE ON PRESCRIBING

General guidance

The general principle of prescribing for animals is that no medicinal product should be administered to a patient unless specifically indicated. In all cases the benefit of administering the medicine should be considered in relation to the risks involved, particularly in food animals.

Administration and owner compliance. Ease of administration must be assigned a high priority when prescribing medicinal products to be given by the owner. Failure to comply with dose recommendations can often account for an apparently poor response to therapy. It is the responsibility of the veterinary surgeon to prescribe medicinal products that the owner can readily administer to the animal at convenient intervals.

Doses. The doses stated in The Veterinary Formulary are intended for general guidance only and represent, unless otherwise stated, the usual range of doses that are generally regarded as suitable for the species indicated. Doses are given in amounts per kilogram bodyweight wherever possible. Doses of drugs to be administered in the drinking water or feed are usually expressed as amount per 100 litres of drinking water or per tonne of feed. All doses are for administration by mouth, unless otherwise stated. The doses are expressed in terms of the drug substance indicated by the monograph title unless otherwise specified. For the purposes of The Veterinary Formulary 'small animals' are considered to be dogs and cats; 'large animals' to be horses, cattle, sheep, and pigs.

Some proprietary and non-proprietary medicines licensed for human use have been included in The Veterinary Formulary. These particular preparations are known to be used in veterinary medicine and have been included when no similar licensed veterinary product is available. Readers should be aware that dosages for drugs that have no veterinary licensed products are commonly used doses. Such doses may not have been derived from research in the particular species being treated; they are to be used when no suitable veterinary product is available and the responsibility for their use lies with the veterinary surgeon.

Drug monograph titles. The drug titles used in The Veterinary Formulary are British Approved Names (BAN) or International Nonproprietary Names (INN), wherever possible. The British Pharmacopoeia Commission has approved several names for substance-combinations. They are identified by the co- prefix. It should be noted that the strengths of ingredients in the combination follow the order of ingredients expressed in the title. For example, co-amoxiclav 40/10 is amoxycillin (as trihydrate) 40 mg with clavulanic acid (as potassium salt) 10 mg. The strength of the ingredients is always listed in the same units; co-trimazine 200/1000, for example, consists of trimethoprim 200 mg and sulphadiazine 1 g.

The licensed indications listed under a drug monograph title may not apply to all preparations of that substance.

Proprietary titles. Names followed by the symbol ™ are or have been used as proprietary names in the UK. These names may in general be applied only to products supplied by the owners of the trade marks.

Licence to manufacture substances or products protected by Letters Patent is neither conveyed, nor implied, by the inclusion of information on such substances in The Veterinary Formulary.

Adverse drug reactions. Any drug may produce unwanted or unexpected adverse reactions. Detection and recording of these are important and veterinarians are urged to help by reporting suspected adverse reactions to:

The Veterinary Medicines Directorate
Woodham Lane,
New Haw, Weybridge, Surrey
KT15 3NB

Form MLA 252A is available on request from the VMD. The form is shown below.

Ministry of Agriculture, Fisheries and Food

In Confidence

Veterinary Medicines – Report on Suspected Adverse Reactions

- This form should be completed whenever a suspected adverse reaction is observed in animals (including birds and fish) during the use of a veterinary medicinal product.
- Suspected adverse reactions to veterinary medicinal products in operators or members of the public should also be reported on this form.
- Please send the completed form to the **Veterinary Medicines Directorate, FREEPOST, Central Veterinary Laboratory, New Haw, Weybridge, Surrey KT15 3NB.** For further information please write to us at this address.
- *Please use BLOCK LETTERS*   *Tick box if extra forms are required*

Name of product

Batch No. of product _____ Product Licence No. _____

Address where
reaction(s) occurred _____
_____ County _____

Name and address of
person reporting the
adverse reaction(s) to
Veterinary Medicines
Directorate
_____ Telephone No. _____

Name and address of
veterinarian involved
(if not given above)
_____ Telephone No. _____

Has the Product Licence holder been informed?   *Please tick appropriate box:*   Yes ☐   No ☐

No. of animals treated _____ No. of animals reacting _____ No. of deaths _____

Dosage (in mg / kg body weight if applicable) _____
Route of administration used
and duration of treatment _____

DETAILS OF REACTION(S) IN ANIMALS *(Please continue on a separate sheet if necessary)*

Date of reaction(s)	Species / Breed	Sex (M / F)	Age	Nature of reaction and diagnosis obtained

Were any other products given concurrently?   *Please tick appropriate box:*   Yes ☐   No ☐
If the answer is **Yes**, please give details:

Please attach results from PM or other relevant diagnostic tests.
Are any results to follow?   *Please tick appropriate box:*   Yes ☐   No ☐
Any other comments you may wish to make:

DETAILS OF SUSPECTED REACTION(S) IN MAN
(If more than one person, please give details on a separate sheet)

Name _____ Age _____ Sex _____

Nature of exposure and reaction (symptom(s), duration): _____

Name of doctor /
hospital (if consulted) _____ Telephone No. _____

For Official Use Only

Adverse Reaction No. _____ VLM file _____ Date arrived in Office | | | | |

MLA 252A(Revised 8/89)   Acknowledgment sent | | | | |

Suspected adverse reactions in animals as well as in any persons who handle the medicines should be reported. Lack of efficacy of a product may be considered an adverse reaction. Adverse drug reports will be considered by the Veterinary Products Committee. When reporting, details of the brand name and batch number of the preparation should be given and a copy of the report should also be sent to the drug manufacturer or licence holder.

Drug storage and dispensing. A code of practice for storage and dispensing of medicines by veterinary surgeons has been approved by the BVA and the RCVS (Code of practice. Sale or supply of animal medicines by veterinary surgeons. *The Veterinary Record* 1990; **127:** 236-40). This code includes advice on premises for storing medicines, storage and display of medicines, dispensing, and labelling of medicines. It includes a recommendation that tablets and capsules that are repacked from bulk containers should be dispensed in child-resistant containers. Preparations for external application should be dispensed in coloured fluted bottles while oral liquids should be dispensed in plain glass bottles.

The person having possession or control of the animal or herd must be warned to keep all medicines out of the reach of children.

Controlled drugs. Controlled drugs are subject to the provisions of the Misuse of Drugs Act 1971 (see Legal aspects of prescribing).

Health and safety. The Control of Substances Hazardous to Health (COSHH) Regulations 1988 relate to work involving substances hazardous to health. Employers are responsible for identifying hazardous substances used in practice, assessing the degree of risk, and taking appropriate measures to contain the risk at acceptable levels.

When handling chemical or biological materials particular attention should be given to the possibility of allergy or poisoning in the operator. Reactions in humans preparing and giving medicines may be caused by direct contact with drugs such as penicillins or prostaglandins, by the injection of etorphine or oil-based solutions, or by the inhalation of substances containing organophosphorus compounds. For the *BVA Code of Practice for using prostaglandins in cattle and pigs*, see *The Veterinary Record* 1987; **120:** 511-12. Accidental self-injection with oil-based preparations can cause severe vascular spasm and prompt medical attention should be sought.

Care should be taken not to dispose of chemicals into ditches or waterways as they may be harmful to fish and invertebrates. Advice on the disposal of chemicals such as spent sheep dips can be sought from the National Rivers Authority, the local Ministry agricultural advisor, or the product manufacturer. The main aim is to ensure that water resources are not polluted. Prescribers are advised to consult the MAFF/HSC. *Pesticides: code of practice for the safe use of pesticides on farms and holdings*. London: HMSO, 1990 and other relevant information. NOAH have issued interim *Guidelines for the disposal of used sheep dip and containers*.

Withdrawal periods. The withdrawal period is the time interval after cessation of treatment and before the animal or any of its products can be used as human food. With increasing public awareness of the use of drugs such as hormones and antimicrobials in animals that may enter the human food chain, it is essential that veterinarians play an active part in ensuring that medicines are administered according to their directions and that withdrawal periods are strictly followed.

Right to prescribe. Due to increased licensing costs and legislation, many useful medicines have not received a product licence or manufacturers have not renewed the licence for animal use. The veterinarian has a right to prescribe human licensed medicines (printed in smaller-than-text typeface in The Veterinary Formulary) or animal medicines with unlicensed indications (marked with ✦ in The Veterinary Formulary) for 'animals under his care'. An interpretation of 'animals under his care' is described in the *Guide to Professional Conduct* (RCVS, 1990).

The Presidents of the RCVS, BVA, the Chief Veterinary Officers of the Ministry of Agriculture, Fisheries and Food, the Department of Agriculture for Northern Ireland, and the Director of the Veterinary Medicines Directorate have issued the following statement of advice on the use of medicines in animals:

"Introduction

1. This letter is issued jointly by the President of the Royal College of Veterinary Surgeons, the President of the British Veterinary Association, the Chief Veterinary Officers of the Ministry of Agriculture, Fisheries and Food and the Department of Agriculture for Northern Ireland, and the Director of the Veterinary Medicines Directorate. With changes in EC legislation and public attitudes and sensitivities, the use of medicines has been under close scrutiny. This letter reviews the general principles which should guide veterinary surgeons in treating animals (which includes birds, fish or reptiles) and reminds them of the strict limitations to the use of unlicensed medicines."

"General Principles

2. The general principles to be followed are that-
(a) No-one should manufacture, sell or supply a medicinal product unless it is licensed.
(b) Food producing animals should be treated only with medicinal products licensed for animal use.
(c) Non-food producing animals may be treated with unlicensed veterinary medicinal products or human medicinal products only when no equivalent licensed veterinary product is available.
(d) Unlicensed medicinal products should only be used on one particular animal or small number of animals. A small number of animals does *not* mean a flock or herd or other similar group of animals."

"3. *Advice to the Profession*

In addition to the General Principles, we take this opportunity to advise and remind the profession of the following:
(a) The veterinary surgeons' exemption

from the licensing system (Section 9(2) – Medicines Act 1968) is to be interpreted very narrowly. It is available *only* for products which the veterinary surgeon manufactures for him/herself or which are manufactured to his/her special order for administration to a particular animal or animals under his/her care. Repackaging or re-labelling does not constitute manufacture to a veterinary surgeon's special order. Clearly the exemption does not apply to ready-made products which a veterinary surgeon may buy off the shelf. A veterinary surgeon does not require a product licence to procure the manufacture or assembly of a stock of a medicinal product specially prepared by him or to his order for administration to one or more animals under his care. Veterinary surgeons are reminded that under SI 1972/1200 they may hold in stock no more than 5 litres of fluid or 2.5 kg of solids of all such medicinal products.
(b) The Veterinary Medicines Directive 81/851/EEC has the effect of prohibiting the administration of unlicensed veterinary medicines to animals. The only exemption relates to the treatment of one individual animal or a small number of animals. These provisions were incorporated into UK law by the Medicines (Restrictions on the Administration of Veterinary Medicinal Products) Regulations 1983 (SI No 1732 of 1983).
(c) When veterinary medicinal products are incorporated into feedingstuffs, medication must be in accordance with the Medicated Feedingstuffs Regulations.
(d) When prescribing for horses, veterinary surgeons will have to consider whether there is any likelihood of the individual animal being used for human consumption within two months. If so, the guidance on food animals must be followed (i.e. only products licensed for use in animals should be prescribed for or administered to the horse). If not, guidance for non-food animals should be followed.
(e) When prescribing veterinary medicinal products outwith the rec-

ommendations specified on the data sheet, or whose data sheets do not specify withdrawal periods the following minimum standard withdrawal periods should be used:-

Eggs	7 days
Milk	7 days
Meat from poultry and mammals[1]	28 days
Meat from Fish[1]	500 degree days[2]

[1] includes muscle, fat, liver etc.

[2] cumulative sum of mean daily water temperatures in degrees Celsius following the last treatment.

(f) There are a number of long established substances which are still employed or supplied as traditional remedies and those that are GSL category. Veterinary surgeons may continue to prescribe and supply these substances and also mineral supplements, vitamins and trace elements for animals.

(g) Where the absence or limited availability of a licensed medicinal product for the treatment or prevention of disease would lead to animal health or welfare problems the Licensing Authority is prepared to consider issuing a simplified product licence. This will apply to products where the pharmacological properties and clinical use of the active ingredients are well known and safe, or where appropriate conditions can be agreed which will safeguard animals, humans (who may come into contact with the product or who may consume meat, eggs or milk from treated or in-contact animals) and the environment.

The Veterinary Surgeon's Responsibility

In January 1988 statutory slaughterhouse sampling of meat commenced, and from 1 January 1989 the number of carcases being examined for residues under the statutory scheme has been increased to 40,000 per year. Now, for the first time, extensive numerical data will be available on residues in meat from cattle, sheep, pigs and horses. Poultry meat is also monitored. Both poultry meat and fish will be brought within the statutory scheme within the next few years. Irresponsible or illegal use of medicinal substances in animals will be detected with a high degree of certainty.

The veterinary surgeon has an important part to play in ensuring that all medicinal substances (whether PoM, P or PML) are responsibly used. This letter should be used as the basis for administration of medicines to animals."

Legal aspects of prescribing

Veterinary drug classification

Veterinary drugs are classified into pharmacy medicines (P), general sale list medicines (GSL), pharmacy and merchants list medicines (PML), and prescription-only medicines (PoM), which include controlled drugs (CD). Drug preparations without a legal category such as nutritional feed supplements are classified as non-medicinal.

In the Misuse of Drugs Regulations 1985, controlled drugs are divided into 5 schedules, in decreasing order of stringency of control.

Schedule 1 includes cannabis and hallucinogenic drugs such as LSD, which are not normally used therapeutically. Veterinarians have no general authority to possess and use them.

Schedule 2 drugs that may be used in veterinary practice include etorphine, fentanyl, morphine, pethidine, the amphetamines, and quinalbarbitone. These drugs are subject to special prescription requirements, and to legislation on requisition, record keeping, safe custody, except quinalbarbitone, and destruction of unwanted stock.

Schedule 3 includes butobarbitone, pentobarbitone, and phenobarbitone. These drugs are subject to prescription and requisition requirements, but transactions do not have to be recorded in the controlled drugs register. The safe custody requirements apply to preparations of diethylpropion or buprenorphine but not to other S3 drugs.

Schedule 4 includes the benzodiazepines such as diazepam. When used in normal veterinary practice they are exempt from most restrictions as controlled drugs.

Schedule 5 includes certain preparations of cocaine, codeine, and morphine that contain less than a specified amount of the drug. They are exempt from all CD requirements pertaining to veterinary practice other than the need to keep relevant invoices for 2 years.

Prescription writing

There are specific legal requirements for prescriptions for schedule 2 and 3 controlled drugs, and rather less stringent requirements for all other prescription-only medicines. Prescriptions for GSL, P, and PML products are not subject to any mandatory constraints. However, to avoid ambiguity it is good practice to write all prescriptions legibly in a standard manner (see Figure 1). The prescription should include:

- the name and address of the prescriber, which may be printed on practice forms. The name and address of the client and the date of prescription issue. It is good practice to indicate the species or animal name/number and to add the words 'for animal treatment only'
- the name(s) and strength(s) of drugs(s) to be dispensed. Usually this will be a pre-prepared formulation. Medicinal products may be prescribed using the generic name or specifying a proprietary preparation. In the former case only, the pharmacist may dispense any suitable product
- the formulation of any preparation that needs to be extemporaneously prepared. All prescriptions should indicate the quantity to be dispensed. The total quantity must be written in words and figures for schedule 2 or 3 controlled drugs
- the directions that the prescriber wishes to appear on the labelled product. It is good practice to include here the words 'for animal treatment only', the dose and directions for use, and any precautions relating to the use of the product
- the prescriber's signature and qualifications, which are required for all POMs
- a declaration that 'This prescription is issued in respect of an animal under my care' or words to that effect. This statement is required for all POMs

- any instructions for repeating the prescription. Repeat prescriptions for controlled drugs are not permitted.

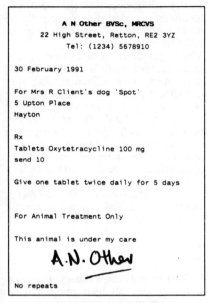

```
        A N Other BVSc, MRCVS
      22 High Street, Retton, RE2 3YZ
         Tel: (1234) 5678910


30 February 1991

For Mrs R Client's dog 'Spot'
5 Upton Place
Hayton


Rx
Tablets Oxytetracycline 100 mg
send 10


Give one tablet twice daily for 5 days


For Animal Treatment Only

This animal is under my care

   A.N. Other


No repeats
```

Fig. 1. Sample prescription

Prescriptions for POMs must be written indelibly and contain the prescriber's name and address, signature, qualifications, and declaration as outlined above. A PoM prescription must be dispensed within 6 months of the date issued and will not be repeated unless it contains a specific direction for further dispensing.

Prescribing controlled drugs

Prescriptions for schedule 2 and 3 controlled drugs must be indelible and conform with particular requirements in addition to those for POMs. To minimise the possibility of forgery, the following particulars must be in the **veterinarian's own handwriting** (except for phenobarbitone and phenobarbitone sodium):

- the name and address of the owner of the animal. The date on which the prescription was signed
- the form and strength of the preparation

- the total quantity, in both words and figures, to be dispensed
- the dosage details
- prescriber's signature and qualifications.

A pharmacist must not dispense a prescription for an S2 or S3 CD unless it complies with the above requirements and the prescriber's address is in the UK. The prescription must be dispensed within 13 weeks of the date of issue. The pharmacist should have no reason to suppose that the signature is not genuine.

Storing controlled drugs

Great care should be taken to ensure safe storage of all medicinal products. Schedule 2 and some Schedule 3 controlled drugs must be kept in a locked receptacle within the meaning of the Misuse of Drugs (Safe Custody) Regulations. A locked car is not considered to be such a receptacle and veterinarians are advised to provide additional locked units within any vehicles used for the transport of medicinal products.

Labelling of dispensed animal medicines

Medicines should be dispensed correctly labelled (see Figure 2). Dispensing veterinarians should ensure that the label includes:

- the name of the person who has possession or control of the animal or herd and the address of the premises where the animal or herd is kept

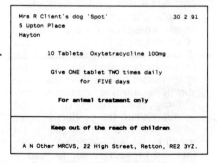

```
Mrs R Client's dog 'Spot'                    30 2 91
5 Upton Place
Hayton

      10 Tablets  Oxytetracycline 100mg

      Give ONE tablet TWO times daily
             for  FIVE days

          For animal treatment only


     Keep out of the reach of children

A N Other MRCVS, 22 High Street, Retton, RE2 3YZ.
```

Fig. 2. Sample label

- the name and address of the veterinarian
- the date of dispensing
- the words 'for animal treatment only', unless the container or package is too small for it to be practicable to do so
- the words 'keep out of the reach of children' or words having a similar meaning
- the words 'for external use only' for medicines that are only for topical use
- the relevant withdrawal period should always be stated on medicinal products for food animals
- (included at the discretion of the veterinarian) the name and the strength of the product, pack size, directions for use, precautions relating to the use of the product, and the name or description of animals to be treated.

Although not mandatory, it is good practice to include the drug name, drug concentration and amount dispensed, and to use mechanically printed lettering.

Veterinary drugs which are General Sales List Medicines or Pharmacy Medicines, when sold or supplied by retail, must where appropriate bear cautionary labels as follows:

- if containing aspirin, with the words 'unsuitable for cats' and (unless 'aspirin' is included in the name of the product) 'contains aspirin', enclosed within a ruled rectangle
- if containing aloxiprin, with the words 'unsuitable for cats' and 'contains an aspirin derivative', enclosed within a ruled rectangle
- if containing salicylamide, with the words 'unsuitable for cats' within a ruled rectangle
- if containing hexachlorophane for oral administration in the prevention or treatment of liver fluke disease in sheep, a warning that protective clothing must be worn by the operator when the product is being administered. If the product is for use in cattle, an additional warning that the product is not for use in lactating cattle.

Medicated animal feeding stuffs

Legislation controlling medicated animal feeding stuffs is to be found in *The Medicines (Medicated Animal Feeding Stuffs) Regulations* 1989 (SI 2320). The legislation is designed principally to protect the public against medicinal residues in food animals.

The Regulations apply to anyone who incorporates a medicinal product of any description in an animal feeding stuff including liquid feed such as whey or skimmed milk, 'in the course of business carried on by him'. Therefore, home-mixers such as farmers, and keepers of zoo animals and dogs for business purposes are affected as well as commercial feed compounders. However, the legislation does not affect a companion animal owner administering a medicinal product mixed in the feed, since no business is involved. Nor does it affect a farmer 'top dressing' feed or medicating via the drinking water.

Registered feed compounders. The regulations require all feed compounders, that is commercial and home-mixers, who add medicines to feeds to register with the Royal Pharmaceutical Society of Great Britain (RPSGB) or the Department of Agriculture for Northern Ireland (DANI). The RPSGB and DANI enforce the legislation and associated Codes of Practice as stated below.

Part A of the Register relates to feed compounders proposing to include medicinal products at an incorporation rate of less than 2 kg/tonne of feed. The registration requirements are aimed primarily at commercial feed compounders. Persons registered in Part A have to comply with the requirements of a stringent Category A Code of Practice, which includes premises, equipment, personnel and training, documentation, and quality assurance. Failure to observe any of the provisions of the Code may lead to removal from the Register.

Part B of the Register relates to manufacturers and home-mixers including medicinal products at an incorporation rate of 2 kg or more/ tonne. They have to comply with the requirements of a Category B Code of Practice, which are generally less stringent than those for Category A. They are designed to ensure that the minimum EC and UK standards are satisfied. Again, failure to comply with the requirements of the Code may lead to registration refusal or removal from the Register.

The regulations exempt fish farmers from registration.

Those dealing with intermediate medicated feeds are also required to register with the RPSGB or DANI and to comply with a Code of Practice. For registration purposes they are designated Category II agricultural merchants. Intermediate medicated feeds are feeding stuffs used as ingredients in preparing final feeds and although classed as medicinal products they are exempt from licensing requirements and from certain aspects of prescription only control.

Authority to medicate feeding stuffs. A PML or PoM medicinal product may be incorporated in an animal feeding stuff by an appropriately registered person only if the product has a relevant product licence (PL) or an animal test certificate (ATC) providing specifications for incorporation. Otherwise, incorporation must be in accordance with a veterinary written direction (VWD) issued by a veterinarian for the treatment of animals 'under his care'.

PML products are primarily intended for incorporation at specified concentrations for particular species, and a VWD is not mandatory for the incorporation or subsequent supply of the final feed. However, if they are to be incorporated in any way not in accordance with the product licence, for example at higher levels or not as shown on the label, a VWD is required. A VWD is generally

necessary for incorporation of a PoM product into a feeding stuff and it is certainly required before such medicated feed is supplied to a farmer.

Veterinary Written Direction. Medicinal products to be included in feed must, by law, be licensed for in-feed use, although the veterinarian may authorise use for species or conditions other than those specified in the product licence.

The MAFF, RCVS, and BVA have issued a joint statement which emphasises that the choice of any medicinal product should be restricted to licensed products. They should, wherever possible, be used in accordance with data sheet recommendations as regards inclusion rates, target species, and withdrawal periods.

All VWDs for medicated feed should follow the form specified in the 1989 Regulations (see below).

Section 1 of the schedule requests details on the amount of product to be incorporated in the feed, the number and species to which it is to be administered, details of the recipient of the medicated feed and how it should be used, and the name and address of the prescribing veterinarian.

Section 2 requests the name and address of the supplier who should be a person registered with the RPSGB or DANI (refer to notes above).

Section 3 need only be completed in 2 emergency situations stated below:

- if incorporation of a product is required at less than 2 kg/tonne and the compounder or farmer is not on Part A of the register. The person incorporating the medicinal product must send a copy of the VWD to the RPSGB or DANI within 28 days of incorporation
- if the compounder is not on Part A or B of the register.

SCHEDULE

Regulation 5

DIRECTION FOR THE INCORPORATION OF A MEDICINAL PRODUCT IN AN ANIMAL FEEDING STUFF OR FOR THE SALE, SUPPLY OR IMPORTATION OF MEDICATED ANIMAL FEEDING STUFFS

REFERENCE NUMBER

SECTION I – TO BE COMPLETED IN ITS ENTIRETY BY VETERINARY SURGEON OR VETERINARY PRACTITIONER

1. Please manufacture/sell/supply/import*.......tonnes/kg* of (name/type of feed)........meal/pellets/crumbs* containing-

................}
................} g/tonne (mg/kg)* of ....} product licence number(s)
................}   ....} and/or generic name(s))

to give-

................}   ....} (precise description of
            g/tonne (mg/kg)* of
................}   ....} active substance(s))

in the final medicated feeding stuff for administration to the following animals which are under my care:
Species .... Approx. number............................

2. The medicated feeding stuff must be sold/supplied* to (name of farmer and address of farm)...

Recommendations For Use On The Farm
(i)   Quantity of medicated feeding stuff to be given daily...................
(ii)   Duration of treatment..
(iii)   Animals must not be slaughtered for human consumption until.............
        after the last treatment
        Milk/eggs* must not be taken for human consumption until................
        after the last treatment
(iv)   Special precautions..

3. This direction is valid for 30 days from the date of signature.

Signature of Veterinary Surgeon or Veterinary Practitioner.................................	**SECTION II–TO BE COMPLETED BY VETERINARY SURGEON OR VETERINARY PRACTITIONER OR**
Name in block letters........................	**FARMER**
Practice Address...........................	Name and address
....	manufacturer/seller/supplier/
....	importer*......................
....	
Date...........Telephone No................	....

*Delete as appropriate

SECTION III–IF APPLICABLE, TO BE COMPLETED BY VETERINARY SURGEON OR VETERINARY PRACTITIONER

1. Reason(s) for authorising incorporation by a manufacturer (including an on-farm mixer) not in Part A of the Register......................................
....

2. Reason(s) for authorising a manufacturer not in Part A or B of the Register...
....

NOTES

1. This form must be completed in triplicate, in ink or by other indelible means, and signed in ink in his own name by the Veterinary Surgeon or Veterinary Practitioner, who will retain one copy and give one copy each to the manufacturer and farmer.

2. If any part of Section III has been completed, the manufacturer must send a copy of the form to RPSGB, 1 Lambeth High Street, London, SE1 7JN, or DANI, "Duniris", 15 Galway Park, Dundonald, Belfast, BT16 0AN, within 28 days of incorporation.

Prescribing for animals used in competitions

When prescribing for animals engaged in competitive activities, it is necessary not only to consider the therapeutic aspects of any drug treatment, but also to ensure that the rules of the controlling body of the sport are not contravened. It is the purpose of such rules to encourage fair competition with animals being judged on their inherent merits, unaided by drugs. This can present a dilemma, for there is a fine distinction between legitimate therapy and unacceptable drug administration, particularly in competitions with more than one stage, such as Three-Day Eventing. Some controlling bodies allow the use of certain medications, designate threshold levels for concentrations of certain substances in body fluids, or require competitors to have undergone a strict vaccination programme against specified diseases.

It is essential to be aware that rules need not be permanent. Legislators are conscious that approaches to therapy can change and that rules may be modified in the light of new developments and scientific discovery. Information on prescribing for animals used in competitions is included in:

- Fédération Equestre Internationale. *Veterinary regulations*
- National Greyhound Racing Club Limited. *Rules of racing and directions*
- Royal College of Veterinary Surgeons. *Guide to professional conduct*
- The Kennel Club. *Rules and regulations*
- The Jockey Club. *Rules of racing and instructions*
- Dyke, TM. Pharmacokinetics of therapeutic substances in racehorses. *Australian Equine Veterinarian* 1989; 7 (suppl 1).

Therapeutic considerations

Ingredients. The contents of any proprietary mixture should be disclosed and the actions known. An apparently harmless tonic may contain a prohibited substance such as caffeine. Traces of caffeine metabolites have been detected in the urine for up to 10 days after administration, and it is advisable to discontinue treatment with caffeine-containing mixtures at least 14 days before competition.

Formulation. Some drugs are specifically formulated to prolong their action. Particular care needs to be taken with hormonal implants and long-acting antibiotic preparations. Although specific information is not available for horses or dogs, it is likely that absorption of drug from slow-release implants will be essentially complete in 6 months.

The local anaesthetic procaine is used in procaine penicillin to prolong the duration of antibiotic activity. Since procaine is a basic drug, its urinary concentration is governed by the pH of the urine, and it may be detected in this medium for up to 18 days after injection in horses. If treatment against penicillin-sensitive infections is necessary, benzylpenicillin sodium may be administered intramuscularly, up to 72 hours before competing.

Pharmacokinetics. Delayed absorption and excretion may occur following intramuscular injection or oral administration. Acepromazine may be excreted sporadically and, in horses, metabolites have been detected in urine many weeks after dosing. Since absorption is related to vascularity and lipid solubility, inadvertent injection into fatty tissue or between fascial planes may lead to prolonged excretion.

Lipid-soluble substances such as corticosteroids and local anaesthetics are well absorbed following intra-articular injection and may be detected in the urine.

Absorption of drugs across mucous membranes can be rapid. Camphor and other ingredients of many traditional inhalants may be detectable in urine. Nebulisation can produce high plasma-drug concentrations due to absorption through the alveolar surface.

The intact epidermis acts as a barrier to absorption and even highly lipid-soluble substances only penetrate skin slowly. If the barrier is damaged, the permeable underlying dermis allows the passage of lipid-soluble and water-soluble molecules. Care must be taken with topical applications such as oil of wintergreen, which contains methyl salicylate, especially when abrasions are present.

Dimethyl sulphoxide (DMSO) possesses pharmacological properties of its own, but can also act as a vehicle for other drugs whose transcutaneous absorption may be enhanced. This is particularly applicable to substances with a molecular weight of less than 3000.

There are too many variable factors involved to offer precise advice on *elimination times* for drugs. Apparent 'clearance times' are influenced by the sensitivities of the analytical techniques used.

With important exceptions (see above), the RCVS recommends the discontinuance of drugs for racehorses not less than 8 days before racing, even though such a period is longer than is necessary in many instances (*Guide to professional conduct*. London: The Royal College of Veterinary Surgeons, 1990). The Royal College make it clear in issuing its advice, that they cannot accept responsibility for the possibility that an atypical horse may take longer than normal to clear a drug, even if the drug is not formulated for sustained release.

Desensitised and hypersensitised limbs. The Fédération Equestre Internationale (FEI) states that no horse shall be allowed to compete following neurectomy on a limb nor when any limb has been temporarily or permanently desensitised by any means (*Veterinary regulations*. 6th ed. Switzerland: Fédération Equestre Internationale, 1990).

Oxygen and intravenous fluid therapy. FEI rules govern the use of oxygen by inhalation, and the parenteral administration of substances including sodium chloride solutions, electrolyte solutions, and glucose.

Oxygen administration is forbidden throughout the period of the event except by intubation as first-aid after Phase D at Three-Day Events and after the Marathon at Driving Events, with the approval of the Veterinary Commission. Under the rules of Long Distance Riding (a discipline of the British Horse Society), fluid therapy by nasogastric intubation or rectal infusion is also forbidden throughout the period of the ride.

Medication in equine competitions

Several autonomous bodies produce their own rules on medication control based on a list of prohibited substances. In essence these can be regarded as variations on the rules of the Jockey Club (The Stewards of the Jockey Club. *Rules of racing 1990 and instructions*. London: Jockey Club, 1990) or of the Fédération Equestre Internationale (FEI). An exception to this is the Hurlingham Polo Association Directive 9001 (Misuse of Drugs), which includes a list of permitted substances (see below).

The Jockey Club describe a prohibited substance as "A substance originating externally whether or not it is endogenous to the horse which falls in any of the categories contained in the List of Prohibited Substances... 'Substance' includes the metabolites of the substance".

Maximum permitted concentrations have been established for certain substances that are commonly detected in equine urine samples. Such substances may occur in ordinary diets, or may be endogenous to the horse, or may arise as a result of contamination.

Salicylic acid can be derived directly from ingested plant materials. Lucerne, in particular, is rich in salicylic acid.

Theobromine and **arsenic** can arise as a result of feed contamination. Theobromine from cocoa products is often introduced into compound feeds during manufacture.

The estranediol:estrenediol ratio in

urine is used to distinguish between endogenous **nandrolone** (detectable in normal stallion urine) and administered nandrolone.

Jockey Club list of prohibited substances

Substances acting on the nervous system
Substances acting on the cardiovascular system
Substances acting on the respiratory system
Substances acting on the digestive system
Substances acting on the urinary system
Substances acting on the reproductive system
Substances acting on the musculoskeletal system
Substances acting on the blood system
Substances acting on the immune system
Substances acting on the endocrine system, endocrine secretions and their synthetic counterparts
Anti-infectious (including antiparasitic) substances
For the purposes of clarity these include:
Antipyretics, analgesics and anti-inflammatory substances
Cytotoxic substances
Antihistamines
Diuretics
Local anaesthetics
Muscle relaxants
Respiratory stimulants
Sex hormones, anabolic agents and corticosteroids
Substances affecting blood coagulation

Jockey Club list of maximum permissible concentrations of prohibited substances

Arsenic, 300 nanograms/mL in urine
Nandrolone free and conjugated 5α-estrane-3β, 17α-diol to $5(10)$-estrene-3β, 17α-diol in urine at a ratio of 1
Salicylic acid, 750 micrograms/mL in urine
Theobromine, 2 micrograms/mL in urine

FEI list of prohibited substances

Substances acting on the nervous system
Substances acting on the cardiovascular system

Substances acting on the respiratory system
Substances acting on the alimentary system
Substances acting on the urinary system
Substances acting on the musculoskeletal system
Substances acting on the immune system
Antibiotics, antibacterial, and antiviral substances
Antiparasitic substances
Antipyretics, analgesics and anti-inflammatory substances other than phenylbutazone and oxyphenbutazone
Endocrine secretions and their synthetic counterparts
Substances affecting blood coagulation
Cytotoxic substances

FEI list of maximum permissible concentrations of prohibited substances

Arsenic, 200 nanograms/mL of urine
Oxyphenbutazone, 2 micrograms/mL of plasma
Phenylbutazone, 2 micrograms/mL of plasma
Salicylic acid, 750 micrograms/mL of urine
Theobromine, 2 micrograms/mL of urine

The Hurlingham Polo Association list of permitted substances

Antibiotics except procaine penicillin
Flunixin
Isoxsuprine
Phenylbutazone
Regumate™ [altrenogest]
Sputolosin™ [dembrexine hydrochloride]
Ventipulmin™ [clenbuterol hydrochloride]
Vi-Sorbin™ [iron and vitamin B substances]
The following drugs are only permitted if prior declaration of their administration has been made:
Diuretics
Local anaesthetics

The Hurlingham Polo Association list of maximum permissible concentrations

Phenylbutazone with oxyphenbutazone 10 micrograms/mL of plasma
Flunixin 10 micrograms/mL of plasma

Note. If phenylbutazone and flunixin are used together the concentration of either must be less than 5 micrograms/mL

Vaccination of horses

All competing horses should be protected against tetanus, although this is not a mandatory requirement under any rules. However, the Jockey Club and the FEI insist that horses or ponies that compete under their regulations are vaccinated against equine influenza.

Many showgrounds require entrants to be adequately vaccinated against influenza, whether or not such a requirement is incorporated into the rules of the organising authority. This also applies to any horse or pony entering property owned, used or controlled by the horseracing authorities, unless the property is common ground. Foals less than 4 months old are exempt, providing the dam is fully vaccinated before foaling.

There must be irrefutable evidence that the vaccination record applies to the animal presented and all entries must be signed and stamped by a veterinary surgeon. For racehorses, the Jockey Club require entries to be endorsed in the horse's passport, and does not accept entries which have been altered in any way. An incorrect endorsement must be completely deleted and a new endorsement of the whole entry made. FEI and Jockey Club rules differ, but any vaccination programme which follows the vaccine manufacturer's recommendations will satisfy both sets of rules.

Jockey Club rules. Two injections for primary vaccination must be given not less than 21 days and no more than 92 days apart. Horses foaled on or after January 1st 1980 should have received a booster between 150 and 215 days after the second injection of the vaccine. Following the initial course (primary vaccination and first booster), a booster injection must be given each year. For horses foaled before January 1st 1980, the interval between boosters given before March 16th 1981 should have been not more than 14 months.

FEI rules. Two injections for primary vaccination must be given no less than 21 days and no more than 92 days apart. A booster injection must be given each succeeding 12 months, subsequent to the second injection of the primary course. Prior to January 1st 1980, the interval between booster injections should have been no more than 14 months.

Under both sets of rules, vaccinations given by a veterinary surgeon, who is the owner of the horse at the time of vaccination, are not accepted. The Jockey Club extend this to exclude vaccinations given by a veterinary surgeon who is the trainer or who is named on the Register of Stable Employees as being employed by the trainer of the horse.

No horse may compete or enter competition premises until 7 days after vaccination. When calculating this interval, the day of vaccination should not be included. Horses need only have completed a primary vaccination course before competition. It is not necessary to wait until after the first booster. Annual boosters may be given on the same day in consecutive years.

Medication in greyhound racing

The National Greyhound Racing Club (NGRC) rules of racing do not contain a list of prohibited substances, but disciplinary measures may be taken when a sample has been produced which shows the presence of any quantity of any substance or metabolite, the origin of which cannot be traced to normal and ordinary feeding or care and which by its nature could affect the performance of a greyhound (*Rules of racing and directions*. London: Stewards of the National Greyhound Racing Club Ltd, 1989).

Any tonic, medicament, or other substance administered or applied to a greyhound must be recorded in the (NGRC) Trainer's Greyhound Treatment Book.

Except for drugs used for oestrus control, no substance should be used for at least 7 days before a trial or race. This avoids the possibility of the constituents of tonics or other medicaments being excreted in the urine, and interfering with the interpretation of · tests.

Vaccination of greyhounds

The NGRC state that racing greyhounds are required to have had initial inoculations with approved vaccines against distemper, viral hepatitis, *Leptospira canicola*, *Leptospira icterohaemorrhagiae*, and parvovirus and to have had booster inoculations at 12-monthly intervals from the date of the initial puppy inoculations. Additional inoculations against these and other diseases may be given at the discretion of the veterinary surgeon in charge of the greyhound.

Medication for show animals

The Kennel Club consider that nothing may be done which is calculated to deceive. No substance which alters the natural colour, texture, or body of the coat may be used in preparing a dog for exhibition. Dogs are judged against a 'breed standard' and action may be taken should a dog act in a way markedly different from that described as its normal temperament. Although no specific vaccination programmes are cited, dogs should not have had a

communicable disease in the previous 6 weeks.

At major livestock shows, similar rules apply and action will be taken against any exhibitor who is found to have administered, or permitted the administration of, any tranquilliser or other drugs, which may in any way affect the performance of the animal, or have the effect of making it behave in the show in a manner which is not natural.

Testing of animals

Forensic analysis of urine or blood samples from competing animals is undertaken at designated laboratories. Any other body fluid or biological material, such as vomit from greyhounds, may also be examined if necessary. Typically, samples are collected after performance but rules do not preclude examination at any stage of competition. Greyhounds are frequently sampled before racing, and a positive result may lead to the animal being withdrawn.

Generally, the amount of a substance found in a sample taken from a competing animal is irrelevant in determining whether or not there has been a breach of the rules, except for those substances with limits specified in the Jockey Club, FEI, and Hurlingham Polo Association rules (see above).

Prescribing for horses, cattle, sheep, goats, deer, and pigs

Cattle, sheep, goats, deer, pigs, and in some countries horses, constitute the food-producing animals providing meat, milk, or both, for human consumption. Standard withdrawal periods (see General guidance on prescribing) should be adhered to unless otherwise stated by the manufacturer. Drugs may be prescribed as group medication for administration in the feed or drinking water or for individual animal treatment. Ruminal boluses that provide continuous or pulsatile release of a drug over a prolonged period have been developed for use in cattle and sheep for the delivery of anthelmintics and trace elements.

There is wide variation in drug absorption and metabolism among these species. Absorption from the gastro-gintestinal tract in ruminant species is influenced by the volume and pH of the ruminal contents and whether the drug is subject to metabolism by ruminal micro-organisms. Pigs are monogastric and absorption takes place mainly from the small intestine.

In horses, an orally administered drug may be partly absorbed from the small intestine with further absorption occurring 8 to 12 hours later from the large intestine. Absorption of some drugs administered in the feed or after feeding can be delayed for several hours, since unabsorbed drug may be conveyed to the large intestine where further absorption takes place.

Drugs that are extensively metabolised by hepatic microsomal oxidative reactions are, in general, metabolised more rapidly in ruminant animals and horses than in pigs. Phenylbutazone is a notable exception in that the half-life of this drug in cattle is many times longer than in horses. The dose of xylazine administered to cattle is one-fifth of that used in horses.

Horses are particularly sensitive to certain drugs and drug formulations. Oil-based formulations may cause tissue irritation and damage at the site of injection.

Orally administered broad-spectrum antimicrobials may disturb bacterial fermentation in the caecum and colon in horses and the rumen in animals with a functional rumen resulting in severe digestive disturbances. Tetracyclines may cause severe enterocolitis in horses exposed to stress and rapid intravenous injection to cattle may cause cardio-vascular collapse, due to chelation of calcium and consequent vasodilatation and myocardial depression.

Phenothiazines such as acepromazine should be used with caution in male horses as these drugs may cause paralysis of the retractor penis muscle. The hypotensive effect of acepromazine makes its use in horses with colic questionable. Acepromazine causes reduction in packed cell volume, which is attributed to splenic sequestration of red blood cells. This may lead to misinterpretation of laboratory diagnostic data.

Prescribing for dogs and cats

Drug absorption from the gastro-intestinal tract and from parenteral injection sites is related to drug formulation, and is generally similar in dogs and cats. The rate of percutaneous absorption of highly lipid-soluble drugs may be more rapid in cats.

Dogs and cats differ markedly in their capacity to eliminate drugs by certain metabolic pathways. Glucuronide synthesis is an important metabolic pathway for the elimination of a variety of therapeutic agents. The cat has a relative deficiency in hepatic microsomal glucuronyl transferase activity. Therefore, drugs that are metabolised by this pathway will usually be eliminated at a slower rate and should be used with caution in cats in order to avoid toxic effects.

Renal excretion of drugs is similar in dogs and cats. Drugs that are eliminated unchanged in the urine may be administered at the same dose per kg bodyweight for both species.

There are many dog breeds and, as a general rule, for larger breeds calculation of the total dose should be based at the lower end of the recommended range. Salicylates such as aspirin may cause gastric ulceration, particularly at high doses. Tetracycline antibacterials may cause staining of the teeth in offspring if given in pregnancy. A similar effect may occur if tetracyclines are administered to puppies. Sulphonamides and sulphasalazine, administered systemically, may cause keratoconjunctivitis sicca and potentiated sulphonamides may cause an immune-mediated polyarthritis in Dobermann Pinschers. Phenothiazines such as acepromazine should be used with caution in brachycephalic breeds as spontaneous fainting may be precipitated. Barbiturates such as thiopentone may have prolonged action in coursing hounds due to limited redistribution of the drug into fatty tissue in these breeds.

Pharmaceutical adjuvants may also induce adverse reactions in some species. Polyoxyl 35 castor oil, the solubilising constituent of Saffan™ (alphaxalone and alphadolone acetate), causes the release of histamine and histamine-like substances in dogs and therefore the preparation should not be used in this species.

There are specific problems related to drug use in cats. Drugs conjugated with glucuronide in the liver such as organophosphorus compounds, aspirin, chloramphenicol, phenytoin, and griseofulvin (see also Prescribing in hepatic impairment) should be avoided or used with caution. Antiseptics and disinfectants such as iodine and its derivatives, benzyl benzoate, and phenols and cresol are particularly toxic to cats due to increased drug ingestion because of the animal's grooming habits as well as prolonged drug metabolism. Opioid analgesics including morphine, butorphanol, pethidine, and pethidine derivatives such as diphenoxylate hydrochloride may cause violent excitatory activity at high doses. Phenothiazines such as acepromazine may cause paradoxical excitement in some cats. Xylazine may cause emesis in dogs and cats and may be used therapeutically for this purpose. High doses of aminoglycoside antibacterials such as gentamicin, streptomycin, and neomycin are particularly toxic in cats, causing ototoxicity, nephrotoxicity, or both.

Prescribing for birds

Poultry, game birds, and pigeons are kept in the UK. Although similar diseases and conditions may affect these species, methods of housing and rearing and whether the birds are farmed for production of meat or eggs or kept for exhibition or racing, leads to varying treatment regimens.

Poultry

Poultry are farmed domestic birds, which include fowl, turkeys, ducks, and geese.

The influence of management procedures on the presenting disease should be investigated before medicating the flock. An undesirable environment can nullify the benefits of medication and may be the cause of illness. In some circumstances it may be more economical to slaughter the flock earlier than planned because of the costs of treatment.

Administration of drugs in the drinking water is always preferable as birds will drink when they will not eat. However, fluid intake by the birds may vary due to the climate, to the ease of access or hygiene of drink dispensers, or to the unpalatability of the water due to the drug incorporated. Care must be taken that the medication does not block the water system.

Alternatively, the feed may be medicated. This is convenient for the farmer but it may take time getting feed mixed at the mill and mills may find making special mixes uneconomical. Absorption of the drug may be unpredictable because of binding to feed ingredients. Some birds may have a reduced feed intake and may require adjustment of the drug concentration in their feed. Medicated feed may only be sold from mills on authorisation of a Veterinary Written Direction (see Legal aspects of prescribing) supplied by a veterinarian who has the birds 'under his care'.

Treatment by injection is the most predictable method of drug administration but is only practicable where there are sufficient staff available and the birds are of high monetary value such as turkeys and breeding stock.

Many antibacterials are licensed for use in poultry for the treatment of enteric and respiratory disease. Information on dosage and preparations available is found in section 1.1.1. Some antibacterials may be used as growth promoters (see section 17.1). Coccidiosis is a common infection in poultry flocks and medication is usually administered prophylactically to control the disease (see section 1.4.1). Anticoccidials such as monensin, narasin, or salinomycin should not be administered concurrently with tiamulin as toxic effects are often fatal. Erythromycin and sulphonamides have also been reported to cause toxic effects when administered with monensin.

Infection with the gapeworm, *Syngamus trachea*, and intestinal nematodes such as *Capillaria*, *Heterakis*, and *Ascaridia* may be treated with licensed preparations including mebendazole and piperazine (see section 2.1). Lice, mites, and fleas may affect poultry and preparations licensed for treatment include cypermethrin (see section 2.2). Poultry houses may also be treated to ensure insect eradication (see section 2.2.2.8).

Many vaccines are available to provide protection against avian viruses and these are described in section 18.6.

Game birds

Game birds include pheasants, quail, partridges, grouse, and guinea fowl, which are essentially wild birds that are hatched and reared in small, often isolated groups. The diseases of game birds are not unique, although management practices do have an influence on the occurrence and type of diseases observed in these species.

Drugs may be administered to game

birds in the drinking water or in the feed for mass medication, or by injection of individual birds. In the earlier stages of rearing and before release, the birds are fairly easily handled and treated with medication being administered via the drinking water. Fluid intake may vary due to climatic conditions or if the medicated drinking water is unpalatable. Feed medication is usually impractical as the quantity of feed required is much smaller than the usual minimum amount supplied by the larger mills as a single mix batch. Drug inclusion in feed has to be prescribed under a Veterinary Written Direction (see Legal aspects of prescribing).

Few drugs are licensed for use in game birds and therefore most drugs must be prescribed by a veterinarian who has the birds 'under his care' (see General guidance on prescribing).

Antimicrobial doses of drugs used in game birds are listed in Table 1. Infections caused by *Escherichia coli*, *Salmonella*, and *Staphylococcus* are commonly seen in game birds. *Salmonella* usually causes enteric disease, which under stress may lead to septicaemia. This condition has a high mortality rate. Antibacterials should be given although they will only reduce the degree of infection rather than eliminate it. Neomycin is the drug of choice for enteric salmonellosis, while potentiated sulphonamides are effective for the systemic disease caused by *Salmonella*, and colibacillosis. Furazolidone may be more effective for *E. coli* infections if the birds are over 3 weeks of age but this drug may have a toxic effect on the nervous system and it must be used with care in young birds. Drugs used for the treatment of staphylococcal infections include chlortetracycline for infection within the joints and amoxycillin when the infection causes acute toxaemia.

Mycoplasma infection commonly occurs in conjunction with *E. coli* infection, causing severe respiratory problems in the younger birds and reduced production in the older breeding birds. The disease is egg transmitted and it is impracticable to eradicate the condition from any one flock. Treatment for

Table 1 Antimicrobial doses of drugs unlicensed for use in game birds

Drug	By addition to drinking water	By addition to feed
Amoxycillin	4–20 mg/kg	—
Chlortetracycline	4–12 g/100 L	200–600 g/tonne
Clopidol	—	125 g/tonne†
Co-trimazine	10.7 g/100 L	—
Dimetridazole	Treatment. 27 g/100 L† Prophylaxis. 12.5 g/100 L†	Treatment. 500 g/tonne† Prophylaxis. 125–150 g/tonne†
Furaltadone	20–40 g/100 L	—
Furazolidone	—	200–400 g/tonne
Halofuginone	—	3 g/tonne†
Lasolocid	—	90–125 g/tonne†
Neomycin	12.6 g/100 L	220 g/tonne
Tetracycline	4–12 g/100 L	200–600 g/tonne
Tiamulin	Treatment. 25 g/100 L Prophylaxis. 12.5 g/100 L	—
Tylosin	50 g/100 L	—

† preparations licensed for use in this species now available

Mycoplasma can be given by injection to young birds and via the drinking water to any older, rearing, or laying birds. Tiamulin may be used for treatment but must not be given in combination with ionophore anticoccidials, such as monensin or salinomycin, as concurrent administration may exacerbate toxic effects. Tetracyclines may be used for prophylaxis in breeding stock to reduce the level of infection present in the parent birds, maintain a good production rate, and reduce the level of egg-borne trans-mission.

Coccidiosis is a common problem in game birds, which may lead to high mortality rates. *Eimeria colchici* is the main protozoon causing mortality. Infections occur at around 20 days of age when treatment with potentiated sulphonamides is relatively easy and effective. All birds under approximately 8 weeks of age are given anticoccidials in the feed for prophylaxis.

Infection with flagellate parasites such as *Hexamita meleagridis* and *Trichomonas phasioni* may lead to unthrifty birds. Clinical signs are usually seen early in rearing and infections are treated with dimetridazole or tetracyclines. Dimetridazole is given in the feed as a prophylactic against histomoniasis.

The gapeworm, *Syngamus trachea*, affects game birds by causing an obstruction of the trachea characterised by 'gaping' respiration. Differential diagnosis for these clinical signs include aspergillosis, which affects the air sacs. Other worms affecting game birds are the common intestinal roundworms and the much smaller *Capillaria* worm. *Capillaria* affects adult breeding stock causing a delay in onset of laying and reduced egg production. Treatment of helminth infection is based on the use of benzimidazoles such as fenbendazole and mebendazole. Repeated doses may

Table 2 Parasiticide doses of drugs licensed for use in game birds

Drug	By addition to drinking water	By addition to feed
Fenbendazole	—	7–10 mg/kg body-weight (grouse); 12 mg/kg body-weight (partridges, pheasants)
Mebendazole	—	120 g/ tonne feed
Nitroxynil	24 mg/kg	—

be given every 6 to 8 weeks for prevention of helminth infection. Breeding birds should be treated before commencement of lay to ensure maximum production and fertility. Parasiticide doses of drugs used in game birds are listed in Table 2.

Viral diseases seen in game birds include Newcastle disease, which can be a fatal condition in pheasants. Licensed vaccines are available (see section 18.6.11). There are no licensed vaccines available for protection against other viral diseases such as marble spleen disease caused by an adenovirus.

As few medications are licensed for use in game birds, veterinary involvement in this field is essential to ensure that both legal and welfare aspects are adequately covered.

Pigeons

In the UK, pigeons are mainly kept for racing or showing (fancy pigeons). Pigeons are usually medicated individually by mouth with tablets or capsules, or by group medication via the drinking water. Medication of feed is not used for pigeons.

Knowledge of the care and treatment of pigeons and diseases which affect these birds is growing and it should be noted that all prescription-only medicines (PoM) may only be prescribed by a veterinarian who has the birds 'under his care'. The management and hygiene of the loft is important to ensure prevention of infection from contact with birds from other lofts.

Coccidiosis is seen in pigeon flocks and anticoccidials such as amprolium may be given prophylactically to control infection. Drugs used for treatment and prophylaxis of trichomoniasis (canker) caused by *Trichomonas gallinae* (*T. columbae*) include carnidazole and dimetridazole. Antibacterials that are not available as licensed preparations for pigeons may be administered at approximately the same dosage in mg/kg as for poultry.

Gastro-intestinal roundworms found in pigeons include *Ascaridia* and *Capillaria* species. Treatment by mouth with cambendazole or levamisole given routinely is effective. Pigeon tapeworm infection is treated with dichlorophen. A combination preparation containing methyridine and piperazine citrate for the control of roundworm and hairworm is also available. Loft hygiene is important in the control of external parasites and pesticides such as malathion are used for routine disinfection of the pigeon loft.

Other preparations licensed for use in pigeons include bromhexine and phenylephrine employed for respiratory-tract disorders.

Pigeons may be vaccinated for protection against pigeon paramyxovirus (see section 18.6.14).

Prescribing for laboratory animals

Animals used in research include guinea pigs, mice, rats and other small rodents, rabbits, primates, dogs, cats, farm animals, and a range of less familiar species such as amphibians, reptiles, and fish.

The Animals (Scientific Procedures) Act 1986 requires that all premises registered under the Act employ a 'named veterinary surgeon' to advise on the health and welfare of all laboratory animals. The animals are under the care of the named veterinary surgeon and it is appropriate that he or she should take responsibility for prescribing all required medication and formulating preventive health control programmes.

Before giving any medication, it is necessary to determine whether the animals are being or will be used for any experimental procedures. If so, the proposed therapy should be discussed with the 'named person in day to day care' and the personal licensee responsible for the animals, as well as the project licence holder. The welfare of the animals concerned must be the most important consideration. Although treatment may interfere with an experiment, this should not be a total contra-indication for the use of medication.

In many instances it will be found that treatment cannot be undertaken as it could influence the results of the proposed or current study and in these circumstances it may be necessary to kill the animals humanely. In other instances, for example when deciding whether to administer analgesics, the research worker should be required to provide specific scientific evidence that the drug should be withheld. If the veterinary surgeon is still uncertain as to the correct action to be taken the Home Office Inspectorate may be consulted.

Treatment may require medication of an individual animal or mass medication. Drugs may be administered to groups of animals via the feed or drinking water. Antibiotics administered in the drinking water may be ineffective due to reduction in water consumption as a consequence of the disease process or unpalatability of the water due to addition of the drug. It is preferable, although very labour intensive, to administer preparations by injection or gavage to each individual animal.

Although the majority of preparations which have a veterinary product licence have not been approved for use in laboratory rodents or rabbits, most products licensed for human use will have been administered to laboratory species to assess their safety and efficacy. Therefore drug information may be obtained from scientific literature or pharmaceutical companies. See Prescribing for rabbits and rodents for specific drug information.

Prescribing for rabbits and rodents

In this section, prescribing for gerbils, guinea pigs, hamsters, mice, rabbits, and rats is discussed (see also Prescribing for laboratory animals).

Administration of medication to these species may be by mouth or by injection. Before treatment, animals should be accurately weighed in order to determine the correct dose of a drug. Many drug preparations will have to be diluted to obtain the required dose. Some drugs are not water soluble and may require dilution in other solvents. These species will more readily accept oral medication if either palatable veterinary preparations or human paediatric sugar-based formulations are used.

The use of antimicrobial drugs in rabbits and rodents is associated with a high incidence of undesirable side-effects. Clindamycin, lincomycin, erythromycin, and narrow-spectrum penicillins can produce fatal adverse reactions through an indirect effect on gastro-intestinal micro-organisms. Alteration of the normal bacterial flora in the intestine results in proliferation of organisms such as *Clostridium* species and the production of an often fatal entero-toxaemia. Antibiotics such as streptomycin and dihydrostreptomycin have been reported to have a toxic effect in rats, mice, and gerbils. For specific antimicrobial drug dosages, see Table 3.

Parenteral and topical ectoparasiticides may be used for the treatment of mites in rabbits and rodents. Endoparasites may be a problem in large groups of animals and treatment is administered in the feed or drinking water. For specific parasiticide doses, see Table 4.

Many anaesthetics and analgesics are used in rodents and rabbits. A drug may be used alone or in combination, and specific drug regimens are given in Table 5. Parenteral fluids may be administered to aid recovery.

Licensed preparations of buserelin and gonadorelin are available for the induction of ovulation in rabbits (see section 8.1.2).

Vaccines are not commonly used to prevent disease in rabbits and rodents. Rabbits may be vaccinated against infectious myxomatosis (see section 18.7).

Table 3 Antimicrobial doses of drugs unlicensed for use in rabbits and rodents

Drug	Gerbil	Guinea pig	Hamster	Mouse	Rabbit	Rat
Amoxycillin	—	—	—	100 mg/ kg s.c. once daily	—	150 mg/ kg i.m. once daily
Ampicillin	—	—	—	150 mg/ kg s.c. twice daily	25 mg/kg s.c. twice daily	150 mg/ kg s.c. twice daily
Benzylpenicillin	—	—	—	60 mg/kg i.m. twice daily	—	12 mg/kg p.o. once daily
Cephalexin	25 mg/kg i.m. once daily	25 mg/kg i.m. once daily	—	60 mg/kg p.o. 30 mg/kg i.m. once daily	15 mg/kg s.c. twice daily	60 mg/kg p.o. 15 mg/kg s.c. once daily

Table 3 Antimicrobial doses of drugs unlicensed for use in rabbits and rodents (*continued*)

Chloramphenicol	30 mg/kg i.m. once daily	50 mg/kg p.o. 3 times daily 20 mg/kg i.m. twice daily	30–100 mg/kg s.c.	200 mg/kg p.o. 3 times daily 50 mg/kg s.c. twice daily	50 mg/kg p.o. once daily 15 mg/kg i.m. twice daily	20–50 mg/kg p.o. twice daily 10 mg/kg i.m. twice daily
Chlortetracycline	—	—	—	—	1 g/L drinking water†	—
Clopidol	—	—	—	—	200 g/tonne feed†	—
Co-trimazine	—	0.5 mL/kg s.c. once daily	0.2 mL/kg s.c.	—	0.2 mL/kg s.c. once daily	0.5 mL/kg s.c. once daily
Dimetridazole	—	—	500 mg/L drinking water	1 g/L drinking water	100 mg/L drinking water	1 g/L drinking water
Furazolidone	—	—	30 mg/kg p.o. once daily	—	100 g/tonne feed†	—
Gentamicin	5 mg/kg i.m. once daily	—	—	5 mg/kg i.m. once daily	4 mg/kg i.m. once daily	4.4 mg/kg i.m. twice daily
Griseofulvin	15–25 mg/kg p.o.	25 mg/kg p.o. 800 micrograms/kg feed	25–30 mg/kg p.o.	25 mg/kg p.o.	25 mg/kg p.o.	25 mg/kg p.o.
Neomycin	100 mg/kg p.o.	5 mg/kg p.o. twice daily	250 mg/kg p.o.	2.5 g/L drinking water	—	2 g/L drinking water
Oxytetracycline	5 g/L drinking water 20 mg/kg s.c. once daily	—	5 g/L drinking water 20 mg/kg s.c. once daily	400 mg/L drinking water	30 mg/kg p.o. twice daily 15 mg/kg i.m. twice daily	800 mg/L drinking water
Robenidine	—	—	—	—	50–66 g/tonne feed†	—
Streptomycin	—	—	25 mg/kg s.c. once daily	—	50 mg/kg i.m. once daily	—

Table 3 Antimicrobial doses of drugs unlicensed for use in rabbits and rodents (*continued*)

Drug	Gerbil	Guinea pig	Hamster	Mouse	Rabbit	Rat
Sulphadimidine	—	20 g/L drinking water	—	500 mg/L drinking water	100–233 mg/L drinking water†	200 mg/L drinking water
Tetracycline	20 mg/kg p.o. twice daily	—	10 mg/kg p.o. once daily	500 mg/L drinking water	30 mg/kg p.o. twice daily	15–20 mg/kg p.o. twice daily
Tylosin	10 mg/kg s.c. once daily	—	500 mg/L drinking water 10 mg/kg s.c. once daily	—	—	10 mg/kg i.m. once daily

† preparations licensed for use in these species are now available

Table 4 Parasiticide doses of drugs unlicensed for use in rabbits and rodents

Drug	Gerbil	Guinea pig	Hamster	Mouse	Rabbit	Rat
Ivermectin	200 micrograms/ kg s.c.	200 micrograms/ kg s.c.	200 micrograms/ kg s.c.	200 micrograms/ kg s.c.	200 micrograms/ kg s.c.	—
Niclosamide	100 mg/kg p.o.	—	100 mg/kg p.o.	100 mg/kg p.o.	150 mg/kg p.o.	100 mg/ kg p.o.
Piperazine	5 g/L drinking water for 7 days	3 g/L drinking water for 7 days	10 g/L drinking water for 7 days	5 g/L drinking water for 7 days	500 micrograms/ kg p.o.	2 g/L drinking water for 7 days
Thiabend-azole	—	100 mg/kg p.o.	3 mg/g feed for 7–10 days	100 mg/kg p.o. weekly for 4 weeks	25 mg/kg p.o.	200 mg/ kg p.o. for 5 days

Table 5 Doses of analgesics, anaesthetics, and associated drugs unlicensed for use in rabbits and rodents

Drug	Gerbil	Guinea pig	Hamster	Mouse	Rabbit	Rat
Alphadolone/ alphaxalone	—	40 mg/kg i.p.	—	10–15 mg/ kg i.v.	6–9 mg/kg i.v.	10–12 mg/ kg i.v.
Atropine	40 micrograms/ kg s.c., i.m.	50 micrograms/ kg s.c., i.m.	40 micrograms/ kg s.c., i.m.	40 micrograms/ kg s.c., i.m.	50 micrograms/ kg s.c., i.m.	40 micrograms/ kg s.c., i.m.
Buprenorphine	—	50 micrograms/ kg s.c.	—	100 micrograms/ kg s.c.	50 micrograms/ kg s.c., i.v.	100 micrograms/ kg s.c.
Butorphanol	—	—	—	400 micrograms/ kg s.c.	250 micrograms/ kg s.c., i.v.	400 micrograms/ kg s.c.
Doxapram	5–10 mg/kg i.v.	5–10 mg/kg i.v.	5–10 mg/kg i.v.	5–10 mg/kg i.v.	5–10 mg/kg i.v.	5–10 mg/kg i.v.
Fentanyl citrate/ fluanisone	0.5–1.0 mL/kg i.m.	1 mL/kg i.m. 0.5 mL/kg i.m.†	1 mL/kg i.m., i.p.	0.3 mL/kg i.m., i.p.	0.5 mL/kg i.m.†	0.4 mL/kg i.m., i.p.
Fentanyl citrate/ fluanisone + diazepam	0.3 mL/kg + 5 mg/kg i.p.	1 mL/kg i.m. + 2.5 mg/kg i.p.	1 mL/kg + 5 mg/kg i.p.	0.3 mL/kg + 5 mg/kg i.p.	0.3 mL/kg i.m. + 2 mg/kg i.p., i.v.	0.3 mL/kg i.m. + 2.5 mg/kg i.p.
Ketamine	200 mg/kg i.m., i.p.	100 mg/kg i.m., i.p.	200 mg/kg i.m., i.p.	150 mg/kg i.m., i.p.	50 mg/kg i.m.	100 mg/kg i.m., i.p.
Ketamine + xylazine	50 mg/kg + 2 mg/kg i.m.	40 mg/kg + 5 mg/kg i.m.	200 mg/kg + 10 mg/ kg i.p.	200 mg/kg + 2 mg/kg i.p.	35 mg/kg + 5 mg/kg i.m.	90 mg/kg + 10 mg/kg i.p.
Methohexitone	—	30 mg/kg i.p.	—	6 mg/kg i.v.	10 mg/kg i.v.	7–10 mg/kg i.v.
Morphine	—	10 mg/kg s.c.	—	10 mg/kg s.c.	5 mg/kg s.c.	10 mg/kg s.c.
Pentazocine	—	—	—	10 mg/kg s.c.	5 mg/kg i.v.	10 mg/kg s.c.
Pentobarbitone	60–80 mg/ kg i.p.	37 mg/kg i.p. 13–30 mg/ kg i.v.†	50–90 mg/ kg i.p.	40 mg/kg i.p. 37 mg/kg i.v.†	45 mg/kg i.v.†	40 mg/kg i.p. 24 mg/kg i.v.†
Pethidine	—	10 mg/kg s.c., i.m.	—	10 mg/kg s.c., i.m.	10 mg/kg s.c., i.m.	10 mg/kg s.c., i.m.
Thiopentone	—	—	—	30–40 mg/ kg i.v.	30 mg/kg i.v.	30 mg/kg i.v.

† preparations licensed for use in these species are now available

Prescribing for fish

Fish are farmed as food-producing animals and also kept by enthusiasts as a hobby. Atlantic salmon and rainbow trout are the fish most commonly farmed in the UK. Species kept by enthusiasts include marine fish such as clownfish and wrasse and freshwater fish such as goldfish and koi (Japanese carp).

Preventive medicine is extremely important for fish health. Fish live in a 'bacterial soup' and poor water quality or frank infection may quickly lead to an acute cascade of disease within a cage, pond, or tank. Maintenance of good water quality, adequate feeding but not overfeeding, long quarantine, and generous stocking densities will aid the production of healthy fish.

The majority of bacterial infections affecting fish are caused by Gram-negative organisms such as *Aeromonas*, *Vibrio*, and *Pseudomonas* species, which cause septicaemia, furunculosis, and ulcer disease. *Yersinia ruckeri* infection causes enteric redmouth disease.

Antibiotics given to farmed fish are usually formulated as in-feed medications. The drugs are combined with food by admixture with fish oil, corn oil, or gelatin, or are incorporated into the pelleting process at the feed mill. Proprietary oil-based preparations containing added vitamins are also available. Fish should be starved for 12 to 24 hours before treatment. Initially, only a few fish in a group, as a representative sample, should be treated. After observing these fish for good recovery over a few hours the rest of the fish can be treated similarly. Adequate oxygenation should always be provided in treatment tanks.

Licensed preparations are available containing the broad-spectrum antibacterials **amoxicillin**, **oxytetracycline**, **oxolinic acid**, and **co-trimazine**, which are administered in the feed. It is imperative that licensed veterinary products are prescribed for fish if the fish are intended for human consumption. Oxytetracycline is chelated in hard water.

When administering antibiotics to farmed fish, the appropriate withdrawal periods should be observed. Since fish are poikilothermic their basal metabolic rate varies with water temperature. Therefore withdrawal periods, stated in degree days, vary with ambient water temperature. For example 400 degree days is 20 days at a water temperature of 20°C or 40 days at 10°C. The standard withdrawal period for fish is 500° days unless otherwise indicated in the product data sheet.

In general, treatment with antibiotics or methylene blue should not be carried out in tanks with biological filters. Although some drugs are claimed not to disturb biological filters, many do so according to the dose used. It is preferable to administer the treatment in a quarantine tank without filtration.

AMOXYCILLIN TRIHYDRATE

Indications. Amoxycillin-sensitive infections

Dose. *Fish: by addition to feed*, 40 mg/kg body-weight daily for 10 days

PoM **Vetremox™** (Vetrepharm)
Powder, for addition to feed, amoxicillin trihydrate, for *Atlantic salmon*; 400 g, 1 kg, other sizes available
Withdrawal Periods. *Fish*: slaughter 500° days

CO-TRIMAZINE

Preparations of trimethoprim 1 part and sulphadiazine 5 parts

Indications. Co-trimazine-sensitive infections

Dose. Expressed as trimethoprim + sulphadiazine
Fish: by addition to feed, 30 mg/kg body-weight daily for 7–10 days

PoM **Sulphatrim** (Hand/PH)
Powder, for addition to feed, co-trimazine 83/417 [trimethoprim 83.3 g, sulphadiazine 416.7 g]/kg, for *salmon*; 2 kg
Withdrawal Periods. *Fish:* slaughter 500° days

PoM **Tribrissen™ 40% Powder** (Coopers Pitman-Moore)
Powder, for addition to feed, co-trimazine 67/333 [trimethoprim 67 g, sulphadiazine 333 g]/kg, for *Atlantic salmon, rainbow trout*; 3.75 kg
Withdrawal Periods. *Salmon*: slaughter 350° days. *Trout*: slaughter 500° days

OXOLINIC ACID

Indications. Oxolinic acid-sensitive infections
Dose. *Fish*: *by addition to feed*, 10 mg/kg body-weight daily for 10 days

PoM **Aqualinic™** (Vetrepharm)
Powder, for addition to feed, oxolinic acid 100%, for *Atlantic salmon, rainbow trout, brown trout*; 2 kg, 4 kg
Withdrawal Periods. *Fish*: slaughter 500° days

PoM **Aquinox™** (Hand/PH)
Powder, for addition to feed, oxolinic acid 500 g/kg, for *salmon*; 1 kg, 2 kg, 20 kg
Withdrawal Periods. *Fish*: slaughter 30 days
Note. Aquiflake (Hand/PH) medicated feed preparation contains Aquinox™ at an inclusion of 2 g/kg of finished feed

OXYTETRACYCLINE

Indications. Oxytetracycline-sensitive infections
Warnings. Chelated in hard water
Dose. *Fish*: *by addition to feed*, 75 mg/kg body-weight daily for 5–10 days

PoM **Tetraplex™** (Hand/PH)
Powder, for addition to feed, oxy-tetracycline 500 g/kg, for *Atlantic salmon*; 2 kg, 25 kg
Withdrawal Periods. *Fish*: slaughter 400° days
Note. Tetraflake (Hand/PH) medicated feed preparation contains Tetraplex™ at an inclusion of 15 g/kg of finished feed

Ornamental fish may be treated by in-feed medication but antibiotics are more commonly given by intramuscular or preferably by intraperitoneal injection (see Figure 3). The needle should be carefully angled so as not to remove scales when injecting.

Doses of antibiotics unlicensed for use in fish are listed in Table 6. A preparation licensed for use in fish containing buserelin is available. This may be used to facilitate stripping in male and female rainbow trout in spawning condition and to reduce mortality due to egg binding (see section 8.1.2).

Topical drug therapy is used on fish to control ectoparasites and external fungal infections. The common protozoal infections include white spot caused by *Ichthyophthirius multifiliis*, slime disease due to *Chilodonella*, *Costia* (*Ichthyobodo*), and *Trichodina*, velvet disease caused by *Oodinium* species, and fin rot caused by *Epistylis* and traumatic injury. Other ectoparasites causing lesions include flukes such as *Gyrodactylus*, which attach onto the skin and *Dactylogyrus*, which affect the gills, and the

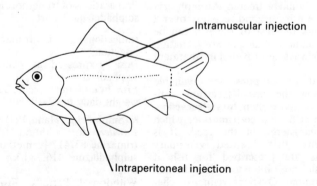

Fig. 3 Injection sites for fish

Table 6 Antimicrobial doses of drugs unlicensed for use in fish

Drug	By addition to water	By addition to feed	By injection
Amoxy-cillin	—	40 mg/kg body-weight†	—
Co-trimazine	—	30 mg/kg body-weight†	125 micrograms/ kg i.p.
Furalta-done	2–5 g/100 litres for 24 hours	—	—
Furazoli-done	—	75 mg/kg body-weight	—
Genta-micin	500 mg/ 100 litres	—	4–5 mg/ kg i.m.
Neomycin	3–5 g/100 litres for 24–48 hours	—	—
Oxolinic acid	—	10 mg/kg body-weight†	—
Oxytetra-cycline	—	75 mg/kg body-weight†	25 mg/kg i.p.

† licensed preparations available

anchor worm *Lernaea*. *Saprolegnia* is a common fungal infection in fish.

The drugs are added to the water, which is used as a bath, a flush, or a dip. To prepare a **bath**, a low concentration of drug is added to the water and the fish are placed in the solution for 30 to 60 minutes, or longer for prolonged immersion. When given as a **flush**, a higher concentration of drug is added to the water which is then flushed through with fresh incoming water. This usually means the fish remain in contact with the drug for 15 to 20 minutes. In a **dip**, a very concentrated solution of the drug is prepared and fish are netted into the solution for 30 to 60 seconds and then replaced in their original tank.

The organophosphorus pesticide **dichlorvos** is used for the treatment of salmon infected by the sea louse, *Lepeophtheirus salmonis*, before the stage at which serious skin damage is evident. Water aeration should be provided when using this drug. Gasping and rolling are signs of toxicity and asphyxiation of the fish.

DICHLORVOS

Indications. Sea lice infection
Warnings. Organophosphorus compounds may be toxic to animals and the operator. Care should be taken with dosage and handling of the product. The recommendations for storage, use, and disposal of waste or unused materials and containers should be followed (MAFF/HSC. *Pesticides: code of practice for the safe use of pesticides on farms and holdings*. London: HMSO, 1990).

PoM **Aquagard**™ (Ciba-Geigy)
Liquid, dichlorvos 500 g/litre, for *salmon*; 1 litre
Withdrawal Periods. *Fish*: slaughter 4 days
Dose. *Fish*: *by bath*, 0.2 mL/100 litres for 30-60 minutes

Suppliers of chemicals used in the treatment of fish diseases include:
• Aqua Med
• AVL
• Micro-Biologicals.
Addresses for these companies may be found in the Index of manufacturers
Malachite green is used as a general ectoparasiticide. A zinc-free grade should be used as other grades may be lethal to fish. Low doses should be used at low pH and higher doses used at high pH. **Formaldehyde** solutions are often used for more resistant infections and fluke infections due to *Gyrodactylus*. The dose of formaldehyde should be adjusted according to the pH; low doses should be used at low pH and higher doses used at high pH. Toxic precipitates of paraformaldehyde form on storage which should be filtered off prior to use. Formaldehyde actively depletes water oxygen and adequate aeration must

therefore be provided. Malachite green and formaldehyde are often used in combination (**Leteux-Meyer mixture**) as an ectoparasiticide particularly for white spot and slime disease.

Chloramine is effective against flukes and fin rot. This chemical is more toxic in soft water with a low pH. **Potassium permanganate** is toxic in water of high pH as manganese dioxide may precipitate onto the gills.

Copper sulphate is used for velvet disease but is very toxic. It is inadvisable to use this compound where other treatments are available or where the fishkeeper is inexperienced. The dose of copper sulphate in freshwater depends on the water hardness. It should be used with caution if the calcium carbonate level in the water is less than 50 mg/litre such as in soft water.

Sodium chloride is used as a general ectoparasiticide and for supportive therapy.

Iodine compounds are used for disinfection of fish eggs and also for direct application to lesions. These compounds are toxic to newly hatched fish. **Benzalkonium chloride** (see section 14.6) is used as a general ectoparasiticide and antibacterial at the rates of 1 g/100 litres for 5 minutes, or 500 mg/100 litres for 30 minutes, or 100 to 400 mg/100 litres for 1 hour. It acts as a surfactant, removing excess mucus and slime containing parasites and bacteria from the fish. Benzalkonium chloride tends to be more toxic in soft water and lower doses should then be used. It is less toxic but also less effective in hard water.

Potassium permanganate acts by liberating oxygen and has been used in situations of intensive fish stocking in earth ponds where emergency aeration is needed. **Methylene blue** is also used in cases of respiratory distress. It is absorbed through the skin regardless of the condition of the gills. It is easily removed by charcoal filtration.

CHLORAMINE
(Chloramine-T)

Indications. Ectoparasite and fungal infections; disinfection

Warnings. High doses may be toxic to koi carp. Should not be used with formaldehyde or benzalkonium chloride; avoid contact with metal

Dose. *By bath*, dose dependent on pH and water hardness as indicated in the following table:

pH of the water	Dose (g/100 litres)	
	Soft water	Hard water
6.0	0.25	0.7
6.5	0.5	1.0
7.0	1.0	1.5
7.5	1.8	1.8
8.0	2.0	2.0

The doses are suggested for systems with a 4 hour turnover and where appropriate they can be repeated 3 times at 4 hour intervals

COPPER SULPHATE

Indications. Ectoparasite and fungal infections

Warnings. Very toxic, see notes above; most toxic in low salt mixtures; kills marine invertebrates

Dose. *By prolonged immersion*, 10-40 mg/100 litres

See section 15.1 for preparation details

FORMALDEHYDE SOLUTION

Formaldehyde solution is generally available as a 34 to 38% w/w solution with methyl alcohol as a stabilising agent to delay polymerisation

Indications. Ectoparasite and fungal infections

Contra-indications. Should not be mixed with potassium permanganate

Warnings. Operators should avoid contact with skin and inhalation of formaldehyde fumes, see notes above

Dose. *By bath*, 25 mL/100 litres (high pH) or 17 mL/100 litres (low pH), for 30 to 60 minutes

By prolonged immersion, 2 mL/100 litres for 12 hours

See section 15.1 for preparation details

FORMALDEHYDE AND MALACHITE GREEN SOLUTION
(Leteux-Meyer mixture)

A stock solution containing malachite green 3.3 g/litre in formaldehyde solution

Indications. Ectoparasite and fungal infections, particularly white spot infection

Contra-indications. Warnings. See under Malachite Green and Formaldehyde

Dose. *By bath*, 2.5 mL/100 litres for 1 hour

By prolonged immersion, 1.5 mL/100 litres given as 3 treatments every other day for *Ichthyophthirius* infections

IODINE COMPOUNDS

Indications. Disinfection of fish eggs
Warnings. Toxic to unfertilised ova and live fish

Wescodyne™ (Ciba-Geigy)
Solution, available iodine 1.6%; 25 litres
Dose. *Eggs*: *by bath*, 3 mL/litre for 10 minutes. Rinse ova thoroughly in clean water

See also section 14.6

MALACHITE GREEN
(Zinc-free)

Indications. Ectoparasitic and fungal infections; proliferative kidney disease in rainbow trout; fungal infections in eggs
Contra-indications. Toxic to Tetras, may be toxic to small marine fish
Dose. *Fish*: *by dip*, 5-6 g/100 litres for 10 to 30 seconds
By bath, 100 mg/100 litres (low pH), 200 mg/100 litres (high pH) for 30-60 minutes, see notes above
By prolonged immersion, 10 mg/100 litres for 30 to 96 hours
Proliferative kidney disease in rainbow trout. Double the above dose, repeat weekly for 3 weeks
Eggs: *by bath*, 500 micrograms/litre for 1 hour

METHYLENE BLUE

Indications. Ectoparasite and fungal infections
Contra-indications. Toxic to scaleless fish
Warning. May inhibit bacterial filters
Dose. *By prolonged immersion*, 20-40 mL/100 litres of a stock solution containing 10 g/litre. Dose may be doubled

POTASSIUM PERMANGANATE

Indications. Ectoparasite and fungal infections, emergency aeration
Contra-indications. Should not be mixed with formaldehyde
Warnings. See notes above
Dose. Treatment. *By bath*, 500 mg/100 litres for 1 hour
By dip, 100 g/100 litre for 10-40 seconds. If organic loading is high, repeat treatment after 24 hours
Oxygen depletion. *By permanent bath*, 200 mg/100 litres or 300-400 mg/100 litres if a high organic load is present

SODIUM CHLORIDE
(Iodine-free)

Indications. Ectoparasitic and fungal infections in freshwater fish
Contra-indications. Saltwater fish; galvanised zinc containers
Dose. *By bath*, 1.0-1.5 kg/100 litres for 20 minutes
By dip, 2-3 kg/100 litres until fish show signs of distress

Anaesthetics

Anaesthetics should be administered to fish preferably after they have been starved for 12 to 14 hours. Constant aeration and a recovery tank of clean water should be available in case the fish become over anaesthetised. If this happens fish should be pushed through the water manually so that fresh water passes across their gills in an antero-posterior direction. **Never push the fish backwards through the water so water enters the gills from the posterior end first.** This will severely damage the delicate structure of the gills and the fish will almost certainly die from the trauma.

A few fish are anaesthetised as a sample group. Tranquillisation or anaesthesia should take 45 to 90 seconds to develop. Fish placed in a clean tank following anaesthesia usually recover within 60 seconds.

The anaesthetics most commonly used in fish are **tricaine mesylate** and **benzocaine**. They are used for tranquillisation of fish for transport, for minor procedures such as treating a surface lesion, and for anaesthesia prior to drug administration by injection. Tranquillising doses may be given by merely reducing the amount of anaesthetic which is placed in the bath. Tricaine mesylate can reduce the pH of the water to about 3.8, which may constitute a stressor when given to fish. Therefore, the pH of the water should be buffered to approximately pH 7 by the addition of phosphate-buffered saline (0.1M). Benzocaine should be dissolved in an organic solvent before use (see below).

BENZOCAINE

Indications. Tranquillisation and anaesthesia of fish

Warnings. Care should be taken when handling the organic solvent. Solutions should be stored protected from light

Dose. Reconstitute 100 g benzocaine in 1 litre ethanol or acetone (benzocaine 100 mg/mL) as stock solution. *By bath*, 30-50 mL stock solution/100 litres

TRICAINE MESYLATE

Indications. Tranquillisation and anaesthesia of fish

Warnings. Use in a buffered solution when giving to fish, see notes above

Dose. *Fish*: *by bath*, 5-10 g/100 litres

PML **MS-222 Sandoz**™ (Thomson and Joseph)

Powder, tricaine mesylate, for *fish*; 25 g, 100 g

Withdrawal Periods. *Fish*: slaughter 3 days

Prescribing for exotic vertebrates

There are over 4000 species of mammals, 9000 species of birds, and 4000 species of reptiles and amphibians. Therapy of exotic species may be based upon extrapolation from treatment regimens that have been studied and found effective in man and the domestic species. Species may be similar enough to justify attempts to extrapolate from one to another, but sufficiently different to make the task difficult and at times hazardous. In addition to the difficulty of dose estimation, the nature of the non-domestic species and the systems of management under which they are kept often set constraints on administration regimens.

In the absence of known contra-indications to drug treatment, dosage may be based on an established dose for a closely related species. Therefore, doses for the horse may be a basis for extrapolating to other Equidae or more broadly to other Perissodactyla. If a drug has been found to be safe and effective in a range of domestic species and man, it is likely to be safe in other species although there may be exceptions. Ivermectin is safe in many species of birds and mammals but is toxic in collie dogs and also Chelonia.

When prescribing a drug for a species in which it has not been evaluated, it is important to consider the taxonomic position of the animal and that rates of drug absorption, metabolism, and excretion tend to increase with body temperature and with decreasing body-size.

Metabolic pathways that are of major importance in one species may be unimportant or non-existent in another. Such variation can influence the kinetics of some drugs. For example, the elimination of salicylates is much slower in the cat than in other domestic species. Closely related species are more likely to have similar metabolic pathways.

Rates of drug metabolism may also be affected by body temperature. The metabolic rate of reptiles is at least 10 times lower than that of mammals of comparable body-size, even when reptiles are kept at high ambient temperatures. This may cause a difference in drug-clearance rate. Therefore it may be appropriate, in the absence of specific information, to reduce the frequency of drug administration in reptiles compared to that used in mammals.

The rates of many physiological processes are also dependent on body-size. For example, the rate of energy expenditure is proportional to the three-quarter power of body-weight ($W^{0.75}$). In general, volume per time functions, such as volume of urine produced per hour, increase with $W^{0.75}$ and the duration of physiological events, such as blood circulation time or the time taken for the clearance of substances from the circulation, increases with $W^{0.25}$. It could be predicted that, if all else is equal, the half-life of a drug would be 10 times shorter in an animal of 5 g than one of 50 kg.

Estimation of dosage regimen. The dangers of extrapolating dosage from one species to another have been well documented, but until there has been more research into drug kinetics in all species of terrestrial vertebrates, there is no alternative but to extrapolate.

The dose required, in mg/kg, to produce a given peak plasma-drug concentration may vary in proportion with body-size. There are indications that smaller doses in mg/kg of drugs such as ketamine may be required in larger-sized animals than in smaller individuals but this has not been fully substantiated.

The dose frequency may be more readily predicted. Suppose it is well established that for one species the dose of a drug needed to sustain therapeutic levels is 10 mg/kg. Therefore, assuming that drug clearance is related to $W^{0.25}$ and that all else is equal, it would be appropriate to adjust the frequency of administration of a 10 mg/kg dose to an animal of a different species using the following equation:

$$F_2 = F_1\frac{W_1^{0.25}}{W_2^{0.25}}$$

where W_1 and F_1 are the body-weight (kg) and recommended dose frequency for the species for which dosage is known, and W_2 and F_2 are body-weight and estimated dose frequency for the animal for which the information is required. Therefore, if W_2 is 10 000 times less than W_1, the dose frequency, if all else is assumed to be equal, should be 10 times greater.

Table 7 indicates how the predicted dose frequency alters with the weight ratio W_1/W_2. In estimating the dose frequency for poikilothermic animals, the lower metabolic rate should be borne in mind.

Table 7 The ratio of the predicted dose frequency F_2, for an animal of body-weight W_2, to the recommended dose frequency F_1, for an animal of body-weight W_1

W_1/W_2	F_2/F_1
10 000	10.0
1 000	5.6
100	3.2
10	1.8
1.0	1.0
0.1	0.56
0.01	0.32
0.001	0.18
0.0001	0.10

Prescribing for exotic birds

Exotic birds include passerines, psittacines, and raptors. No drug preparations licensed for use in exotic avian species are available. Preparations licensed for use in other species may be administered under the responsibility of the veterinarian who has the animal 'under his care'.

Disease in these birds may be influenced by nutrition, housing, and stress. It is often advisable to treat them under hospital care where an ambient temperature of 29°C to 32°C and supportive therapy, such as fluids, can be provided. Lactated Ringer's solution given by intravenous injection or into the cloaca often produces considerable clinical improvement.

Drugs may be administered to exotic avian species by addition to drinking water or feed. The drug dose is mixed in half the daily ration, which should be consumed before offering any further water or feed. This method is non-stressful and convenient for dosing large groups of birds on either a therapeutic or prophylactic basis. Often the correct dose may not be consumed as sick birds may be anorexic or polydipsic leading to under or overdosage. Palatability of drugs, such as chlortetracycline or ivermectin, may be improved by mixing with honey, syrup, or fruit juice or, alternatively, a sweetened paediatric preparation may be used where available.

Drugs may be given by gavage using a metal tube for parrots, although plastic catheters are normally suitable for other birds. This direct method of medication is more reliable but requires frequent handling, which may cause stress. Capsules or tablets can be given to birds of pigeon size and larger.

Therapy may also be administered by parenteral injections but frequent handling of the patient is necessary. Subcutaneous injections may be given in the 'groin' and over the breast, but are most readily given at the back of the base of the neck. Care should be taken not to puncture the crop or the cervical-cephalic air sac, both of which may extend into this area. For critically ill birds, intramuscular or intravenous injection is preferred. Intramuscular injections are given in the posterior part of the pectoral muscles or the quadriceps muscle. Birds have a renal-portal system and some fraction of a medicament may therefore be excreted before reaching the systemic circulation when the drug is given into the leg muscles. Intravenous injections are given into the right jugular or the brachial vein.

Nebulisation may be used for treatment of respiratory-tract disease. This requires specialised equipment and that produced for human use may be employed, although the droplet size of the aerosol produced may be too large to penetrate sufficiently into the avian respiratory system. Drugs used for nebulisation include amphotericin, chloramphenicol, erythromycin, spectinomycin, and tylosin (see Table 8 for dilution details).

Drugs may also be applied topically although preparations should be used sparingly. Ointments and creams used in excess are easily spread through preening and may damage plumage, which can lead to loss of body heat. Some drugs, such as ivermectin, are absorbed percutaneously.

Many antimicrobial drugs are used in avian medicine and suggested doses are listed in Table 8. The aminoglycoside antibiotics are nephrotoxic. Calcium and magnesium found in bird grit may affect the efficacy of tetracyclines.

Overgrowth of *Candida* in the gastrointestinal tract may occur with prolonged antibiotic therapy or vitamin A deficiency. Nystatin is effective against candidiasis. Treatment of aspergillosis includes amphotericin in combination with fluid therapy and immunostimulants such as levamisole 2 mg/kg by subcutaneous injection every 4 days for a total of 3 doses. Amphotericin is hepatotoxic and should not be used in birds that are dehydrated or have renal impairment. Ketoconazole and

Table 8 Antimicrobial doses of drugs unlicensed for use in exotic birds

Drug	By mouth	By addition to drinking water	By addition to feed	By injection	Other methods of administration
Amoxycillin	150 mg/kg 3 times daily	200–400 mg/L	300–500 mg/kg soft feed	250 mg/kg i.m. daily (long-acting preparation)	—
Amphotericin	—	—	—	1.5 mg/kg i.v. daily for 7 days	By oral topical application, 10% solution By nebulisation, 100 mg diluted in 15 mL of saline solution By intratracheal administration, 1 mg/kg daily for 12 days then every other day for 5 weeks
Cephalexin	35–50 mg/kg, repeat 4 times daily (more than 500 g body-weight); 35–50 mg/kg repeat 8 times daily (less than 500 g body-weight)	—	—	—	—
Chloramphenicol	—	—	—	—	By nebulisation, 200 mg diluted in 15 mL of saline solution
Chlortetracycline	190 mg/kg 4 times daily	Treatment. 5 g/L for 30 days Prophylaxis. 1 g/L for 30 days	Treatment. 5 g/kg soft feed for 30 days Prophylaxis. 1 g/kg soft feed for 30 days	—	—

Table 8 Antimicrobial doses of drugs unlicensed for use in exotic birds (*continued*)

Drug	By mouth	By addition to drinking water	By addition to feed	By injection	Other methods of administration
Co-amoxiclav (Dose expressed as amoxycillin)	125 mg/kg 4 times daily	—	—	—	—
Co-trimazine	12–60 mg/kg	—	—	30 mg/kg s.c., i.m.	—
Dimetridazole	50 mg/kg daily	100 mg/L (finches); 100–250 mg/L (other species)	—	—	—
Doxycycline	10 mg/kg daily (parrots); 25 mg/kg twice daily (other species)	500 mg/L	—	—	—
Erythromycin	—	125 mg/L for 3–5 days	200 mg/kg soft feed	20 mg/kg s.c., i.m. twice daily	By injection into infra-orbital sinus, 44–88 mg/kg twice daily for 5–7 days By nebulisation, 200 mg diluted in 15 mL saline solution
Gentamicin	—	—	—	2.5 mg/kg i.m. 3 times daily (raptors); 5–10 mg/kg i.m. 2–3 times daily (other species)	By intratracheal administration 10 mg/kg daily
Ketoconazole	25–30 mg/kg 3 times daily for 2 weeks	200 mg/L for 1–2 weeks	—	—	—
Metronidazole	20–50 mg/kg twice daily for 7 days	100 mg/L	—	5 mg/kg i.m. twice daily	—

Table 8 Antimicrobial doses of drugs unlicensed for use in exotic birds (*continued*)

Drug	By mouth	By addition to drinking water	By addition to feed	By injection	Other methods of administration
Miconazole	—	—	—	10 mg/kg i.m. daily for 6–12 days (raptors); 20 mg/kg i.m. daily for 8–10 days (psittacines)	—
Nystatin	300 000–600 000 units/kg 2–3 times daily for 1–2 weeks	100 000 units/L for 3–6 weeks	200 000 units/kg soft feed for 3–6 weeks	—	—
Oxytetra-cycline	—	Treatment. 2.5 g/L Prophylaxis. 250 mg/L	Treatment. 5 g/kg Prophylaxis. 50 mg/kg soft feed	58 mg/kg i.m. daily (more than 400 g body-weight); 100 mg/kg i.m. daily (less than 400 g weight)	—
Spectino-mycin	—	—	—	—	By nebulisation, 200 mg diluted in 15 mL saline solution
Sulpha-dimidine	50 mg/kg	220 mg/L for 3 days, repeat after 2 days	—	30 mg/kg s.c., i.m.	—
Tobramycin	—	—	—	10 mg/kg i.m. 2–3 times daily	—
Tylosin	—	500 mg/L	—	60 mg/kg i.m. 3 times daily (50–250 g body-weight); 25 mg/kg i.m. 3 times daily (0.25–1 kg body-weight); 15 mg/kg i.m. 3 times daily (more than 1 kg weight)	By nebulisation, 100 mg diluted in 5 mL DMSO and 10 mL saline solution

miconazole are also hepatotoxic with prolonged therapy.

Metronidazole is used for *Trichomonas* infections and dimetridazole for *Giardia* infections. Coccidiosis may occasionally be a problem, particularly in finches, budgerigars, and parrots. Sulphadimidine is an effective treatment.

Parasiticides administered to exotic avian species are listed in Table 9. The benzimidazole endoparasiticides may cause feather abnormalities in some birds during the moult, and may lead to vomiting and death in nestlings if used during the breeding season. Levamisole gives a bitter taste when added to drinking water and the addition of sweeteners may improve palatability. This drug may be toxic to finches and budgerigars. Ectoparasiticides are used in birds to control *Cnemidocoptes* and lice infestations.

Medroxyprogesterone acetate, by subcutaneous or intramuscular injection, at a dose of 5 to 10 mg/kg may be used to stop persistent egg laying due to ovarian

Table 9 Parasiticide doses of drugs unlicensed for use in exotic birds

Drug	By mouth	By addition to drinking water	By injection	Other methods of administration
Endoparasiticides				
Fenbendazole	10–50 mg/kg, repeat: —after 10 days (nematodes); —daily for 3 days (microfilaria and trematodes); —daily for 5 days (*Capillaria*)	50 mg/L (finches)	—	—
Ivermectin	200 micrograms/ kg diluted in propylene glycol	—	200 micrograms/ kg s.c., i.m.	By topical application, one drop of 1% solution
Levamisole	10–20 mg/kg, repeat after 2 weeks	80 mg/L (finches); 100–200 mg/L daily for 3 days (other species)	10 mg/kg s.c. (not finches)	—
Niclosamide	100 mg/kg	—	—	—
Praziquantel	5–10 mg/kg, repeat after 2–4 weeks	—	7.5 mg/kg s.c., i.m., repeat after 2–4 weeks	—
Ectoparasiticides				
Dichlorvos-impregnated strips	—	—	—	Minimum air space 30 m³, use for up to 3 days
Pyrethrins	—	—	—	Dusting powder

Table 10 Anaesthetic doses of drugs unlicensed for use in exotic birds

Drug	Dose
Alphadolone/ alphaxalone	10–36 mg/kg i.v. May be administered by subcutaneous or intramuscular injection. but not as effective by these routes
Ketamine	50 mg/kg i.m.
Ketamine + acepromazine	25–50 mg/kg i.m. 0.5–1.0 mg/kg
Ketamine + diazepam	10–40 mg/kg i.m. 1.0–1.5 mg i.m.
Ketamine + xylazine	20 mg/kg i.m. 4 mg/kg i.m.

cysts. Medical treatment for egg binding includes oxytocin 3 to 5 units/kg given by intramuscular injection in combination with calcium gluconate 10% solution at 10 to 20 mL/kg administered by the same route.

Birds normally excrete uric acid but renal impairment or incorrect diet may lead to retention and hence gout. Allopurinol 10 to 15 mg/kg orally may aid recovery, although it is not effective in reducing uric acid tophi already present in joints and other tissues. Bromhexine 3 to 6 mg/kg by intramuscular injection or 6.5 mg/litre by addition to the drinking water, with concurrent vitamin A therapy, may aid therapy of disorders of the respiratory system. Bird seed often does not supply adequate vitamin A, which may need to be supplemented (see section 16.5.1).

Inhalational and injectable anaesthetics are used in exotic avian practice (see Table 10). Ketamine, given alone or in combination with sedatives, is the injectable drug of choice. Isoflurane, halothane, and methoxyflurane are used for inhalational anaesthesia.

Prescribing for reptiles

Reptiles kept in captivity usually belong to the order Squamata which includes lizards and snakes, or the order Chelonia consisting of tortoises, terrapins, and turtles. There are no drug preparations licensed for use in reptiles. Drugs licensed for use in other species may be administered under the responsibility of the veterinarian who has the animal 'under his care'. Reptiles are poikilothermic and their metabolic rate is affected by ambient temperature. Thus the pharmacokinetics of any drug administered will vary with temperature changes.

All reptiles have a preferred body temperature (PBT) range, which is the range at which that animal thrives best (see Table 11). This range may vary at different seasons of the year, or even different times of the day. Knowing the PBT range of a reptile is important when administering drugs.

A drop of 6°C, for example, doubles the elimination half-life of an antibiotic in a reptile, resulting in a cumulative effect with subsequent doses, which may lead to toxicity. For most drugs, an optimum temperature-dependent dose is stated. Therefore, when medicating reptiles, environmental temperature before, during, and after treatment should be considered.

Medication may be administered to reptiles by mouth or stomach tube or by subcutaneous, intramuscular, intravenous, intracoelomic, or intratracheal injection. In an iguana with hypocalcaemic tetany it is advantageous to correct the calcium imbalance as quickly as possible, therefore the intravenous route is preferred to intramuscular injection. For rehydration of reptiles that are severely dehydrated, the intracoelomic route is preferred to administration by mouth or stomach tube. However, if repeated fluid therapy is required, then oral administration or gastric intubation is used rather than repeated injections into the coelomic cavity.

The majority of bacterial infections in reptiles are from Gram-negative microorganisms, particularly Enterobacteriaceae. Reptiles are especially prone to infections due to *Pseudomonas*, *Aeromonas*, and *Proteus* species. Protozoal infection due to *Entamoeba* and *Balantidium* species also occurs. Table 12 lists doses for commonly used antimicrobials in reptilian medicine.

Terrestrial reptiles produce uric acid as their main excretory waste product. Dehydration, and liver or kidney damage may result in uricaemia and tophi formation in the joints or visceral organs. Any antibiotic therapy, but particularly when using gentamicin, should be accompanied by fluids to maintain adequate renal function and reduce the possibility of nephrotoxicity.

As most of the diseases that affect reptiles are related to their environment, supportive therapy alone will often aid recovery. Using antibiotics in debilitated animals may cause further deterioration due to excessive bacterial endotoxin release.

Table 11 Examples of preferred body temperature ranges for different species

Species	Preferred body temperature (PBT) °C
Boa (*Constrictor constrictor*)	26–34°
Garter snake (*Thamnophis sirtalis*)	20–35°
American chameleon (*Anolis carolinensis*)	22.6–30.4°
Greek tortoise (*Testudo graeca*)	22–30°
Red eared terrapin (*Pseudemys scripta elegans*)	24–30°
Bell's hinged back tortoise (*Kinixys belliana*)	25–27°
Common agama (*Agama agama*)	26–30°
Slow worm (*Anguis fragilis*)	15–22°
Corn snake (*Elaphe guttata*)	25–30°
Rat snake (*Elaphe obsoleta*)	25–30°

Table 12 Antimicrobial doses of drugs unlicensed for use in reptiles

Drug	Dose	Maintenance temperature °C
Amikacin	2.5–5.0 mg i.m. every 3 days	25°
Ampicillin	3–6 mg/kg s.c., i.m. daily	26°
Carbenicillin	200–400 mg/ kg i.m. daily	30°
Ceftazidime	20 mg/kg i.m. every 3 days	30°
Cefuroxime	50 mg/kg i.m. every other day	30°
Cephalothin	40–80 mg/kg i.m. every other day	30°
Co-trimazine	15 mg/kg i.m. daily	24°
Dimetridazole	40 mg/kg p.o. daily for 5 days	Preferred body temperature
Gentamicin	2.5 mg/kg s.c. every 3 days	24°
Kanamycin	10 mg/kg s.c., i.m. daily	24°
Metronidazole	100–275 mg/ kg p.o. as a single dose	Preferred body temperature
Tobramycin	2 mg/kg i.m. daily	26°
Tylosin	25 mg/kg i.m. daily	30°

Parasitic infections including helminths, mites, and ticks are common in reptiles and parasiticides are listed in Table 13. Parasites may prove difficult to eliminate where there is environmental contamination. Wherever possible, a snake being treated for external parasites should be put into a hospital vivarium while the original environment is treated with, for example, a dichlorvos-impregnated strip (Vapona™ (Nicholas Laboratories Ltd)).

Some nematodes, such as *Kalicephalus* species, have larvae that are capable of penetrating the skin and migrating through the body. Therefore worming should be repeated until recurrent faecal samples are negative of larvae or larvated eggs.

Reptiles are particularly susceptible to parasiticide toxicity, which may manifest as seizures. This is commonly seen in

Table 13 Parasiticide doses of drugs unlicensed for use in reptiles

Drug	Dose
Endoparasiticides	
Albendazole	50–75 mg/kg p.o. as a single dose
Bunamidine	150–300 mg/kg p.o. as a single dose
Fenbendazole	100 mg/kg p.o. as a single dose
Ivermectin	200 micrograms/kg s.c. as a single dose (not for use in Chelonia)
Levamisole	200 mg/kg p.o. as a single dose
Mebendazole	20–25 mg/kg p.o. as a single dose
Niclosamide	150–300 mg/kg p.o. as a single dose
Oxfendazole	68 mg/kg p.o. as a single dose
Praziquantel	3.5–7.5 mg/kg s.c. as a single dose
Thiabendazole	50 mg/kg p.o. as a single dose
Ectoparasiticides	
Coumaphos	0.1% wash
Dichlorvos-impregnated strip	1 cm of strip/30 cm³ for 3–5 days

Table 14 Anaesthetic doses of drugs unlicensed for use in reptiles

Drug	Dose
Alphadolone/ alphaxalone	6–9 mg/kg i.v. up to 15 mg/kg i.m. in incremental doses every 30 minutes according to the animal's response
Etorphine	up to 1 mg/kg for terrapins
Ketamine	10–100 mg/kg s.c., i.m. in incremental doses every 30 minutes according to the animal's response
Pentobarbitone	10–30 mg/kg i.m., i.p.
Propofol	14 mg/kg i.v. for Chelonia 10 mg/kg i.v. for Squamata Additional doses of 10% of the original dose may be administered
Thiopentone	20–30 mg/kg i.p.

snakes that are fed while a dichlorvos-impregnated strip is present in the vivarium. Ivermectin is effective in Squamata but highly toxic in Chelonia.

Other problems encountered in reptilian medicine include egg binding, which is treated with calcium gluconate 10% 1 to 2 mL/kg daily for 4 days, followed by 2 to 10 units/kg oxytocin, both by intramuscular injection. Hypovitaminosis A may be treated with vitamin A 100 000 units/kg weekly for 3 weeks, by intramuscular injection.

Anaesthesia may be induced in reptiles by using inhalational or injectable anaesthetics (see Table 14). Inhalational anaesthesia may involve the use of nitrous oxide, methoxyflurane, or isoflurane. Adult reptiles often have liver impairment. Therefore, isoflurane is the preferred inhalational anaesthetic as it is less hepatotoxic than methoxyflurane or halothane.

Propofol is the injectable anaesthetic of choice due to its rapid induction and recovery time. Anaesthetic drugs given by intramuscular injection have a longer induction time than drugs given intravenously. The recovery times for the different anaesthetic drugs vary considerably. The recovery time for thiopentone is approximately 2 to 6 hours whereas for ketamine and pentobarbitone it may be up to several days. Ketamine should be used with caution in debilitated reptiles.

Prescribing in hepatic impairment

Liver disease can influence the pharmacological effects of a drug depending on the nature and severity of the disease. The liver is the principal organ for metabolism of lipid-soluble drugs and for the production of plasma proteins and coagulation factors.

Altered response to drugs in animals with liver disease is mainly caused by a decreased rate of drug metabolism, thereby increasing the duration of drug action. Fasting may decrease the rate of hepatic metabolism. Hypoalbuminaemia causes reduced protein binding and increased toxicity of highly protein-bound drugs such as phenytoin and prednisolone.

The occurrence of drug-induced hepatotoxicity is more commonly associated with chronic medication or overdosage of certain drugs than with short courses of therapy. The halogenated anaesthetic agents, paracetamol, antiepileptics, and corticosteroids are among the most significant causes of drug-related hepatotoxicity encountered in veterinary practice.

Routine liver function tests poorly correlate liver dysfunction and drug metabolising activity. In chronic liver disease, serum-albumin concentration might serve as a crude index of hepatic drug-metabolising activity. Therefore, it is not possible to predict the extent to which the metabolism of a particular drug will be impaired or any dosage adjustment that may be necessary.

A general recommendation is that drugs which depend on hepatic metabolism for elimination should be given in reduced doses to animals with liver impairment. Whenever alternative therapy is feasible, the use of drugs which undergo extensive hepatic metabolism should be avoided.

Table 15 includes drugs that should be avoided or used with caution in liver impairment. This list is not comprehensive; absence from the table does not imply safety.

Table 15 Drugs to be avoided or used with caution in animals with hepatic disease

Anaesthetics, halogenated
Antiepileptics
Beta blockers
Butorphanol
Chloramphenicol
Chlorpromazine
Corticosteroids
Doxapram
Doxorubicin
Ethyloestrenol
Fentanyl citrate + fluanisone [Hypnorm™]
Flucytosine
Griseofulvin
Heparin
Ketamine
Ketoconazole
Lignocaine
Lincosamides
Meclofenamic acid
Pancuronium
Pentobarbitone
Phenylbutazone
Polysulphated glycosaminoglycan
Propofol
Quinidine
Sulphonamides
Suxamethonium
Tubocurarine
Vecuronium

Prescribing in renal impairment

Renal excretion is the principal process of elimination for drugs that are predominantly ionised at physiological pH and for drug metabolites with low lipid solubility. Renal impairment decreases the rate of excretion of these substances causing drug accumulation and a greater risk of toxicity. Hypoalbuminaemia, which occurs in the nephrotic syndrome, and uraemia may further enhance the severity of the condition by causing an increase in the plasma concentration of the unbound fraction of drugs such as phenylbutazone, frusemide, and phenytoin.

Reduced renal function is commonly assessed from the concentrations of blood urea nitrogen (BUN) or serum creatinine. Increased BUN and creatinine concentrations result from moderate to severe renal impairment but may be complicated by diet and protein metabolism. Creatinine clearance may be more indicative of the degree of renal impairment but is more difficult to measure.

Nephrotoxic renal failure is most commonly associated with injury to the proximal tubules. It may be caused by certain antimicrobial drugs such as aminoglycosides, polymyxins, cephaloridine, and amphotericin, and by heavy metals including mercuric salts, arsenic salts, bismuth, and copper.

Nephrotoxicity of aminoglycosides is dose-related; the total amount of drug administered is probably more important than the daily dose in determining toxicity. Dehydration due to sodium deprivation or frusemide administration increases the nephrotoxic potential of aminoglycosides. Neonatal animals are more susceptible than adult animals to aminoglycoside nephrotoxicity.

In general, dosage may be adjusted by decreasing the dose or lengthening the dosing interval. Drugs that are excreted mainly unchanged in the urine should be avoided in animals with renal impairment.

Table 16 includes drugs that should be avoided or used with caution in renal impairment. This is not a comprehensive list; absence from the table does not imply safety.

Table 16 Drugs to be used with caution in animals with renal impairment

Acepromazine
Alcuronium
Allopurinol
Amphotericin
Aminoglycosides
Captopril
Cardiac glycosides
Cisplatin
Cephalosporins
Chlorpromazine
Doxapram
Fentanyl citrate + fluanisone [Hypnorm™]
Flucytosine
Fluorouracil
Gallamine
Hydroxyurea
Ketamine
Meclofenamic acid
Methotrexate
Methoxyflurane
Nitrofurantoin
Non-steroidal anti-inflammatory drugs
Pancuronium
Pethidine
Piperazine
Polysulphated glycosaminoglycan
Procainamide
Propofol
Spironolactone
Sulphonamides
Tetracyclines (except doxycycline)
Thiazides
Tubocurarine

Prescribing for pregnant animals

Drugs can have harmful effects on the fetus at any time during pregnancy, although only limited data are available. Manufacturer information on the effect of drugs in laboratory animals may be helpful when assessing drug safety in other species.

Drugs may cause congenital malformations (teratogenesis) or neonatal disease if administered during pregnancy. Drugs that are known to cause teratogenesis in animals include some benzimidazoles such as albendazole, cambendazole, and oxfendazole, particularly at high doses; corticosteroids; griseofulvin; ketoconazole; and methotrexate. Many drugs may cross the placental barrier and affect the fetus or neonate. Opioids and barbiturates may affect respiration. Chlorpropamide and tolbutamide may cause hypoglycaemia. Salicylates are teratogenic and prolonged use may also increase risk of haemorrhage. Tetracyclines may cause dental discoloration in the offspring. Corticosteroids may cause teratogenesis and also affect skeletal calcification. Steroid hormones including androgens, anabolic steroids, and progestogens may affect antenatal sexual development of the offspring.

Drugs may cause pregnancy termination or premature parturition. Abortion may be induced by corticosteroids, some prostaglandins, and alpha$_2$-adrenergic receptor agonists such as xylazine. Prostaglandins are used therapeutically to terminate early pregnancy in cattle, and to induce parturition in cattle and pigs. When drugs are used to induce early parturition, the length of gestation should be calculated to minimise the risk of non-viable offspring.

Drugs may also prolong normal delivery. Clenbuterol is used as a bronchodilator and also to reduce uterine motility. When used to treat a respiratory condition, therapy should be discontinued prior to parturition.

Tables 17 and 18 include drugs which should, if at all possible, be avoided during pregnancy or at parturition respectively. These lists are not comprehensive; absence from the table does not imply safety.

Table 17 Drugs to be avoided or used with caution in pregnant animals

Some benzimidazoles
Corticosteroids
Cytotoxic drugs
Griseofulvin
Ketoconazole
Prostaglandins
Salicylates
Sex hormones
Tetracyclines
Vaccines, living

Table 18 Drugs to be avoided or used with caution at parturition

Barbiturates
Chlorpropamide
Clenbuterol
Opioid analgesics
Tolbutamide
Xylazine

Prescribing for lactating animals

During lactation lipid-soluble drugs pass from the systemic circulation into milk. The concentration of drug attained in the milk is influenced by the extent of plasma protein-binding, the lipid-solubility of the drug, and the degree of ionisation of the drug. Milk is separated from the general circulation by an intact membrane through which only the non-ionised lipophilic form of a drug may pass. When the non-ionised form of a basic drug such as a macrolide enters the relatively acid milk it dissociates and so becomes trapped resulting in high concentrations in milk – the so called 'ion-trap'. Polar organic bases, such as aminoglycosides, and organic acids are less concentrated in milk than in plasma. There are limited data available on the effect of drugs on the suckling offspring. Danthron preparations, for example, should not be administered to lactating mares as the drug may affect the nursing foal. In general, any treatment given to the dam during lactation should be used with caution.

Drugs such as atropine, bromocriptine, and frusemide may inhibit lactation and cause agalactia.

Prescribing for neonates

The neonatal period is generally defined as the first month of postnatal life. However, it may be considered to vary with the species; from one week in foals to 6 to 8 weeks in calves and puppies. Physiological systems that affect drug absorption and disposition differ during the neonatal period and undergo rapid development during the first 24 hours after birth. Characteristics of the neonatal period include more efficient absorption from the gastro-intestinal tract compared to older animals, lower binding to plasma proteins, increased volume of distribution, increased permeability of the blood-brain barrier, and slower elimination of many drugs. These differences largely account for the clinical observation that neonates are often more sensitive to the effects of some drugs.

Some antimicrobial agents that are poorly absorbed after oral administration to adult animals may attain effective systemic concentrations in neonates. The absorption pattern of drugs in young ruminants is similar to that in monogastric species since it takes 8 to 12 weeks, depending on dietary composition, for a functional rumen to develop.

There is wide variation among species in the rate of development of hepatic microsomal oxidative reactions, which constitute the principal pathways of metabolism for various lipid-soluble drugs. Until the pathways are fully developed at between 1 and 8 weeks of age, depending on the species, drugs are metabolised at a slower rate. Most other hepatic metabolic pathways develop rapidly within the first 1 to 2 weeks after birth.

Renal excretion mechanisms are poorly developed in neonates, particularly in puppies, kittens, and piglets. In calves and foals, glomerular filtration reaches functional maturity 24 to 48 hours after birth, whereas in puppies it may take 2 weeks.

Neonates of all species produce acidic urine, which promotes tubular reabsorption of lipid-soluble organic acids further prolonging the duration of action of these drugs. The combined effect of slow hepatic metabolic reactions and inefficient renal excretion in very young animals may considerably decrease the elimination of lipid-soluble drugs and their metabolites.

Precise recommendations cannot be made on dosage adjustment of drugs for neonates. In general, the dosing interval, which is based on the rate of elimination, may need to be increased. In The Veterinary Formulary the dose for young animals, in mg/kg, is the same as that given for adults, unless otherwise stated.

The oral route is preferable to parenteral administration but when the latter is required it may be best to administer the drug by slow intravenous infusion to avoid circulatory overload.

Emergency treatment of poisoning

Diagnosis of poisoning is not easy and can seldom be made from a single observation. The primary aims of the treatment of poisoning in all species are to prevent further exposure and absorption of the toxin, to hasten elimination of absorbed poison, and to provide supportive therapy. If specific poisons are known to be implicated, antidotes may be available. Advice may be sought from the National Poisons Information Services (NPIS). The telephone numbers of centres are given below.

National Poisons Information Services	
Belfast	0232 240503
Birmingham	021-554 3801
Cardiff	0222 709901
Dublin	0001 379964
	0001 379966
Edinburgh	031-229 2477
	031-228 2441 (Viewdata)
Leeds	0532 432799
	0532 430715
London	071-635 9191
	071-955 5095
Newcastle	091-232 5131

Animals should be removed from the contaminated area and any suspected material such as half-eaten food withdrawn. Any vomitus should be kept, together with a sample of the suspected poison and its packaging, for subsequent examination, identification, and possible analysis. Wash any contaminants from the skin, fur, or fleece with running water. Oily materials, paint, or tar should be removed with rags or paper towels and then the area cleaned using cooking oil or margarine. Commercial grease solvents or hand cleaners may be used sparingly, provided they are washed off with plenty of water, and the animal then washed using soap or liquid detergent. If the animal has been in contact with strong alkalis, wash with copious amounts of water, and vinegar or lemon juice. If acids are implicated,

wash with water and a weak solution of sodium bicarbonate. The owner should be advised to be careful of self-exposure to the toxicant and to wear protective clothing if necessary.

In dogs and cats, ingested materials may be removed by inducing vomiting (see section 3.4). Vomiting should not be induced if the poison has been ingested for more than 2 to 3 hours or if the ingesta is thought to contain paraffin or petroleum products due to the risk of inhalation. Ingesta containing strong acids or alkalis may cause further oesophageal damage if emesis is attempted. Ingested alkalis can be partly neutralised using lemon juice or vinegar diluted one part with 4 parts water. Ingested acids should not be neutralised with sodium bicarbonate because of gas formation; magnesium hydroxide mixture is preferable. Gastric lavage with water, saline solution, or a slurry of **activated charcoal** may be carried out. Some activated charcoal should be left in the stomach after lavage. Saline or oily laxatives may also aid elimination of the toxin.

In large animal practice, emesis and gastric lavage are not used. Laxatives may be used to eliminate toxin from the gastro-intestinal tract. In ruminants, gastric emptying may only be performed by rumenotomy. If the ruminal contents are removed, they should be replaced by suitable fluids and roughage, and the bacterial microflora re-established.

Antidotes (see below) act in a variety of ways. They may antagonise the toxin, react with it to form less active or inactive complexes, or interfere with the metabolism of the poison. Other techniques intended to enhance the elimination of poisons include intravenous fluids (see section 16.1.2) and diuretics (see section 4.2).

Supportive therapy including warmth, intravenous fluids, analgesics, and antiepileptics may be necessary until the toxin has been metabolised or eliminated.

CHARCOAL, ACTIVATED

Indications. See notes above
Dose. *By gastric lavage*, two to five 5-mL spoonfuls/200 mL water

P **Carbomix**™ (Penn)
Oral powder, activated charcoal; 50 g

P **Medicoal**™ (Torbet)
Oral granules, effervescent, activated charcoal; 5 g

See section 3.1.1 for Antidiarrhoeal adsorbent preparations containing charcoal

Antidotes

Drug poisoning

Poisoning with *anaesthetics* or *analgesics* may occur from overdosage or from ingestion of human medication. If an anaesthetic overdose is given, artificial respiration should be provided and **doxapram hydrochloride** (see section 5.5) administered. Intravenous fluid therapy may facilitate clearance of the toxin.
Salicylates such as aspirin may have an irritant effect on the gastric mucosa in the dog. Clinical symptoms include vomiting followed by incoordination and lethargy. *Aspirin* is particularly toxic to cats due to the very slow elimination of the drug in this species. **Sodium bicarbonate** is given by gastric lavage with **compound sodium lactate intravenous infusion** (Lactated Ringer's solution) (see section 16.1.2) given by intraperitoneal injection to correct the fluid and pH imbalance.
Paracetamol poisoning occurs most commonly in the cat due to prolonged drug metabolism in this species. **Acetylcysteine** may help to prevent hepatic and possibly renal damage. **Ascorbic acid** (see section 16.5.3) 30 mg/kg by mouth should be given with each dose of acetylcysteine.
Poisoning with *caffeine* or 'doping' may be seen in horses or dogs used in competitions. In dogs, **pentobarbitone sodium** (see section 6.6.2) 20 mg/kg by intravenous injection is used to control the clinical symptoms of excitement, incoordination, and convulsions.
For reference to poisoning with carbamates, chlorinated hydrocarbons, and organophosphorus compounds, see below, under Pesticides.

ACETYLCYSTEINE

Indications. Paracetamol poisoning
Dose. *Cats*: *by intravenous injection*, 140 mg/kg. Repeat every 6 hours at 70 mg/kg for 7 treatments. Ascorbic acid (see notes above) is given concurrently.

PoM **Parvolex**™ (DF)
Injection, acetylcysteine 200 mg/mL; 10 mL

Poisonous plants

Plants may be ingested from roadsides, neglected pastures, or dried in hay. Plants infected with fungi such as ergot may also cause poisoning.
Sweet vernal grass *Anthoxanthum odoratum* contains *coumarin*, which may cause clinical signs in cattle similar to warfarin poisoning. **Phytomenadione** (vitamin K_1) (see section 16.5.6) is given by intramuscular injection at a dose of 1 to 3 mg/kg body-weight.
Cyanogenetic glycosides found in plants such as cherry laurel, linseed, and some grasses are toxic and may affect cattle and sheep. Treatment includes sodium nitrite injection followed by sodium thiosulphate injection. See below under Minerals and inorganic substances.
The *nitrite* and *nitrate* content of various plants is influenced by climate and use of nitrogenous fertilisers. The toxin converts haemoglobin to methaemoglobin in the body causing hypoxia. **Methylene blue** is used as an antidote as it converts methaemoglobin to haemoglobin.
Beet tops should be introduced into the diet slowly as these and other plants such as *Oxalis* species may be toxic due to their *oxalate* content. *Rhubarb* leaves commonly cause oxalate poisoning in goats kept in gardens. Clinical signs are those of hypocalcaemia and treatment is by subcutaneous or intravenous injection of **calcium borogluconate** (see section 16.4.1).

Bracken and *Equisetum* species contain thiaminases, which may cause thiamine deficiency. **Thiamine** (see section 16.5.2) 100 mg daily by intramuscular or intravenous injection is used for the treatment of thiaminase poisoning in horses and pigs.

METHYLENE BLUE

Indications. Nitrite and nitrate poisoning; chlorate poisoning (see below)
Dose. *Cattle, sheep, pigs, dogs, cats: by intravenous injection*, 5-10 mg/kg

PoM **Methylene Blue** (Farillon)
Injection, methylene blue 10 mg/mL; 10 mL

Pesticides

Many *rodenticides* contain warfarin or other anticoagulants, which act by inhibiting the production of prothrombin and thus interfering with the clotting mechanism. Animals are poisoned by direct ingestion of the anticoagulant or ingestion of a poisoned rodent. Dogs and cats are the main species affected. Similar clinical signs of pallor, lameness, and haemorrhage are seen in cattle poisoned by sweet vernal grass. Therapy includes **phytomenadione** (vitamin K_1) (see section 16.5.6) and blood transfusions if necessary. Phytomenadione is administered by intramuscular injection 0.5 to 1.0 mg/kg to horses and pigs, and at a dose of 2.5 to 5.0 mg/kg daily in divided doses to dogs and cats.
Paraquat preparations available to farmers and horticulturalists are extremely toxic. Early treatment is essential and **fuller's earth** or **bentonite** may be given by mouth to reduce absorption of the drug from the gastro-intestinal tract. In conjunction with supportive therapy, excretion is accelerated by forced diuresis. Oxygen therapy should not be used.
Organophosphorus compounds and *carbamates* are used as pesticides and parasiticides, which may be toxic to animals, and humans handling the drugs. Organophosphorus compounds and carbamates form a stable complex with cholinesterases therefore prolonging and intensifying the effects of acetylcholine. **Atropine** (see section 6.6.1) 0.25 to 1.0 mg/kg, by subcutaneous injection, is used to control the muscarinic effects produced. In severe cases, one third of the initial dose may be given intravenously as a dilute solution (2%) and the remainder of the dose administered by subcutaneous or intravenous injection. The dose may be repeated at 3 to 6 hour intervals for 24 hours or more. Organophosphorus compounds inhibit cholinesterase by phosphorylation and **pralidoxime** is able to combine with the fixed molecule allowing regeneration of the active enzyme. Similarly carbamates such as carbaryl and propoxur inhibit cholinesterase but by carboxylation rather than phosphorylation. Therefore pralidoxime is an ineffective antidote for carbamate poisoning.
There are no specific antidotes for poisoning by *organochlorines* including lindane, *metaldehyde* used as a molluscicide, or *fluoroacetates*. These compounds cause central nervous system stimulation; **pentobarbitone sodium** (see section 6.6.2) is used to control convulsions.
Poisoning with *sodium chlorate*, which is used as weedkiller, causes conversion of haemoglobin to methaemoglobin. **Methylene blue** is administered as the antidote.
Thallium salts have been used as rodenticides. Orally administered **prussian blue** forms a non-absorbable complex with the thallium ion in the gastro-intestinal tract, which is then excreted in the faeces.

PRALIDOXIME MESYLATE

Indications. Adjunct to atropine in organophosphorus poisoning
Dose. *By slow intravenous injection*, 40 mg/kg

PoM **Pralidoxime Mesylate** (Non-proprietary)
Injection, pralidoxime mesylate 200 mg/mL; 5 mL
Information on availability from National Poisons Information Service

PRUSSIAN BLUE

Indications. Thallium poisoning
Dose. *Dogs, cats*: *by mouth*, 150 micrograms/kg 3 times daily

Information on availability from National Poisons Information Service

Minerals and inorganic substances

Arsenic, *cyanide*, *copper*, *mercury*, and *nitrite* and *nitrate* (see under Poisonous plants) are inorganic compounds contained in pesticides, plants, and therapeutic preparations.
Sodium thiosulphate in conjunction with **sodium nitrite** is given in the treatment of cyanide poisoning. In the body sodium nitrite converts some haemoglobin to methaemoglobin. The lethal cyanide ion binds with methaemoglobin forming cyanomethaemoglobin. This is converted to the readily eliminated thiocyanate following sodium thiosulphate administration. Sodium thiosulphate is also used in the treatment of poisoning by *arsenic* and *mercury*. Dimercaprol is a chelating agent that has been used as an alternative antidote for arsenic or mercury poisoning. It is now considered too toxic for routine use.
Sodium sulphate in combination with **ammonium molybdate** is used for *copper* poisoning in sheep. **Penicillamine** (see section 8.7.3) 10 to 15 mg/kg twice daily by mouth may be of benefit in copper poisoning in dogs.
Lead poisoning occurs from ingestion of old paint, batteries, sump oil, lead shot, or lead weights. Cattle, dogs, and birds are most commonly affected. **Sodium calciumedetate** is a chelating agent used in the treatment of lead poisoning. It mobilises lead from bone and tissues and aids elimination from the body by forming a stable, water-soluble lead complex that is readily excreted by the kidneys. **Penicillamine** (see section 8.7.3) is a chelating agent used in the treatment of lead poisoning. Doses of 33 to 55 mg/kg have been used in dogs. Animals may exhibit signs of *molybdenum* poisoning when grazing on pastures deficient in copper and having high

sulphate levels. Copper supplements (see section 16.4.3) are used in the treatment of molybdenosis.

AMMONIUM MOLYBDATE

Indications. Copper poisoning
Dose. *Sheep*: *by mouth*, 100 mg ammonium molybdate with 1 g sodium sulphate daily
Ammonium molybdate is available from Aldrich, BDH, and other chemical suppliers

SODIUM CALCIUMEDETATE

Indications. Lead poisoning
Dose. *Cattle, dogs, cats*: *by intravenous infusion*, 75 mg/kg, administered as a 5% solution
Birds: *by intramuscular injection*, 38 mg/100 g daily for 4 days

PoM **Sodium Calcium Edetate** (Animalcare)
Injection, sodium calciumedetate 250 mg/mL; 100 mL. To be diluted before use

SODIUM NITRITE

Indications. Cyanide poisoning
Dose. *Cattle, sheep*: *by intravenous injection*, sodium nitrite 1% injection, 22 mg/kg, followed by sodium thiosulphate 25% injection, 660 mg/kg, with sodium thiosulphate 30 g by mouth every hour to prevent further absorption of cyanide
Dogs, cats: *by intravenous injection*, sodium nitrite 1% injection, 25 mg/kg, followed by sodium thiosulphate 25% injection, 1.25 g/kg

PoM **Sodium Nitrite** (Non-proprietary)
Injection, sodium nitrite 30 mg/mL
Available by special order from Martindale, Penn, etc.

SODIUM SULPHATE

Indications. Copper poisoning (in combination with ammonium molybdate)
Crystalline sodium sulphate is available from Loveridge and other wholesalers

SODIUM THIOSULPHATE

Indications. Arsenic, mercury, cyanide poisoning (in combination with sodium nitrite)

PoM **Sodium Thiosulphate** (Non-proprietary)
Injection, sodium thiosulphate 500 mg/mL
Available as a special order from Martindale, Penn, etc.
Crystalline sodium thiosulphate is available from Loveridge and other wholesalers

Snake and insect bites

The only venomous snake indigenous to the UK is the common adder *Vipera berus*. Dogs are the main species affected and are usually bitten on the head or neck. **Snake antivenom**, available through National Poisons Information Service, is the antidote. **Glucocorticoids** (see section 7.2.1) may be of some benefit.

Localised swelling occurs after bee, hornet, or wasp stings. Insect stings around the larynx may cause respiratory distress. **Glucocorticoids** (see section 7.2.1) and **antihistamines** (see section 5.2.1) are used as therapy.

Miscellaneous poisons

The common toad *Bufo vulgaris* secretes venom from glands within the skin. Dogs and cats may be poisoned when they 'mouth' the amphibian and will show clinical symptoms of profuse salivation. Mouth-washes containing **sodium bicarbonate** and administration of **atropine** (see section 6.6.1) are used as therapy.

There is no specific antidote for *strychnine* poisoning. Seizures may be controlled by **pentobarbitone sodium** (see section 6.6.2).

Ethylene glycol is used as antifreeze in cars. An intravenous injection of **ethanol 20%** 5.5 mg/kg, followed by an intra-peritoneal injection of **sodium bicarbonate intravenous infusion 5%** (see section 16.1.2) 8.8 mg/kg are given as antidotes. Surgical spirit should not be used.

CLASSIFIED NOTES ON DRUGS AND PREPARATIONS

1 Drugs used in the treatment of

BACTERIAL, FUNGAL, VIRAL, and PROTOZOAL INFECTIONS

1.1 Antibacterial drugs
1.2 Antifungal drugs
1.3 Antiviral drugs
1.4 Antiprotozoal drugs

1.1 Antibacterial drugs

1.1.1 Beta-lactam antibacterials
1.1.2 Tetracyclines
1.1.3 Aminoglycosides
1.1.4 Macrolides and lincosamides
1.1.5 Chloramphenicol
1.1.6 Sulphonamides and potentiated sulphonamides
1.1.7 Nitrofurans
1.1.8 Nitroimidazoles
1.1.9 Oxolinic acid
1.1.10 Compound antibacterial preparations
1.1.11 Compound preparations for bacterial enteritis

SELECTION OF A SUITABLE DRUG

Bacterial sensitivity. Antibacterial drugs are often used unnecessarily and sometimes (as in uncomplicated diarrhoeas) when they are clearly contra-indicated. However, when antibacterial therapy is essential, there is now a rational basis for deciding which antibacterial drug to use in a specific case. The aim of antibacterial therapy is to maintain an effective concentration of the drug at the site of infection for as long as possible. An effective concentration may be defined as that which is sufficiently in excess of the minimum inhibitory concentration (MIC) of the drug appropriate for the causal micro-organisms. Effective therapy is thus dependent on the susceptibility of the micro-organisms to the drug and the pharmacokinetics which determine its ability to attain and maintain effective concentrations at the infection site.

Except in the rare cases where sensitivity data are available, assessment of the potential sensitivity of the micro-organisms concerned depends firstly upon accurate clinical diagnosis and secondly upon the knowledge that these are the micro-organisms likely to be implicated and their susceptibility to antibacterial drugs. Fortunately, detailed knowledge of MIC values is not required as microbial sensitivity to a drug can be expressed in terms of the concentrations attained in body tissues. In this 'chapter', an organism will be deemed 'sensitive' to a drug if, following administration according to the recommended dosage regimen, tissue concentrations are likely to be in excess of the MIC for that micro-organism for a major part of the time between doses. Having narrowed the list of possible drugs to those likely to be active against the micro-organism or micro-organisms concerned, the final choice is based on the following criteria.

Species and breed. Species differ in their ability to eliminate antibacterial drugs. The cat is less able than other species to metabolise chloramphenicol, which may accumulate following prolonged administration in this species. The young of all species are similarly deficient in their ability to metabolise drugs. Bacterial fermentation is an obvious target for antibiotic action and animals with a functional rumen should not be given broad-spectrum antibiotics by mouth. Tetracyclines by any route may cause a fatal enterocolitis in horses subjected to stress, and penicillins and macrolides should not be used in gerbils, guinea pigs, hamsters, or rabbits in which they are likely to cause a fatal enterotoxaemia.

Predisposition to toxicity. Certain conditions may exacerbate the toxicity of antibacterial drugs. Renal disease may predispose animals, especially cats, to the toxic effects of aminoglycosides since these drugs are eliminated solely by renal excretion and so may accumulate in renal failure. Tetracyclines are contra-indicated in bitches in late pregnancy when they may cause enamel defects and discoloration in the puppies' milk teeth. In calves being introduced to a high barley diet, nitrofurans may cause hyperexcitability.

Site of infection. Special considerations apply to the treatment of infections at particular sites. Antibiotics such as chloramphenicol and the macrolides are extensively metabolised and so are not used to treat urinary-tract infections. In the treatment of urinary-tract infections it is important to choose a drug with actions that are favoured by the prevailing pH to maximise efficacy. In particular, aminoglycosides are much more active in alkaline than in acidic urine and conversely nitrofurantoin and ampicillin are favoured by acidic conditions. Some body compartments, notably the brain and the internal structures of the eye are penetrated only by lipophilic drugs that are able to cross intact cell membranes.

Permeability is increased by inflammation. Although chloramphenicol and sulphonamides normally enter the brain, ampicillin and doxycycline do so only in the presence of inflammation. Similarly, milk is separated from the general circulation by an intact membrane through which only the non-ionised lipophilic form of a drug may pass. When the non-ionised form of a basic drug such as a macrolide enters the relatively acid milk it dissociates and so becomes trapped resulting in high concentrations in milk – the so called 'ion-trap'. Conversely, acidic drugs such as benzylpenicillin are largely excluded from the healthy udder. Both factors cease to operate in the presence of inflammation so that drugs penetrate the acutely inflamed mammary gland to the same extent as any other inflamed tissue.

Mode of antibacterial action. As noted in the sections dealing with individual groups of drugs, some are bactericidal, that is they are able to kill bacteria, while others are bacteriostatic, only inhibiting multiplication and hence relying upon host defences to clear the infection. Although the advantages of bactericidal drugs have probably been exaggerated in the past, there are certain situations in which their use is essential. These include the treatment of endocarditis, and in cases of immunosuppression occurring either naturally or due to concomitant administration of corticosteroids.

Antibiotic policy. It is essential that antibiotics are given according to a predetermined policy in order that efficacy may be monitored. Changes in resistance patterns in a particular area should be noted and therapy altered accordingly. In general, in order to delay the onset of resistance, narrow-spectrum drugs should be used when possible. Benzylpenicillin is still an extremely useful drug, while the newer and broader-spectrum drugs should be reserved for situations where they are specifically indicated. Other considerations include cost and the effect on public health.

BEFORE COMMENCING THERAPY

The **dose** of an antibacterial drug expressed as weight of drug per kg bodyweight will vary with a number of factors including intercurrent disease, severity of the infection, and size of the animal. In serious infections high doses are usually given not less frequently than every 8 hours. 'Depot' preparations are long-acting but attain relatively low plasma-drug concentrations and are not suitable for the treatment of acute severe infections. The aminoglycosides should be given no more frequently than every 12 hours and the interval between doses increased in patients with renal failure. In general, the larger the animal the smaller the dosage per unit body-weight. The **duration of therapy** depends upon the nature of the infection and the response to treatment but is typically 5 to 7 days. In certain infections such as endocarditis and bone and skin infections it is necessary to continue therapy for a considerably longer period.

The **route of administration** depends upon the severity of the disease and ease of administration. In the treatment of severe infections it is advantageous to give the initial dose by the intravenous route in appropriate cases. In companion animals subcutaneous injection may be preferred to the more painful intramuscular route. Intratracheal injection of tetracyclines or aminoglycosides may result in higher concentrations of antibiotic in the lung than are achieved following intramuscular injection. Although oral medication given with food is often convenient, it may considerably reduce the amount of drug absorbed. For example, ampicillin is poorly absorbed in dogs that have recently been fed. Milk, iron salts, and antacids all interfere with the absorption of tetracyclines from the gastro-intestinal tract.

1.1.1 Beta-lactam antibacterials

1.1.1.1 Narrow-spectrum penicillins
1.1.1.2 Beta-lactamase resistant penicillins
1.1.1.3 Broad-spectrum penicillins
1.1.1.4 Antipseudomonal penicillins
1.1.1.5 Cephalosporins

This group comprises the penicillins and the cephalosporins. They are bactericidal by interfering with cell wall synthesis. Beta-lactam antibacterials are not metabolised in the body, but are rapidly excreted unchanged in the urine. Relatively insoluble depot preparations are often used to prolong action, albeit at the expense of concentrations achieved in body fluids. An initial high concentration of drug in body fluids with prolonged activity may be obtained by simultaneous administration of a soluble and a less soluble penicillin salt.

1.1.1.1 NARROW-SPECTRUM PENICILLINS

Benzylpenicillin, also known as penicillin G, was the first of the penicillins, and remains an important and useful antibiotic. It is particularly active against Gram-positive bacteria. Sensitive organisms include Gram-positive aerobes such as *Staphylococcus aureus*, streptoccoci, most *Actinomyces* species, *Erysipelothrix*, and *Bacillus* species. Most anaerobic bacteria including *Clostridium* and some *Bacteroides* species, though not *B. fragilis*, are also sensitive. Benzylpenicillin has activity against the more fastidious Gram-negative aerobes such as *Haemophilus*, *Pasteurella*, *Leptospira*, and some *Actinobacillus* species. Benzylpenicillin is broken down by the beta-lactamase enzymes produced by staphylococci and *Bacteroides*. A high proportion of strains of these organisms are now resistant to benzylpenicillin. Other organisms mentioned retain their sensitivity to benzylpenicillin due to their inability to produce beta-lactamase. Benzylpenicillin is inactivated by gastric acid and so is not given by mouth. It is available as a range of salts which differ in their solubility and hence their duration of action. The sodium and potassium salts are very soluble and therefore rapidly absorbed following subcutaneous or intramuscular injection, but give effective concentrations for no more than 4 hours. The procaine salt is slightly soluble. Following parenteral administration, it forms a 'depot' which slowly releases free benzylpenicillin into the circulation, maintaining effective concentrations against the more susceptible organisms for up to 24 hours. **Benzathine penicillin** is a very slightly soluble salt, which has a prolonged action after intramuscular injection although plasma concentrations produced are low. It is available in combination with procaine penicillin. **Phenoxymethylpenicillin**, or penicillin V, has a similar antibacterial spectrum to benzylpenicillin but is less active. It is gastric acid-stable and thus suitable for oral administration. It should not be used for severe infections because absorption can be unpredictable and plasma-drug concentrations variable.

BENZYLPENICILLIN
(Penicillin G)

Indications. Penicillin-sensitive infections, see notes above
Contra-indications. Penicillin hypersensitivity; should not be administered to gerbils, guinea pigs, hamsters, rabbits
Side-effects. Allergic reactions in animals. Occasional skin sensitisation in operators
Dose. *Horses*: *by intravenous injection*, 10 mg/kg twice daily for 1 day

PoM **Crystapen**™   (Coopers Pitman-Moore)
Injection, powder for reconstitution, benzylpenicillin (as sodium salt) 3 g, for *horses*
Withdrawal Periods. Should not be used in *horses* intended for human consumption

PHENOXYMETHYLPENICILLIN
(Penicillin V)

Indications. Penicillin-sensitive infections, see notes above
Contra-indications. **Side-effects**. See notes above and under Benzylpenicillin
Dose. *Pigs*: 200 g/tonne feed
Dogs, cats: 8 mg/kg 3 times daily *or* 16 mg/kg twice daily

PoM **Phenoxymethylpenicillin**   (Non-proprietary)
Capsules, phenoxymethylpenicillin (as potassium salt) 250 mg
Tablets, phenoxymethylpenicillin (as potassium salt) 250 mg
Elixir, powder for reconstitution, phenoxymethylpenicillin (as potassium salt) 25 mg/mL, 50 mg/mL; 100 mL

PoM **Potencil**™ (Hand/PH)
Oral powder, for addition to feed, phenoxymethylpenicillin potassium 100 mg/g, for *pigs*; 2 kg, 25 kg
Withdrawal Periods. *Pigs*: slaughter 1 day

PROCAINE PENICILLIN
(Procaine Benzylpenicillin)

Indications. Penicillin-sensitive infections, see notes above
Contra-indications. **Side-effects**. See under Benzylpenicillin
Dose. *Horses, cattle, sheep, goats, pigs, dogs, cats*: *by subcutaneous or intramuscular injection*, 10-15 mg/kg 1-2 times daily

PoM **Depocillin**™ (Mycofarm)
Injection, procaine penicillin 300 mg/mL, for *horses, cattle, sheep, pigs, dogs, cats*; 50 mL, 100 mL
Withdrawal Periods. *Cattle*: slaughter 3 days, milk 48 hours. *Sheep, pigs*: slaughter 3 days

PoM **Duphapen**™ (Duphar)
Injection, procaine penicillin 300 mg/mL, for *horses, cattle, sheep, goats, pigs, dogs, cats*; 40 mL, 100 mL
Withdrawal Periods. *Cattle*: milk 48 hours

PoM **Econopen**™ (BK)
Injection, procaine penicillin 300 mg/mL, for *horses, cattle, sheep, goats, pigs, dogs, cats*; 100 mL
Withdrawal Periods. *Cattle*: milk 48 hours

PoM **Ethacilin**™ (Intervet)
Injection, procaine penicillin 300 mg/mL, for *horses, cattle, sheep, goats, pigs, dogs, cats*; 100 mL
Withdrawal Periods. *Cattle*: slaughter 3 days, milk 48 hours. *Sheep, pigs*: slaughter 3 days

PoM **Lenticillin**™ (RMB)
Injection, procaine penicillin 300 mg/mL, for *horses, cattle, sheep, goats, pigs, dogs, cats*; 100 mL
Withdrawal Periods. *Cattle*: milk 48 hours

PoM **Norocillin**™ (Norbrook)
Injection, procaine penicillin 300 mg/mL, for *horses, cattle, sheep, goats, pigs, dogs, cats*; 50 mL, 100 mL
Withdrawal Periods. *Cattle*: milk 48 hours

PoM **Penillin**™ (Univet)
Injection, procaine penicillin 300 mg/
mL, for *horses, cattle, sheep, pigs, dogs, cats*; 100 mL
Withdrawal Periods. *Cattle*: slaughter 3 days, milk 48 hours. *Sheep, pigs*: slaughter 3 days

PoM **Procillin**™ (Bimeda)
Injection, procaine penicillin 300 mg/
mL, for *cattle, sheep, pigs*; 100 mL
Withdrawal Periods. *Cattle*: slaughter 7 days, milk 72 hours. *Sheep*: slaughter 3 days, milk from treated animals should not be used for human consumption.
Pigs: slaughter 5 days
For intramuscular injection

BENZATHINE PENICILLIN and PROCAINE PENICILLIN

Indications. Penicillin-sensitive infections
Contra-indications. Side-effects. See under Benzylpenicillin
Dose. Expressed for a suspension containing benzathine penicillin 112.5 mg + procaine penicillin 150 mg/mL
Horses, cattle, sheep, goats, pigs: by intramuscular injection, 0.04 mL/kg, repeat after 3-4 days
Dogs, cats: by intramuscular injection, 0.1 mL/kg, repeat after 3-4 days

PoM **Depopen**™-P (BK)
Depot injection, benzathine penicillin 112.5 mg, procaine penicillin 150 mg/
mL, for *horses, cattle, sheep, goats, pigs, dogs, cats*; 100 mL
Withdrawal Periods. *Cattle*: milk 72 hours

PoM **Duphapen**™ LA (Duphar)
Depot injection, benzathine penicillin 112.5 mg, procaine penicillin 150 mg/
mL, for *horses, cattle, sheep, pigs, dogs, cats*; 50 mL, 100 mL
Withdrawal Periods. *Cattle*: slaughter 21 days, milk 72 hours. *Sheep, pigs*: slaughter 21 days

PoM **Duplocillin**™ LA (Mycofarm)
Depot injection, benzathine penicillin 112.5 mg, procaine penicillin 150 mg/
mL, for *horses, cattle, sheep, pigs, dogs, cats*; 50 mL, 100 mL

Withdrawal Periods. *Cattle*: slaughter 4 days, milk 72 hours. *Sheep, pigs*: slaughter 4 days

PoM **Ethacilin**™ P-A (Intervet)
Depot injection, benzathine penicillin 112.5 mg, procaine penicillin 150 mg/
mL, for *horses, cattle, sheep, pigs, dogs, cats*; 50 mL, 100 mL
Withdrawal Periods. *Cattle*: slaughter 4 days, milk 72 hours. *Sheep, pigs*: slaughter 4 days

PoM **Lentrax**™ (RMB)
Depot injection, benzathine penicillin 115 mg, procaine penicillin 150 mg/mL, for *horses, cattle, sheep, pigs, dogs, cats*; 90 mL
Withdrawal Periods. *Cattle*: milk 48 hours

PoM **Norocillin**™ LA (Norbrook)
Depot injection, benzathine penicillin 112.5 mg, procaine penicillin 150 mg/
mL, for *horses, cattle, sheep, pigs, dogs, cats*; 50 mL, 100 mL
Withdrawal Periods. Should not be used in *horses* intended for human consumption. *Cattle*: slaughter 14 days, milk 72 hours. *Sheep*: slaughter 14 days, milk from treated animals should not be used for human consumption. *Pigs*: slaughter 10 days

PoM **Penillin**™ LA (Univet)
Depot injection, benzathine penicillin 112.5 mg, procaine penicillin 150 mg/
mL, for *horses, cattle, sheep, pigs, dogs, cats*; 100 mL
Withdrawal Periods. *Cattle*: slaughter 4 days, milk 72 hours. *Sheep, pigs*: slaughter 4 days

PoM **Procillin LA**™ (Bimeda)
Depot injection, benzathine penicillin 112.5 mg, procaine penicillin 150 mg/
mL, for *cattle, sheep, pigs*; 100 mL
Withdrawal Periods. *Cattle*: slaughter 14 days, milk 10 days. *Sheep*: slaughter 21 days, milk from treated animals should not be used for human consumption.
Pigs: slaughter 21 days

PoM **Propen**™ (Coopers Pitman-Moore)
Depot injection, benzathine penicillin 112.5 mg, procaine penicillin 150 mg/
mL, for *horses, cattle, sheep, goats, pigs, dogs, cats*; 100 mL
Withdrawal Periods. *Cattle*: slaughter 2

days, milk 72 hours. *Sheep, goats, pigs*: slaughter 21 days

PoM **Vetipen**™ (C-Vet)
Depot injection, benzathine penicillin 112.5 mg, procaine penicillin 150 mg/mL, for *horses, cattle, sheep, goats, pigs, dogs, cats*; 100 mL
Withdrawal Periods. *Cattle*: slaughter 4 days, milk 72 hours. *Sheep, goats, pigs*: slaughter 4 days

1.1.1.2 BETA-LACTAMASE RESISTANT PENICILLINS

These have the antibacterial spectrum of benzylpenicillin but in addition are stable in the presence of staphylococcal beta-lactamases. They are effective in infections caused by penicillin-resistant staphylococci, the sole indication for their use. Cloxacillin is commonly incorporated into intramammary and ophthalmic preparations. **Flucloxacillin** is absorbed from the gastro-intestinal tract and is available for oral administration.
See section 11.1 for preparations for the treatment of mastitis and section 12.2.1 for preparations for eyes.

FLUCLOXACILLIN

Indications. Infections due to penicillinase-producing staphylococci
Contra-indications. **Side-effects**. See under Benzylpenicillin (1.1.1.1)
Dose. *Dogs, cats*: 15 mg/kg 4 times daily

PoM **Flucloxacillin** (Non-proprietary)
Capsules, flucloxacillin (as sodium salt) 250 mg, 500 mg
Elixir, powder for reconstitution, flucloxacillin (as sodium salt) 125 mg/5 mL; 100 mL

1.1.1.3 BROAD-SPECTRUM PENICILLINS

Ampicillin and **amoxycillin** have slightly less activity than benzylpenicillin against Gram-positive bacteria and anaerobes but considerably greater activity against Gram-negative bacteria, although their action is poor against *Klebsiella*, some

Proteus species, and *Pseudomonas*. In addition, they are broken down by beta-lactamases, both the staphylococcal enzymes and those produced by Gram-negative organisms such as *E. coli* and *Haemophilus*. Acquired resistance in such organisms has limited the usefulness of these antibiotics.
Amoxycillin is better absorbed following administration by mouth than ampicillin, giving higher plasma and tissue concentrations. Its absorption is less affected by the presence of food in the stomach. Ampicillin and amoxycillin are excreted into both bile and urine.
Depot preparations of both amoxycillin and ampicillin are available. The drug is incorporated into an oily vehicle to prolong the action of the antibiotic. Depot oil-based ampicillin preparations include aluminium monostearate in the formulation.
Clavulanic acid has no significant antibacterial activity, but is a potent beta-lactamase inhibitor. Therefore, its inclusion in preparations of amoxycillin renders the combination active against most strains of *Staph. aureus*, some *E. coli* species, as well as *Bacteroides* and *Klebsiella*.

AMOXYCILLIN

Indications. Amoxycillin-sensitive infections
Contra-indications. **Side-effects**. See under Benzylpenicillin (1.1.1.1)
Dose. *Cattle, sheep, pigs, dogs, cats*: *by mouth*, 10 mg/kg twice daily; *by subcutaneous or intramuscular injection*, 7 mg/kg daily; *by depot subcutaneous or intramuscular injection*, 15 mg/kg, repeat after 2 days
Poultry: *by addition to drinking water*, 20 mg/kg
Fish: see Prescribing for fish

Oral preparations

PoM **Amoxypen**™ (Mycofarm)
Tablets, scored, amoxycillin (as trihydrate) 40 mg, for *dogs, cats*; 100, 500
Tablets, scored, amoxycillin (as trihydrate) 200 mg, for *dogs*; 100, 250
Tablets, scored, amoxycillin (as tri-

hydrate) 400 mg, for *calves*; 50
Withdrawal Periods. *Calves*: slaughter
10 days

PoM **Betamox**™ (Norbrook)
Tablets, scored, amoxycillin (as trihydrate) 40 mg, for *dogs, cats*; 100, 500
Tablets, scored, amoxycillin (as trihydrate) 200 mg, for *dogs*; 100, 250
Tablets, scored, amoxycillin (as trihydrate) 400 mg, for *calves*; 20, 50
Withdrawal Periods. *Calves*: slaughter
10 days

PoM **Betamox**™ **Drops** (Norbrook)
Oral suspension, powder for reconstitution, amoxycillin (as trihydrate)
50 mg/mL, for *dogs, cats*; 15-mL dropper
bottle. Life of reconstituted mixture 7
days

PoM **Clamoxyl**™ (SmithKline Beecham)
Tablets, scored, amoxycillin (as trihydrate) 40 mg, for *dogs, cats*; 100, 500
Tablets, scored, amoxycillin (as trihydrate) 200 mg, for *dogs*; 100, 250
Tablets, scored, amoxycillin (as trihydrate) 400 mg, for *calves*; 60
Withdrawal Periods. *Calves*: slaughter 7
days

PoM **Clamoxyl**™   **Drops**   (SmithKline
Beecham)
Oral suspension, powder for reconstitution, amoxycillin (as trihydrate)
50 mg/mL, for *dogs, cats*; 15-mL dropper
bottle. Life of reconstituted mixture 14
days

PoM **Clamoxyl**™ **Oral Multidoser** (Smith-
Kline Beecham)
Mixture, amoxycillin (as trihydrate)
40 mg/dose, for *lambs, piglets*; 100-dose
applicator
Withdrawal Periods. *Lambs, piglets*:
slaughter 7 days

PoM **Clamoxyl**™ **Soluble Powder** (Smith-
Kline Beecham)
Oral powder, for addition to drinking
water, amoxycillin (as trihydrate)
510 mg/g, for *broiler chickens*; 98 g
Withdrawal Periods. *Poultry*: slaughter
1 day
Note. Should not be used in layer hens

PoM **Duphamox**™ (Duphar)
Tablets, scored, amoxycillin (as tri-

hydrate) 40 mg, for *dogs, cats*; 500
Tablets, scored, amoxycillin (as trihydrate) 200 mg, for *dogs*; 100, 250
Tablets, scored, amoxycillin (as trihydrate) 400 mg, for *calves*; 20, 50
Withdrawal Periods. *Calves*: slaughter
10 days

PoM **Duphamox**™ **Drops** (Duphar)
Oral suspension, powder for reconstitution, amoxycillin (as trihydrate)
50 mg/mL, for *dogs, cats*; 15-mL dropper
bottle. Life of reconstituted mixture 7
days

PoM **Vetremox**™ (Vetrepharm)
See Prescribing for fish for preparation
details

Parenteral preparations

PoM **Amoxypen**™ (Mycofarm)
Injection (oily), amoxycillin (as trihydrate) 150 mg/mL, for *cattle, sheep,
pigs, dogs, cats*; 100 mL
Withdrawal Periods. *Cattle*: slaughter 18
days, milk 24 hours. *Sheep, pigs*:
slaughter 18 days

PoM **Betamox**™ (Norbrook)
Injection, amoxycillin (as trihydrate)
150 mg/mL, for *cattle, sheep, pigs, dogs,
cats*; 50 mL, 100 mL
Withdrawal Periods. *Cattle*: slaughter 18
days, milk 24 hours. *Sheep*: slaughter 18
days, milk from treated animals should
not be used for human consumption.
Pigs: slaughter 18 days

PoM **Clamoxyl**™ (SmithKline Beecham)
Injection, amoxycillin (as trihydrate)
150 mg/mL, for *cattle, sheep, pigs, dogs,
cats*; 100 mL, 250 mL
Withdrawal Periods. *Cattle, sheep*:
slaughter 10 days, milk 24 hours. *Pigs*:
slaughter 10 days

PoM **Duphamox**™ (Duphar)
Injection, amoxycillin (as trihydrate)
150 mg/mL, for *cattle, sheep, pigs, dogs,
cats*; 100 mL
Withdrawal Periods. *Cattle*: slaughter 18
days, milk 24 hours. *Sheep*: slaughter 18
days, milk from treated animals should
not be used for human consumption.
Pigs: slaughter 10 days

PoM **Qualamox**™ **15** (RMB)
Injection, amoxycillin (as trihydrate)
150 mg/mL, for *cattle, sheep, pigs, dogs*

cats; 100 mL
Withdrawal Periods. *Cattle*: slaughter 18 days, milk 24 hours. *Sheep*: slaughter 18 days, milk from treated animals should not be used for human consumption. *Pigs*: slaughter 18 days

Depot injections

PoM **Amoxypen**™ **LA** (Mycofarm)
Depot injection (oily), amoxycillin (as trihydrate) 150 mg/mL, for *cattle, sheep, pigs, dogs, cats*; 100 mL
Withdrawal Periods. *Cattle*: slaughter 21 days, milk 24 hours. *Sheep, pigs*: slaughter 21 days

PoM **Betamox**™ **LA** (Norbrook)
Depot injection, amoxycillin (as trihydrate) 150 mg/mL, for *cattle, sheep, pigs, dogs, cats*; 50 mL, 100 mL
Withdrawal Periods. *Cattle*: slaughter 21 days, milk 60 hours. *Sheep*: slaughter 21 days, milk from treated animals should not be used for human consumption. *Pigs*: slaughter 21 days

PoM **Clamoxyl**™ **LA** (SmithKline Beecham)
Depot injection (oily), amoxycillin (as trihydrate) 150 mg/mL, for *cattle, sheep, pigs, dogs, cats*; 100 mL, 250 mL
Withdrawal Periods. *Cattle, sheep*: slaughter 14 days, milk 72 hours. *Pigs*: slaughter 14 days

PoM **Duphamox**™ **LA** (Duphar)
Depot injection, amoxycillin (as trihydrate) 150 mg/mL, for *cattle, sheep, pigs, dogs, cats*; 100 mL
Withdrawal Periods. *Cattle*: slaughter 14 days, milk 60 hours. *Sheep*: slaughter 14 days, milk from treated animals should not be used for human consumption. *Pigs*: slaughter 14 days

PoM **Qualamox**™ **LA** (RMB)
Depot injection, amoxycillin (as trihydrate) 150 mg/mL, for *cattle, sheep, pigs, dogs, cats*; 100 mL
Withdrawal Periods. *Cattle*: slaughter 21 days, milk 24 hours. *Sheep*: slaughter 21 days, milk from treated animals should not be used for human consumption. *Pigs*: slaughter 21 days

CO-AMOXICLAV
Preparations of amoxycillin and clavulanic acid

Indications. Amoxycillin-sensitive infections
Contra-indications. Side-effects. See under Benzylpenicillin (1.1.1.1)
Dose. Expressed as amoxycillin
Cattle: by subcutaneous or intramuscular injection, 7 mg/kg daily; *calves*: by mouth, 5-10 mg/kg twice daily
Dogs, cats: by mouth, 10-20 mg/kg twice daily; by subcutaneous or intramuscular injection, 7 mg/kg daily

PoM **Synulox**™ (SmithKline Beecham)
Tablets, scored, co-amoxiclav 40/10 [amoxycillin (as trihydrate) 40 mg, clavulanic acid (as potassium salt) 10 mg], for *dogs, cats*; 100, 500
Tablets, scored, co-amoxiclav 200/50 [amoxycillin (as trihydrate) 200 mg, clavulanic acid (as potassium salt) 50 mg]; for *dogs*; 100, 250
Tablets, scored, co-amoxiclav 400/100 [amoxycillin (as trihydrate) 400 mg, clavulanic acid (as potassium salt) 100 mg], for *calves*; 20, 100
Withdrawal Periods. *Calves*: slaughter 4 days

PoM **Synulox**™ **Drops** (SmithKline Beecham)
Mixture, oral powder for reconstitution, co-amoxiclav 40/10 [amoxycillin (as trihydrate) 40 mg, clavulanic acid (as potassium salt) 10 mg]/mL, for *dogs, cats*; 15-mL dropper bottle. Life of reconstituted mixture 7 days

PoM **Synulox**™ (SmithKline Beecham)
Injection, co-amoxiclav 140/35 [amoxycillin (as trihydrate) 140 mg, clavulanic acid (as potassium salt) 35 mg]/mL, for *cattle, dogs, cats*; 40 mL, 100 mL
Withdrawal Periods. *Cattle*: slaughter 14 days, milk 24 hours

AMPICILLIN

Indications. Ampicillin-sensitive infections
Contra-indications. Side-effects. See under Benzylpenicillin (1.1.1.1)
Dose. *Horses*: by subcutaneous or

intramuscular injection, 2-10 mg/kg 1-2 times daily
Cattle, sheep: *by subcutaneous or intramuscular injection*, 2-10 mg/kg 1-2 times daily; *by depot intramuscular injection*, 15 mg/kg, repeat after 2 days; *calves*: *by mouth*, 4-12 mg/kg 1-2 times daily
Pigs: *by mouth*, 4-20 mg/kg 1-2 times daily; *by subcutaneous or intramuscular injection*, 2-10 mg/kg 1-2 times daily; *by depot subcutaneous injection*, 25 mg/kg, repeat after 2 days
Dogs, cats: *by mouth*, 4-20 mg/kg 1-3 times daily; *by subcutaneous or intramuscular injection*, 2-10 mg/kg 1-2 times daily; *by depot subcutaneous injection*, 15-20 mg/kg, repeat after 2 days

Oral preparations

PoM **Amfipen**™ (Mycofarm)
Tablets, ampicillin   50 mg,   125 mg, 500 mg, for *calves, pigs, dogs, cats*; 50-mg tablets 100, 400; 125-mg tablets 100, 400; 500-mg tablets 30
Withdrawal Periods. *Calves, pigs*: slaughter 2 days
Capsules, ampicillin 250 mg, for *calves, pigs, dogs*; 250, 1000
Withdrawal Periods. *Calves, pigs*: slaughter 2 days

PoM **Intacilin**™ (Intervet)
Tablets, ampicillin 50 mg, 125 mg; for *calves, pigs, dogs, cats*; 400
Withdrawal Periods. *Calves, pigs*: slaughter 2 days
Capsules, ampicillin 250 mg, for *calves, pigs, dogs*; 250, 1000
Withdrawal Periods. *Calves, pigs*: slaughter 2 days

PoM **Penbritin**™ (SmithKline Beecham)
Capsules, ampicillin (as trihydrate) 50 mg, for *dogs, cats*; 500

PoM **Vidocillin**™ (BK)
Capsules, ampicillin 250 mg, for *dogs*; 250, 1000

Parenteral preparations

PoM **Amfipen**™ **15%** (Mycofarm)
Injection (oily), ampicillin 150 mg/mL, for *horses, cattle, sheep, pigs, dogs, cats*; 100 mL
Withdrawal Periods. Should not be

used in *horses* intended for human consumption. *Cattle, sheep*: slaughter 6 days, milk 24 hours. *Pigs*: slaughter 12 days

PoM **Amfipen**™ **30%** (Mycofarm)
Injection (oily), ampicillin 300 mg/mL, for *horses, cattle, sheep, pigs*; 100 mL
Withdrawal Periods. Should not be used in *horses* intended for human consumption. *Cattle*: slaughter 6 days, milk 24 hours. *Sheep*: slaughter 6 days. *Pigs*: slaughter 12 days.

PoM **Compropen**™ (Coopers Pitman-Moore)
Injection, ampicillin (as trihydrate) 150 mg/mL, for *horses, cattle, sheep, pigs, dogs, cats*; 100 mL
Withdrawal Periods. *Cattle*: slaughter 9 days, milk 24 hours. *Sheep, pigs*: slaughter 9 days

PoM **Duphacillin**™ (Duphar)
Injection, ampicillin (as trihydrate) 150 mg/mL, for *horses, cattle, sheep, pigs, dogs, cats*; 50 mL, 100 mL
Withdrawal Periods. *Cattle*: slaughter 9 days, milk 24 hours. *Sheep, pigs*: slaughter 9 days

PoM **Embacillin**™ (RMB)
Injection, ampicillin (as trihydrate) 150 mg/mL, for *horses, cattle, sheep, pigs, dogs, cats*; 100 mL
Withdrawal Periods. *Cattle*: slaughter 9 days, milk 24 hours. *Sheep, pigs*: slaughter 9 days

PoM **Intacilin**™ **15%** (Intervet)
Injection (oily), ampicillin 150 mg/mL, for *horses, cattle, sheep, pigs, dogs, cats*; 100 mL
Withdrawal Periods. Should not be used in *horses* intended for human consumption. *Cattle, sheep*: slaughter 6 days, milk 24 hours. *Pigs*: slaughter 12 days

PoM **Intacilin**™ **30%** (Intervet)
Injection (oily), ampicillin 300 mg/mL, for *horses, cattle, sheep, pigs*; 100 mL
Withdrawal Periods. Should not be used in *horses* intended for human consumption. *Cattle*: slaughter 6 days, milk 24 hours. *Sheep*: slaughter 6 days. *Pigs*: slaughter 12 days

PoM **Norobrittin**™ (Norbrook)
Injection, ampicillin (as trihydrate)
150 mg/mL, for *horses, cattle, sheep,
pigs, dogs, cats*; 50 mL, 100 mL
Withdrawal Periods. *Cattle*: slaughter 9
days, milk 24 hours. *Sheep, pigs*:
slaughter 9 days

PoM **Penbritin**™ (SmithKline Beecham)
Injection (oily), ampicillin (as trihydrate)
150 mg/mL, for *cattle, dogs, cats*; 100 mL
Withdrawal Periods. *Cattle*: milk 8 or 12
hours

PoM **Penbritin**™ **Veterinary** (SmithKline
Beecham)
Injection, powder for reconstitution,
ampicillin (as sodium salt) 500 mg, 2 g,
for *horses, dogs, cats*
Withdrawal Periods. See page xiv.
Dose. *Horses, dogs, cats*: *by intramuscular
or intravenous injection*, 2-7 mg/kg 1-2
times daily

PoM **Vidocillin**™ (BK)
Injection, ampicillin (as trihydrate)
150 mg/mL, for *horses, cattle, sheep,
pigs, dogs, cats*; 50 mL, 100 mL
Withdrawal Periods. *Cattle*: slaughter 9
days, milk 24 hours. *Sheep, pigs*:
slaughter 9 days

Depot injections

> Accidental self-injection with oil-based
> preparations can cause severe vascular
> spasm and prompt medical attention is
> essential

PoM **Amfipen**™ **LA** (Mycofarm)
Depot injection (oily), ampicillin 100 mg/
mL with aluminium monostearate, for
cattle, sheep, pigs, dogs, cats; 30 mL,
80 mL
Withdrawal Periods. *Cattle*: slaughter 14
days, milk 72 hours. *Sheep, pigs*:
slaughter 14 days

PoM **Intacilin**™ **LA** (Intervet)
Depot injection (oily), ampicillin 100 mg/
mL with aluminium monostearate, for
cattle, sheep, pigs, dogs, cats; 80 mL
Withdrawal Periods. *Cattle*: slaughter 14
days, milk 72 hours. *Sheep, pigs*:
slaughter 14 days

1.1.1.4 ANTIPSEUDOMONAL PENICILLINS

Carbenicillin and **ticarcillin** are principally indicated for the treatment
of *Pseudomonas aeruginosa* infections
although they are also active against
a number of other Gram-negative
organisms including *Proteus* and *Bacteroides*. Carbenicillin has largely been
replaced by ticarcillin which is more
active against these organisms. Ticarcillin is broken down by the beta-
lactamase produced by some strains
of *Ps. aeruginosa*. Ticarcillin is also
available in preparations to which
clavulanic acid has been added to inhibit
this enzyme.

CARBENICILLIN

Indications. Infections due to *Pseudomonas* species, see notes above
Contra-indications. **Side-effects**. See
under Benzylpenicillin (1.1.1.1)
Dose. *Dogs, cats*: *by intramuscular or
intravenous injection*, 10-20 mg/kg 2-3
times daily

PoM **Pyopen**™ (Beecham)
Injection, powder for reconstitution, carbenicillin (as sodium salt) 1 g, 5 g

TICARCILLIN

Indications. Infections due to *Pseudomonas* species, see notes above
Contra-indications. **Side-effects**. See
under Benzylpenicillin (1.1.1.1)
Dose. *Dogs, cats*: *by intramuscular or
intravenous injection*, 15-25 mg/kg 3
times daily

PoM **Ticar**™ (Beecham)
Injection, powder for reconstitution, ticarcillin (as sodium salt) 1 g, 5 g

Ticarcillin with clavulanic acid

PoM **Timentin**™ (Beecham)
Injection, powder for reconstitution, ticarcillin (as sodium salt) 750 mg, clavulanic acid
(as potassium salt) 50 mg; 800 mg
Injection, powder for reconstitution, ticarcillin (as sodium salt) 1.5 g, clavulanic acid
(as potassium salt) 100 mg; 1.6 g

Injection, powder for reconstitution, ticarcillin (as sodium salt) 3 g, clavulanic acid (as potassium salt) 200 mg; 3.2 g
Dose. Expressed as ticarcillin + clavulanic acid
Dogs, cats: *by intravenous infusion*, 15-25 mg/kg 3 times daily

1.1.1.5 CEPHALOSPORINS

The cephalosporins comprise a large group of antibacterials containing the beta-lactam ring. They are closely related to the penicillins. Like the penicillins they are bactericidal but are relatively non-toxic and less likely to cause allergic reactions. Cephalosporins are suitable for use in rabbits and rodents.
Cephalexin and **cefadroxil** are active against a range of both Gram-positive and Gram-negative organisms comprising staphylococci, including beta-lactamase-producing strains, *Pasteurella*, *Escherichia coli*, *Actinobacillus*, *Actinomyces*, *Haemophilus*, *Erysipelothrix*, *Clostridium*, and *Salmonella*. *Pseudomonas* and many *Proteus* species are resistant. Some 'third-generation' cephalosporins, including cefoperazone, are used in intramammary preparations (see section 11.1). They are more active against Gram-negative organisms. 'Third generation' drugs are not widely used in veterinary medicine because, in general, they are not well absorbed following oral administration and are rapidly excreted.

CEFADROXIL

Indications. Cefadroxil-sensitive infections
Contra-indications. Hypersensitivity to cephalosporins or penicillins
Side-effects. Occasional vomiting, diarrhoea; lethargy
Dose. *Cats*: 22 mg/kg daily

PoM **Cefa-Tabs**™ (Willows Francis)
Tablets, cefadroxil 50 mg, 100 mg, for *cats*; 50, 100, 500

CEPHALEXIN

Indications. Cephalexin-sensitive infections
Contra-indications. Hypersensitivity to cephalexin. Renal impairment
Side-effects. Local tissue reaction
Dose. *Cattle*: *by intramuscular injection*, 7 mg/kg daily
Sheep, pigs: *by intramuscular injection*, 10 mg/kg daily
Dogs, cats: *by mouth*, 10-15 mg/kg twice daily; *by subcutaneous or intramuscular injection*, 10 mg/kg daily

Oral preparations

PoM **Ceporex**™ (Coopers Pitman-Moore)
Tablets, cephalexin 50 mg, 250 mg, for *dogs, cats*; 100

PoM **Ceporex**™ **Oral Drops** (Coopers Pitman-Moore)
Oral suspension, granules for reconstitution, cephalexin 100 mg/mL, for *dogs up to 20 kg, cats*; 10-mL dropper bottle. Life of reconstituted mixture 10 days

Parenteral preparations

PoM **Ceporex**™ (Coopers Pitman-Moore)
Injection (oily), cephalexin (as sodium salt) 180 mg/mL, for *cattle, sheep, pigs, dogs, cats*; 30 mL, 100 mL
Withdrawal Periods. *Cattle*: slaughter 4 days, milk withdrawal period nil. *Sheep*: slaughter 3 days, milk from treated animals should not be used for human consumption. *Pigs*: slaughter 2 days

The following drugs are included in Prescribing for reptiles – see that section for indications and dosage

CEFTAZIDIME

PoM **Fortum**™ (Glaxo)
Injection, powder for reconstitution, ceftazidime (as pentahydrate) 250 mg, 500 mg, other sizes available

CEFUROXIME

PoM **Zinacef**™ (Glaxo)
Injection, powder for reconstitution, cefuroxime (as sodium salt) 250 mg, 750 mg 1.5 g

CEPHALOTHIN

PoM **Keflin**™ (Lilly)
Injection, powder for reconstitution, cephalothin (as sodium salt) 1 g

1.1.2 Tetracyclines

The tetracyclines are broad-spectrum antibiotics that inhibit *Mycoplasma*, *Chlamydia*, and *Rickettsia* as well as bacteria. They are active against a range of Gram-positive and Gram-negative bacteria but have little useful activity against *E. coli*, *Salmonella*, *Proteus* or *Pseudomonas*. Tetracyclines are bacteriostatic and acquired resistance is now widespread among bacteria.

The widely-used **oxytetracycline** and the less often-used **tetracycline** and **chlortetracycline** have similar properties. When given by intramuscular injection they may be irritant, depending on the vehicle used. For this reason some preparations incorporate a local anaesthetic. Depot preparations will maintain effective plasma concentrations for 72 to 96 hours. Some preparations may be given intravenously, but rapid injection by this route in cattle may cause cardiovascular collapse, apparently due to chelation of calcium. Oral administration may cause diarrhoea. Absorption of tetracyclines from the alimentary tract is variable and is reduced by milk (not doxycycline), antacids, and by calcium, iron, magnesium, and zinc salts.

Tetracyclines are deposited in growing teeth by binding to calcium and if given to a bitch in late pregnancy may cause discoloration and defects of the enamel of the puppies' temporary dentition. Horses that are given parenteral tetracyclines and also exposed to stress may suffer a severe enterocolitis, which can prove fatal.

The main excretory routes for tetracyclines are the urinary system and the gastro-intestinal tract via the biliary system.

Doxycycline is more lipophilic than the older tetracyclines and has a number of advantages. Absorption of orally administered doxycycline is better and is less affected by milk and calcium salts.

Doxycycline also penetrates better into several body compartments, notably the brain and cerebrospinal fluid. It enters the gastro-intestinal tract through the bile and is particularly liable to produce enterocolitis in the horse.

CHLORTETRACYCLINE

Indications. Chlortetracycline-sensitive infections; intra-uterine use (8.6)
Contra-indications. Renal impairment
Side-effects. May cause vomiting, diarrhoea
Dose. *Calves, lambs, pigs*: 10-20 mg/kg daily in divided doses
Dogs, cats, mink: 20-50 mg/kg daily in divided doses
Poultry: 14 g/100 litres drinking water; 100-300 g/tonne feed
Rabbits, rodents: 1 g/litre drinking water

PoM **Aureomycin**™ Soluble Oblets (Cyanamid)
Tablets, or to prepare an oral solution, scored, chlortetracycline hydrochloride 500 mg, for *calves, dogs*; 48
Withdrawal Periods. *Calves*: slaughter 30 days
Note. May also be used for intra-uterine administration (see section 8.6)

PoM **Aureomycin**™ Soluble Powder (Cyanamid)
Oral powder, for addition to drinking water, milk, milk replacer, or to prepare an oral solution, chlortetracycline hydrochloride 55 g/kg, for *calves, pigs, chickens, mink, rabbits, laboratory animals*; 225 g, 5 kg
Withdrawal Periods. *Calves*: slaughter 55 days. *Pigs*: slaughter 20 days. *Poultry*: slaughter 7 days, egg withdrawal period nil

PoM **Aureosup 100**™ (Micro-Biologicals)
Premix, chlortetracycline 100 g/kg, for *pigs*; 2 kg, 3 kg, 25 kg
Withdrawal Periods. *Pigs*: slaughter 10 days

PoM **Aurofac**™ **100** (Cyanamid)
Premix, chlortetracycline hydrochloride 100 g/kg, for *pigs, chickens*; 10 kg
Withdrawal Periods. *Pigs*: slaughter 10 days. *Poultry*: slaughter 3 days, egg withdrawal period nil

PoM **Aurofac™ 200 MA** (Cyanamid)
Oral powder, for addition to milk, milk replacer, or to prepare an oral solution, chlortetracycline hydrochloride 200 g/kg, for *calves*; 500 g, 10 kg
Withdrawal Periods. *Calves*: slaughter 60 days

PoM **Auromix™ 100** (Cheminex)
Premix, chlortetracycline hydrochloride 100 g/kg, for *pigs*; 2 kg, 3 kg, 25 kg
Withdrawal Periods. *Pigs*: slaughter 10 days

PoM **CTC on Crystakon™** (Hand/PH)
Oral powder, for addition to feed, chlortetracycline hydrochloride 100 g/kg, for *pigs*; 3 kg, 25 kg
Withdrawal Periods. *Pigs*: slaughter 5 days

PoM **Pharmsure™** **Chlortetracycline** (Hand/PH)
Premix, chlortetracycline hydrochloride 100 g/kg, for *pigs*; 12 kg
Withdrawal Periods. *Pigs*: slaughter 5 days

DOXYCYCLINE

Indications. Doxycycline-sensitive infections
Contra-indications. Side-effects. See under Chlortetracycline
Dose. *Dogs*: 5-10 mg/kg daily

PoM **Doxycycline** (Non-proprietary)
Capsules, doxycycline (as hydrochloride) 100 mg

PoM **Vibramycin™** (Invicta)
Syrup, doxycycline (as calcium chelate) 10 mg/mL; 30 mL

PoM **Vibramycin-D™** (Invicta)
Tablets, dispersible, doxycycline 100 mg; 8

OXYTETRACYCLINE

Indications. Oxytetracycline-sensitive infections; intra-uterine use (8.6)
Contra-indications. Side-effects. See under Chlortetracycline. Avoid subcutaneous injection in horses. Some manufacturers recommend that intravenous injection in dogs is avoided
Dose. *Horses*: *by intramuscular or intravenous injection*, 1.5-5.0 mg/kg daily; *foals*: *by mouth*, 10-20 mg/kg twice daily

Cattle, sheep, goats, red deer, pigs: *by subcutaneous, intramuscular, or intravenous injection*, 5-10 mg/kg daily; *by depot intramuscular injection*, 20 mg/kg, repeat after 2-4 days; *calves, lambs, pigs*: *by mouth*, 10-20 mg/kg twice daily
Dogs, cats: *by mouth*, 20 mg/kg twice daily; *by subcutaneous, intramuscular, or intravenous injection*, 5-10 mg/kg daily
Poultry: 6-25 g/100 litres drinking water; 100-500 g/tonne feed; *by subcutaneous or intramuscular injection*, 25-50 mg/kg daily
Mink: *by subcutaneous or intramuscular injection*, 25-50 mg
Fish: see Prescribing for fish

Oral preparations

PoM **Occrycetin™** (Willows Francis)
Tablets, oxytetracycline dihydrate 100 mg, for *dogs, cats*; 250
Tablets, scored, oxytetracycline hydrochloride 500 mg, for *calves*; 20

PoM **Oxytetracycline** (Animalcare)
Tablets, oxytetracycline hydrochloride 50 mg, 100 mg, 250 mg, for *foals, calves, lambs, pigs, dogs, cats*; 500, 1000

PoM **Oxytetracycline** (Bimeda)
Oral powder, for addition to drinking water or feed, oxytetracycline hydrochloride 56 g/kg, for *calves, lambs, pigs*; 25 g, 250 g, 500 g
Withdrawal Periods. *Cattle, sheep*; slaughter 7 days, milk 48 hours. *Pigs*: slaughter 7 days

PoM **Terramycin™** **Feed** **Supplements** (Pfizer)
Premix, oxytetracycline hydrochloride 100 g/kg, 200 g/kg, for *calves, pigs*; 25 kg
Withdrawal Periods. *Cattle*: slaughter 5 days, milk from treated animals should not be used for human consumption. *Pigs*: slaughter 5 days

PoM **Terramycin™ Soluble Powder** (Pfizer)
Oral powder, for addition to drinking water, feed, or to prepare an oral solution, oxytetracycline hydrochloride 55 g/kg, for *calves, pigs, chickens, turkeys*; 225 g, 2 kg
Withdrawal Periods. *Cattle*: slaughter 10 days, milk withdrawal period nil. *Pigs*:

slaughter 7 days. *Poultry*: slaughter 7 days, eggs 1 day

PoM **Terramycin**™ **Soluble Powder Concentrate** (Pfizer)
Oral powder, for addition to drinking water or to prepare an oral solution, oxytetracycline hydrochloride 200 g/kg, for *calves, pigs, chickens, turkeys*; 225 g, 2 kg
Withdrawal Periods. *Cattle*: slaughter 10 days, milk withdrawal period nil. *Pigs*: slaughter 7 days. *Poultry*: slaughter 7 days, eggs 1 day

PoM **Tetra Tab**™ (Bimeda)
Tablets, scored, oxytetracycline hydrochloride 500 mg, for *calves, lambs, pigs*; 100
Withdrawal Periods. *Cattle*: slaughter 7 days, milk 48 hours. *Sheep, pigs*: slaughter 7 days
Note. May also be used for intra-uterine administration (see section 8.6)

PoM **Tetramin**™ **100** (Cheminex)
Premix, oxytetracycline dihydrate 100 g/kg, 200 g/kg, for *pigs*; 2 kg, 25 kg
Withdrawal Periods. *Pigs*: slaughter 5 days

PoM **Tetraplex**™ (Hand/PH)
See Prescribing for fish for preparation details

Parenteral preparations

PoM **Alamycin**™ (Norbrook)
Injection, oxytetracycline hydrochloride 50 mg/mL, for *horses, cattle, sheep, pigs, dogs, cats*; 50 mL, 100 mL
Withdrawal Periods. *Cattle*: milk 48 hours

PoM **Alamycin**™ **10** (Norbrook)
Injection, oxytetracycline hydrochloride 100 mg/mL, for *cattle, pigs*; 100 mL
Withdrawal Periods. *Cattle*: slaughter 15 days, milk 60 hours. *Pigs*: slaughter 15 days

PoM **BK-Mycen**™ **5** (BK)
Injection, oxytetracycline hydrochloride 50 mg/mL, for *horses, cattle, sheep, pigs, dogs, cats*; 100 mL
Withdrawal Periods. *Cattle*: milk 48 hours

PoM **BK-Mycen**™ **10** (BK)
Injection, oxytetracycline hydrochloride 100 mg/mL, for *cattle, pigs*; 100 mL
Withdrawal Periods. *Cattle*: slaughter 15 days, milk 60 hours. *Pigs*: slaughter 15 days

PoM **Duphacycline**™ **50** (Duphar)
Injection, oxytetracycline hydrochloride 50 mg/mL, for *horses, cattle, sheep, pigs, dogs, cats, ornamental fowl*; 40 mL, 100 mL
Withdrawal Periods. *Cattle*: milk 48 hours

PoM **Duphacycline**™ **100** (Duphar)
Injection, oxytetracycline hydrochloride 100 mg/mL, for *cattle, pigs*; 100 mL
Withdrawal Periods. *Cattle*: slaughter 15 days, milk 60 hours. *Pigs*: slaughter 15 days

PoM **Embacycline**™ **5** (RMB)
Injection, oxytetracycline hydrochloride 50 mg/mL, for *horses, cattle, sheep, pigs, goats, dogs, cats*; 100 mL
Withdrawal Periods. *Cattle*: milk 48 hours

PoM **Engemycin**™ **5%** (Mycofarm)
Injection, oxytetracycline (as hydrochloride) 50 mg/mL, for *horses, cattle, sheep, pigs, dogs, cats, poultry*; 50 mL, 100 mL
Withdrawal Periods. *Cattle*: milk 72 hours

PoM **Engemycin**™ **10%** **(DD)** (Mycofarm)
Injection, oxytetracycline (as hydrochloride) 100 mg/mL, for *horses, cattle, sheep, pigs*; 100 mL
Withdrawal Periods. *Cattle*: slaughter 5 days, milk 60 hours. *Sheep*: slaughter 5 days, milk 48 hours. *Pigs*: slaughter 5 days
Note. May also be given as a Depot intramuscular injection

PoM **Intacycline**™ **5%** (Intervet)
Injection, oxytetracycline (as hydrochloride) 50 mg/mL, for *horses, cattle, sheep, pigs, dogs, cats, poultry*; 100 mL
Withdrawal Periods. Should not be used in *horses* intended for human consumption. *Cattle, sheep*: slaughter 8 days, milk 48 hours. *Pigs*: slaughter 8 days

PoM **Intacycline**™ **10% (DD)** (Intervet)
Injection, oxytetracycline (as hydrochloride) 100 mg/mL, for *horses, cattle, sheep, pigs*; 100 mL
Withdrawal Periods. Should not be used in *horses* intended for human consumption. *Cattle*: slaughter 8 days, milk 60 hours. *Sheep*: slaughter 8 days, milk 48 hours. *Pigs*: slaughter 8 days
Note. May also be given as a Depot intramuscular injection

PoM **Occrycetin**™ (Willows Francis)
Injection, oxytetracycline hydrochloride 100 mg/mL, for *cattle, pigs*; 50 mL, 100 mL
Withdrawal Periods. *Cattle*: slaughter 15 days, milk 60 hours. *Pigs*: slaughter 15 days

PoM **Oxytetrin**™ (Coopers Pitman-Moore)
Injection, oxytetracycline hydrochloride 50 mg/mL, for *horses, cattle, sheep, pigs, dogs, cats*; 100 mL
Withdrawal Periods. *Cattle*: milk 60 hours

PoM **Terramycin**™ **LA** (Pfizer)
See Depot injections below for preparation details
Withdrawal Periods. *Cattle*: slaughter 21 days, milk 7 days
Note. Administered by intravenous injection in cattle for short-acting effect

PoM **Terramycin**™ **Q-50** (Pfizer)
Injection, oxytetracycline hydrochloride (as magnesium complex) 50 mg/mL, for *cattle, sheep, pigs*; 40 mL, 100 mL
Withdrawal Periods. *Cattle*: slaughter 14 days, milk 4 days. *Sheep*: slaughter 14 days, milk from treated animals should not be used for human consumption. *Pigs*: slaughter 14 days

PoM **Terramycin**™ **Q-100** (Pfizer)
Injection, oxytetracycline hydrochloride (as magnesium complex) 100 mg/mL, for *cattle, sheep, pigs*; 100 mL
Withdrawal Periods. *Cattle*: slaughter 14 days, milk 5 days. *Sheep*: slaughter 28 days, milk from treated animals should not be used for human consumption. *Pigs*: slaughter 21 days

PoM **Tetcin**™ **5** (Univet)
Injection, oxytetracycline hydrochloride 50 mg/mL, for *horses, cattle, sheep, pigs, dogs, cats, mink, poultry*; 100 mL

Withdrawal Periods. *Cattle*: milk 48 hours

PoM **Tetroxy**™ **5%** (Bimeda)
Injection, oxytetracycline hydrochloride (as magnesium complex) 50 mg/mL, for *cattle, sheep, pigs*; 100 mL
Withdrawal Periods. *Cattle*: slaughter 7 days, milk 72 hours. *Sheep*: slaughter 5 days. *Pigs*: slaughter 11 days

PoM **Tetroxy**™ **10%** (Bimeda)
Injection, oxytetracycline hydrochloride (as magnesium complex) 100 mg/mL, for *cattle, sheep, pigs*; 100 mL
Withdrawal Periods. *Cattle*: slaughter 7 days, milk 80 hours. *Sheep*: slaughter 5 days, milk from treated animals should not be used for human consumption. *Pigs*: slaughter 11 days

PoM **Vetimycin**™ **5%** (C-Vet)
Injection, oxytetracycline hydrochloride 50 mg/mL, for *horses, cattle, sheep, pigs, dogs, cats*; 100 mL
Withdrawal Periods. *Cattle, sheep*: slaughter 5 days, milk 3.5 days. *Pigs*: slaughter 5 days

Depot injections

PoM **Alamycin**™ **LA** (Norbrook)
Depot injection, oxytetracycline (as dihydrate) 200 mg/mL, for *cattle, sheep, pigs*; 50 mL, 100 mL
Withdrawal Periods. *Cattle, sheep*: slaughter 21 days, milk 7 days. *Pigs*: slaughter 21 days

PoM **BK-Mycen**™ **20** (BK)
Depot injection, oxytetracycline 200 mg/mL, for *cattle, sheep, pigs*; 100 mL
Withdrawal Periods. *Cattle, sheep*: slaughter 21 days, milk 7 days. *Pigs*: slaughter 21 days

PoM **Duphacycline**™ **LA** (Duphar)
Depot injection, oxytetracycline dihydrate 200 mg/mL, for *cattle, sheep, pigs*; 100 mL
Withdrawal Periods. *Cattle, sheep*: slaughter 21 days, milk 7 days. *Pigs*: slaughter 21 days

PoM **Embacycline**™ **LA** (RMB)
Depot injection, oxytetracycline (dihydrate as magnesium complex) 200 mg/mL, for *cattle, sheep, pigs*; 100 mL
Withdrawal Periods. *Cattle, sheep*

slaughter 21 days, milk 7 days. *Pigs*: slaughter 21 days

PoM**Engemycin**™ **10% (DD)** (Mycofarm)
See Parenteral preparations above for preparation details
Withdrawal Periods. *Cattle*: slaughter 10 days, milk 72 hours. *Sheep*: slaughter 10 days, milk 48 hours. *Pigs*: slaughter 10 days

PoM**Engemycin**™ **LA** (Mycofarm)
Depot injection, oxytetracycline 200 mg/mL, for *cattle, sheep, pigs*; 50 mL, 100 mL
Withdrawal Periods. *Cattle, sheep*: slaughter 21 days, milk 7 days. *Pigs*: slaughter 21 days

PoM**Intacycline**™ **10% (DD)** (Intervet)
See Parenteral preparations above for preparation details
Withdrawal Periods. *Cattle*: slaughter 10 days, milk 72 hours. *Sheep*: slaughter 10 days, milk 48 hours. *Pigs*: slaughter 10 days

PoM**Occrycetin**™ **PA** (Willows Francis)
Depot injection, oxytetracycline (as dihydrate) 200 mg/mL, for *cattle, sheep, pigs*; 50 mL, 100 mL
Withdrawal Periods. *Cattle*: slaughter 21 days, milk 7 days. *Sheep, pigs*: slaughter 21 days

PoM**Oxytetrin**™ **LA** (Coopers Pitman-Moore)
Depot injection, oxytetracycline dihydrate 200 mg/mL, for *cattle, sheep, pigs*; 100 mL
Withdrawal Periods. *Cattle*: slaughter 21 days, milk 7 days. *Sheep, pigs*: slaughter 21 days

PoM**Terramycin**™ **LA** (Pfizer)
Depot injection, oxytetracycline (dihydrate as magnesium complex) 200 mg/mL, for *cattle, sheep, red deer, pigs*; 100 mL
Withdrawal Periods. *Cattle*: slaughter 21 days, milk 7 days. *Sheep*: slaughter 21 days, milk from treated animals should not be used for human consumption. *Pigs*: slaughter 21 days. *Red deer*: slaughter 30 days
Note. Administered by intramuscular injection for long-lasting effect

PoM**Tetcin-LA**™ (Univet)
Depot injection, oxytetracycline (as magnesium complex) 200 mg/mL, for *cattle, sheep, pigs*; 100 mL
Withdrawal Periods. *Cattle*: slaughter 35 days, milk intended for manufacturing processes 7 days. *Sheep*: slaughter 21 days, milk from treated animals should not be used for human consumption. *Pigs*: slaughter 35 days

PoM**Tetroxy**™ **LA** (Bimeda)
Depot injection, oxytetracycline (as magnesium complex) 200 mg/mL, for *cattle, sheep, pigs*; 100 mL
Withdrawal Periods. *Cattle, sheep*: slaughter 21 days, milk 7 days. *Pigs*: slaughter 21 days

PoM**Vetimycin**™ **LA** (C-Vet)
Depot injection, oxytetracycline 200 mg/mL, for *cattle, sheep, pigs*; 100 mL
Withdrawal Periods. *Cattle, sheep*: slaughter 21 days, milk 7 days. *Pigs*: slaughter 21 days

Compound oxytetracycline preparations

PoM**Finabiotic**™ (Schering-Plough)
Injection, oxytetracycline (as hydrochloride) 100 mg, flunixin (as meglumine) 20 mg/mL, for *cattle*; 100 mL
Withdrawal Periods. *Cattle*: slaughter 21 days, milk 5 days
Dose. *Cattle*: *by intramuscular or intravenous injection*, 0.1 mL/kg daily for 3-5 days

TETRACYCLINE HYDROCHLORIDE

Indications. Tetracycline-sensitive infections
Contra-indications. **Side-effects**. See under Chlortetracycline
Dose. *Calves*: *by addition to feed*, 9.0-17.5 mg/kg body-weight daily in divided doses
Pigs: *by addition to feed*, 11.0-27.5 mg/kg body-weight daily
Dogs, cats: 50 mg/kg daily in divided doses
Poultry: 33 g/100 litres drinking water

PoM **Panmycin™ Aquadrops** (Upjohn)
Oral suspension, tetracycline hydrochloride 100 mg/mL, for *dogs, cats*; 20-mL dropper bottle

PoM **Tetsol™** (Micro-Biologicals)
Oral powder, for addition to drinking water, tetracycline hydrochloride 500 g/kg, for *chickens*; 120 g
Withdrawal Periods. *Poultry*: slaughter 2 days, egg withdrawal period nil

1.1.3 Aminoglycosides

This group includes **streptomycin** and **dihydrostreptomycin**, **neomycin**, **framycetin**, **gentamicin**, **apramycin**, and **spectinomycin**. All are bactericidal and active against Gram-negative organisms and some Gram-positive organisms, but not streptococci. Only gentamicin is active against *Pseudomonas aeruginosa*. Aminoglycosides are taken up into bacteria by an oxygen-dependent process and are therefore inactive against anaerobic bacteria. They are more active in alkaline than in acidic media, which is of particular importance when treating urinary infections. They show synergism with beta-lactam antibiotics.

Bacteria may rapidly acquire resistance to these antibiotics. Enteric bacteria may gain the ability to produce a range of aminoglycoside-inactivating enzymes particularly if a subtherapeutic dose is given. The different members of the group vary in their susceptibility to these inactivating enzymes.

The aminoglycosides are not absorbed from the gastro-intestinal tract after oral administration and therefore are given by injection to treat systemic infections. They are poorly distributed into body compartments such as the brain, cerebrospinal fluid, and the eye. Elimination is solely by renal excretion. If there is renal impairment, aminoglycosides may accumulate in the body resulting in toxicity, particularly in the cat. The important side-effects are vestibular or auditory ototoxicity, and to a lesser extent nephrotoxicity. Risk of toxicity following systemic administration varies with different members of the group. Neomycin is particularly toxic to the auditory and renal systems. Streptomycin and dihydrostreptomycin are ototoxic and gentamicin is ototoxic and nephrotoxic.

Simultaneous administration with the potentially ototoxic loop diuretics such as frusemide should be avoided (see Drug Interactions – Appendix 1). Aminoglycosides may impair neuromuscular transmission and so are not given to animals with myasthenia gravis. These drugs are well absorbed from the peritoneal cavity and instillation during surgery may result in drug overdose and transient respiratory paralysis.

APRAMYCIN

Indications. Apramycin-sensitive infections
Warnings. Caution in renal impairment. Cats, see notes above
Dose. *Calves: by addition to drinking water, milk, or milk replacer*, 20-40 mg/kg daily; *by intramuscular injection*, 20 mg/kg daily
Lambs: by mouth, 10 mg/kg daily
Pigs: by addition to drinking water, 7.5-12.5 mg/kg daily; 100 g/tonne feed; *piglets: by mouth*, 20-40 mg daily
Poultry: 25-50 g/100 litres drinking water

Oral preparations

PoM **Apralan™ 100** (RMB)
Premix, apramycin (as sulphate) 100 g/kg, for *pigs*; 5 kg
Withdrawal Periods. *Pigs*: slaughter 14 days

PoM **Apralan™ Oral Doser** (RMB)
Mixture, apramycin (as sulphate) 20 mg/dose, for *lambs, piglets*; 150-mL dose applicator (1 dose = 1.1 mL)
Withdrawal Periods. *Lambs*: slaughter 35 days. *Piglets*: slaughter 28 days

PoM **Apralan™ Soluble Powder** (RMB)
Oral powder, for addition to drinking water, milk, or milk replacer, apramycin (as sulphate) 1 g, 50 g, for *calves, pigs, poultry*
Withdrawal Periods. *Calves*: slaughter 28 days. *Pigs*: slaughter 14 days. *Poultry*: slaughter 7 days, eggs from treated birds should not be used for human consumption

Parenteral preparations

PoM **Apralan™ 200** (RMB)
Injection, apramycin (as sulphate)
200 mg/mL, for *calves*; 100 mL
Withdrawal Periods. *Calves*: slaughter
35 days

FRAMYCETIN SULPHATE

Indications. Framycetin-sensitive infections
Warnings. Caution in renal impairment
Side-effects. Ototoxicity; nephrotoxicity
Dose. *Cattle, lambs, pigs*: *by intramuscular injection*, 5-10 mg/kg 1-2 times
daily; *by slow intravenous injection*,
2 mg/kg 1-2 times daily; *calves, pigs*: *by
mouth*, 10 mg/kg daily for treatment,
5 mg/kg daily for prophylaxis
Dogs, cats: *by intramuscular injection*,
10 mg/kg 1-2 times daily
Poultry: *by addition to feed*, 10 mg/kg
body-weight daily for treatment, 5 mg/
kg body-weight daily for prophylaxis

Oral preparations

PoM **Framomycin™ Anti-Scour Paste** (C-Vet)
Oral paste, framycetin sulphate 100 mg/
dose, for *piglets*; 10-dose metered
applicator

PoM **Framomycin™ Feed Additive** (C-Vet)
Premix, framycetin sulphate 100 g/kg,
for *pigs, poultry*; 2 kg

PoM **Framomycin™ Sachets** (C-Vet)
Oral powder, for addition to drinking
water or milk, framycetin sulphate
250 mg, for *calves*

PoM **Framomycin™ Soluble Powder** (C-Vet)
Oral powder, for addition to drinking
water or liquid feed, framycetin sulphate
250 mg/g, for *calves, pigs, poultry*; 300 g

Parenteral preparations

PoM **Framomycin™ 5%** (C-Vet)
Injection, framycetin sulphate 50 mg/
mL, for *lambs, piglets, dogs, cats*; 50 mL
PoM **Framomycin™ 15%** (C-Vet)
Injection, framycetin sulphate 150 mg/
mL, for *cattle, pigs*; 100 mL
Withdrawal Periods. *Cattle*: slaughter

1.5 days, milk 36 hours. *Pigs*: slaughter
1.5 days

GENTAMICIN

Indications. Gentamicin-sensitive infections
Warnings. Caution in renal impairment
Side-effects. May cause imbalance;
ototoxicity; nephrotoxicity
Dose. *Dogs, cats*: *by subcutaneous or
intramuscular injection*, 5 mg/kg twice
daily for 24 hours then once daily

PoM **Pangram™** (Virbac)
Injection, gentamicin (as sulphate)
50 mg/mL, for *dogs, cats*; 50 mL

NEOMYCIN SULPHATE

Indications. Neomycin-sensitive infections
Warnings. Caution in renal impairment
Side-effects. Ototoxicity; nephrotoxicity
Dose. *Foals, calves, pigs*: *by mouth*,
14 mg/kg 1-2 times daily; 12.5 g/
100 litres drinking water; 230 g/tonne
feed
Chickens: 12.5 g/100 litres drinking
water; 230 g/tonne feed
Turkeys: (up to 6 weeks of age) 12.5 g/
100 litres drinking water; (6-26 weeks of
age) 25 g/100 litres drinking water; (all
ages) 230 g/tonne feed

PoM **Neobiotic™ Soluble Powder** (Upjohn)
Oral powder, for addition to drinking
water or feed, neomycin sulphate
700 mg/g, for *calves, pigs, chickens,
turkeys*; 20 g, 500 g

PoM **Orojet™ N** (Willows Francis)
Oral liquid, neomycin sulphate 70 mg/
mL, for *foals, calves, piglets*; 210-mL
dose applicator (1 dose = 1 mL)

SPECTINOMYCIN

Indications. Spectinomycin-sensitive
infections
Warnings. Cautions in renal impairment
Dose. *Horses*: *by intravenous injection*,
10-20 mg/kg daily
Cattle, sheep: *by intramuscular or
intravenous injection*, 10-30 mg/kg daily;
calves, lambs: *by mouth*, 7.5-12.5 mg/
kg body-weight twice daily for treatment,

by addition to feed, 3-5 mg/kg body-weight twice daily for prophylaxis
Pigs: 25 g/100 litres drinking water for treatment, 17 g/100 litres drinking water for prophylaxis; *by intramuscular or intravenous injection*, 10-20 mg/kg daily; **piglets**: *by mouth*, (less than 4.5 kg body-weight) 50 mg twice daily; (more than 4.5 kg body-weight) 100 mg twice daily
Dogs, cats: *by intramuscular or intravenous injection*, 100-300 mg daily
Poultry: 55 g/100 litres drinking water; *by subcutaneous or intramuscular injection*, 10-20 mg/kg daily; *by intrasinal instillation*, 35 mg/kg, 1/3 of dose into each sinus and remainder parenterally

PoM **Spectam™ Scour Halt** (Sanofi)
Mixture, spectinomycin activity (as dihydrochloride pentahydrate) 50 mg/dose, for **piglets**; 100-mL dose applicator (1 dose = 1 mL)
Withdrawal Periods. *Piglets*: slaughter 21 days

PoM **Spectam™ Soluble** (Sanofi)
Oral powder, for addition to drinking water or feed, or to prepare an oral solution, spectinomycin activity (as dihydrochloride) 500 mg/g, for **calves, lambs, pigs, poultry**; 1 g, 100 g, 250 g
Withdrawal Periods. *Calves, lambs, pigs, poultry*: slaughter 5 days

PoM **Spectam™** (Sanofi)
Injection, spectinomycin activity (as dihydrochloride) 100 mg/mL, for **horses, cattle, sheep, pigs, dogs, cats, poultry**; 100 mL
Withdrawal Periods. *Cattle, sheep*: slaughter 5 days, milk 48 hours. *Pigs, poultry*: slaughter 5 days

STREPTOMYCIN SULPHATE

Indications.   Streptomycin-sensitive infections
Warnings. Caution in renal impairment
Side-effects. May cause imbalance; ototoxicity
Dose. *Horses, cattle, sheep, goats, dogs, cats*: *by intramuscular injection*, 10 mg/kg twice daily

PoM **Devomycin™** (Norbrook)
Injection, streptomycin sulphate 250 mg/mL, for **horses, cattle, sheep, goats, dogs, cats**; 100 mL

DIHYDROSTREPTOMYCIN and STREPTOMYCIN

The antibacterial activity of these drugs is similar, but they differ in their toxic effects, dihydrostreptomycin being more likely to cause auditory damage while streptomycin is more likely to produce vestibular damage. Hence, a mixture of the two is claimed to have the same activity as, but may be less toxic than, either alone.

PoM **Devomycin-D™** (Norbrook)
Injection, dihydrostreptomycin sulphate 150 mg, streptomycin sulphate 150 mg/mL, for **horses, cattle, sheep, goats, pigs, dogs, cats**; 100 mL
Dose. *Horses, cattle, sheep, goats, pigs, dogs, cats*: *by intramuscular injection*, 0.042 mL/kg

PoM **Dimycin™** (Coopers Pitman-Moore)
Injection, dihydrostreptomycin (as sulphate) 167 mg, streptomycin (as sulphate) 167 mg/mL, for **horses, cattle, sheep, goats, pigs, dogs, cats**; 100 mL
Dose. *Horses, cattle, sheep, goats, pigs, dogs, cats*: *by intramuscular injection*, 0.015-0.03 mL/kg

Some of the following drugs are included in Prescribing for reptiles and Prescribing for exotic birds – see those sections for indications and dosage

AMIKACIN

PoM **Amikin™** (Bristol-Myers)
Injection, amikacin (as sulphate) 50 mg/mL 250 mg/mL; 2 mL

KANAMYCIN

PoM **Kannasyn™** (Sterling-Winthrop)
Injection, powder for reconstitution, kanamycin (as acid sulphate) 1 g

TOBRAMYCIN

PoM **Nebcin™** (Lilly)
Injection, tobramycin (as sulphate) 10 mg/mL, 40 mg/mL; 10-mg/mL vial 2 mL; 40-mg/mL vial 1 mL, 2 mL

1.1.4 Macrolides and lincosamides

The macrolides include erythromycin, spiramycin, tiamulin, and tylosin, while clindamycin and lincomycin belong to the related lincosamide group. All are basic compounds that are well absorbed following oral administration and inactivated by hepatic metabolism. Due to their basic nature they are concentrated by the 'ion-trap' in acidic fluids such as milk and prostatic fluid. They are usually bacteriostatic in action.

Tylosin has good activity against *Mycoplasma* and *Treponema hyodysenteriae* and a number of Gram-positive aerobes, but little activity against Gram-negative organisms or anaerobes. **Tiamulin** has a broader spectrum of action, which includes more fastidious Gram-negative organisms such as *Haemophilus*, *Bordetella*, *Pasteurella*, *Actinobacillus*, and also a number of anaerobic organisms. **Erythromycin** is active against streptoccoci, *Staph. aureus* including penicillin-resistant strains, the more fastidious Gram-negative bacteria, and anaerobes. It is likely to be the drug of choice for *Campylobacter*. Erythromycin has less activity than tiamulin or tylosin against *Mycoplasma* or *T. hyodysenteriae*.

Lincomycin is effective against Gram-positive bacteria, anaerobes, and *Mycoplasma* but has little activity against Gram-negative organisms. **Clindamycin** has more potent antibacterial activity than lincomycin. It is particularly indicated in staphylococcal osteomyelitis. Lincosamides may cause a fatal enterocolitis in horses, rabbits, and rodents. Accidental oral administration of small amounts of lincomycin to cattle may cause severe toxicity.

CLINDAMYCIN

Indications. See notes above
Contra-indications. Horses, rabbits, and rodents; hepatic impairment; see notes above
Dose. *Dogs*: *by mouth*, 5.5-11.0 mg/kg twice daily; *by intramuscular injection*, 10 mg/kg twice daily
***Cats*:** *by mouth*, 10 mg/kg twice daily; *by intramuscular injection*, 10 mg/kg twice daily

PoM **Antirobe™** (Upjohn)
Capsules, clindamycin (as hydrochloride) 25 mg, 75 mg, 150 mg, for *dogs*; 80

PoM **Dalacin C™** (Upjohn)
Injection, clindamycin (as phosphate) 150 mg/mL; 2 mL, 4 mL

ERYTHROMYCIN

Indications. Erythromycin-sensitive infections, especially *Campylobacter*
Side-effects. Intramuscular injection may cause pain in dogs and cats
Dose. *Cattle*: *by intramuscular injection*, 2-4 mg/kg daily
***Sheep*:** *by intramuscular injection*, 2 mg/kg daily; ***lambs*:** *by intramuscular injection*, 10 mg/kg daily
***Pigs*:** *by intramuscular injection*, 2-6 mg/kg daily; ***piglets*:** (more than 1 week of age) *by intramuscular injection*, 10 mg/kg
***Dogs, cats*:** *by mouth*, 2-10 mg/kg daily; *by intramuscular injection*, 10 mg/kg daily
***Poultry*:** 12.5-25.0 g/100 litres drinking water; *by subcutaneous or intramuscular injection*, 10-20 mg/kg daily

Oral preparations

PoM **Erythromycin** (Non-proprietary)
Tablets, e/c, erythromycin 250 mg, 500 mg

PoM **Erythromycin Stearate** (Non-proprietary)
Tablets, erythromycin (as stearate) 250 mg, 500 mg

PoM **Erythrocin™ Proportioner** (Sanofi)
Oral powder, for reconstitution and then addition to drinking water, erythromycin activity 300 mg/g, for *poultry*; 78 g
Reconstitute erythromycin 23.12 g (78 g powder) in 1.1 litres water

PoM **Erythrocin™ Soluble** (Sanofi)
Oral powder, for reconstitution and then addition to drinking water, erythromycin

activity (as thiocyanate) 165 mg/g, for
poultry; 70 g
Reconstitute erythromycin 11.56 g (70 g
powder) in 2.5 litres water

Parenteral preparations

PoM**Erythrocin**™ (Sanofi)
Injection, erythromycin activity 200 mg/
mL, for *cattle, sheep, pigs, dogs, cats,
poultry*; 50 mL
Withdrawal Periods. *Cattle, sheep*:
slaughter 2 days, milk 24 hours. *Pigs*:
slaughter 2 days

LINCOMYCIN

Indications. See notes above
Contra-indications. Horses, rabbits, and
rodents; hepatic impairment; see notes
above
Dose. *Pigs*: 3.3 g/100 litres drinking
water; 110-220 g/tonne feed; *by intramuscular injection*, 4.5-11.0 mg/kg daily
Dogs, cats: *by mouth*, 44-45 mg/kg daily
in divided doses; *by subcutaneous or
intramuscular injection*, 22 mg/kg daily;
by slow intravenous injection, 11-22 mg/
kg 1-2 times daily

PoM**Lincocin**™ (Upjohn)
Tablets, scored, lincomycin (as hydrochloride) 100 mg, 500 mg, for *dogs, cats*;
100-mg tablets 100; 500-mg tablets 50
Syrup, lincomycin (as hydrochloride)
50 mg/mL, for *dogs, cats*; 20-mL dropper
bottle
Oral powder, for addition to drinking
water, lincomycin (as hydrochloride)
400 mg/g, for *pigs*; 7.5 g, 150 g
Withdrawal Periods. *Pigs*: slaughter 1
day
Premix, lincomycin (as hydrochloride)
44 g/kg, for *pigs*; 2.5 kg, 25 kg
Withdrawal Periods. *Pigs*: slaughter 1
day
Injection, lincomycin (as hydrochloride)
100 mg/mL, for *pigs, dogs, cats*; 20 mL,
50 mL, 100 mL
Withdrawal Periods. *Pigs*: slaughter 2
days

PoM**Lincomix**™ (Upjohn)
Premix, lincomycin (as hydrochloride)
44 g/kg, for *pigs*; 5 kg
Withdrawal Periods. *Pigs*: slaughter 3
days

SPIRAMYCIN

Indications. Spiramycin-sensitive organisms
Dose. *Calves, pigs*: *by intramuscular
injection*, 20 mg/kg daily

PoM**Rovamycin**™ (RMB)
Injection, spiramycin 200 mg/mL, for
calves, pigs; 100 mL
Withdrawal Periods. *Calves, pigs*:
slaughter 21 days

TIAMULIN FUMARATE

Indications. Tiamulin-sensitive organisms
Side-effects. Rarely, skin erythema
Warnings. Should not be administered
within 7 days of products containing
maduramicin, monensin, narasin, or
salinomycin (see Drug Interactions –
Appendix 1)
Dose. *Pigs*: *by addition to drinking water
or feed*, 8.8 mg/kg body-weight daily;
by intramuscular injection, 10-15 mg/kg
daily

PoM**Tiamutin**™ (Leo)
Oral solution, for addition to drinking
water, tiamulin fumarate 125 mg/mL,
for *pigs*; 20 mL, 250 mL, 1 litre
Withdrawal Periods. *Pigs*: slaughter 5
days
Oral powder, for addition to drinking
water, tiamulin fumarate 450 mg/g, for
pigs; 200 g
Withdrawal Periods. *Pigs*: slaughter 5
days
Premix, tiamulin fumarate 20 g/kg, for
pigs; 1 kg, 5 kg
Withdrawal periods. *Pigs*: slaughter 5
days
Premix, tiamulin fumarate 250 g/kg, for
pigs; 1.2 kg, 24 kg
Withdrawal Periods. *Pigs*: slaughter 5
days
Injection (oily), tiamulin fumarate
200 mg/mL, for *pigs*; 100 mL
Withdrawal Periods. *Pigs*: slaughter 14
days

Accidental self-injection with oil-based preparations can cause severe vascular spasm and prompt medical attention is essential

TYLOSIN

Indications. Tylosin-sensitive organisms; to improve growth-rate and feed conversion efficiency in pigs (17.1)

Dose. *Cattle*: *by intramuscular injection*, 4-10 mg/kg daily

Pigs: 25 g/100 litres drinking water; 100 g/tonne feed; *by intramuscular injection*, 2-10 mg/kg daily

Dogs, cats: *by mouth*, 20-45 mg/kg daily in divided doses; *by intramuscular injection*, 2-10 mg/kg daily

Poultry: 50 g/100 litres drinking water

Oral preparations

PoM **Tylan**™ (Elanco)
Tablets, scored, tylosin 200 mg, for *dogs, cats*; 50
Oral powder, for addition to drinking water, tylosin (as tartrate) 100 g, for *pigs, chickens, turkeys*
Withdrawal Periods. *Pigs*: slaughter withdrawal period nil. *Chickens*: slaughter 1 day, eggs from treated birds should not be used for human consumption. *Turkeys*: slaughter 5 days
Premix, tylosin (as phosphate) 20 g/kg, for *pigs*; 25 kg
Withdrawal Periods. *Pigs*: slaughter withdrawal period nil

Parenteral preparations

PoM **Bilosin**™ (Bimeda)
Injection, tylosin (as tartrate) 200 mg/mL, for *cattle, pigs*; 50 mL, 100 mL
Withdrawal Periods. *Cattle*: slaughter 8 days, milk 4 days. *Pigs*: slaughter 21 days

PoM **Tylan**™ (Elanco)
Injection, tylosin 50 mg/mL, for *cattle, pigs, dogs, cats*; 50 mL
Withdrawal Periods. *Cattle*: slaughter 7 days, milk 4 days. *Pigs*: slaughter 7 days
Injection, tylosin 200 mg/mL, for *cattle, pigs, dogs, cats*; 100 mL
Withdrawal Periods. *Cattle*: slaughter 7 days, milk 4 days. *Pigs*: slaughter 7 days

PoM **Tyluvet-20** (Univet)
Injection, tylosin 200 mg/mL, for *cattle, pigs*; 100 mL
Withdrawal Periods. *Cattle*: milk 4 days

1.1.5 Chloramphenicol

Chloramphenicol is a broad-spectrum bacteriostatic antibiotic. It is active against rickettsial and chlamydial infections, the majority of anaerobes, most Gram-positive aerobes, and non-enteric aerobes including *Actinobacillus*, *Bordetella*, *Haemophilus*, and *Pasteurella*. Enterobacteriaceae including *Escherichia* and *Salmonella* are intrinsically susceptible but plasmid-mediated resistance is widespread. Chloramphenicol has activity against *Mycoplasma* and *Proteus* but is unreliable. It is inactive against *Pseudomonas*. As chloramphenicol has broad-spectrum activity it is often used for suppression of secondary bacterial invaders in viral infections such as feline panleucopenia.

Chloramphenicol is used in the treatment of human *Salmonella typhi* infection. It is recommended that the use of chloramphenicol in veterinary medicine be restricted to infections such as systemic salmonellosis and respiratory disease in calves or where no other antibiotic would be effective and after bacterial sensitivity testing confirms susceptibility. The drug is contraindicated in lactating animals where the milk is intended for human consumption. Operators must wear impervious gloves and avoid drug-skin contact.

Chloramphenicol is a simple uncharged lipid-soluble compound which readily crosses cellular barriers. Either chloramphenicol or palmitate ester is used for oral administration, and for intravenous injection the soluble succinate is employed. Chloramphenicol diffuses throughout the body and reaches sites of infection inaccessible to many other antibacterial drugs including cerebrospinal fluid, brain, and internal structures of the eye. It is inactivated in the liver by conjugation and then excreted in urine and bile.

Drug metabolism is particularly rapid in the horse. Hence, this antibiotic is of limited use in this species. In newborn animals conjugation mechanisms take several weeks to mature and dosage intervals should therefore be increased in neonates. Due to limited drug metabolism in the cat, chloramphenicol may accumulate giving rise to reversible bone-marrow suppression. Treatment should be restricted to one week in this species.

The bacteriostatic action of chloramphenicol may inhibit the bactericidal action of beta-lactam antibiotics and these drugs should not therefore be used concurrently. Chloramphenicol may inhibit metabolism of certain barbiturates and hence greatly prolong pentobarbitone anaesthesia.

CHLORAMPHENICOL

Indications. See notes above
Contra-indications. Hepatic impairment. See Drug Interactions – Appendix 1; see notes above
Warnings. Administer with caution to cats and neonates. Should not be administered intravenously unless indicated
Dose. *Cattle*: by intramuscular injection, 10-25 mg/kg twice daily; *calves*: by intramuscular injection, 11.25 mg/kg daily
Pigs: by intramuscular injection, 11.25 mg/kg daily
Dogs: by mouth or by subcutaneous, intramuscular, or slow intravenous injection, 50 mg/kg twice daily
Cats: by mouth or by subcutaneous, intramuscular, or slow intravenous injection, 25 mg/kg twice daily

Oral preparations

PoM **Chloramphenicol** (Willows Francis)
Tablets, chloramphenicol 100 mg, for *dogs, cats*; 250

PoM **Chloromycetin**™ (Parke-Davis)
Capsules, chloramphenicol 250 mg, for *dogs*; 100
Oral suspension, chloramphenicol (as palmitate) 125 mg/5 mL, for *dogs, cats*; 100 mL

Parenteral preparations

PoM **Chloramphenicol** (Willows Francis)
Injection, chloramphenicol 150 mg/mL, for *calves, pigs, dogs, cats*; 50 mL, 100 mL
Withdrawal Periods. *Calves, pigs*: slaughter 10 days
Note. Should not be used in lactating cattle. For intramuscular injection

PoM **Chloromycetin**™ **Succinate** (Parke-Davis)
Injection, powder for reconstitution, chloramphenicol (as sodium succinate) 300 mg, 1.2 g, for *dogs, cats*
For subconjunctival, subcutaneous, intramuscular, or intravenous injection

PoM **Intramycetin**™ (Parke-Davis)
Injection, chloramphenicol 150 mg/mL, for *cattle, dogs*; 30 mL, 75 mL
Withdrawal Periods. *Cattle*: slaughter 28 days, milk from treated animals should not be used for human consumption
For intramuscular injection

1.1.6 Sulphonamides and potentiated sulphonamides

1.1.6.1 Sulphonamides
1.1.6.2 Potentiated sulphonamides

1.1.6.1 SULPHONAMIDES

The sulphonamides form an extensive series of drugs that differ more in their physicochemical characteristics and hence in mode of administration and pharmacokinetics than they do in their antibacterial activity. They are bacteriostatic to a range of Gram-positive and Gram-negative bacteria. They inhibit aerobic Gram-positive cocci and some rods and many Gram-negative rods including Enterobacteriaceae. *Leptospira* and *Pseudomonas* species are resistant. Sulphonamides are also active against *Chlamydia*, *Toxoplasma*, and *Coccidia* (see section 1.4). Acquired resistance to sulphonamides is widespread. They act by competing with tissue factors, notably *p*-aminobenzoic acid, and are therefore inactive in the presence of necrotic tissue.

The sodium salts are alkaline and hence irritant by intramuscular injection and so are often given intravenously. Sulphonamides are well absorbed following oral administration. They diffuse well into body tissues and are partly inactivated in the liver, mainly by acetylation. The acetylated derivatives are relatively insoluble in acidic urine and so may precipitate in the renal tubules of carnivores leading to crystalluria and renal failure.

The sulphonamides include **sulphadimidine** and **sulphamethoxypyridazine**. The 'bowel-active' sulphonamide **phthalylsulphathiazole** when given orally is retained in the bowel and so is used for enteric infection where systemic activity is not required (see section 1.1.11). Sulphamethoxypyridazine is highly bound to plasma proteins and hence is slowly excreted. It is given every 24 hours.

Prolonged administration of certain sulphonamides may cause keratoconjunctivitis sicca (dry eye) in dogs, and sulphadiazine-containing preparations may promote a reversible immune-mediated sterile polyarthritis in Dobermann Pinschers. Sulphonamides may cause petechial haemorrhages in poultry due to vitamin K antagonism.

SULPHADIMIDINE

Indications. Sulphadimidine-sensitive infections
Contra-indications. Renal or hepatic impairment
Side-effects. Transient irritation at injection site
Dose. *Cattle*: *by subcutaneous or intravenous (preferred) injection*, initial dose 100-200 mg/kg then 50-100 mg/kg daily; *calves*: *by mouth or by subcutaneous injection*, initial dose 100-200 mg/kg then 50-100 mg/kg daily
Sheep: *by subcutaneous or intravenous (preferred) injection*, initial dose 100-200 mg/kg then 50-100mg/kg daily
Pigs: *by mouth or by subcutaneous or intravenous (preferred) injection*, initial dose 100-200 mg/kg then 50-100 mg/kg daily; 100 g/tonne feed

See section 1.4.1 for dose for coccidiosis

Oral preparations

PoM **Bimadine**™ (Bimeda)
Tablets, scored, sulphadimidine 5 g, for *calves*; 100
Withdrawal Periods. *Cattle*: slaughter 8 days
Oral powder, to prepare an oral solution, sulphadimidine, for *calves*; 25 g, 500 g, other sizes available
Withdrawal Periods. *Cattle*: slaughter 21 days

PoM **Micro-Bio**™ **Sulphadimidine** (Micro-Biologicals)
Oral powder, for addition to feed, pure sulphadimidine, for *pigs*; 25 kg
Withdrawal Periods. *Pigs*: slaughter 7 days
Premix, sulphadimidine 100 g/kg, for *pigs*; 25 kg
Withdrawal Periods. *Pigs*: slaughter 7 days

See under Parenteral preparations below for oral solutions for poultry

Parenteral preparations

PoM **Bimadine**™ **33 1/3** (Bimeda)
Injection, sulphadimidine sodium 333 mg/mL, for *milking cows*, *calves*; 500 mL, 2.5 litres
Withdrawal Periods. Should not be used in *adult cattle* intended for human consumption. *Cattle*: milk 72 hours. *Calves*: slaughter 7 days

For intravenous injection in adult cattle. For subcutaneous injection in calves.

PoM **Intradine**™ (Norbrook)
Injection, sulphadimidine sodium 333 mg/mL, for *cattle*, *sheep*, *pigs*; 500 mL
Withdrawal Periods. *Cattle*: slaughter 7 days, milk 72 hours. *Sheep*: slaughter 7 days, milk from treated animals should not be used for human consumption. *Pigs*: slaughter 7 days

PoM **Sulfoxine**™ **33** (Univet)
Injection or oral solution, for addition to drinking water, sulphadimidine sodium 333 mg/mL, for *cattle*, *sheep*, *pigs*, *poultry* (see section 1.4.1); 400 mL
Withdrawal Periods. *Cattle*, *sheep*:

slaughter 7 days, milk 72 hours. *Pigs, poultry*: slaughter 7 days

PoM **Sulphamezathine 33⅓%** (Coopers Pitman-Moore)
Injection, sulphadimidine sodium 333 mg/mL, for *cattle;* 500 mL
Withdrawal Periods. *Cattle*: slaughter 14 days, milk 60 hours

PoM **Vesadin™** (RMB)
Injection, sulphadimidine sodium 333 mg/mL, for *cattle, sheep, pigs*; 500 mL
Withdrawal Periods. *Cattle*: slaughter 7 days, milk 72 hours. *Sheep*: slaughter 7 days, milk from treated animals should not be used for human consumption. *Pigs*: slaughter 7 days

SULPHAMETHOXYPYRIDAZINE

Indications. Sulphamethoxypyridazine-sensitive infections
Contra-indications. **Side-effects**. See under Sulphadimidine
Dose. *Cattle, sheep, pigs*: *by subcutaneous, intramuscular, intraperitoneal, or intravenous injection*, 20 mg/kg daily

PoM **Bimalong™** (Bimeda)
Injection, sulphamethoxypyridazine (as sodium salt) 250 mg/mL, for *cattle*; 100 mL, 400 mL
Withdrawal Periods. *Cattle*: slaughter 21 days, milk 48 hours
For subcutaneous or intravenous injection

PoM **Midicel™** (Parke-Davis)
Injection, sulphamethoxypyridazine 250 mg/mL, for *cattle, sheep*; 100 mL, 250 mL
Withdrawal Periods. *Cattle*: slaughter 7 days, milk 48 hours. *Sheep*: slaughter 7 days, milk from treated animals should not be used for human consumption

PoM **Sulfoxine™ LA** (Univet)
Injection, sulphamethoxypyridazine (as sodium salt) 250 mg/mL, for *cattle, sheep, pigs*: 100 mL, 400 mL
Withdrawal Periods. *Cattle, sheep*: slaughter 7 days, milk 48 hours. *Pigs*: slaughter 7 days

1.1.6.2 POTENTIATED SULPHONAMIDES

Sulphonamides may be combined with the folate reductase inhibitor **trimethoprim**. These drugs block sequential stages in the synthesis of tetrahydrofolate and thus have a synergistic antibacterial action. This combination may be bactericidal and allows a smaller dose of sulphonamide to be used. The antibacterial spectrum of the combination is broad and includes a high proportion of anaerobic bacteria, *Nocardia*, *Chlamydia*, and *Toxoplasma*. Plasmid-mediated resistance to trimethoprim occurs.

The compound preparations contain 5 parts sulphonamide and one part trimethoprim. The sulphonamides most commonly used in conjunction with trimethoprim are sulphadiazine (co-trimazine) and sulphadoxine, the latter acting for a longer period.

Trimethoprim, like the sulphonamides, diffuses well into body tissues and so the combination is the treatment of choice for cases such as coliform meningitis. Unfortunately, in domesticated animals, trimethoprim is more rapidly inactivated than the sulphonamide component so that useful ratios are present in the body for a short time only.

CO-TRIMAZINE

Preparations of trimethoprim 1 part and sulphadiazine 5 parts

Indications.   Co-trimazine-sensitive infections; intra-uterine use (8.6)
Warnings. Concomitant administration of potentiated sulphonamides and detomidine increases the risk of cardiac arrhythmias (see Drug Interactions – Appendix 1)
Dose. Expressed as trimethoprim + sulphadiazine
Horses, cattle, sheep: *by mouth*, 30 mg/kg; *by intramuscular or slow intravenous injection*, 15-24 mg/kg daily
Pigs: *by mouth*, 30 mg/kg body-weight; 300-450 g/tonne feed; *by intramuscular or slow intravenous injection*, 15-24 mg/kg daily

Dogs, cats: *by mouth or by subcutaneous injection*, 30 mg/kg daily
Poultry: *by addition to drinking water*, 15 mg/kg body-weight daily; 300 g/tonne feed
Fish: see Prescribing for fish

Oral preparations

PoM **Delvoprim**™ (Mycofarm)
Tablets, co-trimazine 20/100 [trimethoprim 20 mg, sulphadiazine 100 mg], for *dogs, cats*; 100, 1000
Tablets, scored, co-trimazine 80/400, [trimethoprim 80 mg, sulphadiazine 400 mg], for *dogs*; 100, 1000
Tablets, scored, co-trimazine 200/1000 [trimethoprim 200 mg, sulphadiazine 1 g], for *calves*; 20
Withdrawal Periods. *Calves*: slaughter 28 days

PoM **Delvoprim**™ **Piglet Suspension** (Mycofarm)
Oral suspension, co-trimazine 10/50 [trimethoprim 10 mg, sulphadiazine 50 mg]/dose, for *piglets*; 250-mL dose applicator (1 dose = 1.1 mL)
Withdrawal Periods. *Piglets*: slaughter 28 days

PoM **Delvoprim**™ **Horse Paste** (Mycofarm)
Oral paste, co-trimazine 250/1250 [trimethoprim 260 mg, sulphadiazine 1.3 g]/division, for *horses*; 45-g metered-dose applicator
Withdrawal Periods. Should not be used in *horses* intended for human consumption

PoM **Duphatrim**™ (Duphar)
Tablets, co-trimazine 20/100 [trimethoprim 20 mg, sulphadiazine 100 mg], for *dogs, cats*; 100
Tablets, scored, co-trimazine 80/400 [trimethoprim 80 mg, sulphadiazine 400 mg], for *dogs*; 100, 500
Tablets, scored, co-trimazine 200/1000 [trimethoprim 200 mg, sulphadiazine 1 g], for *foals, calves, lambs*; 10
Withdrawal Periods. *Calves, lambs*: slaughter 5 days
Note. Duphatrim 200/1000 tablets may also be used for intra-uterine administration (see section 8.6)

PoM **Duphatrim**™ **Equine Formula** (Duphar)
Oral paste, co-trimazine 250/1250 [trimethoprim 250 mg, sulphadiazine 1.25 g]/division, for *horses*; 37.5-g metered-dose applicator
Withdrawal Periods. Should not be used in *horses* intended for human consumption

PoM **Duphatrim**™ **Piglet Suspension** (Duphar)
Oral suspension, co-trimazine 10/50 [trimethoprim 10 mg, sulphadiazine 50 mg]/dose, for *piglets*; 200-mL dose applicator (1 dose = 1.1 mL)
Withdrawal Periods. *Piglets*: slaughter 5 days

PoM **Duphatrim**™ **Poultry Suspension** (Duphar)
Oral suspension, for addition to drinking water, co-trimazine 80/400 [trimethoprim 80 mg, sulphadiazine 400 mg]/mL, for *poultry*; 200 mL
Withdrawal Periods. *Poultry*: slaughter 5 days, eggs from treated birds should not be used for human consumption

PoM **Equitrim**™ **Equine Paste** (Boehringer Ingelheim)
Oral paste, co-trimazine 250/1250 [trimethoprim 260 mg, sulphadiazine 1.3 g]/division, for *horses*; 45-g metered-dose applicator
Withdrawal Periods. Should not be used in *horses* intended for human consumption

PoM **Norodine**™ (Norbrook)
Tablets, co-trimazine 20/100 [trimethoprim 20 mg, sulphadiazine 100 mg], for *dogs, cats*; 100
Tablets, scored, co-trimazine 80/400 [trimethoprim 80 mg, sulphadiazine 400 mg], for *dogs*; 100, 500
Tablets, scored, co-trimazine 200/1000 [trimethoprim 200 mg, sulphadiazine 1 g], for *calves*; 20
Withdrawal Periods. *Calves*: slaughter 28 days

PoM **Norodine**™ **Equine Paste** (Norbrook)
Oral paste, co-trimazine 250/1250 [trimethoprim 260 mg, sulphadiazine 1.3 g]/division, for *horses*; 45-g metered-dose applicator
Withdrawal Periods. Should not be

used in *horses* intended for human consumption

PoM Norodine™ Oral Piglet Suspension (Norbrook)
Oral suspension, co-trimazine 10/50 [trimethoprim 10.01 mg, sulphadiazine 50.05 mg]/dose, for *piglets*; 250-mL dose applicator (1 dose = 1.1 mL)
Withdrawal Periods. *Piglets*: slaughter 28 days

PoM Scorprin™ (Willows Francis)
Capsules, co-trimazine 20/100 [trimethoprim 20 mg, sulphadiazine 100 mg], for *dogs, cats*; 80
Capsules, co-trimazine 80/400 [trimethoprim 80 mg, sulphadiazine 400 mg], for *dogs*; 80
Tablets, scored, co-trimazine 200/1000 [trimethoprim 200 mg, sulphadiazine 1 g], for *calves*; 20
Withdrawal Periods. *Calves*: slaughter 5 days

PoM Scorprin™ Suspension (Willows Francis)
Oral suspension, co-trimazine 10/50 [trimethoprim 10 mg, sulphadiazine 50 mg, for *piglets*; 100-mL dose applicator (1 dose = 1.1 mL)
Withdrawal Periods. *Piglets*: slaughter 10 days

PoM Sulfatrim™ (Hand/PH)
See Prescribing for fish for preparation details

PoM Synutrim™ (Hand/PH)
Premix, for addition to feed, co-trimazine 50/250 [trimethoprim 50 g, sulphadiazine 250 g]/kg, for *chickens*; 3 kg, 25 kg
Withdrawal Periods. *Poultry*: slaughter 5 days, eggs from treated birds should not be used for human consumption

PoM Tribrissen™ (Coopers Pitman-Moore)
Tablets, co-trimazine 20/100 [trimethoprim 20 mg, sulphadiazine 100 mg], for *dogs, cats*; 100
Tablets, scored, co-trimazine 80/400 [trimethoprim 80 mg, sulphadiazine 400 mg], for *dogs*; 100, 500
Tablets, scored, co-trimazine 200/1000 [trimethoprim 200 mg, sulphadiazine 1 g], for *foals, calves*; 10
Withdrawal Periods. Should not be

used in *horses* intended for human consumption. *Calves*: slaughter 8 days

PoM Tribrissen™ 40% Powder (Coopers Pitman-Moore)
See Prescribing for fish for preparation details

PoM Tribrissen™ Oral Paste (Coopers Pitman-Moore)
Oral paste, co-trimazine 250/1250 [trimethoprim 250 mg, sulphadiazine 1.25 g]/division, for *horses*; 37.5-g metered dose applicator
Withdrawal Periods. Should not be used in *horses* intended for human consumption

PoM Tribrissen™ Piglet Suspension (Coopers Pitman-Moore)
Oral suspension, co-trimazine 10/50 [trimethoprim 10 mg, sulphadiazine 50 mg]/dose, for *piglets*; 200-mL dose applicator (1 dose = 1.1 mL)
Withdrawal Periods. *Piglets*: slaughter 5 days

PoM Trimediazine™ 15 (Univet)
Premix, co-trimazine 25/125 [trimethoprim 25 g, sulphadiazine 125 g]/kg, for *pigs*; 2 kg, 25 kg
Withdrawal Periods. *Pigs*: slaughter 5 days

PoM Trimediazine™ 30 (Univet)
Oral powder, for addition to feed, co-trimazine 50/250 [trimethoprim 50 mg, sulphadiazine 250 mg]/g, for *horses*; 50 g
Withdrawal Periods. Should not be used in *horses* intended for human consumption

PoM Trimedoxine™ (Univet)
Tablets, co-trimazine 357/1786 [trimethoprim 357 mg, sulphadiazine 1786 mg], for *calves*; 20
Withdrawal Periods. *Calves*: slaughter 28 days

PoM Trimedoxine™ Piglet Suspension (Univet)
Oral suspension, co-trimazine 10/50 [trimethoprim 10.01 mg, sulphadiazine 50.05 mg]/dose, for *piglets*; 250-mL dose applicator (1 dose = 1.1 mL)
Withdrawal Periods. *Pigs*: slaughter 28 days

PoM **Uniprim™ 150** (Cheminex)
Oral powder, for addition to feed, co-trimazine 25/125 [trimethoprim 25 g, sulphadiazine 125 g]/kg, for *pigs, chickens*; 2 kg, 12 kg
Withdrawal Periods. *Pigs*: slaughter 5 days. *Poultry*: slaughter 1 day
Note. Not for use in layer hens

PoM **Uniprim™ for Horses** (Cheminex)
Oral powder, for addition to feed, co-trimazine 5/25 [trimethoprim 5 mg, sulphadiazine 25 mg]/kg, for *horses*; 37.5 g
Withdrawal Periods. Should not be used in *horses* intended for human consumption

Parenteral preparations

PoM **Delvoprim™ Coject** (Mycofarm)
Injection, co-trimazine 40/200 [trimethoprim 40 mg, sulphadiazine 200 mg]/mL, for *horses, cattle, sheep, pigs, dogs, cats*; 100 mL
Withdrawal Periods. Should not be used in *horses* intended for human consumption. *Cattle*: slaughter 18 days, milk 60 hours. *Sheep, pigs*: slaughter 18 days

PoM **Duphatrim™** (Duphar)
Injection, co-trimazine 40/200 [trimethoprim 40 mg, sulphadiazine 200 mg]/mL, for *dogs, cats*; 50 mL
Injection, co-trimazine 80/400 [trimethoprim 80 mg, sulphadiazine 400 mg]/mL, for *horses, cattle, sheep, pigs*; 100 mL
Withdrawal Periods. *Cattle*: slaughter 28 days, milk 72 hours. *Sheep, pigs*: slaughter 28 days

PoM **Equitrim™** (Boehringer Ingelheim)
Injection, co-trimazine 40/200 [trimethoprim 40 mg, sulphadiazine 200 mg]/mL, for *horses, cattle, sheep, pigs, dogs*; 100 mL
Withdrawal Periods. *Cattle*: slaughter 18 days, milk 60 hours. *Sheep, pigs*: slaughter 18 days

PoM **Norodine 24™** (Norbrook)
Injection, co-trimazine 40/200 [trimethoprim 40 mg, sulphadiazine 200 mg]/mL, for *horses, cattle, sheep, pigs, dogs, cats*; 50 mL, 100 mL
Withdrawal Periods. Should not be used in *horses* intended for human consumption. *Cattle*: slaughter 18 days, milk 60 hours. *Sheep, pigs*: slaughter 18 days

PoM **Scorprin™ 240** (Willows Francis)
Injection, co-trimazine 40/200 [trimethoprim 40 mg, sulphadiazine 200 mg]/mL, for *horses, cattle, sheep, pigs, dogs, cats*; 50 mL, 100 mL
Withdrawal Periods. Should not be used in *horses* intended for human consumption. *Cattle*: slaughter 18 days, milk 48 hours. *Sheep, pigs*: slaughter 18 days

PoM **Tribrissen™** (Coopers Pitman-Moore)
Injection, co-trimazine 40/200 [trimethoprim 40 mg, sulphadiazine 200 mg]/mL, for *dogs, cats*; 50 mL
Injection, co-trimazine 80/400 [trimethoprim 80 mg, sulphadiazine 400 mg]/mL, for *horses, cattle, pigs*; 100 mL
Withdrawal Periods. *Cattle*: slaughter 28 days, milk 48 hours. *Pigs*: slaughter 28 days

CO-TRIMOXAZOLE

Preparations of trimethoprim 1 part and sulphamethoxazole 5 parts

Indications.   Co-trimoxazole-sensitive infections
Warnings. See under Co-trimazine
Dose. Expressed as trimethoprim + sulphamethoxazole
Dogs, cats: 30 mg/kg daily

PoM **Co-trimoxazole** (Non-proprietary)
Tablets, co-trimoxazole 80/400 [trimethoprim 80 mg, sulphamethoxazole 400 mg]
Tablets, dispersible, co-trimoxazole 80/400 [trimethoprim 80 mg, sulphamethoxazole 400 mg]
Oral suspension, co-trimoxazole 8/40 [trimethoprim 8 mg, sulphamethoxazole 40 mg]/mL; 100 mL
Oral suspension, co-trimoxazole 16/80 [trimethoprim 16 mg, sulphamethoxazole 80 mg]/mL; 100 mL

SULFADOXINE with TRIMETHOPRIM

Indications. Sulfadoxine/trimethoprim-sensitive infections
Contra-indications. Side-effects. See under Sulphadimidine
Warnings. See under Co-trimazine
Dose. Expressed as sulfadoxine + trimethoprim
Horses: by intramuscular or intravenous (preferred) injection, 15 mg/kg daily
Cattle: by subcutaneous, intramuscular, or intravenous injection, 15 mg/kg daily
Pigs: by subcutaneous or intramuscular injection, 15 mg/kg daily
Dogs: by mouth, 15-20 mg/kg daily; *by subcutaneous, intramuscular, or intravenous injection*, 15 mg/kg daily
Cats: by subcutaneous or intramuscular injection, 15 mg/kg daily

PoM **Borgal**™ (Hoechst)
Tablets, sulfadoxine 250 mg, trimethoprim 50 mg, for *dogs*; 50
Injection, sulfadoxine 62.5 mg, trimethoprim 12.5 mg, lignocaine hydrochloride 1 mg/mL, for *dogs, cats*; 50 mL
Injection, sulfadoxine 200 mg, trimethoprim 40 mg/mL, for *horses, cattle*; 100 mL
Withdrawal Periods. Should not be used in *horses* intended for human consumption. *Cattle*: slaughter 8 days, milk from treated animals should not be used for human consumption

PoM **Trivetrin**™ (Coopers Pitman-Moore)
Injection, sulfadoxine 200 mg, trimethoprim 40 mg/mL, for *horses, cattle, pigs, dogs*; 100 mL
Withdrawal Periods. Should not be used in *horses* intended for human consumption. *Cattle*: slaughter 5 days, milk 48 hours. *Pigs*: slaughter 5 days

SULFAQUINOXALINE with TRIMETHOPRIM

Indications. Sulfaquinoxaline/trimethoprim-sensitive infections
Contra-indications. Side-effects. See under Sulphadimidine
Warnings. See under Co-trimazine
Dose. Expressed as sulfaquinoxaline + trimethoprim

Poultry: by addition to drinking water or feed, 30 mg/kg body-weight

PoM **Duphatrim**™ Poultry Formula (Duphar)
Oral granules, for addition to drinking water or feed, sulfaquinoxaline (as sodium salt) 500 mg, trimethoprim 165 mg/g, for *broiler chickens, turkeys*; 500 g
Withdrawal Periods. *Broiler chickens*: slaughter 7 days. *Turkeys*: slaughter 9 days

SULFATROXAZOLE with TRIMETHOPRIM

Indications. Sulfatroxazole/trimethoprim-sensitive infections
Contra-indications. Side-effects. See under Sulphadimidine
Warnings. See under Co-trimazine
Dose. Expressed as sulfatroxazole + trimethoprim
Cattle, sheep, pigs: by intramuscular or intravenous injection, 15 mg/kg daily; *calves: by mouth*, 20 mg/kg daily

PoM **Leotrox**™ (Leo)
Tablets, scored, sulfatroxazole 667 mg, trimethoprim 133 mg, for *calves*; 50
Withdrawal Periods. *Calves*: slaughter 10 days
Injection, sulfatroxazole 200 mg, trimethoprim 40 mg/mL, for *cattle, sheep, pigs*; 100 mL
Withdrawal Periods. *Cattle*: slaughter 10 days (after intravenous administration), 16 days (after intramuscular administration), milk 60 hours. *Sheep*: slaughter 16 days, milk from treated animals should not be used for human consumption. *Pigs*: slaughter 9 days

SULPHACHLORPYRIDAZINE with TRIMETHOPRIM

Indications. Sulphachlorpyridazine/trimethoprim-sensitive infections
Contra-indications. See under Sulphadimidine
Warnings. See under Co-trimazine
Dose. Expressed as sulphachlorpyridazine + trimethoprim
Calves, pigs, poultry: by addition to

drinking water or feed, 24 mg/kg body-weight

PoM **Cosumix™ Plus** (Ciba-Geigy)
Oral powder, for addition to drinking water, feed, milk, milk replacer, or to prepare an oral solution, sulpha-chlorpyridazine (as sodium salt) 100 g, trimethoprim 20 g/kg, for *calves, pigs, broiler chickens*; 250 g, 5 kg
Withdrawal Periods. *Calves*: slaughter 5 days. *Pigs*: slaughter 3 days. *Poultry*: slaughter 1 day
Note. Should not be used in layer hens

1.1.7 Nitrofurans

The nitrofurans, which include furaltadone, furazolidone, and nitrofurantoin, are relatively broad-spectrum bactericidal drugs. Their use is limited by their toxicity and insolubility. They are active against *Salmonella*, coliforms, *Mycoplasma*, *Coccidia*, and some other protozoa. Resistance is by chromosomal mutation. Plasmid-mediated transmissible resistance is rare.

Furazolidone and **furaltadone** are too toxic for systemic use but are normally poorly absorbed following oral administration and may be given by this route for the treatment of intestinal colibacillosis and salmonellosis. In calves, sufficient drug may be absorbed to cause an encephalitis manifesting as hyperaesthesia.

Nitrofurantoin is absorbed following oral administration and rapidly excreted in the urine. Although blood and tissue concentrations are too low for the treatment of systemic infections, it may be used for urinary-tract infections.

FURALTADONE

Indications. Furaltadone-sensitive infections; coccidiosis in chickens (see section 1.4.1) and histomoniasis in chickens and turkeys (see section 1.4.2)
Dose. *Poultry*: 10-40 g/100 litres drinking water

PoM **Furasol™** (SmithKline Beecham)
Oral powder, for addition to drinking water, furaltadone 200 g/kg, for *chickens, turkeys, ducks*; 2 kg, 10 kg

Withdrawal Periods. *Poultry*: slaughter withdrawal period nil

FURAZOLIDONE

Indications. Furazolidone-sensitive infections; intra-uterine use (see section 8.6)
Side-effects. Overdosing can cause hyperaesthesia in calves
Warnings. Should not be administered to calves in the process of being introduced to a high concentrated barley diet. This does not apply once diet is stabilised.
Dose. *Calves*: by mouth, 10 mg/kg daily; 400 g/tonne feed
Pigs: 15-25 g/100 litres drinking water; 200-600 g/tonne feed; *piglets*: by mouth, 50-200 mg daily
Chickens, turkeys: 15-25 g/100 litres drinking water; 100-400 g/tonne feed
Ducks, rabbits: 100 g/tonne feed

PoM **Furazolidone** (Hand/PH)
Premix, furazolidone 200 g/kg, for *calves, pigs, poultry*; 2 kg, 25 kg
Withdrawal Periods. *Calves, pigs*: slaughter 7 days. *Poultry*: slaughter withdrawal period nil
Premix, furazolidone, for *calves, pigs, poultry*; 25 kg
Withdrawal Periods. *Calves, pigs*: slaughter 7 days. *Poultry*: slaughter withdrawal period nil

PoM **Micro-Bio™ Furazolidone** (Micro-Biologicals)
Oral powder, for addition to drinking water, furazolidone 60 g/kg, for *calves, pigs, poultry*; 227 g
Withdrawal Periods. *Calves, pigs, poultry*: slaughter 7 days
Premix, furazolidone 200 g/kg, for *pigs, poultry*; 2 kg, 25 kg
Withdrawal Periods. *Pigs, poultry*: slaughter 7 days

PoM **Neftin™ 200** (SmithKline Beecham)
Oral powder, for addition to feed, furazolidone 200 g/kg, for *pigs, chickens, turkeys, ducks, rabbits*; 25 kg
Withdrawal Periods. *Pigs*: slaughter 7 days

PoM **Neftin™ Calf Doser** (SmithKline Beecham)
Oral suspension, furazolidone 258 mg/dose, for *calves*; 227-mL dose applicator (1 dose = 3.4 mL)
Withdrawal Periods. *Calves*: slaughter 7 days

PoM **Neftin™ Piglet Medicator** (SmithKline Beecham)
Mixture, furazolidone 50 mg/dose, for *piglets*; 100-mL dose applicator (1 dose = 1 mL)
Withdrawal Periods. *Piglets*: slaughter 7 days

PoM **Nifulidone™** (Duphar)
Oral powder, for addition to drinking water, furazolidone 55 g/kg, for *pigs, poultry*; 1.05 kg

PoM **Nifulidone™ 20%** (Salsbury)
Premix, furazolidone 200 g/kg, for *pigs, poultry*; 25 kg

NITROFURANTOIN

Indications. Nitrofurantoin-sensitive urinary infections and respiratory infections
Contra-indications. Renal impairment
Side-effects. Occasional nausea and vomiting
Dose. *Horses*: initial dose 4.4 mg/kg then 2.2 mg/kg 3 times daily

PoM **BK-Furin E™** (BK)
Oral powder, for addition to feed, nitrofurantoin 500 mg/g, for *horses*; 2 g
Withdrawal Periods. Should not be used in *horses* intended for human consumption

1.1.8 Nitroimidazoles

The nitroimidazoles include dimetridazole and metronidazole, which are bactericidal to most Gram-negative and many Gram-positive anaerobic bacteria but have negligible activity against aerobic bacteria. They are active against *Treponema hyodysenteriae* and a variety of protozoa. Acquired resistance among susceptible organisms is rare.
Dimetridazole is mainly used for the prevention and treatment of swine dysentery and for blackhead in turkeys (see section 1.4.2). **Metronidazole** is well absorbed by mouth and penetrates

tissues throughout the body including the brain and cerebrospinal fluid. It is administered for a variety of anaerobic infections including gingivitis and empyema. The injectable solution may also be used for local irrigation of wounds. The action of metronidazole is restricted to anaerobic organisms but infections are often mixed. Therefore, it may be necessary to administer concurrently a drug which is active against aerobic organisms.

DIMETRIDAZOLE

Indications. Swine dysentery; treatment and prophylaxis of histomoniasis (1.4.2); trichomoniasis in pigeons◆ (1.4.3)
Dose. Treatment. *Pigs*: *by mouth*, 50-100 mg/kg (maximum 300 mg) daily; 26.7 g/100 litres drinking water; 500 g/tonne feed
Prophylaxis. *Pigs*: 13.3 g/100 litres drinking water; 200 g/tonne feed

See section 1.4.2 for preparation details

METRONIDAZOLE

Indications. Infections caused by anaerobic bacteria
Dose. *Horses*: *by slow intravenous injection or infusion*, 20 mg/kg daily
Dogs, cats: *by mouth or by subcutaneous injection or intravenous infusion*, 20 mg/kg daily
Birds, rodents: *by addition to drinking water*, 20 mg/kg

PoM **Metronidazole** (Non-proprietary)
Tablets, metronidazole 200 mg, 400 mg

PoM **Metronex™** (Cheminex)
Oral paste, metronidazole 500 mg/g, for *horses*; 20-g metered dose applicator (1 dose = metronidazole 1.1 g)
Withdrawal Periods. Should not be used in *horses* intended for human consumption

PoM **Torgyl™** (RMB)
Injection, metronidazole 5 mg/mL, for *horses, dogs, cats, birds, rodents*; 50 mL
Withdrawal Periods. Should not be used in *horses, birds* intended for human consumption. Eggs from treated *birds* should not be used for human consumption

Use undiluted for irrigations or wound dressings

1.1.9 Oxolinic acid

Oxolinic acid is used in the treatment of furunculosis caused by *Aeromonas salmonicida*, vibriosis, and enteric redmouth in fish.

OXOLINIC ACID

Indications. Oxolinic acid-sensitive infections
Dose. *Fish*: see Prescribing for fish

PoM **Aqualinic**™ (Vetrepharm)
See Prescribing for fish for preparation details

PoM **Aquinox**™ (Hand/PH)
See Prescribing for fish for preparation details

1.1.10 Compound antibacterial preparations

1.1.10.1 Oral compound antibacterial preparations
1.1.10.2 Parenteral compound antibacterial preparations

1.1.10.1 ORAL COMPOUND ANTIBACTERIAL PREPARATIONS

Although in principle the use of antibacterial mixtures is not to be encouraged, in some cases two antibacterials may be used in combination for their activity against two specific and co-existing infections, for example, a mixture of a macrolide and a sulphonamide for enteric and respiratory disease in pigs.

PoM **Cyfac**™ **HS** (Cyanamid)
Oral powder, for addition to feed, chlortetracycline hydrochloride 73.2 g, procaine penicillin 36.6 g, sulphadimidine 73.2 g/kg, for *pigs*; 2.25 kg, 18 kg
Withdrawal Periods. *Pigs*: slaughter 15 days
Dose. *Pigs*: 2.25 kg/tonne feed

PoM **Linco-Spectin**™ **100** (Upjohn)
Oral powder, for addition to drinking water, lincomycin (as hydrochloride) 33.3 g, spectinomycin (as sulphate) 66.7 g/150 g, for *poultry*; 150 g
Withdrawal Periods. *Poultry*: slaughter 2 days
Dose. *Poultry*: 150 g/120-180 litres drinking water

PoM **Microfac HP**™ (Micro-Biologicals)
Oral powder, for addition to feed, chlortetracycline 82 g, procaine penicillin 41 g, sulphadimidine 82 g/kg, for *pigs*; 2 kg, 20 kg
Withdrawal Periods. *Pigs*: slaughter 15 days
Dose. *Pigs*: 2 kg/tonne feed

PoM **Orojet**™ **N/S** (Willows Francis)
Oral liquid, neomycin sulphate 70 mg, streptomycin sulphate 70 mg/dose, for *foals, calves, piglets*; 210-mL metered-dose applicator (1 dose = 1 mL)
Dose. *Foals, calves*: 1 mL/7 kg twice daily
Piglets: 1-6 mL daily according to age

PoM **Tylasul**™ (Elanco)
Oral powder, for addition to drinking water, sodium sulphathiazole sesquihydrate 750 mg, tylosin (as tartrate) 250 mg/g, for *pigs*; 100 g
Withdrawal Periods. *Pigs*: slaughter 5 days
Dose. *Pigs*: 50 g/100 litres drinking water
Premix, sulphadimidine 50 g, tylosin (as phosphate) 50 g/kg, for *pigs*; 2 kg
Withdrawal Periods. *Pigs*: slaughter 9 days
Dose. *Pigs*: 2 kg/tonne feed
Premix, sulphadimidine 100 g, tylosin (as phosphate) 100 g/kg, for *pigs*; 25 kg
Withdrawal Periods. *Pigs*: slaughter 9 days
Dose. *Pigs*: 1 kg/tonne feed

1.1.10.2 PARENTERAL COMPOUND ANTIBACTERIAL PREPARATIONS

A combination of different salts of benzylpenicillin with a range of solubilities may give initial high plasma-penicillin concentrations from the soluble sodium salt and more prolonged concentrations from the less soluble procaine and benzathine salts. Such combinations are not recommended for severe infections, where repeat administration of a short-acting preparation is preferred.

Procaine penicillin and a streptomycin in combination are complementary, having bactericidal activity against Gram-positive and Gram-negative organisms respectively and may be synergistic. Unfortunately, while the procaine penicillin component may remain effective for up to 24 hours, the streptomycin component is only effective for up to 12 hours.

The use of combination antibacterial and corticosteroid preparations is thought not to be generally justified.

PoM **Depomycin™** (Mycofarm)
Injection, dihydrostreptomycin (as sulphate) 250 mg, procaine penicillin 150 mg/mL, for *horses, cattle, sheep, pigs, dogs, cats*; 100 mL
Withdrawal Periods. *Cattle*: slaughter 3 days, milk 48 hours. *Sheep, pigs*: slaughter 3 days
Dose. *Horses, cattle, sheep, pigs*: by *intramuscular injection*, 0.04 mL/kg
Dogs, cats: by *intramuscular injection*, 0.1 mL/kg

PoM **Depomycin™ Forte** (Mycofarm)
Injection, dihydrostreptomycin (as sulphate) 250 mg, procaine penicillin 200 mg/mL, for *horses, cattle, sheep, pigs, dogs, cats*; 100 mL
Withdrawal Periods. *Cattle*: slaughter 3 days, milk 48 hours. *Sheep, pigs*: slaughter 3 days
Dose. *Horses, cattle, sheep, pigs*: by *intramuscular injection*, 0.04 mL/kg
Dogs, cats: by *intramuscular injection*, 0.1 mL/kg

PoM **Dipen™** (Bimeda)
Injection, dihydrostreptomycin (as sulphate) 150 mg, procaine penicillin 150 mg/mL, for *cattle, sheep, pigs*; 100 mL
Withdrawal Periods. *Cattle*: slaughter 21 days, milk 72 hours. *Sheep*: slaughter 28 days, milk from treated animals should not be used for human consumption. *Pigs*: slaughter 35 days

Dose. *Cattle, sheep, pigs*: by *intramuscular injection*, 0.04 mL/kg

PoM **Duphapen™ + Strep** (Duphar)
Injection, dihydrostreptomycin sulphate 250 mg, procaine penicillin 200 mg/mL, for *horses, cattle, sheep, pigs, dogs, cats*; 40 mL, 100 mL
Withdrawal Periods. *Cattle*: milk 48 hours
Dose. *Horses, cattle*: by *intramuscular injection*, 0.04 mL/kg
Sheep, pigs: by *intramuscular injection*, 0.06 mL/kg
Dogs, cats: by *intramuscular injection*, 0.1 mL/kg

PoM **Milimycin™** (Intervet)
Injection, dihydrostreptomycin (as sulphate) 250 mg, procaine penicillin 200 mg/mL, for *horses, cattle, sheep, pigs, dogs, cats*; 100 mL
Withdrawal Periods. *Cattle*: slaughter 3 days, milk 48 hours. *Sheep, pigs*: slaughter 3 days
Dose. *Horses, cattle, sheep, pigs*: by *intramuscular injection*, 0.04 mL/kg
Dogs, cats: by *intramuscular injection*, 0.1 mL/kg

PoM **Neomycin   Penicillin   100/200** (Intervet)
Injection, neomycin (as sulphate) 100 mg, procaine penicillin 200 mg/mL, for *horses, cattle, sheep, goats, pigs, dogs, cats*; 100 mL
Withdrawal Periods. *Cattle*: milk 72 hours
Dose. *Horses, cattle, sheep, goats, pigs*: by *intramuscular injection*, 0.05 mL/kg
Dogs, cats: by *intramuscular injection*, 0.1 mL/kg

PoM **Pen & Strep** (Norbrook)
Injection, dihydrostreptomycin sulphate 250 mg, procaine penicillin 200 mg/mL, for *horses, cattle, sheep, goats, pigs, dogs, cats*; 50 mL, 100 mL
Withdrawal Periods. *Cattle*: milk 48 hours
Dose. *Horses, cattle, sheep, goats, pigs, dogs, cats*: by *intramuscular injection*, 0.04 mL/kg

PoM **Penicillin/Streptomycin** (BK)
Injection, dihydrostreptomycin sulphate 250 mg, procaine penicillin 200 mg/mL,

for *horses, cattle, sheep, goats, pigs, dogs, cats*; 100 mL
Withdrawal Periods. *Cattle*: milk 48 hours
Dose. *By intramuscular injection. Horses, cattle*: 10-20 mL
Foals, calves, sheep, goats, pigs: 3-10 mL
Dogs: 0.5-5.0 mL
Cats: 0.5-1.0 mL

PoM **Penillin™-S** (Univet)
Injection, dihydrostreptomycin sulphate 250 mg, procaine penicillin 200 mg/mL, for *horses, cattle, sheep, goats, pigs, dogs, cats*; 100 mL
Withdrawal Periods. *Cattle*: milk 48 hours
Dose. *Horses, cattle*: by intramuscular injection, 0.02 mL/kg; *foals, calves*: by intramuscular injection, 0.04-0.06 mL/kg
Sheep, goats, pigs: by intramuscular injection, 0.04-0.06 mL/kg
Dogs, cats: by intramuscular injection, 0.06 mL/kg

PoM **Penstrep™** (C-Vet)
Injection, dihydrostreptomycin 250 mg, procaine penicillin 150 mg/mL, for *horses, cattle, sheep, goats, pigs, dogs, cats*; 100 mL
Withdrawal Periods. *Cattle*: slaughter 3 days, milk 48 hours. *Sheep, goats, pigs*: slaughter 3 days
Dose. *By intramuscular injection. Horses, cattle*: 10-20 mL; *foals, calves*: 3-8 mL
Sheep, goats: 3-5 mL
Pigs: 3-8 mL
Dogs: 1-4 mL
Cats: 0.5-1.0 mL

PoM **Streptopen™** (Coopers Pitman-Moore)
Injection, dihydrostreptomycin (as sulphate) 250 mg, procaine penicillin 250 mg/mL, for *horses, cattle, sheep, goats, pigs, dogs, cats*; 30 mL, 100 mL
Withdrawal Periods. *Cattle*: milk 36 hours
Dose. *Horses, cattle, sheep, goats, pigs, dogs, cats*: by intramuscular injection, 0.02-0.04 mL/kg

PoM **Strypen™** (RMB)
Injection, dihydrostreptomycin sulphate 250 mg, procaine penicillin 200 mg/mL,

for *horses, cattle, sheep, goats, pigs, dogs, cats*; 100 mL
Withdrawal Periods. *Cattle*: milk 48 hours
Dose. *Horses, cattle, sheep, pigs, dogs, cats*: by intramuscular injection, 0.04 mL/kg

1.1.11 Compound preparations for bacterial enteritis

Antibacterial drugs are unnecessary in most cases of bacterial gastro-enteritis and may be contra-indicated. Anti-diarrhoeal drugs may give symptomatic relief but should not distract from the importance of giving oral or parenteral fluids (see section 16.1).

PoM **Kaobiotic™** (Upjohn)
Tablets, scored, neomycin (as sulphate) 5.68 mg, sulphadiazine 16.25 mg, sulphaguanidine 244 mg, sulphamerazine 16.25 mg, sulphathiazole 16.25 mg, kaolin 729 mg, pectin 16.25 mg, for *dogs, cats*; 500
Dose. *Dogs, cats*: 1 tablet/4 kg daily in divided doses

PoM **Neobiotic-P™** (Upjohn)
Tablets, scored, neomycin (as sulphate) 175 mg, hyoscine methobromide 2.5 mg, for *foals, calves, pigs*; 20
Dose. *Foals, calves, pigs*: 1 tablet/22-44 kg daily

PoM **Neobiotic-P™ Aquadrops** (Upjohn)
Oral solution, neomycin (as sulphate) 35 mg, hyoscine methobromide 250 micrograms/mL, for *dogs, cats*; 20-mL dropper bottle
Dose. *Dogs, cats*: 0.1 mL/kg twice daily

PoM **Neobiotic-P™ Pump** (Upjohn)
Oral solution, neomycin (as sulphate) 35 mg, hyoscine methobromide 250 micrograms/dose, for *foals, calves, lambs, pigs, dogs, cats*; 120-mL dose applicator (1 dose = 1 mL)
Dose. *Foals, calves, lambs*: 0.2 mL/kg
Pigs: (up to 7 kg body-weight) 1 mL; (7-11 kg body-weight) 2 mL
Dogs, cats: 0.2 mL/kg

PoM **Neo-Sulphentrin™** (Willows Francis)
Tablets, scored, neomycin sulphate 8 mg, phthalylsulphathiazole 60 mg,

streptomycin sulphate 21 mg, sulphaguanidine 100 mg, sulphathiazole 83 mg, light kaolin 180 mg, for *dogs, cats*; 100, 500
Dose. *Dogs, cats*: 1 tablet/3.5 kg twice daily
Tablets, scored, neomycin sulphate 100 mg, phthalylsulphathiazole 700 mg, streptomycin sulphate 250 mg, sulphaguanidine 1.2 g, sulphathiazole 1 g, light kaolin 1.96 g, for *foals, calves, pigs, dogs*; 20
Dose. *Foals, calves, pigs, dogs*: 1 tablet/45 kg twice daily

1.2 Antifungal drugs

Antifungal drugs are used for the treatment of systemic infections such as aspergillosis, yeast infections including candidiasis and cryptococcosis, and dermatophytosis (ringworm). Topical antifungal drugs are used for the treatment of fungal infections of the skin (see section 14.3), ear (see section 13.1), and eye (see section 12.2.2).
Griseofulvin is an antifungal antibiotic that is deposited in keratin precursor cells and concentrated in the stratum corneum of skin, hair, and nails thus preventing fungal invasion of newly formed cells. Griseofulvin is metabolised in the liver. In the dog and cat, absorption of griseofulvin is enhanced by the administration of a fatty meal. Manufacturers may recommend treatment for 7 days but usually treatment for 3 to 4 weeks is required and extended periods of up to 12 weeks are often necessary.
Griseofulvin may be teratogenic and therefore should not be administered to pregnant animals.
Ketoconazole, an imidazole compound, is active against fungi and yeasts and also against some Gram-positive bacteria. Ketoconazole is well absorbed by mouth and is the treatment of choice for systemic candidiasis and refractory dermatophyte infections. Administration of ketoconazole with food may reduce the nausea associated with the drug. Prolonged administration of ketoconazole may cause liver damage and the drug may be teratogenic.
Nystatin is not absorbed from the alimentary tract and may be given orally for the treatment of alimentary candidiasis. **Amphotericin** is active against yeasts and fungi. Amphotericin may cause renal damage and blood-urea-nitrogen (BUN) concentration should be monitored regularly during treatment.
Flucytosine is effective against systemic yeast infections but not against fungal infections. Resistance develops rapidly and therefore the use of flucytosine is restricted to combination therapy with amphotericin. Flucytosine and amphotericin are synergistic and may be given concurrently to delay the onset of resistance to flucytosine and for the treatment of systemic cryptococcosis. The dose of amphotericin should be halved when used in combination with flucytosine.
Flucytosine is distributed throughout the body and diffuses into the cerebrospinal fluid and thus is active against intracranial organisms.

AMPHOTERICIN

Indications. Systemic yeast and fungal infections
Contra-indications. Renal impairment, see notes above
Side-effects. Nephrotoxicity
Dose. *Dogs, cats*: *by intravenous infusion*, 0.15-1.0 mg/kg, given as amphotericin 200 micrograms/mL solution, 3 times weekly

PoM **Fungizone**™ (Squibb)
Intravenous infusion, powder for reconstitution, amphotericin (as sodium deoxycholate complex) 50 mg

FLUCYTOSINE

Indications. Systemic yeast infections
Contra-indications. Renal and hepatic impairment, pregnant animals
Dose. *Dogs, cats*: 100-200 mg/kg daily in 3-4 divided doses

PoM **Alcobon**™ (Roche)
Tablets, scored, flucytosine 500 mg; 100
Note. Preparations of flucytosine are no generally available. A written order, statin

case details, should be sent to the manufacturer to obtain a supply of the preparation.

GRISEOFULVIN

Indications. Dermatophyte infections
Contra-indications. Hepatic impairment; pregnant animals
Side-effects. High doses may cause hepatotoxicity, particularly in cats
Warnings. Preparations should be handled with caution by women of childbearing age
Dose. *Horses, donkeys*: 10 mg/kg daily
Cattle: 7.5 mg/kg daily
Dogs, cats: 15-20 mg/kg daily

PoM **Dufulvin™** (Duphar)
Oral paste, griseofulvin 333 mg/g, for *horses*; 70-g metered-dose applicator (1 dose = griseofulvin 1.5 g)
Withdrawal Periods. Should not be used in *horses* intended for human consumption
Oral granules, for addition to feed, griseofulvin 75 mg/g, for *cattle*; 1 kg, 3.5 kg
Withdrawal Periods. *Cattle*: slaughter 5 days, milk 48 hours

PoM **Equifulvin™** (Boehringer Ingelheim)
Oral paste, griseofulvin 333 mg/g, for *horses*; 70-g metered-dose applicator
Withdrawal Periods. Should not be used in *horses* intended for human consumption
Oral granules, for addition to feed, griseofulvin 75 mg/g, for *horses, cattle*; 1 kg
Withdrawal Periods. Should not be used in *horses* intended for human consumption. *Cattle*: slaughter 5 days, milk 48 hours

PoM **Fulcin™** (Coopers Pitman-Moore)
Oral powder, for addition to feed, griseofulvin 75 mg/kg, for *horses, donkeys, cattle*; 20 g, 1 kg, 3.5 kg
Withdrawal Periods. *Horses, donkeys*: slaughter 7 days. *Cattle*: slaughter 1 day, milk 72 hours

PoM **Grisol-V™** (Univet)
Oral paste, griseofulvin 333 mg/g, for *horses*; 70-g metered-dose applicator
Withdrawal Periods. Should not be used in *horses* intended for human consumption

Oral granules, for addition to feed, griseofulvin 75 mg/g, for *horses, cattle*; 1 kg, 2.5 kg
Withdrawal Periods. Should not be used in *horses* intended for human consumption. *Cattle*: slaughter 5 days, milk 48 hours

PoM **Grisovin™** (Coopers Pitman-Moore)
Tablets, griseofulvin 125 mg, for *dogs, cats*; 100, 1000
Oral powder, for addition to feed, griseofulvin 75 mg/g, for *horses, cattle*; 500 g, 2.5 kg
Withdrawal Periods. Should not be used in *horses* intended for human consumption. *Cattle*: slaughter 1 day, milk from treated animals should not be used for human consumption

PoM **Norofulvin™** (Norbrook)
Oral paste, griseofulvin 333 mg/g, for *horses*; 70-g metered-dose applicator (1 dose = griseofulvin 1.5 g)
Withdrawal Periods. Should not be used in *horses* intended for human consumption
Oral granules, for addition to feed, griseofulvin 75 mg/kg, for *horses, cattle*; 20 g, 1 kg, 3.5 kg
Withdrawal Periods. Should not be used in *horses* intended for human consumption. *Cattle*: slaughter 5 days, milk 48 hours

KETOCONAZOLE

Indications. Systemic candidiasis, dermatophyte infections
Contra-indications. Hepatic impairment; pregnant animals
Side-effects. Hepatotoxicity, anorexia particularly in cats
Dose. *Dogs, cats*: 5-10 mg/kg daily

PoM **Nizoral™** (Janssen)
Tablets, scored, ketoconazole 200 mg; 30
Oral suspension, ketoconazole 20 mg/mL; 100 mL

NYSTATIN

Indications. Alimentary candidiasis
Dose. *Dogs, cats*: 100 000 units 4 times daily

PoM **Nystatin** (Non-proprietary)
Mixture, nystatin 100 000 units/mL; 30 mL

PoM **Nystan**™ (Squibb)
Tablets, nystatin 500 000 units; 28
Oral suspension, nystatin 100 000 units/mL;
30 mL

PoM **Nystatin-Dome**™ (Lagap)
Oral suspension, nystatin 100 000 units/mL;
30 mL

The following drug is included in Prescribing for exotic birds – see that section for indications and dosage

MICONAZOLE

PoM **Daktarin**™ (Janssen)
Intravenous infusion, miconazole 10 mg/mL;
20 mL

1.3 Antiviral drugs

Antiviral compounds find their chief application in ophthalmology (see section 12.2.3). Idoxuridine, as eye ointment or eye drops, is the treatment of choice for ocular feline herpes infections. Various synthetic interferon-inducing compounds have been used in an attempt to limit the spread of infection under herd or flock conditions but none is currently available in the UK.

1.4 Antiprotozoal drugs

1.4.1 Anticoccidials
1.4.2 Drugs for histomoniasis
1.4.3 Trichomonacides
1.4.4 Drugs for babesiosis

1.4.1 Anticoccidials

Coccidiosis is of major economic importance in the poultry industry, but other animals including calves, lambs, dogs and rabbits may also be affected by the disease. The principal species of enteric coccidia affecting animals are *Eimeria*. The protozoa invade the gut where development stages damage the intestinal mucosa causing diarrhoea. Intestinal damage may occur before diagnosis of coccidiosis is possible. Disease prevention involves good husbandry and the use of anticoccidials. Anticoccidials suppress development of asexual stages, sexual stages, or both.

Different drugs may act at different stages of the protozoal life-cycle. In the poultry industry, the disease is prevented in broiler birds and layer replacement stock. In broilers, anticoccidials are administered continuously until just prior to slaughter. In replacement stock, pullets that are reared on litter but are housed in cages for the laying cycle, are medicated continuously until commencement of egg laying. Anticoccidials may interfere with egg quality and production, and with fertility. Prophylactic medication is therefore discontinued from the commencement of egg laying and some anticoccidials may only be indicated for use in broilers. In pullet rearing, where the birds are to be raised on litter, the use of subtherapeutic doses of anticoccidials allows a degree of parasite development enabling the birds to acquire immunity to reinfection. Continuous use of anticoccidials may cause therapy to become ineffective due to drug-resistance in the parasite populations. Various strategies are employed in the poultry industry to avoid this problem, such as shuttle programmes using different drugs in the starter and grower rations, and rotation of drugs after several crops of broilers. In lambs, calves, and rabbits, continuous anticoccidial medication is used during periods of increased risk and stress. Drugs may also be administered to the ewe at the time of lambing to aid control of coccidiosis in the young.

Treatment of coccidiosis in all species involves restoring body fluids, when practicable, and combating the causal organism with a suitable anticoccidial. The sulphonamides **sulfaquinoxaline** and **sulphadimidine** were amongst the first anticoccidials and are still used for treatment and prevention of the disease in poultry, cattle, sheep, and rabbits. Currently the most widely used compounds are the ionophore antibiotics **Monensin**, **narasin**, and **salinomycin** prevent the development of first generation schizonts. These compounds are used in poultry, cattle, and sheep. They are extremely toxic to horses and cause severe growth depression when administered with tiamulin. **Lasalocid** and **maduramicin** are related compounds used in broilers. Subtherapeutic doses of monensin and lasalocid allow birds to develop immunity to coccidial protozoa and are used in replacement stock to be housed on litter.

Clopidol and **decoquinate** are quinolones which act on first generation schizonts. Clopidol is used for prevention of coccidiosis in poultry and rabbits. Decoquinate is used to control the disease in lambs.

Dinitolmide and **nicarbazin** are dinitro compounds used to prevent coccidiosis in poultry. Dinitolmide affects first generation schizonts and nicarbazin affects second generation schizonts.

Robenidine affects the late first generation and second stage schizonts and is used to control coccidiosis in poultry and rabbits.

Furaltadone is an antimicrobial used to prevent coccidiosis in chickens as well as histomoniasis and bacterial diseases of poultry. **Halofuginone** is available for control of coccidiosis in chickens and turkeys. It affects first and second generation schizonts.

Amprolium is used as an anticoccidial for pigeons. It is also used in combination with **ethopabate** to achieve a broader spectrum of activity, effective for the prevention and treatment of clinical outbreaks of coccidiosis in poultry.

AMPROLIUM HYDROCHLORIDE

Indications. Treatment of coccidiosis

ᴳˢˡ **Coxoid** (Harkers)
Oral solution, for addition to drinking water, amprolium hydrochloride 8.4 mg/mL, for *pigeons*; 112 mL, 500 mL
Dose. Pigeons: by addition to drinking water, 112 mL for treatment of 30 birds

CLOPIDOL

Indications. Prophylaxis of coccidiosis
Contra-indications. Layer replacement stock from commencement of egg laying.

Replacement stock to be housed on litter
Side-effects. Overdosage may cause anorexia
Warnings. Should not be mixed with other anticoccidials
Dose. *Poultry, game birds*: 125 g/tonne feed
Rabbits: 200 g/tonne feed

ᴾᴹᴸ **Clopidol** (Hand/PH)
Premix, clopidol, for *chickens, rabbits*; 25 kg
Withdrawal Periods. *Poultry, rabbits*: slaughter 5 days

ᴾᴹᴸ **Clopidol-250** (Hand/PH)
Premix, clopidol 250 g/kg, for *chickens, pheasants, partridges, rabbits*; 25 kg
Withdrawal Periods. *Poultry, rabbits*: slaughter 5 days. *Game birds*: slaughter 7 days

ᴾᴹᴸ **Coyden**™ (RMB)
Premix, clopidol 250 g/kg, for *broiler chickens, guinea fowl, pheasants, partridges, rabbits*; 25 kg
Withdrawal Periods. *Poultry, guinea fowl, rabbits*: slaughter 5 days. *Pheasants, partridges*: slaughter 7 days

DECOQUINATE

Indications. Treatment and prophylaxis of coccidiosis
Warnings. See under Clopidol
Dose. *Ewes*: 50 g/tonne feed. If feed is administered on a restricted basis, it may be necessary to increase the dosage so that each animal receives a dose of decoquinate 500 micrograms/kg body-weight daily; *lambs*: 100 g/tonne feed. If feed is administered on a restricted basis, it may be necessary to increase the dosage so that each animal receives a dose of decoquinate 1 mg/kg body-weight daily

ᴾᴹᴸ **Deccox**™ (RMB)
Premix, decoquinate 60 g/kg, for *sheep*; 10 kg
Withdrawal Periods. *Sheep*: slaughter 3 days, milk from treated animals should not be used for human consumption

DINITOLMIDE

Indications. Prophylaxis of coccidiosis
Contra-indications. Side-effects. Warnings. See under Clopidol
Dose. *Poultry*: 62.5-125.0 g/tonne feed

PML **Dinitolmide** (AB Pharmaceuticals)
Oral powder, for addition to feed,
dinitolmide 980 g/kg, for *chickens*; 25 kg
Withdrawal Periods. *Poultry*: slaughter
3 days

PML **Salcostat™ Concentrate** (Salsbury)
Oral powder, for addition to feed,
dinitolmide 980 g/kg, for *chickens*; 25 kg
Withdrawal Periods. *Poultry*: slaughter
3 days

PML **Salcostat™ Premix 25%** (Salsbury)
Premix, dinitolmide 250 g/kg, for
chickens; 25 kg
Withdrawal Periods. *Poultry*: slaughter
3 days

FURALTADONE

See section 1.1.7

HALOFUGINONE

Indications. Prophylaxis of coccidiosis
Contra-indications. Side-effects. Warnings. See under Clopidol. Should not be
used in poultry over 12 weeks of age,
pheasants over 8 weeks of age
Dose. *Poultry, game birds*: 3 g/tonne feed

PML **Halofuginone-3** (Hand/PH)
Premix, halofuginone 3 g/kg, for *broiler
chickens, turkeys*; 25 kg
Withdrawal Periods. *Chickens*: slaughter
5 days. *Turkeys*: slaughter 7 days

PML **Stenorol™** (Hoechst)
Premix, halofuginone hydrobromide
6 g/kg, for *broiler chickens, turkeys*;
20 kg
Withdrawal Periods. *Chickens*: slaughter
5 days. *Turkeys*: slaughter 7 days
Premix, halofuginone hydrobromide
6 g/kg, for *pheasants*; 20 kg
Withdrawal Periods. Should not be
used in *pheasants* intended for human
consumption
Note. Not for use in other game birds,
ducks, or geese

LASALOCID SODIUM

Indications. Prophylaxis of coccidiosis
Contra-indications. Side-effects. Warnings. See under Clopidol
Dose. *Chickens*: 75-125 g/tonne feed
Turkeys, game birds: 90-125 g/tonne feed

PML **Avatec™** (Roche)
Premix, lasalocid sodium 150 g/kg, for
chickens, turkeys, pheasants; 20 kg
Withdrawal Periods. *Poultry*: slaughter
5 days. *Game birds*: slaughter 7 days

MADURAMICIN AMMONIUM

Indications. Prophylaxis of coccidiosis
Contra-indications. Side-effects. Warnings. See under Clopidol. Should not be
given 7 days before or after the
administration of tiamulin (See Drug
Interactions – Appendix 1). Toxic to
horses
Dose. *Poultry*: 5 g/tonne feed

PML **Cygro™** (Cyanamid)
Premix, maduramicin ammonium 10 g/
kg, for *broiler chickens*; 25 kg
Withdrawal Periods. *Poultry*: slaughter
7 days

MONENSIN

Indications. Prophylaxis of coccidiosis
in poultry; to improve growth-rate and
feed conversion efficiency in cattle (17.1)
Contra-indications. Side-effects. Warnings. See under Clopidol. Should not be
given within 7 days before or after the
administration of tiamulin (See Drug
Interactions – Appendix 1). Toxic to
horses
Dose. *Chickens*: 100-120 g/tonne feed
Turkeys: 90-100 g/tonne feed

PML **Elancoban™** (Elanco)
Premix, monensin 200 g/kg, for
chickens, turkeys; 25 kg
Withdrawal Periods. *Poultry*: slaughter
3 days
Note. For broiler chickens and replacement chickens intended for use as cage
layers

PML **Monensin-50 Poultry** (Hand/PH)
Premix, monensin (as sodium salt) 50 g/
kg, for *chickens, turkeys*; 2 kg

Withdrawal Periods. *Poultry*: slaughter
3 days

PML **Monensin 100** (AB Pharmaceuticals)
Premix, monensin 100 g/kg, for
chickens, turkeys; 25 kg
Withdrawal Periods. *Poultry*: slaughter
3 days

PML **Monensin-100 Poultry** (Hand/PH)
Premix, monensin (as sodium salt) 100 g/
kg, for *chickens, turkeys*; 25 kg
Withdrawal Periods. *Poultry*: slaughter
3 days

PML **Monensin-200** (Hand/PH)
Premix, monensin (as sodium salt) 200 g/
kg, for *chickens, poultry*; 25 kg
Withdrawal Periods. *Poultry*: slaughter
3 days

NARASIN

Indications. Prophylaxis of coccidiosis
**Contra-indications. Side-effects. Warn-
ings**. See under Clopidol. Should not be
given within 7 days before or after the
administration of tiamulin (see Drug
Interactions – Appendix 1). Toxic to
horses
Dose. *Poultry*: 70 g/tonne feed

PML **Monteban™ 100** (Elanco)
Premix, narasin 100 g/kg, for *broiler
chickens*; 25 kg
Withdrawal Periods. *Poultry*: slaughter
5 days

NICARBAZIN

Indications. Prophylaxis of coccidiosis
**Contra-indications. Side-effects. Warn-
ings**. See under Clopidol
Dose. *Poultry*: 125 g/tonne feed

PML **Nicarbazin** (Hand/PH)
Premix, nicarbazin 250 g/kg, for *broiler
chickens*; 25 kg
Withdrawal Periods. *Poultry*: slaughter
9 days

PML **Nicrazin™** (MSD Agvet)
Premix, nicarbazin 250 g/kg, for *broiler
chickens*; 25 kg
Withdrawal Periods. *Poultry*: slaughter
9 days

ROBENIDINE

Indications. Prophylaxis of coccidiosis
**Contra-indications. Side-effects. Warn-
ings**. See under Clopidol
Dose. *Poultry*: 33 g/tonne feed
Rabbits: 50-66 g/tonne feed

PML **Cycostat™** (Cyanamid)
Premix, robenidine 66 g/kg, for *broiler
chickens, turkeys, rabbits*; 20 kg
Withdrawal Periods. *Poultry, rabbits*:
slaughter 5 days

SALINOMYCIN SODIUM

Indications. Prophylaxis of coccidiosis
in poultry; to improve growth rate and
feed conversion in pigs (see section 17.1)
**Contra-indications. Side-effects. Warn-
ings**. See under Clopidol. Not be given
within 7 days before or after the
administration of tiamulin (see Drug
Interactions – Appendix 1). Toxic to
horses. Should not be used in turkeys
Dose. *Poultry*: 60 g/tonne feed

PML **Sacox™** (Hoechst)
Premix, salinomycin sodium 120 g/kg,
for *broiler chickens*; 25 kg
Withdrawal Periods. *Poultry*: slaughter
5 days

PML **Salgain-60** (Hand/PH)
Oral powder, for addition to feed,
salinomycin sodium 60 g/kg, for *broiler
chickens*; 3 kg, 25 kg
Withdrawal Periods. *Poultry*: slaughter
5 days

SULPHADIMIDINE

Indications. Prophylaxis and treatment
of coccidiosis in poultry; treatment of
coccidiosis in cattle, sheep and rabbits
**Contra-indications. Side-effects. Warn-
ings**. See under Clopidol
Dose. *Calves, lambs*: *by mouth or by
subcutaneous or intravenous injection*,
initial dose 100-200 mg/kg then 50-
100 mg/kg daily
Rabbits, poultry: 100-233 g/100 litres
drinking water

See section 1.1.6.1 for preparation
details and additional doses

COMPOUND ANTICOCCIDIAL PREPARATIONS

PML **Amprolmix-UK**™ (MSD Agvet)
Premix, amprolium hydrochloride 250 g, ethopabate   16 g/kg,   for   *chickens, turkeys*; 25 kg
Withdrawal Periods. *Poultry*: slaughter 3 days
Contra-indications. See under Clopidol
Dose. *Poultry*: 250-500 g premix/tonne feed

PML **Amprol-Plus**™ (MSD Agvet)
Oral solution, for addition to drinking water, milk replacer, or to prepare an oral solution, amprolium hydrochloride 76.8 mg, ethopabate 4.9 mg/mL, for *calves, lambs, chickens, turkeys*; 1 litre, 9.1 litres
Dose. *Poultry*: 156-312 mL/100 litres drinking water
Calves, lambs: 1-2 mL/kg of diluted solution. Dilute 1 part with 6 parts water before use

PML **Lerbek**™ (RMB)
Premix, clopidol 200 g/kg, methyl-benzoquate 16.7 g/kg, for *chickens, turkeys, rabbits*; 25 kg
Withdrawal Periods. *Poultry, rabbits*: slaughter 5 days
Dose. *Poultry*: 500 g premix/tonne feed
Rabbits: 1 kg premix/tonne feed

PoM **Microquinox**™ (Micro-Biologicals)
Oral liquid, for addition to drinking water, pyrimethamine 9 mg, sulpha-quinoxaline sodium 32.2 mg/mL, for *chickens*; 1 litre, 5 litres
Withdrawal Periods. *Poultry*: slaughter 6 days, eggs from treated birds should not be used for human consumption
Dose. *Poultry*: 150 mL/100 litres drinking water for 3 days, then provide unmedicated drinking water for 2 days. Repeat dosage regimen 2-3 times depending on the severity of the infection.

1.4.2 Drugs for histomoniasis

Dimetridazole is used to prevent and treat infections of *Histomonas meleagridis* (blackhead) in poultry and game birds. The disease is now most likely to be encountered in game birds after they

have been released. Dimetridazole is metabolised in the liver.
Furaltadone is also used to prevent histomoniasis in chickens and turkeys when given at a dose of 10-40 g per 100 litres of drinking water for 7 days.

DIMETRIDAZOLE

Indications. Treatment and prophylaxis of histomoniasis, swine dysentery (see section 1.1.8), and trichomoniasis in pigeons♦ (see section 1.4.3)
Contra-indications. Layer replacement stock from commencement of egg laying
Warnings. It should not be administered concurrently with other drugs for histomoniasis
Dose. Treatment. *Poultry, game birds*: 26.7 g/100 litres drinking water; 500 g/tonne feed
Prophylaxis. *Poultry*: 13.3 g/100 litres drinking water; 100-200 g/tonne feed
Game birds: 13.3 g/100 litres drinking water; 125-150 g/tonne feed

PML **Dazole**™ (Hand/PH)
Premix, dimetridazole 200 g/kg, for *turkeys, guinea fowl, pheasants, partridges*; 25 kg
Withdrawal Periods. *Turkeys, guinea fowl*: slaughter 6 days. *Pheasants, partridges*: slaughter 7 days

PoM **Dazole**™ Prescription (Hand/PH)
Premix, dimetridazole 200 g/kg, for *pigs* (see section 1.1.8), *chickens, turkeys, game birds*; 2 kg, 20 kg
Withdrawal Periods. *Pigs, poultry*: slaughter 28 days

PML **Emtryl**™ Premix (RMB)
Premix, dimetridazole 225 g/kg, for *turkeys, guinea fowl, pheasants, partridges*; 10 kg
Withdrawal Periods. *Turkeys, guinea fowl*: slaughter 6 days. *Pheasants, partridges*: slaughter 7 days

PoM **Emtryl**™ Prescription Premix (RMB)
Premix, dimetridazole 225 g/kg, for *pigs* (see section 1.1.8), *chickens, turkeys, game birds*; 10 kg
Withdrawal Periods. *Pigs, poultry, game birds*: slaughter 6 days

PoM **Emtryl™ Prescription Pure** (RMB)
Oral powder, for addition to feed, pure
dimetridazole, for *pigs* (see section
1.1.8), *chickens, turkeys, game birds*; 25
kg
Withdrawal Periods. *Pigs, poultry, game
birds*: slaughter 6 days

PoM **Emtryl™ Prescription Soluble** (RMB)
Oral powder, for addition to drinking
water, dimetridazole 400 g/kg, for *pigs*
(see section 1.1.8), *chickens, turkeys,
game birds*; 500 g
Withdrawal Periods. *Pigs, poultry, game
birds*: slaughter 6 days

PML **Emtryl™ Pure** (RMB)
Oral powder, for addition to feed, pure
dimetridazole, for *turkeys, guinea fowl,
pheasants, partridges*; 25 kg
Withdrawal Periods. *Turkeys, guinea
fowl*: slaughter 6 days. *Pheasants,
partridges*: slaughter 7 days

PML **Emtryl™ Soluble** (RMB)
Oral powder, for addition to drinking
water, dimetridazole 400 g/kg, for
*chickens, turkeys, guinea fowl, pheasants,
partridges*; 500 g
Withdrawal Periods. *Poultry, guinea
fowl*: slaughter 6 days. *Pheasants,
partridges*: slaughter 7 days

PoM **Lutrizol™ Swine and Turkeys** (BASF)
Oral powder, for addition to feed,
dimetridazole, for *pigs* (see section
1.1.8), *chickens, turkeys, game birds*;
25 kg
Withdrawal Periods. *Pigs*: slaughter 6
days. *Poultry, game birds*: slaughter 6
days, eggs from treated birds should not
be used for human consumption

PML **Lutrizol™ Turkeys** (BASF)
Oral powder, for addition to feed,
dimetridazole, for *turkeys, guinea fowl*;
25 kg
Withdrawal Periods. *Turkeys, guinea
fowl*: slaughter 6 days, eggs from treated
birds should not be used for human
consumption

PML **Microvet™** (Micro-Biologicals)
Premix, dimetridazole 250 g/kg, for
turkeys, guinea fowl; 25 kg
Withdrawal Periods. *Poultry, game birds*:
slaughter 6 days
Note. Should not be administered to
birds from commencement of laying

FURALTADONE

See section 1.1.7

1.4.3 Trichomonacides

Dimetridazole♦ (see section 1.4.2)
administered in the drinking water at a
dose of 25-50 grams per 100 litres for 7
days provides effective treatment for
Trichomonas gallinae (*T. columbae*)
(canker) in pigeons. The drug may
be used at monthly intervals for
prophylaxis.
Carnidazole is also used for prophylaxis
and treatment of trichomoniasis infection in individual birds.

CARNIDAZOLE

Indications. Treatment and prophylaxis
of trichomoniasis
Dose. *Pigeons*: (adult birds) 10 mg;
(young birds) 5 mg

P **Spartrix™** (Harkers)
Tablets, scored, carnidazole 10 mg, for
pigeons; 50
Withdrawal Periods. *Pigeons*: Should
not be used in *pigeons* intended for
human consumption

1.4.4 Drugs for babesiosis

Bovine babesiosis (redwater fever) is
characterised by fever and intravascular
haemolysis. Transmission of the protozoa is by ticks and ectoparasitic control
(see section 2.2.2) may assist in
prevention of the disease in cattle.
Imidocarb is effective against *Babesia
divergens* infection. The drug appears
to act directly on the parasite leading to
an alteration in morphology. Imidocarb
is excreted unchanged mainly in the
urine. It is used for the prevention and
treatment of babesiosis. Prophylactic
doses are effective for up to 4 weeks
depending on the severity of challenge.

IMIDOCARB DIPROPIONATE

Indications. Treatment and prophylaxis
of babesiosis in cattle
Contra-indications. Repeated doses

Side-effects. Cholinergic signs. Anaphylactic reactions have been recorded following use

Dose. *Cattle*: treatment, *by subcutaneous injection*, 1.2 mg/kg as a single dose; prophylaxis, *by subcutaneous injection*, 3 mg/kg as a single dose

PoM **Imizol™** (Coopers Pitman-Moore)
Injection, imidocarb dipropionate 120 mg/mL, for *cattle*; 100 mL
Withdrawal Periods. *Cattle*: slaughter 90 days, milk 21 days
Note. The DVO should be informed when treated animals are to go for slaughter or milk is to used for human consumption

2 Drugs used in the treatment of

PARASITIC INFECTIONS

Parasitic infections are caused by helminths, arthropods, and protozoa. The latter group is considered in section 1.4. In this chapter, drug treatment is discussed under the following headings:

2.1 Endoparasiticides
2.2 Ectoparasiticides

2.1 Endoparasiticides

2.1.1 Drugs for roundworms (nematodes)
2.1.2 Drugs for tapeworms (cestodes)
2.1.3 Drugs for flukes (trematodes)
2.1.4 Compound anthelmintics

Control of endoparasites is essential for both animal welfare and to optimise production. Some infections should be controlled for public health reasons, for example, if they have zoonotic potential or cause condemnation of offal or carcasses at the slaughterhouse.

Anthelmintics are used to treat acute infections, but more often they are used prophylactically. Control measures reduce worm burdens, enhance productivity, and substantially reduce the build-up of infective worm larvae on the pasture.

Some endoparasiticides contain cobalt and selenium as nutritional additives. These should be regarded as an adjunct to, rather than a substitute for, other measures to correct mineral deficiencies. The three major groups of helminths are the roundworms (nematodes), tapeworms (cestodes), and flukes (trematodes). The biological characteristics of these groups are often sufficiently disparate to necessitate anthelmintics with different modes of action. Even within a group there is sufficient diversity to limit the spectrum of activity of many drugs, the choice being further complicated by the fact that the various developmental stages of the parasites may not be equally susceptible. The nature and composition of the target population must therefore be known in order to select the most appropriate preparation.

Table 2.1 outlines drugs that are effective against common endoparasitic infections in horses, ruminants, pigs, dogs, cats, poultry, game birds, and pigeons. Different formulations of a preparation may be indicated for different parasites.

2.1.1 Drugs for roundworms (nematodes)

2.1.1.1 Avermectins
2.1.1.2 Benzimidazoles
2.1.1.3 Imidazothiazoles
2.1.1.4 Organophosphorus compounds
2.1.1.5 Tetrahydropyrimidines
2.1.1.6 Other drugs for roundworms

Roundworm infections should be controlled by suitable hygiene and strategic prophylactic treatment based on a knowledge of the epidemiology of the infection.

The roundworms form a large and complex group and infections may be caused by a single or multiple species. Therefore, both specific and broad-spectrum treatments (see section 2.1.4) are used. The latter are also used in cases where it is difficult to make a definitive diagnosis without undue delay or to maximise the production benefits of prophylactic treatment.

Equidae harbour a wider variety of nematodes than any other domesticated animal. Strongylid and ascarid infections commonly cause ill-thrift, diarrhoea, and sometimes colic in the horse and donkey. Migrating *Strongylus vulgaris* larvae damage the cranial mesenteric artery causing equine verminous arteritis. *Dictyocaulus* infection may cause lung lesions.

Control methods include treating newly acquired animals with a broad-spectrum anthelmintic as well as regular dosing of

Table 2.1 Drugs effective against common endoparasitic infections†

Parasite		Endoparasiticides
HORSES		
Gastro-intestinal roundworms	*Parascaris, Strongylus,* Cyathostominae, *Oxyuris*	febantel, fenbendazole, haloxon, ivermectin, mebendazole, oxfendazole, oxibendazole, piperazine (*Parascaris*)◆, pyrantel, thiabendazole
	Strongyloides	fenbendazole, ivermectin, oxibendazole, thiabendazole
	Migratory strongyles	fenbendazole, ivermectin, oxfendazole
Horse bot	*Gasterophilus*	haloxon, ivermectin
Lungworm	*Dictyocaulus*	febantel, fenbendazole, ivermectin, mebendazole (donkeys)
Tapeworm	*Anoplocephala*	pyrantel, praziquantel◆
Liver fluke	*Fasciola*	triclabendazole◆

RUMINANTS (some products not suitable for all ruminant species, please consult individual monographs)

Parasite		Endoparasiticides
Gastro-intestinal roundworms	*Bunostomum, Chabertia, Cooperia, Haemonchus, Nematodirus, Oesophagostomum, Ostertagia, Strongyloides, Trichostrongylus*	albendazole, closantel (*Haemonchus* only), febantel, fenbendazole, ivermectin, levamisole, mebendazole, morantel, netobimin, nitroxynil (narrow spectrum), oxfendazole, oxibendazole, thiabendazole, thiophanate
	Type II ostertagiasis	albendazole, fenbendazole, ivermectin, levamisole, netobimin, oxfendazole, thiophanate
Lungworms	*Dictyocaulus*	albendazole, febantel, fenbendazole, ivermectin, levamisole, mebendazole, netobimin, oxfendazole, thiabendazole, thiophanate
	Protostrongylus	levamisole
Sheep nasal bot	*Oestrus ovis*	closantel, ivermectin, rafoxanide
Tapeworm	*Moniezia*	albendazole, febantel, fenbendazole, mebendazole, netobimin, oxfendazole, oxyclozanide
Liver flukes	*Fasciola* 1–5 weeks	closantel, diamphenethide, oxyclozanide, nitroxynil, rafoxanide, triclabendazole
	6–12 weeks	closantel, diamphenethide, nitroxynil, oxyclozanide, rafoxanide, triclabendazole

Table 2.1 Drugs effective against common endoparasitic infections† (continued)

Parasite		Endoparasiticides
	adult	albendazole, closantel, diamphenethide, netobimin, nitroxynil, oxyclozanide, rafoxanide, triclabendazole
	Dicrocoelium	netobimin
PIGS		
Gastro-intestinal roundworms	Oesophagostomum, Ascaris	febantel, fenbendazole, flubendazole, ivermectin, levamisole, oxibendazole, piperazine (Ascaris), tetramisole, thiophanate
	Hyostrongylus	febantel, fenbendazole, flubendazole, ivermectin, levamisole, oxibendazole, tetramisole, thiophanate
	Trichuris	febantel, fenbendazole, flubendazole, levamisole, oxibendazole, thiophanate
Lungworm	Metastrongylus	febantel, fenbendazole, flubendazole, ivermectin, levamisole, tetramisole

DOGS and CATS (some preparations not suitable for both species, please consult individual monographs)

Gastro-intestinal roundworms	Toxocara, Toxascaris	fenbendazole, mebendazole, nitroscanate, oxfendazole, piperazine, pyrantel
	Uncinaria, Ancylostoma	fenbendazole, mebendazole, nitroscanate, oxfendazole, piperazine, pyrantel
	Trichuris	fenbendazole, mebendazole
	Transplacental roundworm transmission in dogs	fenbendazole, oxfendazole
Lungworms	Filaroides	albendazole◆, fenbendazole◆
	Angiostrongylus	levamisole◆
	Aelurostrongylus	fenbendazole◆
Tapeworms	Echinococcus	bunamidine, mebendazole, praziquantel
	Dipylidium	bunamidine, dichlorophen, nitroscanate, oxfendazole, praziquantel
	Taenia	bunamidine, dichlorophen, fenbendazole, mebendazole, nitroscanate, oxfendazole, praziquantel

Table 2.1 Drugs effective against common endoparasitic infections† (continued)

	Parasite	Endoparasiticides
Heartworm	*Dirofilaria*	
	treatment in imported dogs	**(seek specialist advice before treatment)**
	adults	thiacetarsamide◆, levamisole◆
	microfilariae	dithiazanine◆, levamisole◆
	prophylaxis in dogs for export	diethylcarbamazine◆, ivermectin◆
POULTRY		
Gastro-intestinal roundworms	*Amidostomum, Capillaria, Heterakis*	mebendazole
	Ascaridia	mebendazole, piperazine
Gapeworm	*Syngamus*	mebendazole
Tapeworm	*Hymenolepsis*	mebendazole
GAME BIRDS		
Gastro-intestinal roundworms	*Amidostomum, Ascaridia, Capillaria, Heterakis*	mebendazole
	Trichostrongylus	fenbendazole
Gapeworm	*Syngamus*	fenbendazole, mebendazole, nitroxynil
Tapeworm	*Hymenolepsis*	mebendazole
PIGEONS		
Gastro-intestinal roundworms	*Ascaridia, Capillaria*	cambendazole, levamisole
Tapeworms	*Cotugnia, Hymenolepsis, Raillietina*	dichlorophen

◆ Denotes unlicensed indication in the UK
† Some drugs are only available as a constituent of a compound preparation. See section 2.1.4 for indications for compound preparations

all animals every 8 weeks throughout spring, summer, and autumn, and every 3 months during winter. More frequent administration may be required in places with higher stocking rates such as riding stables or studs.

Although parasitic infections may be the same in domestic Equidae, often different therapy is required in different species. For example, lungworm infection may be treated by fenbendazole or ivermectin in horses, and mebendazole in donkeys.

In *ruminants*, parasitic gastro-enteritis and parasitic bronchitis are the main clinical disorders caused by adult nematodes. *Ostertagia* larvae may undergo an arrested development within the host when environmental conditions are adverse to the survival of free-living stages. Type II ostertagiasis is caused by these larvae emerging from a prolonged hypobiotic state. They have a reduced metabolic rate and are relatively resistant to anthelmintic attack.

Most forms of parasitic gastro-enteritis

in ruminants tend to occur in the second half of the summer, although Type II ostertagiasis occurs in late winter and spring, and nematodiriasis in lambs occurs in late spring. Routine control entails repeated use of anthelmintics during spring and early summer. Alternately a mid-July dose may be given and animals moved to aftermath grazing. When calves are given 2 or 3 strategic anthelmintic doses after turnout, there is a substantial reduction in the build up of infective gastro-intestinal larvae on the pasture.

Other methods of treatment have been developed to facilitate the administration of anthelmintics and to reduce the associated work-load. Sustained-release intra-ruminal devices that provide medication over a period of 90 to 105 days, 'pour-on' formulations, or medicated feed blocks may be used. All these systems will break down if treated animals are subsequently put onto contaminated pasture or if untreated stock are later grazed on clean pasture.

Preventive measures in sheep are more complicated and often less satisfactory. The ewe acts as an extra source of infection to the lamb and treatment is therefore necessary to eliminate the peri-parturient rise in faecal egg-counts. Additional treatment of lambs in spring may be necessary to prevent nematodiriasis, especially if a high-risk season is forecast due to climatic conditions.

In *pigs*, *Hyostrongylus*, *Trichuris*, and lungworms are almost exclusively found in animals kept outdoors. *Ascaris* and *Oesophagostomum* are common even in intensively kept pigs, the former mainly in younger animals, and the latter particularly in breeding stock. They can both cause production losses.

The choice of drug for roundworms affecting extensively farmed animals is restricted, but a wider variety is available for housed stock. For convenience and economy, pig anthelmintics are usually administered as a single dose in the form of a feed dressing or in medicated feed over a period of days. Ivermectin is given by injection. Weaners are dosed before moving to fattening pens and again 8 weeks later. Sows are dosed shortly before farrowing and again at weaning. Boars are dosed regularly at intervals of about 6 months.

Roundworm infections are common in *dogs* and *cats*. Virtually all puppies carry prenatally acquired *Toxocara* infection. As this roundworm is of zoonotic importance as well as being harmful to the puppy, routine worming from an early age is essential. Puppies are dosed fortnightly from 2 weeks of age until 12 weeks, then monthly until 6 months of age. Ease of application is an important criterion for the choice of product in very young pups. Alternatively, nursing bitches may be treated with fenbendazole or oxfendazole (see section 2.1.1.2) to prevent transplacental migration of larvae. Fenbendazole will also prevent the transfer of *Ancylostoma* larvae via the milk, but this parasite is rare in the UK.

Toxascaris, *Uncinaria*, and *Trichuris* are acquired later in life and are associated mainly with large kennel establishments and contaminated exercise areas. *Trichuris*, which causes intermittent diarrhoea, is particularly difficult to treat and repeated dosing may be necessary. For routine control of common gastro-intestinal roundworms, adults should be treated every few months, although from late pregnancy until the offspring are weaned, treatment at least every month is necessary.

At present there are no drug preparations with product licences for lungworm control in dogs and cats. *Angiostrongylus* infections usually respond to levamisole♦, but no effective treatment is known for *Filaroides*, which can be a serious pathogen provoking a dry cough. Some success has been achieved with both albendazole♦ and fenbendazole♦, but in either case, the course of treatment often has to be repeated. Similarly, for the control of *Aelurostrongylus* infections in cats, fenbendazole♦ may be used.

Fortunately, canine heartworm disease (dirofilariasis) is not endemic in the UK but cases do occur among quarantine dogs. Although thiacetarsamide♦ and dithiazanine♦ are used overseas for treatment, only levamisole♦ is readily available in the UK. **Specialist advice should be sought before treating** *Dirofilaria* infections. Dogs travelling to affected countries can be protected with daily doses of diethylcarbamazine♦, or by monthly treatments with ivermectin♦, during the mosquito season.

Poultry, and *game birds* are treated for gastro-intestinal roundworm, gapeworm, and tapeworm infections. Breeding birds are treated before laying and in autumn. Rearing birds are dosed 3 weeks after placing on infected ground, maintenance doses being given every 6 to 8 weeks. *Pigeons* are treated for gastro-intestinal roundworm and tapeworm infections.

2.1.1.1 AVERMECTINS

Ivermectin is a mixture of two avermectin derivatives and is effective against most species of nematodes and horse bots, but its use in dogs♦ is restricted to the control of migrating heartworm larvae. It is also used for the control of ectoparasites (see section 2.2) such as lice, mites, warble fly larvae in cattle, and sheep nasal bot. Ivermectin is not ovicidal and is ineffective against tapeworms and flukes. It interferes with parasite nerve transmission by being an agonist of gamma-aminobutyric acid.

Ivermectin persists in plasma and tissues for prolonged periods and therefore it is not recommended for use in cows for the 28 days prior to calving or for lactating cattle. When ivermectin is used prophylactically to control parasite infections in recently turned out calves, it is administered at 3 and 8 weeks post turnout, while an additional treatment at 13 weeks will also assist in protecting against lungworm infection.

In dogs, ivermectin should not be used at doses greater than those recommended for heartworm prophylaxis as it may cause toxicity with certain blood-lines, particularly rough-haired collies.

Horses carrying heavy infections of *Onchocerca* may develop transient oedema and pruritus following treatment. This may be due to the sudden death of large numbers of microfilariae.

IVERMECTIN

Indications. Gastro-intestinal roundworms and lungworms in horses, ruminants, and pigs; Type II ostertagiasis in ruminants; horse bots; lice and mites on cattle and pigs; warble fly larvae in cattle, nasal bots in sheep; heartworm prophylaxis in dogs♦

Contra-indications. High doses in collie-type dogs, see notes above

Dose. *Horses*: *by mouth*, 200 micrograms/kg

Cattle: *by 'pour-on' application*, 500 micrograms/kg (see section 2.2.1 for notes on method of administration); *by subcutaneous injection*, 200 micrograms/kg

Sheep, goats: *by mouth*, 200 micrograms/kg

Pigs: *by subcutaneous injection*, 300 micrograms/kg

Dogs♦: heartworm prophylaxis, *by mouth*, 6 micrograms/kg every month

Oral preparations

PML **Eqvalan**™ (MSD Agvet)
Oral paste, ivermectin 20 mg/division, for *horses*; 6.42-g metered-dose applicator
Withdrawal Periods. *Horses*: slaughter 21 days

PML **Oramec**™ (MSD Agvet)
Oral solution, ivermectin 800 micrograms/mL, for *sheep, goats*; 1 litre, 2.5 litres, 5 litres
Withdrawal Periods. *Sheep, goats*: slaughter 14 days, milk 14 days but milk from animals treated within 28 days of commencement of lactation should not be used for human consumption

Parenteral preparations

PML **Ivomec**™ (MSD Agvet)
Injection, ivermectin 10 mg/mL, for *cattle*; 50 mL, 200 mL, 500 mL
Withdrawal Periods. *Cattle*: slaughter 21 days, milk from animals treated within 28 days before calving and during lactation should not be used for human consumption
Injection, ivermectin 10 mg/mL, for *pigs*; 100 mL, 500 mL

Withdrawal Periods. *Pigs*: slaughter 28 days
See also section 2.1.4

'Pour-on' preparations

PML **Ivomec**™ (MSD Agvet)
Solution, 'pour-on', ivermectin 5 mg/mL, for *cattle*; 250 mL, 1 litre, 2.5 litres
Withdrawal Periods. *Cattle*: slaughter 28 days, milk from animals treated within 28 days before calving and during lactation should not be used for human consumption

2.1.1.2 BENZIMIDAZOLES

Benzimidazoles such as **albendazole, cambendazole, fenbendazole, flubendazole, mebendazole, oxfendazole, oxibendazole, thiabendazole**, and **triclabendazole** (see section 2.1.3) disrupt parasite energy by binding to tubulin, a protein required for the uptake of nutrients. **Febantel, netobimin**, and **thiophanate** are probenzimidazoles, which are converted to benzimidazole carbamates in the body.
The anthelmintic activity of the benzimidazoles is related to the duration of therapeutic blood concentrations. Doses may need to be repeated in pigs, dogs, and cats, while single doses are sufficient in ruminants and horses as the rumen or large intestine acts as a drug reservoir.
Most benzimidazoles are effective against larval and adult roundworms, and albendazole, febantel, fenbendazole, oxfendazole, and oxibendazole are also ovicidal. Albendazole♦ and fenbendazole♦ have been used for lungworm infection in dogs and cats.
Albendazole, febantel, fenbendazole, mebendazole, netobimin, and oxfendazole are also effective against tapeworms (see section 2.1.2), and some are also active against liver flukes at a higher dosage (see section 2.1.3). Triclabendazole is effective against both immature and adult flukes (see section 2.1.3). Fenbendazole is used in pregnant and lactating bitches to reduce roundworm infection in puppies.
Some benzimidazoles such as albendazole, cambendazole, and oxfendazole have been found to be teratogenic in the early stages of pregnancy. They should not be used at mating or during early pregnancy, or during the pigeon breeding season.
Organisms have been found in the UK that are resistant to benzimidazoles, notably *Haemonchus* in sheep and *Cyathostoma* in horses. Continuing research will provide guidelines as to how current products can best be used to delay the onset of resistance. Resistance to one benzimidazole may also confer resistance to other drugs in the same chemical group. However, it should be remembered that apparent lack of efficacy is often found to be due to inappropriate or inadequate dosing.

ALBENDAZOLE

Indications. Gastro-intestinal roundworms, lungworms, tapeworms (2.1.2), and adult *Fasciola* (2.1.3) in ruminants; Type II ostertagiasis; *Filaroides* in dogs♦
Warnings. Teratogenic, see notes above
Dose. *Cattle*: roundworms and tapeworms, 7.5 mg/kg
Adult flukes, 10 mg/kg
Sheep: roundworms and tapeworms, 5 mg/kg
Adult flukes, 7.5 mg/kg
Dogs♦: 25 mg/kg twice daily for 5 days

PML **Allverm**™ (Crown)
Oral liquid, albendazole oxide 40 mg, hydrated cobalt sulphate 28.8 mg, hydrated sodium selenate 3 mg/mL, for *sheep*; 1 litre, 2.5 litres
Withdrawal Periods. *Sheep*: slaughter 10 days
Oral liquid, albendazole oxide 150 mg/mL, for *cattle*; 1 litre, 2.5 litres
Withdrawal Periods. *Cattle*: slaughter 14 days, milk 72 hours

PML **Bental**™ **2.5%** (C-Vet)
Oral suspension, albendazole oxide 25 mg, hydrated cobalt sulphate 18 mg, sodium selenate 1.9 mg/mL, for *sheep*; 1 litre, 2.5 litres, 10 litres
Withdrawal Periods. *Sheep*: slaughter 10 days, milk from treated animals should not be used for human consumption

PML **Bental**™ **7.5%** (C-Vet)
Oral suspension, albendazole oxide 75 mg, hydrated cobalt sulphate 54 mg,

hydrated sodium selenate 5.7 mg/mL, for *cattle*; 1 litre, 2.5 litres
Withdrawal Periods. *Cattle*: slaughter 14 days, milk 72 hours

PML **Powacide**™ (SmithKline Beecham)
Oral suspension, albendazole 75 mg, hydrated cobalt sulphate 13 mg, sodium selenate 2.38 mg/mL, for *sheep*; 1 litre, 2.5 litres
Withdrawal Periods. *Sheep*: slaughter 10 days

PML **Rycoben**™ **2.5%** (Young's)
Oral suspension, albendazole oxide 25 mg, hydrated cobalt sulphate 18 mg, hydrated sodium selenate 1.9 mg/mL, for *sheep*; 2.5 litres, 10 litres
Withdrawal Periods. *Sheep*: slaughter 10 days, milk from treated animals should not be used for human consumption

PML **Rycoben**™ **7.5%** (Young's)
Oral suspension, albendazole oxide 75 mg, hydrated cobalt sulphate 54 mg, hydrated sodium selenate 5.7 mg/mL, for *cattle*; 1 litre, 2.5 litres
Withdrawal Periods. *Cattle*: slaughter 14 days, milk 72 hours

PML **Valbazen**™ **2.5%** (SmithKline Beecham)
Oral suspension, albendazole 25 mg/mL, for *cattle, sheep*; 1 litre, 2.5 litres, 5 litres
Withdrawal Periods. *Cattle*: slaughter 14 days, milk 72 hours. *Sheep*: slaughter 10 days

PML **Valbazen**™ **10%** (SmithKline Beecham)
Oral suspension, albendazole 100 mg/mL, for *cattle*; 1 litre, 2.5 litres, 5 litres
Withdrawal Periods. *Cattle*: slaughter 14 days, milk 72 hours

PML **Valbazen**™ **Lamb Dose** (SmithKline Beecham)
Oral suspension, albendazole 75 mg, hydrated copper sulphate 13 mg, sodium selenate 2.38 mg/mL, for *lambs*; 1.1 litres
Withdrawal Periods. *Lambs*: slaughter 10 days

PML **Valbazen**™ **SC 2.5%** (SmithKline Beecham)
Oral suspension, albendazole 25 mg, cobalt 630 micrograms, selenium 270 micrograms/mL, for *sheep*; 2.5 litres, 5 litres
Withdrawal Periods. *Sheep*: slaughter 10 days

PML **Valbazen**™ **SC 10%** (SmithKline Beecham)
Oral suspension, albendazole 100 mg, hydrated cobalt sulphate 13 mg, sodium selenate 5.16 mg/mL, for *cattle*; 5 litres
Withdrawal Periods. *Cattle*: slaughter 14 days, milk 72 hours

PML **Valbazen**™ **Total Spectrum Wormer** (SmithKline Beecham)
Pellets, albendazole 30 mg/g, for *cattle, sheep*; 2 kg, 5 kg, 10 kg
Withdrawal Periods. *Cattle*: slaughter 14 days, milk 72 hours. *Sheep*: slaughter 10 days

CAMBENDAZOLE

Indications. Gastro-intestinal roundworms in pigeons
Warnings. Teratogenic, see notes above. Clean and disinfect loft when deworming, see section 2.2.2.8 for preparation details
Dose. *Pigeons*: (up to 400 g body-weight) 30 mg daily for 2 days; (more than 400 g body-weight) 60 mg daily for 2 days

GSL **Ascapilla**™ (Univet)
Capsules, cambendazole 30 mg, for *pigeons*; 100

FEBANTEL

Indications. Gastro-intestinal roundworms and lungworms in horses, ruminants, and pigs; tapeworm in sheep (2.1.2)
Dose. *Horses*: 6 mg/kg
Cattle: 7.5 mg/kg
Sheep, pigs: 5 mg/kg

PML **Bayverm**™ **2.5%** (Bayer)
Oral suspension, febantel 25 mg/mL, for *cattle, sheep*; 1 litre, 2.5 litres, 5 litres
Withdrawal Periods. *Cattle, sheep*: slaughter 8 days, milk 48 hours

PML **Bayverm**™ **10%** (Bayer)
Oral suspension, febantel 100 mg/mL, for *cattle*; 1 litre, 2.5 litres
Withdrawal Periods. *Cattle*: slaughter 8 days, milk 48 hours

PML **Bayverm Armadose**™ (Bayer)
Oral suspension, febantel 100 mg/mL, for *sheep*; 500 mL
Withdrawal Periods. *Sheep*: slaughter 8 days, milk from treated animals should not be used for human consumption

PML **Bayverm**™ **Pellets 1.9%** (Bayer)
Pellets, for use alone or by addition to feed, febantel 19 mg/g for *horses, cattle, sheep, pigs*; 200 g, 2 kg, 10 kg
Withdrawal Periods. Should not be used in *horses* intended for human consumption. *Cattle, sheep*: slaughter 8 days, milk 48 hours. *Pigs*: slaughter 10 days

PML **Bayverm**™ **SC 2.5%** (Bayer)
Oral suspension, febantel 25 mg, cobalt 600 micrograms, selenium 400 micrograms/mL, for *cattle, sheep*; 1 litre, 2.5 litres, 5 litres
Withdrawal Periods. *Cattle, sheep*: slaughter 8 days, milk 48 hours

FENBENDAZOLE

Indications. Gastro-intestinal roundworms in horses, ruminants, pigs, dogs, and cats; Type II ostertagiasis; transplacental roundworm transmission in dogs; lungworms in horses, ruminants, pigs, and dogs♦; gapeworms in game birds; *Trichostrongylus tenuis* in grouse; tapeworms (2.1.2) in sheep, goats, and dogs

Dose. *Horses, donkeys*: roundworms, lungworms, 7.5 mg/kg as a single dose
Larval *Trichonema*, 30 mg/kg as a single dose
Migrating strongyles, 60 mg/kg as a single dose
Cattle: 7.5 mg/kg as a single dose
Sheep, goats: 5 mg/kg as a single dose
Pigs: roundworms, lungworms, 5 mg/kg in divided doses over 6 days
Metastrongylus apri, 25 mg/kg as a single dose
Dogs, cats: roundworms, tapeworms, 20 mg/kg daily for 5 days
Transplacental transmission, 50 mg/kg from day 40 of pregnancy until 14 days post partum
Lungworms♦, 50 mg/kg daily for 7 days
artridges, pheasants: *by addition to eed*, 12 mg/kg body-weight

Grouse: *by addition to feed*, 7-10 mg/kg body-weight; 1 kg/tonne feed

PML **Panacur**™ **1.5%** (Hoechst)
Pellets, fenbendazole 15 mg/g, for *cattle, sheep, goats, pigs*; 2.5 kg, 5 kg, 10 kg
Withdrawal Periods. *Cattle, sheep, goats*: slaughter 14 days, milk 72 hours. *Pigs*: slaughter 14 days

PML **Panacur**™ **2.5%** (Hoechst)
Oral suspension, fenbendazole 25 mg/mL, for *cattle, sheep, goats, pigs, dogs, cats*; 250 mL, 1 litre, other sizes available
Withdrawal Periods. *Cattle, sheep, goats*: slaughter 14 days, milk 72 hours. *Pigs*: slaughter 14 days

PML **Panacur**™ **4%** (Hoechst)
Oral powder, for addition to feed, fenbendazole 40 mg/g, for *horses, cattle, sheep, goats, pigs, dogs, cats, grouse*; 18.75 g, 500 g, 2.5 kg
Withdrawal Periods. *Cattle, sheep, goats*: slaughter 14 days, milk 72 hours. *Pigs*: slaughter 14 days

PML **Panacur**™ **10%** (Hoechst)
Oral suspension, fenbendazole 100 mg/mL, for *horses, cattle, sheep, goats, dogs, cats*; 100 mL, 1.25 litres, other sizes available
Withdrawal Periods. *Cattle, sheep, goats*: slaughter 14 days, milk 72 hours

PML **Panacur**™ **22%** (Hoechst)
Oral granules, for addition to feed, fenbendazole 220 mg/g, for *horses, donkeys, cattle, sheep, goats, dogs, cats*; 1 g, 3 g, other sizes available
Withdrawal Periods. *Horses*: slaughter 14 days. *Cattle, sheep*: slaughter 14 days, milk 72 hours. *Goats*: milk 72 hours

PML **Panacur**™ **Paste** (Hoechst)
Oral paste, fenbendazole 187 mg/g, for *horses, cattle, sheep, goats*; 20-g dose applicator
Withdrawal Periods. *Cattle, sheep, goats*: slaughter 14 days, milk 72 hours

PML **Panacur**™ **SC** (Hoechst)
Oral suspension, fenbendazole 25 mg, cobalt 950 micrograms, selenium 400 micrograms/mL, for *sheep*; 1 litre, 2 litres, other sizes available
Withdrawal Periods. *Sheep*: slaughter 14 days, milk 72 hours

PML **Wormex**™ (Hoechst)
Oral suspension, fenbendazole 20 mg/mL, for *pheasants, partridges*; 200 mL
Withdrawal Periods. *Game birds*: slaughter 30 days, eggs from treated birds should not be used for human consumption

FLUBENDAZOLE

Indications. Gastro-intestinal roundworms and lungworms in pigs
Dose. *Pigs*: *by mouth*, 4-5 mg/kg bodyweight; 30 g/tonne feed

PML **Flubenol**™ (Janssen)
Pellets, flubendazole 5 mg/g, for *pigs*; 10 kg
Withdrawal Periods. *Pigs*: slaughter 14 days
Premix, flubendazole 50 mg/g, for *pigs*; 600 g, 25 kg
Withdrawal Periods. *Pigs*: slaughter 14 days

MEBENDAZOLE

Indications. Gastro-intestinal roundworms in horses, donkeys, ruminants, dogs, and cats; lungworms in donkeys and ruminants; tapeworms (2.1.2) in sheep and goats; *Echinococcus* and *Taenia* in dogs and cats; gastrointestinal roundworms, gapeworms, and tapeworms in poultry and game birds
Contra-indications. Administration during first 4 months of pregnancy in donkeys treated for *Dictyocaulus*. Manufacturer does not recommend administration to pigeons or parrots
Side-effects. Occasional mild diarrhoea
Warnings. May temporarily affect egg laying and egg fertility in breeding birds
Dose. *Horses, donkeys*: roundworms, 5-10 mg/kg
Dictyocaulus arnfieldi in donkeys, 15-20 mg/kg daily for 5 days
Sheep: 15 mg/kg
Goats: 15-30 mg/kg
Dogs, cats: (less than 2 kg body-weight) 50 mg twice daily for 5 days; (more than 2 kg body-weight) 100 mg twice daily for

5 days; (dogs more than 30 kg bodyweight) 200 mg twice daily for 5 days
Poultry: 60 g/tonne feed
Game birds: 120 g/tonne feed

PML **Equivurm**™ **Plus** (Crown)
Oral paste, mebendazole 200 mg/g, for *horses, donkeys*; 20-g dose applicator
Withdrawal Periods. Should not be used in *horses* intended for human consumption
Oral granules, for addition to feed, mebendazole 100 mg/g, for *horses, donkeys*; 20 g
Withdrawal Periods. Should not be used in *horses* intended for human consumption

PML **Mebenvet**™ **1.2%** (Janssen)
Oral powder, for addition to feed, mebendazole 12 mg/g, for *partridges, pheasants, water fowl*; 250 g
Withdrawal Periods. *Game birds*: slaughter 14 days

PML **Mebenvet**™ **5%** (Janssen)
Oral powder, for addition to feed, mebendazole 50 mg/g; for *chickens, turkeys, partridges, pheasants, water fowl*; 2.4 kg
Withdrawal Periods. *Poultry, game birds*: slaughter 14 days

PML **Multispec**™ (Goat Nutrition)
Tablets, scored, mebendazole 1 g, for *goats*; 5
Withdrawal Periods. *Goats*: slaughter 7 days, milk 24 hours

PML **Ovitelmin**™ **S & C** (Janssen)
Oral suspension, mebendazole 50 mg, cobalt sulphate 2.05 mg, sodium selenite 753 micrograms/mL, for *sheep*; 1 litre, 5 litres
Withdrawal Periods. *Sheep*: slaughter 7 days, milk 24 hours

PML **Telmin**™ (Janssen)
Oral paste, mebendazole 200 mg/g, for *horses, donkeys*; 20-g dose applicator
Withdrawal Periods. Should not be used for *horses* intended for human consumption
Oral granules, for addition to feed, mebendazole 100 mg/g, for *horses, donkeys*; 20 g
Withdrawal Periods. Should not be used in *horses* intended for human consumption

PML **Telmin**™ **KH** (Janssen)
Tablets, mebendazole 100 mg, for *dogs, cats*; 10

NETOBIMIN

Indications. Gastro-intestinal roundworms, lungworms, tapeworms (2.1.2), and adult flukes (2.1.3) in ruminants; Type II ostertagiasis
Contra-indications. Administration during first 7 weeks of pregnancy in cattle; first 5 weeks of pregnancy in sheep
Dose. *Cattle, sheep*: roundworms, tapeworms, 7.5 mg/kg
Type II ostertagiasis, adult flukes, 20 mg/kg

PML **Hapadex**™ (Schering-Plough)
Oral suspension, netobimin 50 mg/mL, for *sheep*; 1 litre, 5 litres
Withdrawal Periods. *Sheep*: slaughter 5 days, milk 72 hours
Oral suspension, netobimin 150 mg/mL, for *cattle*; 1 litre, 5 litres
Withdrawal Periods. *Cattle*: slaughter 10 days, milk 48 hours

OXFENDAZOLE

Indications. Gastro-intestinal roundworms in horses, donkeys, ruminants, and dogs; lungworms and tapeworms (2.1.2) in ruminants; Type II ostertagiasis; transplacental roundworm transmission in dogs; *Dipylidium* and *Taenia* in dogs
Contra-indications. First 35 days of pregnancy in dogs. Administration of ruminal boluses or injection into the rumen in non-ruminating cattle; concurrent administration of other ruminal boluses
Dose. *Horses*: 10 mg/kg as a single dose
Cattle: *by mouth*, 4.5 mg/kg as a single dose; *by intra-ruminal injection*, 4.5 mg/kg; see also sustained-release oral preparations below
Sheep: 5 mg/kg as a single dose
Dogs: 10 mg/kg daily for 3 days
Transplacental transmission, 10 mg/kg daily for 3 days, given within the last 14 days of pregnancy

Oral preparations
(see below for sustained-release oral preparations)

P **Head to Tail Bandit**™ (Coopers Pitman-Moore)
Oral suspension, oxfendazole 22.65 mg/mL, for *dogs*; 6 mL
Oral suspension, oxfendazole 90.6 mg/mL, for *dogs*; 6 mL

PML **Parafend**™ (Norbrook)
Oral suspension, oxfendazole 22.65 mg/mL, for *cattle*, *sheep*; 500 mL, 1 litre, other sizes available
Withdrawal Periods. *Cattle*: slaughter 14 days, milk 48 hours. *Sheep*: slaughter 14 days

PML **Parafend**™ **LV** (Norbrook)
Oral suspension, oxfendazole 90.6 mg/mL, for *cattle*; 500 mL, 1 litre, 2.5 litres
Withdrawal Periods. *Cattle*: slaughter 14 days, milk 48 hours

PML **Synanthic**™ (Coopers Pitman-Moore)
Oral suspension, oxfendazole 22.65 mg/mL, for *cattle*, *sheep*; 500 mL, 1 litre, other sizes available
Withdrawal Periods. *Cattle*: slaughter 14 days, milk 48 hours. *Sheep*: slaughter 14 days

PML **Synanthic**™ **DC** (Coopers Pitman-Moore)
Oral suspension, oxfendazole 90.6 mg/mL, for *cattle*; 500 mL, 1 litre, 2.5 litres
Withdrawal Periods. *Cattle*: slaughter 14 days, milk 48 hours

PML **Synanthic**™ **Horse Paste** (Coopers Pitman-Moore)
Oral paste, oxfendazole 500 mg/division, for *horses*, *donkeys*; 32.5-g metered-dose applicator
Withdrawal Periods. *Horses*: slaughter 20 days

PML **Synanthic**™ **Sel/Co** (Coopers Pitman-Moore)
Oral suspension, oxfendazole 22.65 mg, cobalt 1.67 mg, selenium 500 micrograms/mL, for *sheep*; 2.5 litres, 5 litres, 12.5 litres
Withdrawal Periods. *Sheep*: slaughter 14 days, milk 4 days

PML **Systamex**™ **2.265** (Coopers Pitman-Moore)
Oral suspension, oxfendazole 22.65 mg/mL, for *cattle*, *sheep*; 1 litre, 2.5 litres, 10 litres
Withdrawal Periods. *Cattle*: slaughter 14

days, milk 48 hours. *Sheep*: slaughter 14 days

PML **Systamex**™ **906** (Coopers Pitman-Moore)
Oral suspension, oxfendazole 90.6 mg/mL, for *cattle*; 1 litre, 2.5 litres, 10 litres
Withdrawal Periods. *Cattle*: slaughter 14 days, milk 48 hours

PML **Systamex**™ **Handipack** (Coopers Pitman-Moore)
Oral suspension, oxfendazole 90.6 mg/mL, for *sheep*; 500 mL
Withdrawal Periods. *Sheep*: slaughter 14 days, milk from treated animals should not be used for human consumption

PML **Systamex**™ **Paste 18.5%** (Coopers Pitman-Moore)
Oral paste, oxfendazole 185 mg/g, for *horses, donkeys*; 32.5-g dose applicator
Withdrawal Periods. Should not be used in *horses* intended for human consumption

PML **Systamex**™ **SC** (Coopers Pitman-Moore)
Oral suspension, oxfendazole 22.65 mg, cobalt (as sulphate) 1.67 mg, selenium (as sodium selenate) 500 micrograms/mL, for *sheep*; 2.5 litres, 10 litres
Withdrawal Periods. *Sheep*: slaughter 14 days, milk from treated animals should not be used for human consumption

Sustained-release oral preparations

PML **Autoworm**™ **5 with Systamex**™ (Coopers Pitman-Moore)
Ruminal bolus, s/r, comprising 5 tablets each containing oxfendazole 750 mg (= total oxfendazole 3.75 g), for *cattle in their first grazing season weighing between 100 kg and 200 kg*; 12
Withdrawal Periods. *Cattle*: slaughter 6 months, milk from animals treated within 6 months before calving and during lactation should not be used for human consumption
Dose. *Cattle*: (100-200 kg body-weight) one 3.75-g ruminal bolus

PML **Autoworm**™ **Big 5 with Systamex**™ (Coopers Pitman-Moore)
Ruminal bolus, s/r, comprising 5 tablets each containing oxfendazole 1.25 g (= total oxfendazole 6.25 g), for *grazing cattle weighing between 200 kg and 400 kg*; 12

Withdrawal Periods. *Cattle*: slaughter 6 months, milk from animals treated within 6 months before calving and during lactation should not be used for human consumption
Dose. *Cattle*: (200-400 kg body-weight) one 6.25-g ruminal bolus

PML **Autoworm**™ **Big 6 with Systamex**™ (Coopers Pitman-Moore)
Ruminal bolus, s/r, comprising 6 tablets each containing oxfendazole 1.25 g (= total oxfendazole 7.5 g), for *grazing cattle weighing between 200 kg and 400 kg*; 12
Withdrawal Periods. *Cattle*: slaughter 6 months, milk from animals treated within 6 months before calving and during lactation should not be used for human consumption
Dose. *Cattle*: (200-400 kg body-weight) one 7.5-g ruminal bolus

PML **Synanthic**™ **Multidose 130** (Coopers Pitman-Moore)
Ruminal bolus, s/r, comprising 5 tablets each containing oxfendazole 750 mg (= total oxfendazole 3.75 g), for *cattle in their first grazing season weighing between 100 kg and 200 kg*; 12
Withdrawal Periods. *Cattle*: slaughter 6 months, milk from animals treated within 6 months before calving and during lactation should not be used for human consumption
Dose. *Cattle*: (100-200 kg body-weight) one 3.75-g ruminal bolus

PML **Synanthic**™ **Multidose Plus** (Coopers Pitman-Moore)
Ruminal bolus, s/r, comprising 5 tablets each containing oxfendazole 1.25 g (= total oxfendazole 6.25 g), for *grazing cattle weighing between 200 kg and 400 kg*; 12
Withdrawal Periods. *Cattle*: slaughter 6 months, milk from animals treated within 6 months before calving and during lactation should not be used for human consumption
Dose. *Cattle*: (200-400 kg body-weight) one 6.25-g ruminal bolus

PML **Synanthic**™ **Multidose Extra** (Coopers Pitman-Moore)
Ruminal bolus, s/r, comprising 6 tablets each containing oxfendazole 1.25 g (= total oxfendazole 7.5 g), for *grazing*

cattle weighing between 200 kg and 400 kg;
12
Withdrawal Periods. *Cattle*: slaughter 6
months, milk from animals treated
within 6 months before calving and
during lactation should not be used for
human consumption
Dose. *Cattle*: (200-400 kg body-weight)
one 7.5-g ruminal bolus

Parenteral preparations

PML**Synanthic**™ IR (Coopers Pitman-
Moore)
Intra-ruminal injection, oxfendazole
225 mg/mL, for *cattle*; 500 mL, 1 litre
Withdrawal Periods. *Cattle*: slaughter 14
days, milk 48 hours

OXIBENDAZOLE

Indications. Gastro-intestinal roundworms in horses, ruminants, and pigs
Dose. *Horses*: roundworms, 10 mg/kg
Strongyloides westeri, 15 mg/kg
Cattle, sheep: 10 mg/kg
Pigs: *alone or by addition to feed
(pellets)*, 15 mg/kg body-weight as a
single dose; *by addition to feed (oral
powder)*, 1.6 mg/kg body-weight daily
for 10 days

PML**Equidin**™ (Univet)
Oral paste, oxibendazole 1 g/division,
for *horses*; 16.7-g metered-dose applicator
Withdrawal Periods. Should not be
used in *horses* intended for human
consumption

PML**Equitac**™ (SmithKline Beecham)
Oral paste, oxibendazole 1 g/division,
for *horses*; 16.7-g metered-dose applicator
Withdrawal Periods. Should not be
used in *horses* intended for human
consumption

PML**Lincoln Horse and Pony Wormer**™
(Battle Hayward & Bower)
Oral paste, oxibendazole 300 mg/g, for
horses; 16.7-g metered-dose applicator

PML**Loditac**™ 3% (SmithKline Beecham)
Pellets, for use alone or by addition to
feed, oxibendazole 30 mg/g, for *pigs*;
5 kg
Withdrawal Periods. *Pigs*: slaughter 14
days

PML**Loditac**™ 20 (SmithKline Beecham)
Oral powder, for addition to feed,
oxibendazole 20 mg/g, for *pigs*; 2 kg
Withdrawal Periods. *Pigs*: slaughter 14
days

PML**Loditac**™ 200 (SmithKline Beecham)
Oral powder, for addition to feed,
oxibendazole 200 mg/g, for *pigs*; 10 kg
Withdrawal Periods. *Pigs*: slaughter 14
days

PML**Widespec**™ (C-Vet)
Oral suspension, oxibendazole 50 mg,
hydrated cobalt sulphate 18 mg,
hydrated sodium selenate 1.9 mg/mL,
for *cattle, sheep*; 1 litre, 2.5 litres
Withdrawal Periods. *Cattle*: slaughter 4
days, milk 72 hours. *Sheep*: slaughter 4
days

THIABENDAZOLE

Indications. Gastro-intestinal round-
worms in horses and ruminants; lung-
worms in sheep
Dose. *Horses*: roundworms, 44 mg/kg
Parascaris, 88 mg/kg
Cattle: 66-110 mg/kg depending on the
severity of the infection
Sheep: roundworms, 44 mg/kg
Lungworms, 66 mg/kg
Nematodiriasis in lambs, 88 mg/kg

PML**Equizole**™ (MSD Agvet)
Oral powder, for addition to feed,
thiabendazole 333 mg/g, for *horses*; 30 g
Oral paste, thiabendazole 493 mg/g, for
horses; 34.5-g dose applicator

PML**Thibenzole**™ (MSD Agvet)
Oral suspension, thiabendazole 176 mg/
mL, for *cattle, sheep*; 1 litre, 5 litres,
10 litres

THIOPHANATE

Indications. Gastro-intestinal roundworms in ruminants and pigs; Type II
ostertagiasis; lungworms in ruminants
Dose. See preparation details

PML**Nemafax**™ 14 (RMB)
Oral powder, for addition to feed,
thiophanate 225 mg/g, for *cattle, sheep,
goats, pigs*; 10 kg
Withdrawal Periods. *Cattle, sheep, goats*:
slaughter 7 days, milk 72 hours. *Pigs*:
slaughter 7 days

Dose. *Cattle, sheep, goats*: *by addition to feed*, 67.5 mg of thiophanate/kg body-weight as a single dose *or* 21 mg of thiophanate/kg body-weight daily for 5 days *or* 5.25 mg of thiophanate/kg body-weight daily for 20 days
Pigs: *by addition to feed*, 67.5 mg of thiophanate/kg body-weight as a single dose *or* 6-7 mg of thiophanate/kg body-weight daily for 14 days

PML **Nemafax™ Drench** (RMB)
Oral suspension, thiophanate 200 mg/mL, for *cattle, sheep, goats*; 2.5 litres
Withdrawal Periods. *Cattle, sheep, goats*: slaughter 7 days, milk 72 hours
Dose. *Cattle*: roundworms, 60 mg/kg Type II ostertagiasis, up to 140 mg/kg
Sheep, goats: roundworms, 50 mg/kg Nematodiriasis, severe lungworm infection, 100 mg/kg

PML **Wormalic™** (Dallas Keith)
Oral liquid, thiophanate 12 mg/mL, for *cattle, sheep*; 25 litres
Withdrawal Periods. *Cattle, sheep*: slaughter 7 days, milk 72 hours
Dose. *Cattle*: *by addition to feed*, 2.4-4.8 g per animal daily for 7 days
Sheep: *by addition to feed*, 240-480 mg per animal daily for 7 days

PML **Wormer with Nemafax™** (Colborn-Dawes)
Medicated feed block, thiophanate 3.5 g/kg, for *cattle, sheep*; 20 kg
Dose. *Cattle*: 1 feed block per 2 animals to provide treatment for 20 days
Sheep: 1 feed block per 3 animals to provide treatment for 42 days

2.1.1.3 IMIDAZOTHIAZOLES

Levamisole and **tetramisole** are imidazothiazoles that act by interfering with parasite nerve transmission causing muscular paralysis and rapid expulsion. They are effective against adult and larval gastro-intestinal roundworm and lungworm infection. Levamisole is effective against *Protostrongylus* infection. The therapeutic index of levamisole is low in animals, especially in horses and dogs. The clinical signs of toxicity include salivation and muscle tremors.

LEVAMISOLE HYDROCHLORIDE

Indications. Gastro-intestinal roundworms in ruminants, pigs, and pigeons; Type II ostertagiasis (not pretype II); lungworms in ruminants, pigs, and dogs◆; heartworm treatment in dogs◆ (seek specialist advice)
Contra-indications. Administration within 14 days of treatment with organophosphorus compounds or diethylcarbamazine. Application of 'pour-on' formulations to wet animals
Side-effects. Occasional vomiting in pigs; see notes above
Dose. *Cattle*: *by mouth or by subcutaneous injection*, 7.5 mg/kg; see preparation details below for 'pour-on' application
Sheep, goats: *by mouth or by subcutaneous injection*, 7.5 mg/kg
Pigs: *by subcutaneous injection*, 7.5 mg/kg
Dogs◆: *Angiostrongylus*, *by mouth*, 10 mg/kg daily for 3 days
Pigeons: see preparation details

Oral preparations

PML **Bionem™** (Coopers Pitman-Moore)
See under Parenteral preparations

PML **Cyverm™** (Cyanamid)
Oral solution, levamisole hydrochloride 32 mg/mL, for *cattle, sheep*; 2 litres
Withdrawal Periods. *Cattle, sheep*: slaughter 3 days, milk 36 hours

PML **Levacide™ Low Volume** (Norbrook)
Oral solution, levamisole hydrochloride 75 mg/mL, for *cattle, sheep*; 500 mL, 1 litre, 2.5 litres
Withdrawal Periods. *Cattle, sheep*: slaughter 5 days, milk 36 hours

PML **Levacide™ Worm Drench** (Norbrook)
Oral solution, levamisole hydrochloride 15 mg/mL, for *cattle, sheep, goats*; 1 litre, 2.5 litres, other sizes available
Withdrawal Periods. *Cattle, sheep, goats*: slaughter 3 days, milk 36 hours

PML **Levadin™** (Univet)
Oral solution, levamisole 15 mg/mL, for *cattle, sheep*; 1 litre, 5 litres
Withdrawal Periods. *Cattle, sheep*: slaughter 3 days, milk 36 hours

PML**Nilverm**™ **Gold** (Coopers Pitman-Moore)
Oral solution, levamisole hydrochloride 30 mg/mL, for *cattle, sheep, goats*; 2.5 litres, 5 litres, 25 litres
Withdrawal Periods. *Cattle, sheep, goats*: slaughter 3 days, milk 24 hours

PML**Nilverm**™ **In-feed** (Coopers Pitman-Moore)
Oral granules, for addition to feed, levamisole hydrochloride 25 mg/g, for *cattle, sheep*; 3 kg
Withdrawal Periods. *Cattle, sheep*: slaughter 3 days, milk 24 hours

PML**Nilverm**™ **Super** (Coopers Pitman-Moore)
Oral solution, levamisole hydrochloride 30 mg, cobalt sulphate heptahydrate 7.64 mg, sodium selenate 766 micrograms/mL, for *cattle, sheep, goats*; 2.5 litres, 5 litres
Withdrawal Periods. *Cattle, sheep, goats*: slaughter 3 days, milk 24 hours

PML**Ridaverm**™ (Crown)
Oral solution, levamisole hydrochloride 32 mg/mL, for *cattle, sheep*; 5 litres
Withdrawal Periods. *Cattle, sheep*: slaughter 3 days, milk 36 hours

PML**Ripercol**™ **3.2%** (Janssen)
Oral solution, levamisole hydrochloride 32 mg/mL, for *cattle, sheep*; 1 litre, 5 litres
Withdrawal Periods. *Cattle, sheep*: slaughter 5 days, milk 48 hours

GSL**Spartakon**™ (Harkers)
Tablets, scored, levamisole (as hydrochloride) 20 mg, for *pigeons*; 50
Withdrawal Periods. *Pigeons*: slaughter 28 days
Dose. *Pigeons*: *by mouth*, levamisole 20 mg

PML**Sure**™ (Young's)
Oral solution, levamisole hydrochloride 32 mg/mL, for *cattle, sheep*; 5 litres
Withdrawal Periods. *Cattle, sheep*: slaughter 3 days, milk 36 hours

PML**Vermisole**™ (Bimeda)
Oral solution, levamisole hydrochloride 15 mg/mL, for *cattle, sheep*; 2.5 litres, 5 litres
Withdrawal Periods. *Cattle, sheep*: slaughter 3 days, milk 36 hours

PML**Wormaway**™ (Deosan)
Oral solution, levamisole hydrochloride 15 mg/mL, for *cattle, sheep*; 2.5 litres, 5 litres, 10 litres
Withdrawal Periods. *Cattle, sheep*: slaughter 3 days, milk 36 hours

Parenteral preparations

PML**Bionem**™ (Coopers Pitman-Moore)
Injection or oral solution, levamisole hydrochloride 75 mg/mL, for *cattle, sheep*; 1.5 litres
Withdrawal Periods. *Cattle, sheep*: slaughter 3 days, milk 24 hours

PML**Levacide**™ (Norbrook)
Injection, levamisole hydrochloride 75 mg/mL, for *cattle, sheep, pigs*; 100 mL, 250 mL, 500 mL
Withdrawal Periods. *Cattle, sheep*: slaughter 3 days, milk 36 hours. *Pigs*: slaughter 5 days

PML**Levadin**™ (Univet)
Injection, levamisole hydrochloride 75 mg/mL, for *cattle, sheep, pigs*; 500 mL
Withdrawal Periods. *Cattle, sheep*: slaughter 7 days, milk 60 hours. *Pigs*: slaughter 7 days

PML**Nilvax**™ (Cooper Pitman-Moore)
See section 18.2.3 for preparation details

PML**Nilverm**™ (Coopers Pitman-Moore)
Injection, levamisole hydrochloride 75 mg/mL, for *cattle, sheep, pigs*; 500 mL
Withdrawal Periods. *Cattle, sheep*: slaughter 3 days, milk 24 hours. *Pigs*: slaughter 5 days

PML**Ridaverm**™ (Crown)
Injection, levamisole hydrochloride 75 mg/mL, for *cattle, sheep, pigs*; 500 mL
Withdrawal Periods. *Cattle, sheep*: slaughter 3 days, milk 36 hours. *Pigs*: slaughter 5 days

PML**Ripercol**™ **7.5%** (Janssen)
Injection, levamisole hydrochloride 75 mg/mL, for *cattle, sheep, pigs*; 500 mL
Withdrawal Periods. *Cattle, sheep*: slaughter 5 days, milk 48 hours. *Pigs*: slaughter 5 days

PML**Rycovamisole**™ (C-Vet)
Injection, levamisole hydrochloride 75 mg/mL, for *cattle, sheep, pigs*; 500 mL
Withdrawal Periods. *Cattle, sheep*: slaughter 3 days, milk 36 hours. *Pigs*: slaughter 5 days

PML **Vermisole™** (Bimeda)
Injection, levamisole hydrochloride 75 mg/mL, for *cattle, sheep*; 500 mL
Withdrawal Periods. *Cattle, sheep*: slaughter 3 days, milk 36 hours

PML **Wormaway™** (Deosan)
Injection, levamisole hydrochloride 75 mg/mL, for *cattle, sheep*; 500 mL
Withdrawal Periods. *Cattle, sheep*: slaughter 3 days, milk 36 hours

'Pour-on' preparations

PML **Anthelpor™ 20** (Young's)
Solution, 'pour-on', levamisole 200 mg/mL, for *cattle*; 500 mL, 2.5 litres
Withdrawal Periods. *Cattle*: slaughter 7 days, milk 24 hours
Dose. *Cattle: by 'pour-on' application*, levamisole 10 mg/kg

PML **Levipor™ 20** (C-Vet)
Solution, 'pour-on', levamisole 200 mg/mL, for *cattle*; 500 mL, 2.5 litres
Withdrawal Periods. *Cattle*: slaughter 7 days, milk 24 hours
Dose. *Cattle: by 'pour-on' application*, levamisole 10 mg/kg

PML **Ripercol™ Pour-on** (Janssen)
Solution, 'pour-on', levamisole 200 mg/mL, for *cattle*; 250 mL, 500 mL, other sizes available
Withdrawal Periods. *Cattle*: slaughter 7 days, milk 24 hours
Dose. *Cattle: by 'pour-on' application*, levamisole 10 mg/kg

TETRAMISOLE HYDROCHLORIDE

Indications. Gastro-intestinal roundworms and lungworms in pigs
Side-effects. See under Levamisole
Dose. *Pigs: by addition to feed*, 15 mg/kg body-weight

PML **Nilverm™ Pig Wormer** (Coopers Pitman-Moore)
Oral powder, for addition to feed, tetramisole hydrochloride 170 g/kg, for *pigs*; 10 kg
Oral granules, for addition to feed, tetramisole hydrochloride 100 mg/g, for *pigs*; 205 g, 1.025 kg
Withdrawal Periods. *Pigs*: slaughter 7 days

2.1.1.4 ORGANOPHOSPHORUS COMPOUNDS

Haloxon is an organophosphorus compound. It acts by inhibiting cholinesterase thereby interfering with neuromuscular transmission in the parasite. Haloxon is effective against adult gastro-intestinal roundworms and bots, but ineffective against migrating larvae, tapeworms, or flukes.

Parasiticides may be toxic to animals and the operator. Care should be taken with dosage and handling of the product. The recommendations for storage, use, and disposal of unused materials and containers should be followed

HALOXON

Indications. Gastro-intestinal roundworms and bots in horses
Contra-indications. Concurrent administration of other organophosphorus compounds or other anticholinesterase compounds (see Drug Interactions – Appendix 1)
Dose. *Horses*: 50-70 mg/kg

PML **Multiwurma™** (Day Son & Hewitt)
Oral powder, for addition to feed, haloxon 612 mg/g, for *horses*; 25 g, 500 g, 1 kg
Withdrawal Periods. Should not be used in *horses* intended for human consumption

PML **Ruby Horse Wormer™** (Spencer)
Oral powder, haloxon 500 mg/g, for *horses*; 20 g

2.1.1.5 TETRAHYDRO-PYRIMIDINES

Tetrahydropyrimidines, such as **morantel** and **pyrantel**, interfere with parasitic nerve transmission as cholinergic agonists, leading to neuromuscular paralysis. They are effective against adult and larval gastro-intestinal roundworms. Pyrantel is also effective against tapeworms in horses. Morantel is available as a slow-release ruminal bolus. A negligible amount of drug is absorbed systemically by this route.

MORANTEL

Indications. Gastro-intestinal round-worms in cattle

Contra-indications. Concurrent administration of other ruminal boluses

Dose. See preparation details

PML **Paratect Flex**™ (Pfizer)
Ruminal bolus, s/r, morantel (as tartrate) 11.8 g, for *cattle*; 20
Withdrawal Periods. *Cattle*: slaughter withdrawal period nil, milk withdrawal period nil
Dose. *Cattle*: (more than 100 kg body-weight) one 11.8-g ruminal bolus

PYRANTEL EMBONATE

Indications. Gastro-intestinal round-worms in horses and dogs; tapeworms (2.1.2) in horses

Contra-indications. Administration to pregnant mares, stallions

Dose. *Horses*: roundworms, 19 mg/kg
Anoplocephala, 38 mg/kg
Dogs: 14.4 mg/kg (= 5 mg pyrantel base/kg)

PML **Strongid**™ (Pfizer)
Oral suspension, pyrantel (as embonate) 5 mg/mL, for *dogs*; 60 mL
Oral paste, pyrantel (as embonate) 7.5 mg/g (1 cm of paste = pyrantel 2.5 mg), for *dogs*; 24 g

PML **Strongid**™**-P** (Pfizer)
Oral paste, pyrantel embonate 439 mg/g, for *horses*; 23.6-g dose applicator
Withdrawal Periods. Should not be used in *horses* intended for human consumption
Oral granules, for addition to feed or for administration by gavage, pyrantel embonate 767 mg/g, for *horses*; 6.75 g, 1.5 kg
Withdrawal Periods. Should not be used in *horses* intended for human consumption

---

2.1.1.6 OTHER DRUGS FOR ROUNDWORMS

Piperazine and **diethylcarbamazine** modify neurotransmission in parasites causing relaxation and subsequent expulsion of helminths. Piperazine is effective against some gastro-intestinal round-worms including *Parascaris*, *Triodontophorus*, and *Strongylus vulgaris* in horses, *Ascaris* and *Oesophagostomum* in pigs, *Toxocara*, *Toxascaris*, and *Uncinaria* in dogs and cats, and *Ascaridia* in poultry. Piperazine is not active against lungworms or tapeworms. Large doses of the drug are required for hookworm, *Triodontophorus*, *Strongylus vulgaris*, and *Oesophagostomum* infections.

Nitroscanate is used for the control of roundworms and some tapeworms (see section 2.1.2) in dogs. **Nitroxynil** is used for the treatment of some roundworm and adult and immature fluke infections (see section 2.1.3). **Closantel** has been used for the treatment of benzimidazole-resistant *Haemonchus* infections in sheep (see section 2.1.3).

DIETHYLCARBAMAZINE CITRATE

Indications. Heartworm prophylaxis in dogs

Contra-indications. Administration to microfilaraemic dogs

Dose. *Dogs*: heartworm prophylaxis, *by mouth* 5.5-11.0 mg/kg daily or every other day commencing before exposure and continuing for at least 60 days after exposure

P **Banocide**™ (Wellcome)
Tablets, scored, diethylcarbamazine citrate 50 mg; 100

NITROSCANATE

Indications. Gastro-intestinal round-worms, *Dipylidium* and *Taenia* (2.1.2) in dogs

Side-effects. Occasional vomiting with high dosage

Warnings. Nitroscanate is irritant and tablets should not be crushed

Dose. *Dogs*: 50 mg/kg, given with a little food but on an empty stomach

PoM **Lopatol**™ (Ciba-Geigy)
Tablets, nitroscanate 100 mg, 500 mg, for *dogs*; 100-mg tablets 100; 500-mg tablets 60

PIPERAZINE

Indications. Roundworms in horses, pigs, dogs, cats, and poultry
Contra-indications. Renal impairment
Warnings. Overdosage may cause vomiting, diarrhoea, and ataxia in dogs and cats
Dose. Expressed as piperazine hydrate
Horses♦: *Parascaris*, up to 160 mg/kg
Pigs: *Ascaris*, up to 160 mg/kg
Dogs, cats: *Toxocara, Toxascaris*, 80 mg/kg
Ancylostoma, Uncinaria, 120-240 mg/kg
Poultry: *Ascaridia*, up to 160 mg/kg
Note. 100 mg piperazine hydrate ≡ 120 mg piperazine adipate ≡ 125 mg piperazine citrate ≡ 104 mg piperazine phosphate

GSL **Biozine**™ (Micro-Biologicals)
Oral powder, for addition to drinking water or feed, piperazine (as dihydrochloride) 530 mg/g, for *pigs, chickens, turkeys*; 113.5 g, 25 kg

GSL **Canovel**™ **Palatable Wormer** (SmithKline Beecham)
Tablets, piperazine phosphate 416 mg, for *dogs*; 4, 12, 100

GSL **Catovel**™ **Palatable Wormer** (Smith-Kline Beecham)
Tablets, piperazine phosphate 416 mg, for *cats*; 4

GSL **Citrazine**™ (Duphar)
Tablets, for addition to drinking water or feed, scored, piperazine citrate 500 mg, for *dogs, cats, poultry*; 500

GSL **Companion Roundwormer**™ (Battle Hayward & Bower)
Tablets, piperazine citrate 500 mg, for *dogs, cats*; 6, 24

GSL **Endorid**™ (SmithKline Beecham)
Tablets, scored, piperazine phosphate 416 mg, for *dogs, cats*; 12, 500

GSL **Head-to-tail Roundworm**™ (Coopers Pitman-Moore)
Tablets, piperazine adipate 450 mg, for *dogs, cats*; 500

GSL **Piperazine Citrate** (Animalcare)
Tablets, piperazine citrate 500 mg; 500, 1000

GSL **Piperazine Citrate** (Arnolds)
Tablets, piperazine citrate 500 mg, for *dogs, cats, poultry*; 500

GSL **Piperazine Citrate** (Loveridge)
Tablets, scored, piperazine citrate 500 mg, for *dogs, cats*; 500, 1000

GSL **Piperazine Citrate** (Univet)
Tablets, scored, piperazine citrate 500 mg, for *dogs, cats*; 500

GSL **Piperazine Pig Worm Powders** (Battle Hayward & Bower)
Oral powder, piperazine citrate 99-100%, for *pigs*; 10 doses, 20 doses, other sizes available

GSL **Piperazine Poultry Worm Powders** (Battle Hayward & Bower)
Oral powder, piperazine citrate 99-100%, for *poultry*; 120 doses, 600 doses, 6000 doses

GSL **Ruby Puppy Wormer** (Spencer)
Syrup, piperazine citrate 100 mg/mL, for *puppies*; 50 mL

GSL **Verocid**™ (Willows Francis)
Tablets, scored, piperazine adipate 500 mg, for *dogs, cats*; 500

2.1.2 Drugs for tapeworms (cestodes)

Adult tapeworms do not usually cause discernible disease. Treatment is often necessary for public health purposes, to prevent disease in farm livestock, and to minimise meat inspection losses.
Diagnosis of infected animals is difficult and often relies on the chance observation of a passed segment, the morphology of which is used for generic identification. Care is needed is assessing the success of treatment. A mass of tapeworm strobilae may be passed after use of a relatively ineffective product, but this is of no benefit if the scolices are left to re-grow. Conversely, a lack of evidence may be due to dissolution of the dead tapeworm within the alimentary tract.
All tapeworms have an indirect lifecycle and preventive measures often include control of arthropods. Information on effective drugs for treatment is given in section 2.1 and Table 2.1.
Treatment for *Anoplocephala* in the

horse is not often required, but heavy infections may be a predisposing factor in some colics, particularly those provoked by intussusception. Pasture-living mites are the intermediate hosts and so infection is unlikely in permanently stabled horses. Horses are usually treated in midsummer and again in early autumn.

Moniezia infection is mostly seen in lambs, and calves during their first summer on pasture, but rarely causes ill-effect except perhaps for a marginal influence on growth. Infections are often lost spontaneously in the summer and are not common in older animals. Free-living mites on the pasture are the intermediate hosts and prevention of re-infection is thus impossible. Control of *Moniezia* includes treatment in late spring or early summer and again in autumn.

Dipylidium, *Echinococcus*, and *Taenia* affect dogs. *Dipylidium* and *Taenia* affect cats. The choice of anthelmintic and advice on preventing re-infection are both determined by accurate knowledge of the tapeworm involved. Long-term control of *Dipylidium* includes elimination of fleas and lice (see sections 2.2.1, 2.2.2, and 2.2.4), the intermediate hosts. Most *Taenia* species, and *Echinococcus* have sheep as the intermediate host. Dogs are infected by the feeding of undercooked meat or viscera, while cats become infected by hunting small mammals. *Echinococcus* is zoonotic. Control of *Taenia* and *Dipylidium* infection requires treatment every 6 months. *Echinococcus* treatment should be repeated every 6 weeks.

Praziquantel is effective against all tapeworms in dogs and cats and is preferred in most *Echinococcus* control programmes as it kills all intestinal forms of the parasite. **Bunamidine** is also effective against tapeworms in dogs and cats but only eliminates mature *E. granulosus*. Both drugs act by causing disruption of the parasite integument. Bunamidine may cause vomiting and increased sensitisation of the heart to catecholamines, especially if the animal is exercised within 24 hours of treatment. **Praziquantel♦** and pyrantel (see section

2.1.1.5) may be used in the treatment of tapeworm infections in horses.

Dichlorophen and **nitroscanate** (see section 2.1.1.6) are effective against *Taenia* and *Dipylidium* but have limited efficacy against *Echinococcus*. Dichlorophen is also used in the treatment of tapeworm infection in pigeons.

Various **benzimidazoles** (see section 2.1.1.2), including albendazole, febantel, fenbendazole, mebendazole, netobimin, and oxfendazole are effective for tapeworm control in ruminants. Fenbendazole, mebendazole, and oxfendazole also control some tapeworms in dogs. The fasciolicide, **oxyclozanide** (see section 2.1.3) causes the release of *Moniezia* segments.

Niclosamide acts by uncoupling oxidative phosphorylation, thereby interfering with adenosine triphosphate production.

BUNAMIDINE

Indications. Tapeworms in dogs and cats
Contra-indications. Unweaned puppies or kittens
Side-effects. Overdosage can lead to vomiting and diarrhoea; cardiac failure, see notes above
Dose. *Dogs, cats*: *Dipylidium*, *Taenia*, 20-50 mg/kg as a single dose
Echinococcus, 20-50 mg/kg, repeat dose after 2 days

PML **Head-to-tail™ Tapeworm** (Coopers Pitman-Moore)
Tablets, bunamidine (as hydrochloride) 100 mg, 200 mg, for *dogs, cats*; 100

DICHLOROPHEN

Indications. *Dipylidium* and *Taenia* in dogs and cats; tapeworms in pigeons
Dose. *Dogs, cats*: 200 mg/kg
Pigeons: 100 mg

GSL **Canovel™ Tapewormer** (SmithKline Beecham)
Tablets, dichlorophen 750 mg, for *dogs*; 4

GSL **Catovel™ Tapewormer** (SmithKline Beecham)
Tablets, dichlorophen 750 mg, for *cats*; 4

GSL **Companion™ Tapewormer** (Battle Hayward & Bower)
Tablets, dichlorophen 500 mg, for *dogs, cats*; 6, 24

GSL **Tapeworm Capsules** (Harkers)
Dichlorophen 100 mg, for *pigeons*; 12

PRAZIQUANTEL

Indications. Tapeworms in horses♦, dogs, and cats
Contra-indications. Unweaned puppies or kittens
Dose. *Horses♦: by mouth*, 10 mg/kg
Dogs, cats: by mouth, 5 mg/kg; *by subcutaneous or intramuscular injection*, 3.5-7.5 mg/kg

Droncit™ (Bayer)
GSL *Tablets*, scored, praziquantel 50 mg, for *dogs, cats*; 20

PoM *Injection*, praziquantel 56.8 mg/mL, for *dogs, cats*; 10 mL

The following drug is included in Prescribing for rabbits and rodents, Prescribing for exotic birds, and Prescribing for reptiles—see those sections for indications and dosage

NICLOSAMIDE

P **Yomesan™** (Bayer)
Tablets, niclosamide 500 mg; 4

2.1.3 Drugs for flukes (trematodes)

The liver fluke *Fasciola hepatica* is endemic in many wet regions and affects mainly ruminants kept in or originating from such areas. The intermediate host is a small mud snail, *Lymnaea truncatula*. Horses are more resistant to fascioliasis but occasionally show clinical signs of ill thrift. The acute disease, which occurs in autumn and early winter, is caused by immature *F. hepatica* destroying the liver parenchyma, while the chronic form in the early months of the year results from the feeding activities of adult flukes in the bile ducts. Both acute and chronic forms of fascioliasis occur in sheep, but only the latter in cattle.

Treatment may be therapeutic or prophylactic. For acute disease in young animals the drug dose should be repeated after 5 to 6 weeks. To prevent infection, all animals exposed to fluke-infested pastures should be treated at regular intervals throughout the fluke season, depending on the area and climatic conditions. The risk of disease varies from year to year and MAFF issues a forecast so that the appropriate level of control can be maintained.

Care is required in the choice of fasciolicide as few are active against all stages of parasitic development. See Table 2.1 in the introduction to section 2.1, and drug monographs for information on drug treatment.

The lancet fluke, *Dicrocoelium dendriticum*, passes through various land snails and ants. This fluke affects cattle and sheep although the affected regions in the UK are mainly sheep-rearing areas such as the Hebrides.

Benzimidazoles (see section 2.1.1.2) effective against flukes include albendazole and netobimin, which are effective against adult stages. **Triclabendazole** is effective against immature and adult stages of *Fasciola*.

Diamphenethide is effective against immature flukes and to a lesser extent adult flukes. Diamphenethide is distributed to the liver and gall-bladder where its metabolite is active against immature flukes that are present in the parenchyma. Activity of diamphenethide against adult flukes is poor as limited metabolite reaches the bile duct.

Nitroxynil is effective against adult flukes and at a higher dosage, immature flukes and also *Haemonchus*. **Closantel** is effective against adult and immature flukes, *Oestrus ovis*, and *Haemonchus contortus*. These drugs act by uncoupling oxidative phosphorylation. They bind strongly to plasma proteins and therefore their activity against nematodes is restricted to those that suck blood.

Oxyclozanide is mainly active against adult flukes. Oxyclozanide is distributed to the liver, kidney, and intestines and is excreted in bile. A higher dose is required for treatment of immature stages. **Rafoxanide** is effective against adult and immature flukes, and also against the sheep nasal bot, *Oestrus ovis*.

CLOSANTEL

Indications. Immature and adult *Fasciola*, nasal bot, and *Haemonchus* in sheep
Dose. *Sheep*: 10 mg/kg

PML **Flukiver**™ (Janssen)
Oral suspension, closantel 50 mg/mL, for *sheep*; 2.5 litres
Withdrawal Periods. *Sheep*: slaughter 28 days, milk from treated animals should not be used for human consumption or manufacturing purposes

DIAMPHENETHIDE

Indications. Immature and adult *Fasciola* in sheep
Warnings. Overdosage may cause transient impairment of vision and loss of wool
Dose. *Sheep*: 105 mg/kg

PML **Coriban**™ (Coopers Pitman-Moore)
Oral suspension, diamphenethide 180 mg/mL, for *sheep*; 2.5 litres
Withdrawal Periods. *Sheep*: slaughter 7 days

NITROXYNIL

Indications. Immature and adult *Fasciola* and *Haemonchus* (2.1.1.6) in ruminants; gapeworms in game birds
Side-effects. Solution may stain wool if accidental spillage occurs
Dose. *Cattle*: by subcutaneous injection, 10 mg/kg
Sheep: by subcutaneous injection, 10 mg/kg
Acute fascioliasis, up to 15 mg/kg
Game birds: by addition to drinking water, 24 mg/kg

PML **Gapex**™ (Connan & Wise)
Oral liquid, nitroxynil 200 mg/mL, for *pheasants and red-legged partridges of 3-17 weeks of age*; 60 mL
Withdrawal Periods. *Game birds*: slaughter 30 days

PML **Trodax**™ **20%** (RMB)
Injection, nitroxynil 200 mg/mL, for *sheep*; 250 mL
Withdrawal Periods. *Sheep*: slaughter 30 days

PML **Trodax**™ **34%** (RMB)
Injection, nitroxynil 340 mg/mL, for *cattle, sheep*; 100 mL, 250 mL, 1 litre

Withdrawal Periods. *Cattle*: slaughter 30 days, milk from treated animals should not be used for human consumption. *Sheep*: slaughter 30 days

OXYCLOZANIDE

Indications. Adult *Fasciola* and tapeworms (2.1.2) in ruminants; immature *Fasciola* in sheep
Side-effects. Occasional loose stools and inappetance in cattle
Dose. *Cattle*: 10 mg/kg
Sheep: 15 mg/kg
Acute fascioliasis, 45 mg/kg
Goats: 15 mg/kg

PML **Zanil**™ **Fluke Drench** (Coopers Pitman-Moore)
Oral suspension, oxyclozanide 34 mg/mL, for *cattle, sheep, goats*; 5 litres, 10 litres
Withdrawal Periods. *Cattle, sheep, goats*: slaughter 14 days

RAFOXANIDE

Indications. Immature and adult *Fasciola* in ruminants; sheep nasal bot
Dose. *Cattle*: by mouth, 7.5 mg/kg; by subcutaneous injection, 3 mg/kg
Sheep: 7.5 mg/kg

PML **Flukanide**™ (MSD Agvet)
Oral suspension, rafoxanide 30 mg/mL, for *cattle, sheep*; 5 litres
Withdrawal Periods. *Cattle*: slaughter 28 days, milk from treated animals should not be used for human consumption or for manufacturing purposes. *Sheep*: slaughter 28 days
Injection, rafoxanide 75 mg/mL, for *cattle*; 500 mL
Withdrawal Periods. *Cattle*: slaughter 21 days, milk from treated animals should not be used for human consumption or for manufacturing purposes

PML **Flukol**™ (Young's)
Oral suspension, rafoxanide 37.5 mg, hydrated cobalt sulphate 18 mg, hydrated sodium selenate 1.9 mg/mL, for *cattle, sheep*; 5 litres
Withdrawal Periods. *Cattle, sheep*: slaughter 28 days, milk from treated animals should not be used for human consumption

TRICLABENDAZOLE

Indications. Immature and adult *Fasciola* in horses◆ and ruminants
Dose. *Horses◆, cattle*: 12 mg/kg
Sheep: 10 mg/kg

PML **Fasinex™ 5%** (Ciba-Geigy)
Oral suspension, triclabendazole 50 mg/mL, for *sheep*; 2.5 litres, 5 litres
Withdrawal Periods. *Sheep*: slaughter 28 days, milk from treated animals should not be used for human consumption

PML **Fasinex™ 10%** (Ciba-Geigy)
Oral suspension, triclabendazole 100 mg/mL, for *cattle*; 2.5 litres
Withdrawal Periods. *Cattle*: slaughter 28 days, milk from animals treated within 7 days of calving and during lactation should not be used for human consumption

2.1.4 Compound endoparasiticides

Multiple parasitisms are the rule rather than the exception in domesticated animals. Many preparations are combinations of drugs with complementary properties to attain an extended range of activity. For example, most combination endoparasiticide preparations for ruminants include a fasciolicide. See sections 2.1.1 to 2.1.3 for specific drug information. **Brotianide** and **clorsulon** are only available in compound preparations effective against fluke infections. **Methyridine** is available in a compound preparation for the treatment of roundworms in pigeons.

Many parasitic infections are seasonal and the prescriber should consider if it is pharmacologically sound to use a compound preparation at a time of year when one ingredient is redundant.

Oral preparations

PML **Benafox™** (Young's)
Oral suspension, oxibendazole 50 mg, rafoxanide 37.5 mg, hydrated cobalt sulphate 18 mg, hydrated sodium selenate 1.9 mg/mL, for roundworms and flukes in *cattle*, roundworms, flukes, and nasal bots in *sheep*; 2.5 litres
Withdrawal Periods. *Cattle, sheep*: slaughter 28 days, milk from treated animals should not be used for human consumption
Dose. *Cattle, sheep*: 0.2 mL/kg

PML **Drontal™ Plus** (Bayer)
Tablets, febantel 150 mg, praziquantel 50 mg, pyrantel embonate 144 mg, for roundworms and tapeworms in *dogs*; 2, 20
Dose. *Dogs*: 1 tablet/10 kg

PML **Duospec™** (C-Vet)
Oral suspension, oxibendazole 50 mg, rafoxanide 37.5 mg, hydrated cobalt sulphate 18 mg, hydrated sodium selenate 1.9 mg/mL, for roundworms and flukes in *cattle, sheep*; 1 litre, 2.5 litres
Withdrawal Periods. *Cattle*: slaughter 28 days, milk from treated animals should not be used for human consumption. *Sheep*: slaughter 28 days
Dose. *Cattle, sheep*: 0.2 mL/kg

PML **Flukombin™** (Bayer)
Oral suspension, brotianide 22.5 mg, thiophanate 200 mg/mL, for roundworms and flukes in *sheep*; 1 litre, 2.5 litre, 5 litres
Withdrawal Periods. *Sheep*: slaughter 21 days
Dose. *Sheep*: 0.25 mL/kg

PML **Levadox™** (Univet)
Oral suspension, levamisole hydrochloride 15 mg, oxyclozanide 30 mg/mL, for roundworms and flukes in *cattle, sheep*; 5 litres
Withdrawal Periods. *Cattle*: slaughter 12 days, milk 36 hours. *Sheep*: slaughter 15 days, milk from treated animals should not be used for human consumption
Dose. *Cattle, sheep*: 0.5 mL/kg

PML **Levafas™** (Norbrook)
Oral suspension, levamisole hydrochloride 15 mg, oxyclozanide 30 mg/mL, for roundworms and flukes in *cattle, sheep*; 1 litre, 2.5 litres, other sizes available
Withdrawal Periods. *Cattle*: slaughter 14 days, milk 36 hours. *Sheep*: slaughter 14 days
Dose. *Cattle, sheep*: 0.5 mL/kg

PML **Levafas™ Diamond** (Norbrook)
Oral suspension, levamisole hydrochloride 30 mg, oxyclozanide 60 mg/mL, for roundworms and flukes in *cattle, sheep*; 1 litre, 2.5 litres, 5 litres

Withdrawal Periods. *Cattle*: slaughter 14 days, milk 36 hours. *Sheep*: slaughter 14 days, milk from treated animals should not be used for for human consumption
Dose. *Cattle, sheep*: 0.25 mL/kg

PML **Nilzan**™ **Drench** (Coopers Pitman-Moore)
Oral suspension, levamisole hydrochloride 15 mg, oxyclozanide 30 mg/mL, for roundworms and flukes in *cattle*, *goats*, roundworms, tapeworms, and flukes in *sheep*; 2 litres, 10 litres
Withdrawal Periods. *Cattle, sheep, goats*: slaughter 14 days, milk 24 hours
Dose. *Cattle, sheep, goats*: 0.5 mL/kg (maximum dose–*cattle*: 150 mL; *sheep, goats*: 35 mL)

PML **Nilzan**™ **Drench Super** (Coopers Pitman-Moore)
Oral suspension, levamisole hydrochloride 30 mg, oxyclozanide 60 mg, cobalt sulphate heptahydrate 7.64 mg, sodium selenate 766 micrograms/mL, for roundworms and flukes in *cattle*, *goats*, roundworms, tapeworms, and flukes in *sheep*; 1 litre, 2.5 litres, 5 litres
Withdrawal Periods. *Cattle, sheep, goats*: slaughter 14 days, milk 24 hours
Dose. *Cattle, sheep, goats*: 0.25 mL/kg (maximum dose–*cattle*: 75 mL; *sheep, goats*: 17.5 mL)

PML **Nilzan**™ **Gold** (Coopers Pitman-Moore)
Oral suspension, levamisole hydrochloride 30 mg, oxyclozanide 60 mg/mL, for roundworms and flukes in *cattle*, *goats*, roundworms, tapeworms, and flukes in *sheep*; 1 litre, 2.5 litres, 5 litres
Withdrawal Periods. *Cattle, sheep, goats*: slaughter 14 days, milk 24 hours
Dose. *Cattle, sheep, goats*: 0.25 mL/kg maximum dose–*cattle*: 75 mL; *sheep, goats*: 17.5 mL)

PML **Nilzan**™ **In-Feed** (Coopers Pitman-Moore)
Oral granules, for addition to feed, levamisole hydrochloride 25 mg, oxyclozanide 50 mg/g, for roundworms and flukes in *cattle*, roundworms, tapeworms, and flukes in *sheep*; 3 kg
Withdrawal Periods. *Cattle, sheep*: slaughter 14 days, milk 24 hours
Dose. *Cattle, sheep*: 300 mg Nilzan™ In-Feed/kg body-weight (maximum dose–*cattle*: 90 g; *sheep*: 15 g)

PML **Ranizole**™ (MSD Agvet)
Oral suspension, rafoxanide 30 mg, thiabendazole 176 mg/mL, for roundworms and flukes in *cattle*, roundworms, tapeworms, and nasal bots in *sheep*; 1 litre, 5 litres, 10 litres
Withdrawal Periods. *Cattle*: slaughter 28 days, milk from treated animals should not be used for human consumption.
Sheep: slaughter 28 days
Dose. *Cattle*: 0.38 mL/kg
Sheep: 0.25 mL/kg

PML **Supaverm**™ (Janssen)
Oral suspension, closantel 50 mg, mebendazole 75 mg/mL, for roundworms, tapeworms, flukes, and nasal bots in *sheep*; 2.5 litres, 5 litres
Withdrawal Periods. *Sheep*: slaughter 28 days, milk from treated animals should not be used for human consumption or for manufacturing purposes
Dose. *Sheep*: 0.2 mL/kg

PML **Systamex**™ **Plus Fluke** (Coopers Pitman-Moore)
Oral suspension, oxfendazole 22.65 mg, oxyclozanide 62.5 mg/mL, for roundworms, tapeworms, and flukes in *cattle*, *sheep*; 1 litre, 2.5 litres, 10 litres
Withdrawal Periods. *Cattle*: slaughter 14 days, milk 5 days. *Sheep*: slaughter 14 days, milk from treated animals should not be used for human consumption
Dose. *Cattle*: 0.2 mL/kg
Sheep: 0.22 mL/kg

PML **Vermadex**™ (RMB)
Oral suspension, brotianide 22.5 mg, thiophanate 200 mg/mL, for roundworms and flukes in *sheep*; 1 litre, 2.5 litres, 5 litres
Withdrawal Periods. *Sheep*: slaughter 21 days
Dose. *Sheep*: 0.25 mL/kg

PML **Vermofas**™ (Bimeda)
Oral suspension, levamisole hydrochloride 15 mg, oxyclozanide 30 mg/mL, for roundworms and flukes in *cattle*, *sheep*; 2.5 litres, 4.5 litres
Withdrawal Periods. *Cattle*: slaughter 12 days, milk 36 hours. *Sheep*: slaughter 15 days, milk from treated animals should not be used for human consumption
Dose. *Cattle, sheep*: 0.5 mL/kg

PML **Wormaway Levamisole Oxyclozanide Drench™** (Deosan)
Oral suspension, levamisole hydrochloride 15 mg, oxyclozanide 30 mg/mL, for roundworms, tapeworms, and flukes in *cattle, sheep*; 2.5 litres, 5 litres, 10 litres
Withdrawal Periods. *Cattle*: slaughter 12 days, milk 36 hours. *Sheep*: slaughter 15 days, milk from treated animals should not be used for human consumption
Dose. *Cattle*: 0.5 mL/kg (maximum dose 150 mL)
Sheep: 0.5 mL/kg (maximum dose 35 mL)
Parenteral preparations

PML **Ivomec-F™** (MSD Agvet)
Injection, clorsulon 100 mg, ivermectin 10 mg/mL, for roundworms, flukes, lice, mites, and warble fly larvae in *cattle*; 50 mL, 200 mL, 500 mL
Withdrawal Periods. *Cattle*: slaughter 28 days, milk from animals treated within 28 days before calving and during lactation should not be used for human consumption
Dose. *Cattle*: by subcutaneous injection, 0.02 mL/kg

2.2 Ectoparasiticides

2.2.1 Systemic ectoparasiticides
2.2.2 Topical ectoparasiticides
2.2.3 Sheep dips
2.2.4 Bands, collars, and tags
Ectoparasite challenge may be predicted: for example, a rise in tick population in the spring and autumn, increased numbers of blowfly in late spring and early summer, warble fly oviposition from May to July, and the possible increase of lice on winter-housed stock. Therefore, strategic therapeutic and propylactic use of ectoparasiticides can be employed. In contrast, parasitism of intensively housed stock or companion animals where transmission is by contact is not 'seasonal' and requires diagnosis as infestations may go unnoticed for some time. In these situations, control measures should be included in routine hygiene programmes treating the animal and, where necessary, the housing.

The sheep scab mite, *Psoroptes ovis*, is the most economically important ectoparasite that occurs in *sheep* and has been the subject of a controlled compulsory dipping programme issued by MAFF but its continuation is now under review. The programme had been re-established in an attempt to eradicate the disease, again, from the UK. These mites, like *Chorioptes* suck lymph by piercing the epidermis, causing crust formation. Wool is pulled out by scratching or biting or simply falls out. This is a continuous process as scab mites migrate away from the initial infective foci. Death can result from scab mite infestations. These organisms are most prevalent in autumn and winter.

'Seasonal' parasites of sheep include *Ixodes ricinus* and myiasis larvae of the family *Calliphoridae*. The life-cycle of the sheep tick may extend over 3 years and the location of flocks in the UK is important when considering challenge and treatment. It is generally considered that ticks feed from March until June in north-east England and north-east Scotland but in Wales, Ireland, Cumbria, and western Scotland and western England there appears a tendency to feed also between August and November. Ticks are blood feeders and may transmit louping-ill virus or rickettsial tick-borne fever, affecting young lambs and cattle (see below). Treatment just before the tick population rise is advocated with additional treatments according to the duration of challenge. Lambs should initially be treated twice at an interval of 3 weeks. Calliphorine myiasis of sheep may be complex and an initial strike may lead to further strikes and result in large wounds. Struck sheep have identifiable characteristics and odour. Feed intake is reduced and their condition deteriorate leading to reduced meat, milk, and fleece production. The use of insecticides immediately before fly challenge and certainly during peak challenge in late spring and early summer is advised. Clipping wool from the area around the tail and breech can help reduce fly strike in this area.

The adult muscid *Hydrotoea irritans* is not a biting fly but the female can abrade skin and the fly does cause worry to **cattle**, **sheep**, and **goats** by feeding on ocular and nasal secretions. Skin lesions, weight loss, and mastitis may result. Treatment should be anticipated for peak activity in July and August.

Melophagus ovinus, the sheep ked, lives in the wool and feeds by sucking blood; heavy infestations may cause anaemia. Generally production loss is associated with irritation leading to wool damage and staining. Sucking lice lead to body fluid losses and biting lice to wool damage. Lice and keds are controlled by ectoparasiticides used for fly, tick, and scab control and generally do not need specific treatment unless identified as a major problem.

Cattle are also susceptible to mites belonging to the principal families that parasitise sheep, resulting in production losses. *Sarcoptes* infestations are uncommon. *Chorioptes bovis*, prevalent in winter, spreads over the body from the base of the tail.

Ixodes species also affect cattle and transmit babesiosis and anaplasmosis. Although challenge can be anticipated, the persistence of many ectoparasiticides on hair is less than on wool. Therefore repeat treatments may be required on cattle depending on the level of challenge.

Larvae of *Hypoderma bovis* and *Hypoderma lineatum* penetrate rapidly into the animal and migrate towards the diaphragm spending the winter months in the spinal canal or the oesophageal area. In the following year the mature larvae locate in the back forming a perforated 'warble', which ultimately downgrades the hide. *Hypoderma* is now almost totally eradicated from the UK. Traditionally, treatment is in the autumn when lice may also be controlled. Systemic organophosphorus parasiticides should not be used from December to March due to the location of the parasite within the animal's body.

The **horse** is also susceptible to many of the flies, lice, and mites discussed above. *Culicoides* causes sweet itch, a dermatitis resulting from hypersensitivity to midge bites. Treatment is usually in summer.

Bots, larvae of several species of the genus *Gasterophilus*, are almost exclusively limited to equines. Larvae penetrate the mucosa of the mouth and migrate to attach to the gastro-intestinal tract where they remain for several months. The infection cannot be diagnosed once the larvae are located in the stomach or intestines but areas around the mouth may be examined for parasite eggs and the pharynx for larvae. Treatment of larvae in the stomach is traditionally given twice yearly, initially after adult fly activity has ceased and during late winter. Insecticides applied in warm water may be used for prophylaxis; eggs are encouraged to hatch and the drug then kills the larvae.

There are 2 main ectoparasites of intensively housed **pigs**, the burrowing mange mite *Sarcoptes scabei* var *suis* and the sucking louse *Haematopinus suis*. Both parasites cause tissue damage with loss of body fluids, restlessness, rubbing, and scratching with consequent skin abrasion and hair loss. This can adversely affect production efficiency in growing stock and cause erratic suckling patterns in nursing sows.

Ideally the ectoparasiticides used should control both mange and lice. If no parasite control programme has been used before, or has been allowed to lapse, the whole herd should be treated using a therapeutic regimen. Prophylactic therapy includes treatment of sows as they enter the farrowing house, young pigs at weaning, and boars every 2 to 3 months. All new additions to the herd should be isolated and treated before mixing with established stock. Empty premises should be disinfected.

Control of ectoparasiticides on **dogs** and **cats** is greatly dependent upon the diligence of the owner. Ticks, lice, and fleas may be noticed by the owner. Microscopic parasitic mites or allergic conditions due to ectoparasites are only initially apparent from the dermatological conditions they cause.

Ctenocephalides felis more commonly infects dogs and cats than *C. canis*. The parasite lays eggs in the animal's bedding and housing and only infests the animal's body to feed. Prophylactic measures may need to be carried out routinely throughout the year depending on the degree of challenge. Lice are considered more prevalent on dogs than cats. Ticks (*Ixodes* species) may be found on dogs that are exercised in infected woodland or open areas.

Localised or generalised demodectic mange, transmitted by contact, is severely traumatic to the dog. Sarcoptic mange also occurs in the dog. Other mites infesting companion animals includes notoedric mange, which principally affects cat's ears but may be generalised, and otodectic mange, which affects aural areas of both dogs and cats. It is important to choose an ectoparasiticide that is indicated for use in cats as some drugs, such as benzyl benzoate, are contra-indicated in this species (see Prescribing for dogs and cats).

Common ectoparasites infesting poultry in the UK include poultry red mite *Dermanyssus gallinae*, northern fowl mite *Ornithonyssus*, and the soft tick *Argas persicus*. Since most production involving poultry for meat or eggs is intensive, there is an opportunity to disinfect either broiler houses or laying houses when they are cleared at the end of each batch of birds. Lice and mites affect pigeons, and lofts should be routinely treated.

Table 2.2 outlines drugs that are effective against common ectoparasitic infections in horses, ruminants, pigs, dogs, cats, poultry, and pigeons. Ectoparasiticides are available for application by various methods including by dip, spray, 'pour-on', dusting powder, collar, and tag. Different formulations of a preparation may be indicated for different parasites.

2.2.1 Systemic ectoparasiticides

2.2.1.1 Avermectins
2.2.1.2 Organophosphorus compounds

Ectoparasiticides are available that act systemically and may be given by injection or applied by the 'pour-on' technique such that a solution of the drug is poured along the animal's dorsal midline. Some of the applied drug is absorbed percutaneously and taken up into the circulatory system.

2.2.1.1 AVERMECTINS

Ivermectin is a broad-spectrum drug used mainly as an endoparasiticide in horses, ruminants, and pigs (see section 2.1.1.1). Ivermectin is carried to all parts of the body in the circulation and therefore mange mites and sucking lice are also controlled. Its spectrum of activity includes the parasitic stage of warbles.

IVERMECTIN

See sections 2.1.1.1 and 2.1.4 for preparation details

Parasiticides may be toxic to animals and the operator. Care should be taken with dosage and handling of the product. The recommendations for storage, use, and disposal of unused materials and containers should be followed. For guidance and information, see:

- MAFF/HSC. *Pesticides: code of practice for the safe use of pesticides on farms and holdings*. London: HMSO, 1990
- *The safe storage and handling of animal medicines*. 2nd ed. NOAH, 1990
- Control of Substances Hazardous to Health (COSHH) Regulation 1988.

2.2.1.2 ORGANOPHOSPHORUS COMPOUNDS

Cythioate is an orally administered organophosphorus compound. Organophosphorus compounds inhibit cholinesterase, thereby interfering with neuromuscular transmission in the ecto parasite. Cythioate is absorbed from the gastro-intestinal tract within 2 to 3 hours of administration. Ectoparasites are killed when they ingest body fluid containing cythioate. The drug persists in the circulation for about 8 hours. Therefore, repeated treatments are necessary.

Phosmet is a systemically acting organophosphorus compound. It is applied b

Table 2.2 Drugs effective against common ectoparasitic infections†

	Parasite	Ectoparasiticides
HORSES		
Flies	*Haematobia*, *Hydrotoea*, *Musca*, *Stomoxys*	cypermethrin, pyrethrins
Biting midges	*Culicoides*	benzyl benzoate, permethrin
Lice	*Damalinia*, *Haematopinus*	carbaryl
Mites	*Chorioptes*, *Psoroptes*, *Sarcoptes*	pyrethrins
Horse bot	*Gasterophilus*	see section 2.1

RUMINANTS (Some preparations are not suitable for all ruminant species, please consult individual monographs)

	Parasite	Ectoparasiticides
Flies	*Haematobia*, *Hydrotoea*, *Morellia*, *Musca*, *Simulium*, *Stomoxys*	cypermethrin, deltamethrin, permethrin
Blowfly larvae	*Calliphora*, *Lucilia*	chlorfenvinphos, chlorpyrifos, coumaphos, cypermethrin, cyromazine, diazinon, propetamphos
Warble flies	*Hypoderma*	ivermectin, phosmet
Sheep keds	*Melophagus ovinus*	amitraz, chlorfenvinphos, chlorpyrifos, coumaphos, deltamethrin, diazinon, flumethrin, iodofenphos, propetamphos
Lice	*Damalinia*, *Haematopinus*, *Linognathus*, *Solenopotes*	amitraz, carbaryl, chlorfenvinphos, chlorpyrifos, coumaphos, cypermethrin, deltamethrin, diazinon, flumethrin, iodofenphos, ivermectin, permethrin, phosmet, propetamphos, pyrethrins
Mites	*Chorioptes*, *Sarcoptes*	amitraz, ivermectin, phosmet, pyrethrins
	Psoroptes (Sheep scab)	chlorfenvinphos+ diazinon, diazinon, flumethrin, propetamphos
Ticks	*Ixodes*, *Dermacentor*, *Haemaphysalis*, *Rhipicephalus*	amitraz, chlorfenvinphos, chlorpyrifos, coumaphos, cypermethrin, deltamethrin, diazinon, flumethrin, propetamphos
Sheep nasal bot	*Oestrus ovis*	see section 2.1

PIGS

	Parasite	Ectoparasiticides
Lice	*Haematopinus*	amitraz, carbaryl, coumaphos, deltamethrin, ivermectin, phosmet
Mites	*Sarcoptes*	amitraz, ivermectin, phosmet

DOGS and CATS (Some preparations are not suitable for both species, please consult individual monographs)

	Parasite	Ectoparasiticides
Fleas	*Ctenocephalides*	carbaryl, cythioate, diazinon, permethrin, phosmet, propoxur, pyrethrins

Table 2.2 Drugs effective against common ectoparasitic infections† (continued)

	Parasite	Ectoparasiticides
Lice	Felicola, Trichodectes	carbaryl, pyrethrins
Mites	Demodex (dogs)	amitraz, cythioate, rotenone
	Sarcoptes (dogs)	phosmet, piperonyl butoxide, pyrethrins
	Notoedres (cats)	piperonyl butoxide
	Otodectes, Cheyletiella, Pneumonyssus, Trombicula	piperonyl butoxide
Ticks	Ixodes, Rhipicephalus	carbaryl, cythioate, diazinon, permethrin, phosmet, pyrethrin
POULTRY		
Lice	Goniodes, Menopon, Menacanthus	carbaryl
Mites	Cnemidocoptes, Dermanyssus, Ornithonyssus, Trombicula	cypermethrin
PIGEONS		
Lice	Columbicola	preparations containing bromocyclen
Mites	Falculifer, Cnemidocoptes Dermanyssus	are now discontinued

† Some drugs are only available as a constituent of a compound preparation. See sections 2.2.2.4 and 2.2.2.5 for indications for compound preparations

the 'pour-on' method as described above and is used to control lice, mites, and warble fly larvae. Treatment in cattle should not be carried out between December and March because larvae are in the spinal cord and oesophageal area during this period and destruction of the parasites may cause side-effects.

CYTHIOATE

Indications. Fleas, *Demodex*, and ticks on dogs; fleas on cats
Contra-indications. Manufacturer does not recommend use in pregnant, sick, or stressed animals
Dose. *Dogs*: fleas, ticks, 3 mg/kg twice weekly for 4 weeks. Repeat every other week to control re-infestation
Demodex, 3 mg/kg twice weekly for at least 6 weeks (maximum 24 weeks)
Cats: fleas, 1.5 mg/kg as a single dose, repeat every 7 days for 4 weeks. Repeat every other week to control re-infestation

ᴾ**Cyflee**™ (Cyanamid)
Tablets, scored, cythioate 30 mg, for *dogs, cats*; 25

PHOSMET

Indications. Warble-fly larvae in cattle lice and mites on cattle, and pigs; fleas *Sarcoptes*, and ticks on dogs
Contra-indications. Calves under : months of age. Treatment within 14 day before or after other organophosphoru compounds or other anticholinesteras compounds (see Drug Interactions - Appendix 1), levamisole, or diethyl carbamazine citrate. Treatment betwee December 1 and March 14 in cattle, se notes above
Dose. *Cattle*: by 'pour-on' application. Lice, 10 mg/kg, repeat after 10-14 day Mites and warble-fly larvae, 20 mg/k as a single dose
Pigs: by 'pour-on' application, 20 mg/k as a single dose
Dogs: by sponge application of 0.09⁹ solution, repeat after 16 days if require

PML **Dermol Plus™** (Crown)
Solution, 'pour-on', phosmet 200 mg/
mL, for *cattle*; 1 litre, 2.5 litres
Withdrawal Periods. *Cattle*: slaughter 14
days, milk 6 hours

PML **Nupor™** (C-Vet)
Solution, 'pour-on', phosmet 200 mg/
mL, for *cattle*; 500 mL
Withdrawal Periods. *Cattle*: slaughter 14
days, milk 6 hours

PML **Porect™** (SmithKline Beecham)
Solution, 'pour-on', phosmet 200 mg/
mL, for *pigs*; 500 mL, 1 litre
Withdrawal Periods. *Pigs*: slaughter 28
days

PML **Poron™ 20** (Young's)
Solution, 'pour-on', phosmet 200 mg/
mL, for *cattle*; 1 litre, 2.5 litres
Withdrawal Periods. *Cattle*: slaughter 14
days, milk 6 hours

PoM **Vet-Kem Prolate™** (BK)
Liquid concentrate, phosmet 116 mg/
mL, for *dogs*; 100 mL, 1 litre. To be
diluted before use
Dilute 1 volume in 127 volumes water
(= phosmet 0.09%)

2.2.2 Topical ectoparasiticides

2.2.2.1 Amidines
2.2.2.2 Carbamates
2.2.2.3 Organochlorines
2.2.2.4 Organophosphorus compounds
2.2.2.5 Pyrethrins and synthetic
          pyrethroids
2.2.2.6 Other ectoparasiticides
2.2.2.7 Fly repellents
2.2.2.8 Environmental control of ecto-
          parasites

2.2.2.1 AMIDINES

Amitraz acts at octopamine receptor
sites in ectoparasites giving rise to
increased nervous activity. It is used for
ectoparasite control on cattle, sheep,
pigs, and dogs. There is no requirement
for removal of mange scabs before
treatment.
Idiosyncratic reactions have been
reported in chihuahuas, and amitraz-
containing preparations should not be
used on dogs in heat stress. Amitraz
may cause colic in horses.

AMITRAZ

Indications. Lice, mites, and ticks on
cattle; keds, lice, and ticks on sheep
(see section 2.2.3.1 for use by dip); lice
and mites on pigs; *Demodex* on dogs
Contra-indications. Manufacturer does
not recommend use on horses, Chihuahuas, cats, or dogs in heat stress
Side-effects. Overdosage may cause
transient somnolence or sedation; recovery is spontaneous
Warnings. Maintenance therapy may be
required in immunosuppressed dogs
Dose. *Cattle*: *by spray*, 0.025% solution
Pigs: *by spray*, 0.05% solution; *by
'pour-on' application*, (180-240 kg body-
weight) 60 mL (dorsal midline), and
5 mL into each ear of 2% solution, (100-
180 kg body-weight) 40 mL (dorsal
midline), and 5 mL into each ear of 2%
solution
Dogs: *by wash*, 0.05% solution

PoM **Derasect™ Demodectic Mange Wash**
(SmithKline Beecham)
Liquid concentrate, amitraz 5%, for
dogs; 50 mL. To be diluted before use
Dilute 1 volume in 100 volumes water
(= amitraz 0.05%)

PML **Taktic™** (SmithKline Beecham)
Liquid or dip concentrate, amitraz
12.5%, for *cattle*, *sheep* (2.2.3.1), *pigs*;
1 litre, 5 litres. To be diluted before use
Withdrawal Periods. *Cattle*: slaughter
1 day, milk withdrawal period nil. *Sheep*:
slaughter 7 days, milk withdrawal period
nil. *Pigs*: slaughter 1 day
Dilute 1 volume in 250 volumes water
(= amitraz 0.05%) for *pigs*
Dilute 1 volume in 500 volumes water
(= amitraz 0.025%) for *cattle*

PML **Taktic Topline™** (SmithKline
Beecham)
Solution, 'pour-on', amitraz 2%, for
pigs; 3 litres
Withdrawal Periods. *Pigs*: slaughter
7 days

2.2.2.2 CARBAMATES

Carbaryl and **propoxur** are carbamates.
They cause inhibition of cholinesterase
at the parasite nerve synapses but with

less affinity than organophosphorus compounds.

Carbaryl and propoxur are used for flea and lice control.

Parasiticides may be toxic to animals and the operator. Care should be taken with dosage and handling of the product. The recommendations for storage, use, and disposal of unused materials and containers should be followed. For guidance and information, see:

● MAFF/HSC. *Pesticides: code of practice for the safe use of pesticides on farms and holdings*. London: HMSO, 1990
● *The safe storage and handling of animal medicines*. 2nd ed. NOAH, 1990
● Control of Substances Hazardous to Health (COSHH) Regulation 1988.

CARBARYL

Indications. Lice on horses, cattle, pigs, and poultry; fleas, ticks, and lice on dogs; fleas on cats
Contra-indications. Puppies or kittens less than 4 weeks of age; pregnant animals

GSL **Derasect™ Insecticidal and Conditioning Shampoo** (SmithKline Beecham)
Carbaryl 0.5%, for *dogs, cats*; 175 mL

GSL **Ruby Farmyard Louse Powder** (Spencer)
Dusting powder, carbaryl 2%, for *horses, cattle, pigs, poultry*; 200 g
Dose. *Horses, cattle*: 110 g of powder (= carbaryl 1.1 g)
Pigs: 85 g of powder (= carbaryl 850 mg)
Poultry: 10 g of powder (= carbaryl 100 mg)

GSL **Vet-Kem™ Flea and Tick Powder** (BK)
Dusting powder, carbaryl 5%, for *dogs*; 140 g

PROPOXUR

Indications. Fleas on dogs and cats
Contra-indications. Concurrent use of other insecticides

PML **Negasunt™** (Bayer)
See section 14.2.1 for preparation details

GSL **Vet-Kem™ Pet Spray** (BK)
Aerosol spray, propoxur 0.25%, for *dogs, cats*; 275 g

2.2.2.3 ORGANOCHLORINES

Organochlorines act as contact poisons, causing stimulation of the parasite nervous system leading to incoordination. They are poorly soluble in water but soluble in oils or organic solvents. When applied as a powder or aqueous solution, organochlorines penetrate the cuticle of insects more readily than skin or intestinal mucosae of animals and therefore are more toxic to insects.

Animals may be poisoned by organochlorines by inhalation of the drug as it slowly vaporises from the skin surface; absorption of the drug, in an oil-basis, through intact skin; or ingestion of spilled preparation or contaminated feed. The drug accumulates and persists in adipose tissue within the body. It is metabolised slowly in the liver and excreted in the urine, bile, faeces, and milk. Drug residues may be found in milk, eggs, and meat for many months or even years after ingestion, depending on the age of the animal, the species, the amount of fatty tissue, and the dose received.

Clinical signs of acute toxicity are of nonspecific stimulation of the CNS. There is no specific antidote for organochlorine poisoning (see Emergency treatment of poisoning).

Organochlorines degrade slowly in the environment because they are resistant to decomposition by chemicals or micro organisms. They may be taken up by foliage and the waxy coating of plants can retain the drug.

The use of organochlorines on animals is now limited or banned in most countries due to their toxicity in animals and persistence in the environment and food chain.

Bromocyclen has been shown to be effective against many ectoparasites but not *Demodex* mites causing mange in dogs.

Lindane (gamma benzene hexachloride) is no longer permitted for use in sheep dipping programmes and is being withdrawn from other licensed preparations.

BROMOCYCLEN

Indications. Lice and mites on horses, cattle, pigs, and pigeons; blowfly larvae, keds, and mites on sheep; fleas, lice, *Otodectes*, and *Sarcoptes* on dogs and foxes; mites on cats, ferrets, mink, cage birds, and laboratory animals

PML **Alugan**™ (Hoechst)
This preparation is now discontinued

LINDANE
(Gamma benzene hexachloride)

Indications. Lice on horses, cattle, sheep, pigs, dogs, and poultry
Contra-indications. Calves, turkey poults less than 3 months of age
Side-effects. Overdose may cause convulsions, muscle tremors and respiratory failure; young animals can be sensitive
Warnings. Caution with use in cats, cage birds, and poultry and with use immediately before roosting

PML **Louse Powder** (Crown)
Dusting powder, lindane 1.1%, for *horses, cattle, pigs, poultry*; 850 g, 2.5 kg, other sizes available
Withdrawal Periods. *Cattle*: milk from treated animals should not be used for human consumption

GSL **Quellada**™ **Veterinary Shampoo** (Stafford-Miller)
Lindane 1%, for *dogs, cats*; 100 mL, 500 mL
Contra-indications. Kittens
Warnings. Care with use on cats

2.2.2.4 ORGANOPHOSPHORUS COMPOUNDS

Organophosphorus compounds inhibit cholinesterase, thereby interfering with neuromuscular transmission in the ectoparasite.
Overdosage or overexposure to organophosphorus compounds in animals and humans is characterised by abdominal pain, diarrhoea, salivation, muscular tremors, and pupil constriction. Death may occur from respiratory failure. Acetylcholine accumulates at muscarinic and nicotinic receptors, which are subsequently overstimulated. Treatment is aimed at inhibiting the effect of acetylcholine with the competitive antagonist, atropine (see Emergency treatment of poisoning).
Operators should take care when handling or using preparations containing organophosphorus compounds. Protective clothing such as gloves and bib-apron should be worn. Care should be taken to avoid inhalation of powder or spray and any skin contamination should be washed off immediately.
Although most organophosphorus compounds are not persistent in the environment, they may be toxic to humans, livestock, and wildlife, and adequate precautions should be taken to avoid environmental contamination.

CHLORFENVINPHOS

Indications. Blowfly larvae, keds, lice, and ticks on sheep (see section 2.2.3.3 for use by dip)

PML **Fly Dip** (Coopers Pitman-Moore)
See section 2.2.3.3 for preparation details

COUMAPHOS

Indications. Lice and ticks on cattle and goats; lice on pigs; blowfly larvae, keds, lice, and ticks on sheep (see section 2.2.3.3 for use by dip)
Warnings. Treatment should not be repeated until after 14 days

PML **Asuntol**™ (Bayer)
Liquid or dip concentrate, powder for reconstitution, coumaphos 50%, for *cattle, sheep* (2.2.3.3), *goats*; 230 g, 1.15 kg

Withdrawal Periods. *Cattle, sheep, goats*: slaughter 21 days

Note. Cattle, goats producing milk for human consumption should be treated immediately after milking

Spray. Reconstitute coumaphos 125 g (= 250 g of powder) in 227 litres water (= coumaphos 0.05%)

PML **Negasunt**™ (Bayer)
See section 14.2.1 for preparation details

DICHLORVOS

See Prescribing for fish for preparation details

COMPOUND ORGANOPHOSPHORUS COMPOUNDS

PML **Nuvan**™ **Top** (Ciba-Geigy)
Aerosol spray, dichlorvos 0.2%, fenitrothion 0.8%, for fleas, flies, lice, mites, and ticks on *dogs*, *cats*; 105 g

PML **Zeprox**™ (Coopers Pitman-Moore)
Aerosol spray, dichlorvos 0.2%, fenitrothion 0.8%, for fleas on *dogs*, *cats*; 138 g

---

2.2.2.5 PYRETHRINS AND SYNTHETIC PYRETHROIDS

Natural **pyrethrins** extracted from pyrethrum flowers and the synthetic pyrethroids **cypermethrin, deltamethrin,** and **permethrin** are used for control of biting and nuisance flies, and lice. They exert their action on the sodium channels of parasite nerve axons, causing paralysis. Pyrethrum extract, prepared from pyrethrum flower, contains about 25% of pyrethrins.

Cypermethrin is applied by spraying on horses, cattle, and poultry, or by 'pour-on' application on sheep and goats to the dorsal midline of the animal for control of ticks and lice. For headflies, the solution is applied to the top of the head between and around the base of the horns. For blowfly larvae it is applied directly to lesions.

Deltamethrin is applied to a single site on the dorsal midline behind the shoulders on cattle and pigs. When used for headflies on sheep, it is applied to the back of the poll of the head.

Permethrin is used on horses, cattle, dogs, and cats. For cattle, a 4% solution is applied by 'pour-on' application to the top of the head, and along the dorsal midline of the neck and back. Shampoos, dusting powders, and sprays containing permethrin 1% are used on dogs and cats.

CYPERMETHRIN

Indications. Flies on horses and cattle; lice on cattle and goats; blowfly larvae, biting lice, ticks, and headflies on sheep; red mites on poultry

Contra-indications. Treatment of lambs less than one week of age or during hot weather

Side-effects. 'Pour-on' preparations should not be applied to the tail region of lambs as this could interfere with ewe-lamb recognition

Warnings. Wash udders of sprayed animals before milking and apply only to unbroken lesions

Parasiticides may be toxic to animals and the operator. Care should be taken with dosage and handling of the product. The recommendations for storage, use, and disposal of unused materials and containers should be followed. For guidance and information, see:
- MAFF/HSC. *Pesticides: code of practice for the safe use of pesticides on farms and holdings*. London: HMSO, 1990
- *The safe storage and handling of animal medicines*. 2nd ed. NOAH, 1990
- Control of Substances Hazardous to Health (COSHH) Regulation 1988.

Dose. Horses: *by spray*, 0.1% solution using 125-500 mL per animal
Cattle: *by spray*, 0.1% solution, using 125-500 mL per animal; *by 'pour-on' application*, 10 mL of 5% solution
Sheep: *by 'pour-on' application*.
Blowfly larvae, 5-10 mL of 2.5% solution on affected area
Headflies, 5 mL of 2.5% solution
Lice, 6-12 mg/kg, using a 2.5% solution

Ticks, 12-25 mg/kg, using a 2.5%
solution
Goats: *by 'pour-on' application*, 6-12 mg/
kg using a 2.5% solution
Poultry: *by spray*, 0.05% solution, using
20 mL per bird

PML **Barricade**™ (Lever)
Liquid concentrate, cypermethrin 5%,
for *horses, cattle, poultry*; 1 litre. To be
diluted before use
Withdrawal Periods. *Horses, cattle*:
slaughter 2 days. *Poultry*: slaughter 14
days
Dilute 1 volume with 49 volumes water
(= cypermethrin 0.1%), using 500 mL
per adult animal for *horses, cattle*
Dilute 1 volume with 99 volumes water
(= cypermethrin 0.05%), using 20 mL
per bird for *poultry*

PML **Cypor**™ (Young's)
Solution, 'pour-on', cypermethrin 2.5%,
for *sheep, goats*; 500 mL, 2.5 litres
Withdrawal Periods. *Sheep, goats*:
slaughter 7 days
Note. Animals producing milk for
human consumption should be treated
immediately after milking and at least 6
hours before next milking

PML **Dy-Sect**™ (Deosan)
Liquid concentrate, cypermethrin 5%,
for *horses, cattle, poultry*; 1 litre. To be
diluted before use
Withdrawal Periods. *Cattle*: slaughter 2
days. *Poultry*: slaughter 14 days
Dilute 1 volume with 49 volumes water
(= cypermethrin 0.1%) for *horses, cattle*
Dilute 1 volume with 99 volumes water
(= cypermethrin 0.05%) for *poultry*

PML **Dy-Sect**™ 'Pour-on' (Deosan)
Solution, 'pour-on', cypermethrin 5%,
for *cattle*; 250 mL, 1 litre
Withdrawal Periods. *Cattle*: slaughter
14 days, milk withdrawal period nil

PML **Ovipor**™ (C-Vet)
Solution, 'pour-on', cypermethrin 2.5%,
for *sheep, goats*; 500 mL, 2.5 litres
Withdrawal Periods. *Sheep, goats*:
slaughter 7 days
Note. Animals producing milk for
human consumption should be treated
immediately after milking and at least 6
hours before next milking

PML **Parasol**™ (Ciba-Geigy)
Solution, 'pour-on', cypermethrin 2.5%,
for *sheep, goats*; 1 litre, 5 litres
Withdrawal Periods. *Sheep, goats*:
slaughter 7 days
Note. Animals producing milk for
human consumption should be treated
immediately after milking and at least 6
hours before next milking

DELTAMETHRIN

Indications. Lice on cattle, sheep, pigs;
flies on cattle; headflies, keds, and ticks
on sheep
Side-effects. Minor signs of discomfort
with some cattle up to 48 hours after
treatment
Dose. *Cattle*: by 'pour-on' application,
10 mL of 1% solution
Sheep, pigs: by 'pour-on' application,
5 mL of 1% solution

PML **Spot On Insecticide**™ (Coopers
Pitman-Moore)
Solution, 'pour-on', deltamethrin 1%,
for *cattle, sheep, pigs*; 250 mL, 1 litre
Withdrawal Periods. *Cattle, sheep*:
slaughter 3 days, milk withdrawal period
nil. *Pigs*: slaughter 7 days

PERMETHRIN

Indications. *Culicoides* on horses; flies
and lice on cattle; fleas on dogs and cats
Contra-indications. Treatment of calves
under one week of age
Side-effects. Cats may show signs of
hyperaesthesia with excitability, twitch-
ing, and collapse if overdosage occurs
Dose. See preparation details

GSL **Companion**™ **Insecticidal Shampoo**
(Battle Hayward & Bower)
Liquid concentrate, permethrin 1.05%,
for *dogs*; 240 mL. To be diluted before
use
Dilute 1 volume with 19 volumes water
(= permethrin 0.05%), using 1 litre per
animal

GSL **Head-To-Tail**™ **Flea Preparations**
(Coopers Pitman-Moore)
Dusting powder, permethrin 1.05%, for
dogs, cats; 85 g
Shampoo, permethrin 1.05%, for *dogs*;
100 mL

Aerosol spray, permethrin 1.05%, for *dogs, cats*; 180 g

PML **Ridect™** (SmithKline Beecham)
Solution, 'pour-on', permethrin 4%, for *cattle*; 1 litre
Withdrawal Periods. *Cattle*: slaughter 3 days, milk withdrawal period nil
Note. Animals producing milk for human consumption should be treated immediately after milking
Dose. *Cattle*: by 'pour-on' application, 0.1 mL/kg

PML **Ryposect™** (C-Vet)
Solution, 'pour-on', permethrin 4%, for *cattle*; 1 litre
Withdrawal Periods. *Cattle*: slaughter 3 days, milk withdrawal period nil
Note. Animals producing milk for human consumption should be treated immediately after milking and at least 6 hours before next milking
Dose. *Cattle*: by 'pour-on' application, 0.1 mL/kg

PML **Stomoxin™ Liquid Concentrate** (Coopers Pitman-Moore)
Permethrin 20%, for *horses, cattle*; 500 mL. To be diluted before use
By hand spray. Dilute 1 volume in 200 volumes water (= permethrin 0.1%), using 0.5-1.0 litre for *horses*, 250-500 mL for *cattle*
By spray arch. Dilute 1 volume in 400 volumes water (= permethrin 0.05%), using 1 litre per animal for *horses, cattle*

PML **Swift™** (Young's)
Solution, 'pour-on', permethrin 4%, for *cattle*; 1 litre
Withdrawal Periods. *Cattle*: slaughter 3 days, milk withdrawal period nil
Note. Animals producing milk for human consumption should be treated immediately after milking and at least 6 hours before next milking
Dose. *Cattle*: by 'pour-on' application, 0.1 mL/kg

PYRETHRINS

Indications. Flies and mites on horses; lice and mites on cattle; fleas, lice, mites and ticks on dogs and cats

Canovel Insecticidal Spray (SmithKline Beecham)
Aerosol spray, piperonyl butoxide 1%, pyrethrins 0.1%, for *dogs*; 165 mL

GSL **Dermoline™ Shampoo** (Day Son & Hewitt)
Liquid concentrate, piperonyl butoxide 0.08%, pyrethrum extract 0.04% (= 0.01% pyrethrins), for *horses, dogs*; 500 mL, 1 litre, other sizes available. To be diluted before use
Withdrawal Periods. Should not be used on *horses* intended for human consumption
Dilute 1 volume with 10 volumes water for initial cleansing

GSL **Extra Tail™** (Kalium)
Aerosol spray, diethyltoluamide 4.5%, piperonyl butoxide 0.6%, pyrethrins 0.075%, for *horses*; 200 mL
Liquid, diethyltoluamide 4.5%, piperonyl butoxide 0.6%, pyrethrins 0.075%, for *horses*; 250 mL, 500 mL, 1 litre

Radiol Insecticidal Shampoo (Fisons)
Shampoo, piperonyl butoxide 0.08%, pyrethrins 0.01%, ethoxylated lanolin 0.4%, methyl salicylate 0.1%; for *horses, dogs*; 500 mL

COMPOUND SYNTHETIC PYRETHROIDS

GSL **Willothrin™** (Willows Francis)
Aerosol spray, phenothrin 0.19%, tetramethrin 0.09%, for fleas on *dogs, cats*; 130 g

---

Parasiticides may be toxic to animals and the operator. Care should be taken with dosage and handling of the product. The recommendations for storage, use, and disposal of unused materials and containers should be followed. For guidance and information, see:

● MAFF/HSC. *Pesticides: code of practice for the safe use of pesticides on farms and holdings.* London: HMSO, 1990

● *The safe storage and handling of animal medicines.* 2nd ed. NOAH, 1990

● Control of Substances Hazardous to Health (COSHH) Regulation 1988.

2.2.2.6 OTHER ECTOPARASITICIDES

Benzyl benzoate is used for control of sweet itch caused by hypersensitivity to *Culicoides* midges. The mode of action of **cyromazine** involves the disruption of insect growth regulation. It is effective against blowfly larvae on sheep and lambs. The drug is applied before an anticipated challenge. Other drugs should be used to treat established myiasis.

Piperonyl butoxide inhibits the microsomal system of some arthropods and has been shown to be effective against some mites. It has a synergistic action on pyrethrins (see section 2.2.2.5). Rotenone is the main active ingredient present in the *Derris* plant.

BENZYL BENZOATE

Indications. *Culicoides* on horses
Contra-indications. Should not be used on cats

GSL **Killitch**™ (Cowie)
Lotion, benzyl benzoate 25%, for horses; 500 mL, 1 litre, 2.5 litres
Withdrawal Periods. Should not be used on **horses** intended for human consumption

GSL **Sweet Itch Plus**™ (Pettifer)
Liquid, benzyl benzoate 25%, for **horses**; 500 mL, 1 litre

CYROMAZINE

Indications. Blowfly larvae on sheep
Dose. *Sheep*: by *'pour-on' application*, 15-60 mL of 6% solution depending on body-weight

ML **Vetrazin**™ (Ciba-Geigy)
Solution, 'pour-on', cyromazine 6%, for **sheep**; 2.5 litres, 5 litres
Withdrawal Periods. *Sheep*: slaughter 3 days, milk from treated animals should not be used for human consumption

PIPERONYL BUTOXIDE

Indications. *Otodectes* and *Sarcoptes* on dogs; *Notoedres* and *Otodectes* on cats

PML **Head-to-Tail**™ **PB Dressing** (Coopers Pitman-Moore)
This preparation is now discontinued

ROTENONE

Indications. *Demodex* on dogs

PML **Head-to-Tail**™ **Demodectic Mange Dressing** (Coopers Pitman-Moore)
This preparation is now discontinued

2.2.2.7 FLY REPELLENTS

Citronella oil, diethyltoluamide, and **dimethyl phthalate** are the active ingredients of fly repellents. These preparations are used mainly in horses and cattle to reduce *Culicoides* attack and prevent worry by nuisance flies such as *Musca*.

PML **Banfly**™ (Arnolds)
Cream, amethocaine hydrochloride 0.5%, cetrimide 0.5%, citronella oil 0.25%; 454 g

GSL **Extra Tail**™ (Kalium)
Liquid, diethyltoluamide 10%, dimethyl phthalate 10%, citronella 3%; 250 mL, 500 mL, 1 litre

GSL **Fly Repellent** (Battle Hayward & Bower)
Aerosol spray, diethyltoluamide 2%, dimethyl phthalate 5%, for **horses, cattle**; 400 g
Liquid, diethyltoluamide 6.6%, dimethyl phthalate 16.6%, for **horses, cattle**; 500 mL

GSL **Fly Repellent Plus** (Coopers Pitman-Moore)
Liquid, citronellol 2%, permethrin 1.05%, for **horses**; 600 mL
Withdrawal Periods. Should not be used on **horses** intended for human consumption

Summer Fly Cream (Battle Hayward & Bower)
Diethyltoluamide 5%, for **sheep**; 400 g

2.2.2.8 ENVIRONMENTAL CONTROL OF ECTOPARASITES

These preparations are used to eradicate arthropods from an environment. They are used in poultry houses and refuse depots to control flies, in pigeon lofts to control mites, and in the home mainly to control fleas. Generally, **these preparations are not for use on animals**. Many preparations are available. This is not a comprehensive list.

Acclaim Plus™ Flea Control (Sanofi)
Aerosol spray, methoprene 0.18%, permethrin 0.567%; 340 g
Note. Not for use on animals

Alfacron™ 10WP (Ciba-Geigy)
Solution, powder for reconstitution, azamethipos 10%; 1 kg
Reconstitute 100 g azamethipos (1 kg powder) in 7.5 litres water
Note. Not for use on animals

Dermanol™ (Harkers)
Liquid concentrate, iodofenphos 50%; 100 mL. To be diluted before use
Dilute 100 mL in 9 litres water
Note. Not for use on animals

Durakil™ (Antec)
Solution, powder for reconstitution, fenitrothion 40%; 250 g
Reconstitute 100 g fenitrothion (250 g powder) in 10 litres water

Duramitex™ (Harkers)
Liquid concentrate, malathion 60%; 140 mL. To be diluted before use
Dilute 140 mL in 9 litres water
Note. Not for use on animals

Louse Powder (Battle Hayward & Bower)
Dusting powder, lindane 0.7%; 375 g, 850 g, other sizes available
Note. Not for use on animals

Microcarb™ (Micro-Biologicals)
Solution, powder for reconstitution; carbaryl 50%; 227 g
Reconstitute 227 g of powder in 27 litres water and apply with a knapsack sprayer
Note. Not for use on animals; **Scattercarb™** (Micro-Biologicals) dusting powder contains Microcarb™ 10%

Micromite™ (Micro-Biologicals)
Liquid concentrate, fenitrothion 50%; 5 litres. To be diluted before use
Dilute 1 volume in 50 volumes water
Note. Not for use on animals or eggs

Nuvan™ 500EC (Ciba-Geigy)
Liquid concentrate, dichlorvos 50%, 1 litre. To be diluted before use
Dilute with water according to manufacturer's instructions and apply by spray
Note. Not for use on animals

Nuvan™ Staykil (Ciba-Geigy)
Aerosol spray, dichlorvos 0.5%, iodofenphos 2.0%; 600 g
Note. Not for use on animals

Nuvanol™ N 500FW (Ciba-Geigy)
Liquid concentrate, iodofenphos 50%; 2 litres, 5 litres. To be diluted before use
Dilute with water according to manufacturer's instructions and apply by spray
Note. Not for use on animals

Super Fly Spray™ (Sorex)
Aerosol spray, phenothrin 0.25%, tetramethrin 0.1%; 450 mL
Note. Not for use on animals

PML**Taktic™** (SmithKline Beecham)
See section 2.2.2.1 for preparation details

Turbair™ Kilsect Super (Pan Brittanica)
Solution, bromophos 5%, resmethrin 0.3%; 1 litre
Note. Not for use on animals

Vet-Kem Siphotrol™ (BK)
Aerosol spray, methoprene 0.18%, permethrin 0.567%; 450 g
Note. Not for use on animals

2.2.3 Sheep dips

2.2.3.1 Amidines
2.2.3.2 Organochlorines
2.2.3.3 Organophosphorus compounds
2.2.3.4 Pyrethroids

Dipping is the most common method of applying an ectoparasiticide to sheep.
Dip management. Certain principles need to be followed to ensure the correct use of sheep dips, the most fundamental being to know the capacity of the dip bath.
The dipwash should be prepared according to the manufacturer's directions. The

dipwash should be stirred thoroughly before dipping and on each occasion when dipping is interrupted. Replenishment should be made using volume drop or head count. The dipwash depletion per animal depends upon the fleece length. The volume of the dipwash should not fall below 75% of original volume.

Attention should be paid to the prevention of post-dipping lameness caused by *Erysipelothrix rhusiopathiae*. The dip should be prepared in a clean bath and any surface residues removed at regular intervals. Excessively fouled dipwashes should be discarded and manufacturers may recommend limitation of the number of sheep dipped to one for each 2 litres of dipwash, after which the bath should be emptied and refilled with fresh dipwash. Alternatively, dip formulations may be bacteriostatic or bactericidal, or manufacturers may advise addition of a disinfectant or bacteriostat to the dipwash at the end of a day's dipping. Phenol, thiram, and copper sulphate are commonly used as disinfectants. The manufacturer's advice on the maximum length of time the dipwash can be used should be followed.

Dipping. To ensure a reasonable level of residual protection, sheep should have at least 3 weeks of wool growth before dipping. Extremes of weather should be avoided and dipping is inadvisable when it is raining or the sheep have wet fleeces. Also, sheep that are hot, tired, thirsty, or full of food should be allowed time to stabilise before dipping.

Where possible, lambs should be dipped separately from ewes with attention being paid to pair-up ewes and lambs after dipping. It is recommended that rams and fat sheep are dipped separately. Care should be taken to reduce immersion shock and to ensure that sheep do not swallow or inhale the dipwash.

When dipping for blowfly larvae, keds, lice, mange mites, and ticks, the body of the sheep should be kept immersed until the fleece is completely saturated with the wash. Thirty seconds should be sufficient. The head should be immersed at least twice allowing the animal to breathe between immersions.

Sheep should be allowed to drip in an open space, preferably in the shade, but not in an enclosed building.

In the UK, it has been compulsory to dip all sheep for the prevention of *sheep scab*. This policy may not continue and only flocks confirmed to be infected with sheep scab quarantined and dipped therapeutically. In compulsory dipping campaigns, MAFF authorises specifications on the time and frequency of dipping required. This may be once or twice yearly. In Britain, for the purposes of the Sheep Scab Order 1986, and in Northern Ireland, for the purpose of the Sheep Scab (Northern Ireland) Order 1970, sheep must be totally immersed in a sheep bath and all parts of the sheep, except the head and ears, immersed for not less than one minute. During this time, the head should be immersed at least twice, allowing the animal time to breathe between immersions. When used in scab control, approved dips should not be used in conjunction with any other dip and the dipwash must be prepared and replenished correctly.

Diazinon, propetamphos, and flumethrin are approved for use against sheep scab in the UK.

Parasiticides may be toxic to animals and the operator. Care should be taken with dosage and handling of the product. The recommendations for storage, use, and disposal of unused materials and containers should be followed. For guidance and information, see:

- MAFF/HSC. *Pesticides: code of practice for the safe use of pesticides on farms and holdings*. London: HMSO, 1990
- *The safe storage and handling of animal medicines*. 2nd ed. NOAH, 1990
- Control of Substances Hazardous to Health (COSHH) Regulation 1988
- *Guidelines for the disposal of used sheep dip and containers*. NOAH, 1990.

Storage. All dip concentrates should be stored in their original containers, kept out of reach of children, and not mixed with other dip concentrates or washes unless otherwise directed by the manufacturer. Dips are for external treatment only.

Protection of operators and the environment. A face shield, rubber gloves, and coveralls should be worn by the operator when handling the dip concentrate and contact with skin and eyes should be avoided. Rubber boots and a waterproof bib-apron or coat are advisable when handling the diluted wash or freshly dipped sheep.

2.2.3.1 AMIDINES

AMITRAZ

Indications. Keds, lice, and ticks on sheep; lice, mites, and ticks on cattle (2.2.2.1); lice and mites on pigs (2.2.2.1); *Demodex* on dogs (2.2.2.1)
Dose. *Sheep*: *by dip*, see preparation details

PML **Taktic**™ (SmithKline Beecham)
Liquid or dip concentrate, amitraz 12.5%, for *cattle* (2.2.2.1), *sheep, pigs* (2.2.2.1); 1 litre, 5 litres. To be diluted before use
Withdrawal Periods. *Cattle*: slaughter 1 day, milk withdrawal period nil. *Sheep*: slaughter 7 days, milk withdrawal period nil. *Pigs*: slaughter 1 day
Dipwash. Dilute 1 volume in 250 volumes water (= amitraz 0.05%)
Replenisher. Dilute 1 volume in 167 volumes water and add to dipwash after each fall in volume of 20%

2.2.3.2 ORGANOCHLORINES

BROMOCYCLEN

Preparations containing Bromocyclen are now discontinued

2.2.3.3 ORGANOPHOSPHORUS COMPOUNDS

Chlorfenvinphos is used for protection against fly-strike and the control of keds,

lice, and ticks. **Coumaphos** is active for up to 14 weeks for the prevention of fly-strike and for up to 20 weeks for protection against keds and lice.

For tick control, hoggs should be dipped when returning from wintering or when ticks appear, ewes as close to lambing as possible, and lambs as appropriate. Adult sheep will be protected for about one month after dipping. Repeat dips may be necessary if insect challenge is severe. Young lambs may be dipped individually in a smaller container, such as a 200-litre drum.

Diazinon and **propetamphos** are approved for use in the control of sheep scab in the UK. Both are also effective against blowfly larvae, keds, lice, and ticks.

CHLORFENVINPHOS

Indications. Blowfly larvae, keds, lice, and ticks on sheep
Warnings. Not approved for sheep scab control
Dose. *Sheep*: *by dip*, see preparation details

PML **Fly Dip** (Coopers Pitman-Moore)
Liquid or dip concentrate, chlorfenvinphos 10%, phenols 29-30%, for *sheep*; 2 litres, 10 litres, 20 litres. To be diluted before use
Withdrawal Periods. *Sheep*: slaughter 14 days
Dipwash. Dilute 1 volume in 200 volumes water (= chlorfenvinphos 0.05%)
Replenisher. 1 volume in 133 volumes water and add to dipwash after each fall in volume of 10%
Spray. Dilute 1 volume with 200 volumes water (= chlorfenvinphos 0.05%)
Replenisher. Dilute 1 volume in 80 volumes water and add to reservoir after each fall of 200 litres
By local application. Dilute 1 volume in 167 volumes water (= chlorfenvinphos 0.06%) for blowfly larvae

PML **Fly Dip** (Deosan)
Dip concentrate, chlorfenvinphos 10% phenols 30.5%, for *sheep*; 10 litres

20 litres, 100 litres. To be diluted before use

Withdrawal Periods. *Sheep*: slaughter 14 days, milk from treated animals should not be used for human consumption

Dipwash. Dilute 1 volume in 200 volumes water (= chlorfenvinphos 0.05%)

Replenisher. Dilute 1 volume in 133 volumes water and add to dipwash after each fall in volume of 225 litres

COUMAPHOS

Indications. Blowfly larvae, keds, lice, and ticks on sheep; lice and ticks on cattle and goats (see section 2.2.2.4 for use by spray); lice on pigs (2.2.2.4)

Warnings. Not approved for sheep scab control

Dose. *Sheep*: *by dip*, see preparation details

PML **Asuntol**™ (Bayer)
Liquid or dip concentrate, powder for reconstitution, coumaphos 50%, for *cattle* (2.2.2.4), *sheep, goats* (2.2.2.4); 230 g, 1.15 kg
Withdrawal Periods. *Cattle, sheep, goats*: slaughter 21 days
Note. Cattle, goats producing milk for human consumption should be treated immediately after milking
Dipwash. Reconstitute coumaphos 575 g (1.15 kg of powder) in 1125 litres water (= coumaphos 0.05%) for blowfly larvae, keds, and ticks
Replenisher. Reconstitute coumaphos 115 g (= 230 g of powder) in 225 litres water and add to dipwash after each fall in volume of 225 litres
Dipwash. Reconstitute coumaphos 575 g (1.15 kg of powder) in 2250 litres water (= coumaphos 0.025%) for lice
Replenisher. Reconstitute coumaphos 115 g (= 230 g of powder) in 450 litres water and add to dipwash after each fall in volume of 225 litres
Bacteriostat
Solution, powder for reconstitution, copper sulphate; contained within dip concentrate packaging 35 g, 350 g

DIAZINON

Indications. Blowfly larvae, keds, lice, *Psoroptes*, and ticks on sheep

Warnings. Some diazinon-containing dip concentrates contain epichlorhydrin 1%; adequate ventilation should be provided for operators working continuously with these preparations

Dose. *Sheep*: *by dip*, see preparation details

PML **Diazadip**™ **All Seasons** (Bayer)
Dip concentrate, diazinon 60%, for *sheep*; 2.5 litres, 5 litres. To be diluted before use
Withdrawal Periods. *Sheep*: slaughter 14 days, milk from treated animals should not be used for human consumption
Dipwash. Dilute dip concentrate 1 volume + disinfectant 2.5 volumes in 1500 volumes water (= diazinon 0.04%)
Replenisher. Add dip concentrate 5 mL for each sheep dipped and replenish water to original volume
Disinfectant
Liquid concentrate, phenols; 5 litres, 10 litres. To be diluted before use
Dilute 1 volume in 300 volumes dipwash

PML **Diazinon**™ **Dip** (Deosan)
Dip concentrate, diazinon 60%, for *sheep*; 1 litre, 4 litres. To be diluted before use
Withdrawal Periods. *Sheep*: slaughter 14 days, milk from treated animals should not be used for human consumption
Dipwash. Dilute dip concentrate 1 volume + disinfectant 2.5 volumes in 1500 volumes water (= diazinon 0.04%)
Replenisher. Add dip concentrate 5 mL for each sheep dipped and replenish water to original volume
Disinfectant
Liquid concentrate, phenols 27%; 2.5 litres, 5 litres. To be diluted before use
Dilute 1 volume in 300 volumes dipwash

PML **Golden Fleece**™ (Bimeda)
Dip concentrate, diazinon 60%, for *sheep*; 1 litre, 5 litres. To be diluted before use
Withdrawal Periods. *Sheep*: slaughter

14 days, milk from treated animals should not be used for human consumption
Dipwash. Dilute dip concentrate 1 volume + disinfectant 2.5 volumes in 1500 volumes water (= diazinon 0.04%)
Replenisher. Add dip concentrate 5 mL for each sheep dipped and replenish water to original volume
Disinfectant
Liquid concentrate, phenols 27%; 2.5 litres; 12.5 litres. To be diluted before use
Dilute 1 volume in 300 volumes dipwash

PML **Paracide**™ (Battle Hayward & Bower)
Dip concentrate, diazinon 60%, for *sheep*; 1 litre, 2 litres, 5 litres. To be diluted before use
Withdrawal Periods. *Sheep*: slaughter 14 days
Dipwash. Dilute dip concentrate 1 volume + disinfectant 3.3 volumes in 1500 volumes water (= diazinon 0.04%) for *Psoroptes*, ticks
Replenisher. Add dip concentrate 5 mL for each sheep dipped and replenish water to original volume
Dipwash. Dilute dip concentrate 1 volume + disinfectant 3.3 volumes in 1600 volumes water (= diazinon 0.04%) for blowfly larvae, keds, and lice
Replenisher. Add dip concentrate 2.75 mL for each sheep dipped and replenish water to original volume
Disinfectant
Liquid concentrate, phenols 15-20%; 2.5 litres, 5 litres, 10 litres. To be diluted before use
Dilute 1 volume in 250 volumes dipwash

PML **Paracide**™ **Plus** (Battle Hayward & Bower)
Dip concentrate, diazinon 16%, phenols (as coal tar phenols) 16%, for *sheep*; 2 litres, 5 litres, 10 litres. To be diluted before use
Withdrawal Periods. *Sheep*: slaughter 14 days
Dipwash. Dilute 1 volume in 400 volumes water (= diazinon 0.04%)
Replenisher. Dilute 1 volume in 267 volumes water and add to dipwash after every 20 sheep dipped

PML **Powerpack**™ **Winter Dip** (Coopers Pitman-Moore)
Dip concentrate, diazinon 45%, for *sheep*; 1 litre. To be diluted before use
Withdrawal Periods. *Sheep*: slaughter 14 days
Dipwash. Dilute 1 volume in 1800 volumes water (= diazinon 0.025%)
Replenisher. Automatic, using metering unit
Bacteriostat
Solution, powder for reconstitution; 45 g
Reconstitute 45 g in 225 litres dipwash

PML **Topclip**™ **Gold Shield** (Ciba-Geigy)
Dip concentrate, diazinon 60%, for *sheep*; 1 litre, 2.5 litres, 5 litres. To be diluted before use
Withdrawal Periods. *Sheep*: slaughter 14 days, milk from treated animals should not be used for human consumption or manufacturing purposes
Dipwash. Dilute dip concentrate 1 volume + disinfectant 3 volumes in 1500 volumes water (= diazinon 0.04%) for *Psoroptes*, ticks
Replenisher. Add dip concentrate 5 mL for each sheep dipped and replenish water to original volume after each fall in volume of 25%
Dipwash. Dilute dip concentrate 1 volume + disinfectant 3.2 volumes in 1600 volumes water (= diazinon 0.04%) for blowfly larvae, keds, lice
Replenisher. Add dip concentrate 2.75 mL for each sheep dipped and replenish water to original volume after each fall in volume of 25%
Note. Spray methods may also be used for blowfly larvae, keds, and lice, see manufacturer details
Disinfectant
Liquid concentrate, phenols 15-20%. To be diluted before use
Dilute 1 volume in 250 volumes dipwash

PROPETAMPHOS

Indications. Blowfly larvae, keds, lice. *Psoroptes*, and ticks on sheep
Dose. *Sheep*: *by dip*, see preparation details

PML **Border™ Winter Dip Scab Approved** (Coopers Pitman-Moore)
Dip concentrate, propetamphos 5.6%, phenols 20%, for *sheep*; 5 litres, 20 litres, 100 litres. To be diluted before use
Withdrawal Periods. *Sheep*: slaughter 14 days, milk from treated animals should not be used for human consumption
Dipwash. Dilute 1 volume in 200 volumes water (= propetamphos 0.028%)
Replenisher. Dilute 1 volume in 100 volumes of water and add to dipwash after each fall in volume of 10%

PML **Flyte 1250** (Young's)
Dip concentrate, propetamphos 40%, for *sheep*; 5 litres. To be diluted before use
Withdrawal Periods. *Sheep*: slaughter 21 days, milk from treated animals should not be used for human consumption
Dipwash. Dilute 1 volume in 1250 volumes water (= propetamphos 0.032%)
Replenisher. Dilute 1 volume in 625 volumes of water and add to dipwash after each fall in volume of 10%

PML **Rycovet™ Sheep Dip** (C-Vet)
Dip concentrate, propetamphos 16%, phenols 20%, for *sheep*; 5 litres. To be diluted before use
Dipwash. Dilute 1 volume in 500 volumes water (= propetamphos 0.032%)
Replenisher. Dilute 1 volume in 333 volumes water and add to dipwash after each fall in volume of 10%
Bacteriostat
Solution, powder for reconstitution; 50 g
Reconstitute 50 g of powder in 500 litres dipwash

PML **Scab-Approved Dip (Border Type)™** (Coopers Pitman-Moore)
Dip concentrate, propetamphos 8%, phenols 20%, for *sheep*; 2 litres, 5 litres, other sizes available. To be diluted before use
Withdrawal Periods. *Sheep*: slaughter 14 days, milk from treated animals should not be used for human consumption
Dipwash. Dilute 1 volume in 250 volumes water (= propetamphos 0.032%)

Replenisher. Dilute 1 volume in 167 volumes of water and add to dipwash after each fall in volume of 10%

PML **Scab Approved Ectomort™ Sheep Dip** (Young's)
Dip concentrate, propetamphos 8%, phenols 20%, for *sheep*; 4 litres, 10 litres, other sizes available. To be diluted before use
Withdrawal Periods. *Sheep*: slaughter 14 days, milk from treated animals should not be used for human consumption
Dipwash. Dilute 1 volume in 250 volumes water (= propetamphos 0.032%)
Replenisher. Dilute 1 volume in 167 volumes of water and add to dipwash after each fall in volume of 10%

PML **Scab Approved Jason™ Winter Dip** (Young's)
Dip concentrate, propetamphos 5.6%, phenols 20%, for *sheep*; 10 litres, 25 litres, 100 litres. To be diluted before use
Withdrawal Periods. *Sheep*: slaughter 14 days, milk from treated animals should not be used for human consumption
Dipwash. Dilute 1 volume in 200 volumes water (= propetamphos 0.028%)
Replenisher. Dilute 1 volume in 100 volumes of water and add to dipwash after each fall in volume of 10%

PML **Scab Approved Summer Dip** (Young's)
Dip concentrate, propetamphos 8%, phenols 10%, for *sheep*; 5 litres. To be diluted before use
Withdrawal Periods. *Sheep*: slaughter 14 days, milk 60 hours
Dipwash. Dilute 1 volume in 250 volumes of water (= propetamphos 0.032%)
Replenisher. Dilute 1 volume in 167 volumes of water and add to dipwash after each fall in volume of 10%
Bacteriostat
Solution, powder for reconstitution, thiram 80%; 50 g
Reconstitute 50 g of powder in 500 litres dipwash

PML**Seraphos**™ (Crown)
Dip concentrate, propetamphos 40%, for *sheep*; 1 litre, 2 litres, 5 litres. To be diluted before use
Withdrawal Periods. *Sheep*: slaughter 21 days, milk from treated animals should not be used for human consumption
Dipwash. Dilute 1 volume in 1250 volumes water (= propetamphos 0.032%)
Replenisher. Dilute 1 volume in 625 volumes of water and add to dipwash after each fall in volume of 10%
Bacteriostat
Solution, powder for reconstitution, thiram 80%; 50 g
Reconstitute 50 g of powder in 500 litres dipwash

COMPOUND ORGANOPHOSPHORUS PREPARATIONS

Warnings. Some diazinon-containing dip concentrates contain epichlorhydrin 1%; adequate ventilation should be provided for operators working continuously with these preparations

PML**Powerpack**™ **Summer Dip** (Coopers Pitman-Moore)
Dip concentrate, chlorfenvinphos 45%, diazinon 45%, for *sheep*; 1 litre. To be diluted before use
Withdrawal Periods. *Sheep*: slaughter 21 days
Dipwash. Dilute 1 volume in 1800 volumes water (= chlorfenvinphos 0.025% + diazinon 0.025%)
Replenisher. Automatic, using metering unit
Bacteriostat
Solution, powder for reconstitution; 45 g
Reconstitute 45 g of powder in 225 litres dipwash

PML**Regional Dip**™ (Deosan)
Dip concentrate, in 2 parts, (A) chlorfenvinphos 4%, phenols 32%, (B) diazinon 50%, for *sheep*; (A)5 litres + (B)500 mL; (A)10 litres + (B)1 litre; (A)20 litres + (B)2 litres. To be diluted before use

Withdrawal Periods. *Sheep*: slaughter 18 days, milk from treated animals should not be used for human consumption
Dipwash. Dilute 10 volumes (A) + 1 volume (B) in 2000 volumes water (= chlorfenvinphos 0.02% + diazinon 0.025%)
Replenisher. Add 29 mL (A) + 2.9 mL (B) for each sheep dipped and replenish water to original volume

PML**Traditional Dip**™ (Deosan)
Dip concentrate, in 2 parts, (A) chlorfenvinphos 10%, phenols 30.5%, (B) diazinon 50%, for *sheep*; (A)10 litres + (B)1 litre; (A)20 litres + (B)2 litres. To be diluted before use
Withdrawal Periods. *Sheep*: slaughter 18 days
Dipwash. Dilute 10 volumes (A) + 1 volume (B) in 2000 volumes water (= chlorfenvinphos 0.05% + diazinon 0.025%)
Replenisher. Add 29 mL (A) + 2.9 mL (B) for each sheep dipped and replenish water to original volume

2.2.3.4 PYRETHROIDS

See section 2.2.2.5 for further information.

FLUMETHRIN

Indications. Keds, lice, *Psoroptes*, and ticks on sheep
Warnings. Not for control of blowfly larvae
Dose. *Sheep*: by *dip*, see preparation details

PML**Bayticol**™ **Scab and Tick Dip** (Bayer)
Dip concentrate, flumethrin 6%, for *sheep*; 1 litre. To be diluted before use
Withdrawal Periods. *Sheep*: slaughter withdrawal period nil, milk withdrawal period nil
Note. Animals producing milk for human consumption should be treated immediately after milking

Dipwash. Dilute 1 volume in 1350 volumes water (= flumethrin 0.004%) for *Psoroptes*
Replenisher. Dilute 1 volume in 1350 volumes water and add to dipwash as necessary
Dipwash. Dilute 1 volume in 900 volumes of water (= flumethrin 0.007%) for keds, lice, and ticks
Replenisher. Dilute 1 volume in 900 volumes water and add to dipwash as necessary
Bacteriostat
Solution, powder for reconstitution, copper sulphate; 50 g
Reconstitute 50 g of powder in 225 litres dipwash

2.2.4 Bands, collars, and tapes

2.2.4.1 Carbamates
2.2.4.2 Organophosphorus compounds
2.2.4.3 Synthetic pyrethroids
Tags are attached to one or both ears of cattle. It is preferable to apply tags to the whole herd. The period of fly challenge in the UK is generally from June until September and for optimum protection the tags should be attached to the animal shortly before required. The insecticide is released onto the animal and spread over its surface by body movement. Most tags act for up to 4 to 5 months and they are used in dairy and beef cattle and calves. Tags should be removed at the end of the fly season or before slaughter.
Bands are used on horses. They are attached to the browband or head collar and left in place for approximately 4 months.
Insecticidal **collars** for dogs and cats work on the same principle of insecticide dispersion as tags and should be worn at all times. The collar should be applied so as to fit loosely around the animal's neck. Elasticated collars are available for cats. Children should not be allowed to handle or play with the collar, and animals should not be allowed to chew it.
Occasionally animals show an allergic reaction to collars and the collar should

be removed immediately if this is evident.

2.2.4.1 CARBAMATES

Collars are available containing **propoxur**, which is effective against fleas on dogs and cats.

PROPOXUR

Indications. Fleas on dogs and cats
Contra-indications. Concurrent use of other ectoparasiticides
Side-effects. Occasional skin irritation and alopecia
Warnings. Children should not be allowed to play with collar

GSL **Vet-Kem Breakaway™ Flea and Tick Cat Collar** (BK)
Propoxur 9.4%

GSL **Vet-Kem™ Flea and Tick Dog Collar** (BK)
Propoxur 9.4%

2.2.4.2 ORGANOPHOSPHORUS COMPOUNDS

The organophosphorus compound **diazinon** is used in collars for flea and tick control on dogs and cats. Some collars contain esters of fatty acids as a conditioner. The effect of the drug on fleas can be seen within a few hours and that on ticks within 5 days. Collars are effective for about 4 months.

Parasiticides may be toxic to animals and the operator. Care should be taken with dosage and handling of the product. The recommendations for storage, use, and disposal of unused materials and containers should be followed. For guidance and information, see:
- MAFF/HSC. *Pesticides: code of practice for the safe use of pesticides on farms and holdings*. London: HMSO, 1990
- *The safe storage and handling of animal medicines*. 2nd ed. NOAH, 1990
- Control of Substances Hazardous to Health (COSHH) Regulation 1988.

DIAZINON

Indications. Fleas and ticks on dogs and cats
Contra-indications. Puppies under 8 weeks of age; cats under 6 months of age, aged cats, nursing queens. Concurrent use of other ectoparasiticides
Side-effects. Occasional skin irritation and alopecia
Warnings. Children should not be allowed to play with collar

GSL **Canovel™ Doublecare Insecticidal Collar** (SmithKline Beecham)
Diazinon 15%, essential fatty acid esters 5%, for *dogs*

GSL **Catovel™ Doublecare Elasticated Insecticidal Collar** (SmithKline Beecham)
Diazinon 15%, essential fatty acid esters 5%, for *cats*

GSL **Catovel Prettycare Insecticidal Collar** (SmithKline Beecham)
Diazinon 15%, for *cats*

GSL **Derasect™ Insecticidal Collar** (SmithKline Beecham)
Diazinon 15%, essential fatty acid esters 5%, for *dogs*

GSL **Derasect™ Insecticidal Elasticated Flea Collar** (SmithKline Beecham)
Diazinon 15%, essential fatty acid esters 5%, for *cats*

GSL **Preventef™ Elasticated Flea Collar for Cats** (Virbac)
Diazinon 15%, essential fatty acid esters 5%

GSL **Preventef™ Insecticidal Collar for Dogs** (Virbac)
Diazinon 15%, essential fatty acid esters 5%

GSL **Preventef™ Insecticidal Collar for Large Dogs** (Virbac)
Diazinon 15%, essential fatty acid esters 5%

2.2.4.3 SYNTHETIC PYRETHROIDS

Tags containing second and third generation synthetic pyrethroids are used to control biting and nuisance flies on cattle. Bands are available for horses. **Cypermethrin** and **fenvalerate** ear tags are attached to the back of the ear and 1 or 2 per animal are required depending upon the fly challenge. A single **permethrin** tag per animal protects for up to 4 months. The tag is attached hanging down in the front of the ear. Collars containing permethrin are also available for use on dogs and cats.

CYPERMETHRIN

Indications. Biting and nuisance flies on horses and cattle

GSL **Equivite™ Fly Bands** (Dalgety)
Cypermethrin 8.5%, for *horses*
Withdrawal Periods. Should not be used in *horses* intended for human consumption

PML **Flectron Attachatags™** (Deosan)
Cypermethrin 8.5%, for *cattle*
Withdrawal Periods. *Cattle*: slaughter withdrawal period nil, milk withdrawal period nil

PML **Flectron™ Fly Tags** (Deosan)
Cypermethrin 8.5%, for *cattle*
Withdrawal Periods. *Cattle*: slaughter withdrawal period nil, milk withdrawal period nil

FENVALERATE

Indications. Biting and nuisance flies on cattle
Warnings. See under Cypermethrin

PML **Tirade™ Fly Tags** (Sorex)
Fenvalerate 8.5%, for *cattle*

PERMETHRIN

Indications. Biting and nuisance flies on cattle; fleas and ticks on dogs and cats
Contra-indications. Concurrent use of other ectoparasiticides
Side-effects. Occasional skin irritation and alopecia in animals wearing insecticidal collars
Warnings. Children should not be allowed to play with collar

GSL **Natura™ Elasticated Insecticidal Collar for cats and kittens** (Virbac)
Permethrin 8%, essential fatty acid esters

GSL **Natura™ Insecticidal Collar for dogs and puppies** (Virbac)
Permethrin 8%, essential fatty acid esters

PML **Stomoxin™ Fly Tags** (Coopers Pitman-Moore)
Permethrin 10.53%, for *cattle*
Withdrawal Periods. *Cattle*: slaughter withdrawal period nil, milk withdrawal period nil

3 Drugs acting on the
GASTRO-INTESTINAL SYSTEM

3.1 Antidiarrhoeal drugs

The causative agents of diarrhoea include infections due to bacteria, fungi, viruses (see Chapter 1), or endoparasites (see section 2.1); dietary imbalance or hypersensitivity; ingestion of toxins; stress; and neoplasia. Diarrhoea may cause changes in the gastro-intestinal tract resulting in malabsorption of fluids and reduced digestibility of nutrients. Treatment includes elimination of the causative agent and supportive therapy such as fluid and electrolyte replacement and dietary control. A period of starvation with oral electrolyte supplements is followed by a bland diet and gradual re-introduction to normal feed. Oral electrolyte replacement solutions (see section 16.1.1) should be offered in place of drinking water or milk. Severely dehydrated animals may require parenteral fluids by intravenous or intraperitoneal routes as well as oral solutions.

Bacteria commonly causing diarrhoea include streptococci, staphylococci, *Escherichia coli*, *Salmonella*, and *Campylobacter*. Antibacterials (see section 1.1) that are poorly absorbed from the gastro-intestinal tract, such as neomycin,

some sulphonamides, dihydrostreptomycin, and nitrofurans, are used. These are often included in compound preparations with adsorbents and astringents (see section 1.1.11). Antibacterials that are absorbed systemically are required for diarrhoea complicated by bacteraemia or other systemic conditions. Antibacterials indicated include oral oxytetracycline, parenteral amoxycillin or ampicillin, or erythromycin and tylosin for diarrhoea caused by *Campylobacter*. The use of antibiotics in the treatment of diarrhoea is controversial, but may be life-saving in neonates developing septicaemia from gastro-intestinal bacterial pathogens. Vaccines (see section 18.2.5) are available for the prevention of scouring due to *E. coli* and rotavirus in calves.

3.1.1 Antidiarrhoeal adsorbent mixtures

Adsorbents may form a protective coating on the gastro-intestinal wall and adsorb toxins, thereby preventing irritation and erosion of the mucosa. They may also adsorb other drugs such as lincomycin, and reduce their efficacy (see Drug Interactions – Appendix 1). **Attapulgite**, **bismuth salts**, **charcoal** (see also Emergency treatment of poisoning), and **kaolin** are available in compound preparations with antacids and electrolytes for the treatment of non-specific diarrhoea. Some absorption of salicylate will occur from administration of bismuth salicylate. **Ispaghula husk** and **sterculia** (see section 3.5.2) are used in the treatment of diarrhoea due to their ability to absorb water and increase faecal mass.

GSL **BCK**™ (Duphar)
Oral granules, by addition to feed or to prepare an oral solution, bismuth subnitrate 40 mg, calcium phosphate 50 mg, charcoal 400 mg, light kaolin

430 mg/g, for *horses, cattle, sheep, pigs, dogs, cats*; 300 g
Dose. *Horses, cattle*: 4 tablespoonfuls 2-3 times daily; *calves*: 1-3 tablespoonfuls 2-3 times daily
Sheep, pigs: 1-3 tablespoonfuls 2-3 times daily
Dogs, cats: one-three 5-mL spoonfuls 2-3 times daily

GSL **CD18**™ (Arnolds)
Oral powder, to prepare an oral solution, catechu 71 mg, chalk 286 mg, ginger 71 mg, kaolin 572 mg/g, for *cattle*; 84 g
Dose. *Cattle*: 84 g 2-3 times daily; *calves*: 84 g daily in divided doses

GSL **Colistol**™ (Crown)
Oral suspension, bismuth salicylate, eucalyptus oil, fullersite, kaolin, magnesium trisilicate, sodium salicylate, for *calves*; 500 mL, 2 litres
Dose. *Calves*: 14-28 mL twice daily

GSL **Forgastrin**™ (Arnolds)
Oral powder, by addition to feed or to prepare an oral solution, bismuth subnitrate 25 mg, charcoal 270 mg/mL, for *horses, cattle, sheep, goats, pigs, dogs, cats*; 250 g, 2.5 kg
Dose. *Horses, cattle*: 3-4 tablespoonfuls 3 times daily
Sheep, goats, pigs: 2-3 tablespoonfuls 3 times daily
Dogs, cats: two-three 5-mL spoonfuls 3 times daily

GSL **Kaogel**™ (Parke-Davis)
Oral suspension, light kaolin 200 mg, pectin 4.3 mg/mL, for *horses, cattle, sheep, pigs, dogs, cats, zoo animals*; 2.25 litres
Dose. *Horses, cattle, sheep, pigs, dogs, cats; zoo animals*: 1 mL/kg daily in divided doses

GSL **Kaopectate**™ V (Upjohn)
Oral suspension, kaolin 206 mg/mL, for *dogs, cats*; 500 mL
Dose. *Dogs, cats*: 0.5-1.0 mL/kg daily in 3-4 divided doses

GSL **Stat**™ (Intervet)
Oral suspension, calcium chloride hexahydrate 1.97 mg, dried aluminium hydroxide gel 19.3 mg, light kaolin 108 mg, magnesium chloride 1 mg, potassium acetate 3.3 mg, sodium acetate

19.8 mg, sodium chloride 18.1 mg/mL, for *calves, lambs, dogs, cats*; 1 litre
Dose. *Calves, lambs*: 0.5-2.0 mL/kg 2-3 times daily
Dogs, cats: 2 mL/kg 2-3 times daily

PoM **Zinc Oxide** (UKASTA)
Oral powder, zinc oxide 100%, for *pigs*
Withdrawal Periods. *Pigs*: slaughter 28 days
Dose. *Pigs*: 3.1 kg/tonne feed daily for up to 14 days

> **Proprietary and non-proprietary medicines that are licensed for human use are printed in small type in The Veterinary Formulary**

3.1.2 Antidiarrhoeal drugs that reduce motility

Diphenoxylate and **loperamide** are opioid derivatives that reduce gastro-intestinal motility. They are used in the treatment of non-specific acute and chronic diarrhoea. Diphenoxylate is well absorbed from the gastro-intestinal tract, whereas loperamide is only partially absorbed. Both drugs are metabolised in the liver. Diphenoxylate and loperamide should be used with care in cats as they may cause morphine-like excitability in this species. In dogs these drugs may be sedative; loperamide less so than diphenoxylate.
Diphenoxylate is used in combination with atropine (co-phenotrope).

CO-PHENOTROPE

A mixture of diphenoxylate hydrochloride and atropine sulphate in the mass proportions 100 parts to 1 part respectively

Indications. Non-specific diarrhoea
Side-effects. Constipation
Warnings. Care on administration to cats
Dose. Expressed as diphenoxylate.
Dogs: 60 micrograms/kg daily

PoM **Lomotil**™ (Gold Cross)
Tablets, co-phenotrope 2.5/0.025 [diphenoxylate hydrochloride 2.5 mg, atropine sulphate 25 micrograms]; 100, 500, 1000
Oral liquid, co-phenotrope 500/5 [diphen-

oxylate hydrochloride 500 micrograms, atropine sulphate 5 micrograms]/mL; 100 mL

LOPERAMIDE HYDROCHLORIDE

Indications. Non-specific diarrhoea
Side-effects. **Warnings**. See under Co-phenotrope
Dose. *Dogs*: 100 micrograms/kg

PoM **Loperamide** (Non-proprietary)
Capsules, loperamide hydrochloride 2 mg

PoM **Imodium**™ (Janssen)
Syrup, loperamide hydrochloride 200 micrograms/mL; 100 mL

3.1.3 Drugs used in the treatment of chronic diarrhoea

Chronic diarrhoea may be caused by dietary imbalance, colitis, parasitism, exocrine pancreatic insufficiency (see section 3.9), or occur as a result of other systemic disease.
Sulphasalazine is used in the management of ulcerative colitis. Intestinal bacteria split the compound into 5-aminosalicylate and sulphapyridine. The aminosalicylate becomes concentrated in the gastro-intestinal wall where it exerts its anti-inflammatory activity. The side-effects of sulphapyridine are typical of the sulphonamides (see section 1.1.6) and prolonged use in dogs may cause keratoconjunctivitis sicca.
Corticosteroids are used in the control of eosinophilic ulcerative colitis. **Prednisolone** (see section 7.2.1) is given at a dose of 0.5–1.0 mg/kg twice daily for 5 to 7 days, and reduced to the lowest effective dose administered on alternate days.

SULPHASALAZINE

Indications. Ulcerative colitis
Warnings. Prolonged administration may cause keratoconjunctivitis sicca in dogs
Dose. *Dogs*: 10-15 mg/kg 3 times daily for one week then reduce to 2.5 mg/kg or lowest effective maintenance dose

PoM **Sulphasalazine** (Non-proprietary)
Tablets, sulphasalazine 500 mg

3.2 Drugs used in the treatment of bloat

Acute ruminal distension can result in compromise of respiratory and cardiovascular function, and requires urgent treatment.
Ruminal tympany or bloat is the accumulation of gas in the rumen in a stable foam (frothy bloat) or as free gas. In the majority of cases, free gas bloat is secondary to other diseases such as oesophagitis, vagal nerve lesions, ruminitis, tetanus, acidosis, or oesophageal obstruction. Frothy bloat is dietary in origin and occurs when leguminous plants or high grain diets, which contain foam-forming agents, are ingested. In frothy bloat a stable foam is produced which traps the gases of fermentation. Small gas bubbles are unable to coalesce thereby preventing their removal by eructation. The production of insufficient saliva, which is alkaline, may also exacerbate frothy bloat.
Treatment of free gas bloat includes ruminal intubation or trocharisation to allow the release of gas. Administration of turpentine oil 15 to 30 mL in linseed oil 300 to 600 mL may be given to decrease gas production. Proquamezine (see section 8.5) may be used for relaxation of oesophageal smooth muscle to aid removal of an obstruction.
Medical treatment of frothy bloat requires the administration of an antifoaming agent to break down the stable foam. Oils such as sunflower oil or arachis oil (peanut oil) are given via stomach tube at a dose of 250 mL for cattle and 50 mL for sheep. A dose of 15 to 60 mL of turpentine oil may be given to cattle to relieve frothy bloat. Turpentine oil may taint meat and milk. Turpentine oil may also be used in the treatment of equine colic due to excessive accumulation of gas. It is administered

as a dose of 60 to 120 mL/500 kg body-weight.

Poloxalene is a nonionic surfactant used for the prevention of frothy bloat. Silicones such as **dimethicone** reduce the surface tension of gas bubbles causing them to coalesce. It is used in the treatment of frothy bloat.

Another treatment for frothy bloat is sodium carbonate 150 to 200 g dissolved in one litre of water given via stomach tube to cause alkalosis of ruminal contents.

The prevention and control of bloat includes limited pasture access, avoiding finely milled feeds, and maintaining high fibre content in the diet. Antifoaming substances may be included in the feed or sprayed on the crops.

DIMETHICONE

Indications. Frothy bloat
Dose. See preparation details

PoM **Antibloat**™ (Bimeda)
Oral suspension, dimethicone 25 mg/mL, for *cattle*; 100 mL
Dose. *Cattle*: *by mouth or intra-ruminal injection*, 100 mL

GSL **Birp**™ (Arnolds)
Dimethicone emulsion BVetC, for *cattle, sheep*; 100 mL
Dose. *Cattle*: 100 mL
Sheep: 25 mL

> In The Veterinary Formulary, the ♦ symbol denotes an unlicensed indication for a preparation that is licensed for use in animals in the UK

PoM **Rumoxane**™ (Willows Francis)
Oral suspension, dimethicone 10 mg, light kaolin 140 mg/mL, for *cattle*; 100 mL
Dose. *Cattle*: *by mouth or intra-ruminal injection*, 100 mL

POLOXALENE

Indications. Prevention of frothy bloat
Dose: See preparation details

PML **Bloat Guard**™ (Mill Feed)
Mixture, poloxalene 830 mg/mL, for *cattle*; 60 mL

Dose. *Cattle*: (less than 227 kg body-weight) 30 mL daily; (more than 227 kg body-weight) 60 mL daily
Oral liquid, for addition to feed, poloxalene 995 g/kg, for *cattle*; 205 litres
Dose. *Cattle*: 22-44 mg of poloxalene/kg body-weight daily
Premix, poloxalene 530 g/kg, for *cattle*; 25 kg
Dose. *Cattle*: 22-44 mg of poloxalene/kg body-weight daily

3.3 Anti-emetics

3.3.1 Drugs used in the treatment of gastritis
3.3.2 Drugs used in the treatment of motion sickness

Vomiting follows stimulation of the vomiting centre in the medulla and the closely associated chemoreceptor trigger zone which is sensitive to many drugs and to certain metabolic disturbances. Stimulation of the vomiting centre also occurs following activation of other areas such as the vestibular apparatus of the ear as in motion sickness. Vomiting is frequently a sign of disease or gastric obstruction and the causative agent should be ascertained before treatment is commenced. If vomiting is prolonged, dehydration, hypokalaemia, and alkalosis may occur and replacement fluids and electrolytes may be necessary (see 16.1.2).

3.3.1 Drugs used in the treatment of gastritis

Metoclopramide has a dual mode of action. It possesses parasympatho-mimetic activity and thereby increases the motility of the upper gastro-intestinal tract without affecting gastric acid secretion. It increases gastric peristalsis leading to accelerated gastric emptying. Metoclopramide is also a dopamine receptor antagonist with a direct depressant effect on the chemoreceptor trigger zone. It is used to reduce vomiting in gastritis and following surgery, and in the treatment of ruminal atony or oesophageal reflux. It is of little benefit in prevention of motion sickness in dogs and cats. Metoclopramide may cause restlessness and excitement in some dogs.

METOCLOPRAMIDE HYDROCHLORIDE

Indications. Vomiting due to gastritis, oesophageal reflux, see notes above
Side-effects. Occasional transient incoordination and excitement
Warnings. Antagonised by antimuscarinic drugs (See Drug Interactions – Appendix 1)
Dose. *Dogs, cats: by mouth or by subcutaneous, intramuscular, or intravenous injection,* 0.5-1.0 mg/kg daily

PoM **Emequell**™ (SmithKline Beecham)
Tablets, scored, metoclopramide hydrochloride 10 mg, for *dogs, cats*; 100
Injection, metoclopramide hydrochloride 5 mg/mL, for *dogs, cats*; 2 mL

3.3.2 Drugs used in the treatment of motion sickness

Acepromazine, chlorpromazine, and **prochlorperazine** are phenothiazine derivatives. They are effective against vomiting induced by stimulation of the chemoreceptor trigger zone. Acepromazine and chlorpromazine have marked sedative properties, which may be helpful in controlling motion sickness in animals. Acepromazine 0.5-1.0 mg/kg by mouth, 15 to 30 minutes before a light meal is effective for preventing motion sickness in dogs and cats. Acepromazine is effective for up to 24 hours.
Cyclizine is an antihistamine. It acts directly on the neural pathways arising in the vestibular apparatus. The action of cyclizine may last for 8 to 12 hours.

ACEPROMAZINE
See section 6.1

CHLORPROMAZINE HYDROCHLORIDE

Indications. Prevention of motion sickness

Contra-indications. Renal or hepatic impairment
Side-effects. May cause drowsiness
Warnings. Owing to the risk of contact sensitisation, operators should avoid direct contact with chlorpromazine; tablets should not be crushed and solutions should be handled with care.
Dose. *Dogs, cats: by mouth,* 0.5-2.0 mg/kg 1-4 times daily; *by intramuscular injection,* 0.5-1.0 mg/kg

PoM **Chlorpromazine** (Non-proprietary)
Tablets, chlorpromazine hydrochloride 10 mg, 25 mg, 50 mg, 100 mg
Elixir, chlorpromazine hydrochloride 5 mg/mL; 100 mL

PoM **Largactil**™ (M&B)
Injection, chlorpromazine hydrochloride 25 mg/mL; 2 mL

CYCLIZINE HYDROCHLORIDE

Indications. Prevention of motion sickness
Dose. *Dogs*: 25-100 mg daily in divided doses

P **Valoid**™ (Calmic)
Tablets, scored, cyclizine hydrochloride 50 mg; 100

PROCHLORPERAZINE

Indications. Prevention of motion sickness
Dose. *Dogs, cats: by mouth,* up to 500 micrograms/kg; *by intramuscular injection,* 100 micrograms/kg

PoM **Prochlorperazine** (Non-proprietary)
Tablets, prochlorperazine maleate 5 mg

PoM **Stemetil**™ (M&B)
Injection, prochlorperazine mesylate 12.5 mg/mL; 1 mL, 2 mL

3.4 Emetics

Vomiting is a protective reflex that occurs effectively only in certain species. True emesis is not possible in horses, ruminants, rabbits, and rodents. In other species that have consumed a poisonous or undesirable substance, it is often useful to produce emesis, within 1 to 2 hours of ingestion, in order to empty the stomach and so minimise further absorption.

Ipecacuanha has an irritant action on the gastro-intestinal tract and may be used to induce emesis in dogs and cats. However, its effectiveness is unpredictable. A maximum dose of 15 mL is advised for dogs. In cases of poisoning, ipecacuanha syrup should not be used in association with activated charcoal since the effectiveness of the charcoal is reduced.

A warm, saturated solution of **sodium chloride** may produce emesis in dogs without damaging the gastro-intestinal tract. Crystalline **sodium carbonate** (washing soda) or sodium chloride deposited at the back of the tongue and swallowed can cause vomiting.

Xylazine (see section 6.1) 0.05-1.0 mg/kg by intramuscular injection has been used in dogs and cats for inducing emesis.

IPECACUANHA

Indications. Induction of emesis
Contra-indications. Poisoning with corrosive compounds or petroleum products (risk of aspiration); shock; see notes above
Side-effects. Cardiac effects if absorbed
Dose. *Dogs, cats*: 1-2 mL/kg. Maximum dose 15 mL for dogs

GSL **Paediatric Ipecacuanha Emetic Mixture** (Non-proprietary)
Total alkaloids (as emetine) 1.4 mg/mL; 100 mL

3.5 Laxatives

3.5.1 Lubricant laxatives
3.5.2 Bulk-forming laxatives
3.5.3 Osmotic laxatives
3.5.4 Stimulant laxatives

3.5.1 Lubricant laxatives

Lubricant laxatives soften and lubricate the faecal mass which allows expulsion.

Liquid paraffin and **white soft paraffin** are commonly used and are thought generally safe, although prolonged use may cause problems. Lubricant laxatives line the mucosal surface and may inhibit the absorption of fat-soluble vitamins, other nutrients, or drugs. Absorption of small amounts of paraffin may lead to granulomatous lesions, especially in the liver.

Liquid paraffin in doses of up to 4 litres may be used in the treatment of equine colic due to impaction. When liquid paraffin is administered to large animals it should be mixed with ginger or mustard to prevent inhalation, except when given by stomach tube.

PARAFFINS

Indications. Constipation
Contra-indications. Prolonged use especially in young animals
Side-effects. Reduced absorption of nutrients; granulomatous lesions developing with prolonged use
Warnings. Accidental administration into the trachea and bronchial tree may lead to lipid pneumonitis
Dose. See preparation details

GSL **Katalax™** (C-Vet)
Oral paste, white soft paraffin 474 mg/g, for *cats*; 20 g
Dose. *Cats*: ½-1 inch of paste 1-2 times daily

Liquid Paraffin
Dose. *Horses, cattle*: 0.5-2.0 litres; *calves, foals*: 60-120 mL
Dogs: 2-60 mL
Cats: 2-10 mL

3.5.2 Bulk-forming laxatives

Ispaghula and **sterculia** take up water in the gastro-intestinal tract, thereby increasing the volume of the faeces and promoting peristalsis. They are used in the management of chronic constipation and when excessive rectal straining is to be avoided, such as following surgery for perineal hernia repair or anal gland removal. Due to their ability to increase faecal mass they are also used in the control of diarrhoea.

Unprocessed wheat **bran**, added to the

diet according to response, is also used to treat chronic constipation.

Adequate fluid intake should be provided when using bulk laxatives to avoid intestinal obstruction.

ISPAGHULA HUSK

Indications. Constipation
Contra-indications. Abdominal pain; vomiting
Warnings. Water must be available at all times
Dose. See preparation details

GSL **Isogel™** (A&H)
Granules, ispaghula husk 90%; 200 g
Dose. *Dogs*: *by addition to food*, one-three 5-mL spoonfuls daily
Cats: *by addition to food*, one 5-mL spoonful daily

STERCULIA

Indications. Constipation
Contra-indications. **Warnings**. See under Ispaghula
Dose. See preparation details

GSL **Peridale™** (Arnolds)
Capsules, sterculia 118 mg, for *cats*; 100
Dose. *Cats*: 118 mg twice daily; *kittens*: 118 mg daily
Oral granules, sterculia 980 mg/g, for *dogs*; 175 g
Dose. *Dogs*: 1.5-6.0 g 1-2 times daily
Oral paste, sterculia 120 mg/dose, for *cats*; metered-dose applicator
Dose. *Cats*: 120 mg twice daily; *kittens*: 120 mg daily

3.5.3 Osmotic laxatives

Osmotic laxatives are hypertonic solutions of poorly absorbed substances that retain and absorb water from the tissues into the intestinal lumen. The resulting bowel distension promotes peristalsis. **Magnesium sulphate** (Epsom salts) is effective within 3 to 12 hours in simple-stomached animals and after approximately 18 hours in ruminants. Fluid should be available throughout treatment. Magnesium sulphate is particularly contra-indicated as a laxative in dehydrated animals.

A number of compound preparations contain a range of other constituents of unproven value.

Impacted rectal and colonic contents are best resolved by the use of an enema. Warm, soapy water solutions soften and break up the faecal mass. Intestinal distension will stimulate contractions of the gut wall.

Proprietary enema preparations containing **phosphates** or **sodium citrate** act as osmotic laxatives and are used to treat constipation, and evacuation of the bowel prior to surgery or radiographic examination.

MAGNESIUM SALTS

GSL **Magnesium Hydroxide Mixture (Cream of Magnesia)**
Magnesium oxide (hydrated) about 55 mg/mL
Dose. *Horses, cattle*: 1-4 litres
Dogs: 5-10 mL
Cats: 2-6 mL

GSL **Magnesium Sulphate (Epsom salts)**
Dose. *Horses*: 30-100 g
Cattle: 250-500 g
Pigs: 25-125 g
Dogs: 5-25 g
Cats: 2-5 g

PoM **Bimodrench™** (Bimeda)
Oral powder, to prepare an oral solution, anhydrous sodium sulphate 434 mg, anise 15 mg, camphor 8 mg, dried magnesium sulphate 434 mg, ginger 73 mg, potassium nitrate 35 mg/g, for *cattle, sheep, pigs*; 500 g
Dose. *Cattle*: up to 300 g
Sheep, pigs: 50 g

PHOSPHATE (RECTAL)

Indications. Rectal impaction
Dose. *Dogs, cats*: half to one enema as necessary

P **Fletchers' Phosphate Enema™** (Pharmax)
Sodium acid phosphate 12.8 g, sodium phosphate 10.24 g/128 mL; 128-mL single dose with rectal tube

SODIUM CITRATE (RECTAL)

Indications. Constipation
Dose. *Dogs, cats*: one enema as necessary

PMicralax™ Micro-Enema (Evans Medical)
Sodium citrate 450 mg, sodium alkyl-
sulphoacetate 45 mg, sorbic acid 5 mg/5 mL
with glycerol and sorbitol; 5-mL dose
applicator

3.5.4 Stimulant laxatives

Danthron is an anthraquinone laxative.
Colonic bacteria liberate active anthraquinone from glycosides, which stimulates myenteric plexes. Danthron is
effective within 6 to 14 hours in dogs
and cats, and within 12 to 36 hours in
horses and cattle.

Danthron has been used in veterinary
medicine although prolonged administration may cause degeneration of the
myenteric plexes leading to loss of
intestinal motility, or reversible mela-
nosis coli. Danthron is excreted into the
milk and may affect suckling offspring.

3.6 Modulators of intestinal motility

Diphenoxylate and loperamide (see
section 3.1.2) cause a reduction in
gastro-intestinal motility and are used
in the treatment of diarrhoea.

Atropine (see section 6.6.1), hyoscine,
and ambutonium bromide, are antimuscarinic compounds with antispasmodic activity. Ambutonium is less
lipid soluble than atropine, and therefore
less effectively absorbed and less likely
to cross the blood-brain barrier. Hyoscine
is available, in combination with
dipyrone, for use in the treatment of
spasmodic equine colic.

Carbachol is a quaternary ammonium
parasympathomimetic that increases
intestinal motility. It is a very potent
drug and can cause intestinal rupture.
Conservative therapy, such as mineral
oils for the treatment of intestinal
blockage, is a safer alternative.

ATROPINE SULPHATE

Indications. Adjunct in gastro-intestinal
disorders characterised by smooth
muscle spasm; pre-anaesthetic medication (6.6.1), antidote for organo-
phosphorous poisoning (see Emergency
treatment of poisoning)
Contra-indications. Glaucoma
Side-effects. Dry mouth; dilation of
pupils and photophobia; constipation;
urinary retention; tachycardia
Dose. By subcutaneous injection. Horses,
cattle: 30-60 micrograms/kg
Sheep: 80-160 micrograms/kg
Pigs: 20-40 micrograms/kg
Dogs, cats: 30-100 micrograms/kg
See section 6.6.1 for preparation details

AMBUTONIUM BROMIDE

Indications. Adjunct in gastro-intestinal
disorders characterised by smooth
muscle spasm
Contra-indications. Side-effects. See
under Atropine sulphate
Dose. See preparation details

PoM Aludrox SA™ (Charwell)
Oral suspension, ambutonium bromide
500 micrograms, aluminium hydroxide mixture 0.95 mL, magnesium hydroxide 20 mg/
mL; 100 mL
Dose. Dogs: 2-5 mL 2-3 times daily
Cats: 1.0-2.5 mL 2-3 times daily

COMPOUND PREPARATIONS

PoM Buscopan™ Compositium (Boehringer Ingelheim)
See section 10.3 for preparation details

3.7 Antacids and ulcer-healing drugs

3.7.1 Antacids
3.7.2 Ulcer-healing drugs

3.7.1 Antacids

Antacids are used in the therapy of
gastric ulceration and to prevent and
treat mild ruminal acidosis. Ruminal
acidosis is caused by excessive carbohydrate intake from grain engorgement
which leads to the production of large

quantities of lactic acid in the rumen instead of the normal volatile fatty acids. Antacids neutralise gastric acid and this helps ulcers to heal. They may be combined with bitters and carminatives in compound preparations. **Ammonium bicarbonate** and **sodium bicarbonate** are soluble and act rapidly, producing carbon dioxide which is released by eructation. Gas may accumulate if the rumen is atonic and lead to free gas bloat (see section 3.2). Bicarbonate may be absorbed systemically and produce alkalosis. **Aluminium hydroxide** and **ammonium carbonate** are less soluble and therefore slower acting. Aluminium salts tend to cause constipation. Some compound preparations contain additional ingredients of unproven value.

ALUMINIUM HYDROXIDE

Indications. Gastric acidosis, gastric ulceration (3.7.2)
Side-effects. Constipation
Warnings. Reduces the absorption of other drugs (see Drug Interactions – Appendix 1)
Dose. *Dogs, cats*: 0.5 mL/kg twice daily

GSL **Aluminium Hydroxide** (Non-proprietary)
Mixture (gel), about 40 mg/mL Al_2O_3 in water; 200 mL

COMPOUND ANTACID PREPARATIONS

PoM **Stomach Powder** (Arnolds)
Oral powder, to prepare an oral solution, ammonium bicarbonate 146 mg, gentian 67.5 mg, ginger 17 mg, prepared nux vomica 67.5 mg, sodium bicarbonate 702 mg/g, for *cattle*; 450 g
Dose. *Cattle*: 38 g 3 times daily for 3-4 days

Proprietary and non-proprietary medicines that are licensed for human use are printed in small type in The Veterinary Formulary

3.7.2 Ulcer-healing drugs

Gastric ulceration may occur in all species. Mucosal damage may be caused by parasite invasion, neoplasia, uraemia, or prolonged use of certain anti-inflammatory drugs. Antacids (see 3.7.1) are used alone or as an adjunct to treatment for gastric ulceration. **Cimetidine** and **ranitidine** block H_2-receptors and inhibit the secretion of gastric acid and reduce pepsin output. Reduced gastric acid secretion allows the ulcer to heal.

Cimetidine is used as an adjunct in the treatment of pancreatitis to inhibit acid peptic breakdown of pancreatic enzyme supplements.

CIMETIDINE

Indications. Gastric ulceration; pancreatitis
Dose. *Dogs*: 5-10 mg/kg 2-4 times daily

PoM **Cimetidine** (Non-proprietary)
Tablets, cimetidine 200 mg, 400 mg, 800 mg

PoM **Tagamet**™ (SK&F)
Syrup, cimetidine 40 mg/mL; 600 mL

RANITIDINE

Indications. Gastric ulceration
Dose. *Dogs*: 2 mg/kg twice daily

PoM **Zantac**™ (Glaxo)
Tablets, dispersible, scored, ranitidine (as hydrochloride) 150 mg; 60
Syrup, ranitidine (as hydrochloride) 15 mg/mL; 300 mL

3.8 Choleretics

Choleretics stimulate hepatocytes to secrete bile. **Menbutone**, an oxobutyric acid derivative, is a choleretic used in veterinary medicine. It is indicated for those conditions where a digestive stimulant is required to promote an effect on biliary, pancreatic, and gastric secretion.

MENBUTONE

Indications. See notes above
Contra-indications. Should not be mixed with solutions containing calcium salts, procaine penicillin, or vitamin B complex

(see Drug Incompatibilities – Appendix 2); cardiac degeneration
Side-effects. Defaecation, urination, salivation, sweating, dyspnoea
Dose. Expressed as menbutone.
Horses, cattle, sheep, pigs: *by intramuscular or slow intravenous injection*, 5-10 mg/kg
Dogs, cats: *by mouth*, 20 mg/kg; *by intramuscular or slow intravenous injection*, 5-10 mg/kg

PoM **Genebile**™ (Boehringer Ingelheim)
Injection, menbutone 100 mg/mL, for *horses, cattle, sheep, pigs, dogs, cats*; 100 mL

Quadramax™ (Willows Francis)
P *Tablets*, scored, menbutone 100 mg, thiamine hydrochloride 5 mg, dried yeast 250 mg, for *dogs, cats*; 250

PoM *Injection*, menbutone 100 mg/mL, for *cattle, sheep, pigs, dogs, cats*; 100 mL

3.9 Pancreatin supplements

Pancreatin supplements are given by mouth to supplement reduced or absent exocrine pancreatic secretions in cases of pancreatic hypoplasia, chronic pancreatitis, or pancreatic degenerative atrophy.
The supplements contain enzymes having protease, lipase and amylase activity which are able to assist in the digestion of starch, fat, and protein respectively. Pancreatin is inactivated by gastric acid and therefore supplements are usually given just before or after food. Gastric acid secretion may be reduced by giving cimetidine (see section 3.7.2). Dosage is adjusted according to response of the individual patient. Frequent small amounts of a diet containing low fat, low fibre and highly digestible protein, or special dietary foods (see section 16.7) may aid in the management of pancreatic insufficiency.

PANCREATIN

Indications. Treatment of diarrhoea and indigestion due to exocrine pancreatic deficiency

GSL **Pancreatin BP (Vet)** (Distributed by Millpledge)
Tablets, amylase 5000 units, lipase 5600 units, protease 330 units, for *dogs, cats*; 500
Dose. *Dogs, cats*: 2-4 tablets/100 g of feed consumed

GSL **Pancrex**™-**Vet** (Paines & Byrne)
Capsules, amylase 9000 units, lipase 8000 units, protease 430 units, for *dogs, cats*; 500
Dose. *Dogs, cats*: 1-2 capsules/100 g of feed consumed
Tablets, amylase 5000 units, lipase 5600 units, protease 330 units, for *dogs, cats*; 500
Dose. *Dogs, cats*: 2-4 tablets/100 g of feed consumed
Tablets, e/c, amylase 5000 units, lipase 5600 units, protease 330 units, for *dogs, cats*; 500
Dose. *Dogs, cats*: 2-4 tablets/100 g of feed consumed
Oral granules, e/c, amylase 4000 units, lipase 5000 units, protease 300 units/g, for *dogs, cats*; 500 g
Dose. *Dogs, cats*: 2-4 g/100 g of feed consumed
Oral powder, amylase 30 000 units, lipase 25 000 units, protease 1400 units/g, for *dogs, cats*; 250 g
Dose. *Dogs, cats*: 400-800 mg/100 g of feed consumed

GSL **Pancrin** (Univet)
Tablets, amylase 5000 units, lipase 5600 units, protease 330 units, for *dogs, cats*; 500
Dose. *Dogs, cats*: 2-4 tablets/100 g of feed consumed

PoM **Tryplase**™ (Intervet)
Capsules, amylase 10 000 units, lipase 14 000 units, protease 500 units, for *dogs, cats*; 100, 250
Dose. *Dogs*: 2-5 capsules daily with feed
Cats: 1-2 capsules daily with feed

Compound pancreatin preparations

GSL **Panteric**™ (Parke-Davis)

Tablets, amylase 7200 units, lipase 6000 units, protease 420 units, sodium tauroglycocholate 100 mg, for *dogs, cats*; 100

Dose. *Dogs, cats*: 1-2 tablets/85 g of feed consumed

4 Drugs used in the treatment of disorders of the
CARDIOVASCULAR SYSTEM

4.1 Myocardial stimulants

4.1.1 Cardiac glycosides
4.1.2 Methylxanthines

Congestive heart failure is usually a progressive disease in spite of treatment. Treatment of causative factors such as nutritional imbalance, bacterial endocarditis, or pericardial effusions may produce symptomatic improvement but frequently the pathological changes in valvular or myocardial tissues are irreversible. Diuretics (see section 4.2) are the mainstay of therapy for congestive heart failure where there is pulmonary or systemic fluid retention. Severe or non-responsive cases may additionally require vasodilator therapy, and myocardial stimulants are necessary where myocardial failure is either a primary or secondary problem. In the dog and the cat, management of congestive heart failure can significantly improve longevity and the quality of life. For working animals, therapy is rarely economically viable.

4.1.1 Cardiac glycosides

Cardiac glycosides act as positive inotropes by increasing the force of myocardial contraction by mechanisms that enhance calcium influx into the myocardial cells. These effects produce an increase in the refractory period of the cells and a decrease in conductivity throughout the myocardium. This causes a decrease in the rate of contraction and thus a negative chronotropic effect. The effect of cardiac glycosides on the autonomic nervous system also contributes to the slowed heart-rate. Parasympathomimetic effects cause slowing of the sino-atrial node rate and delayed conduction in the atrio-ventricular (A-V) node. The increase in cardiac output resulting from digoxin treatment may lead to a reduction in sympathetic drive. In dogs and cats the major indication for cardiac glycoside therapy is supraventricular arrhythmias. Their main use in the horse is in the control of atrial fibrillation.

Cardiac glycosides also have a place in the management of congestive heart failure where it is associated with primary or secondary myocardial failure. They are not indicated for the treatment of congestive heart failure caused by valvular insufficiency or intra-cardiac shunts unless there is secondary myocardial failure.

Digoxin clearance is mainly via the kidney, with a plasma half-life of 20 to 35 hours in the dog and 16 to 23 hours in the horse. **Digitoxin** has mainly hepatic clearance and a half-life of 8 to 12 hours in the dog. These drugs have a narrow therapeutic margin and doses should be titrated for each patient. Slow digitalisation is the method of choice and relies on the plateau principle dependent on the half-life of the drug. In the dog therapeutic plasma-drug concentrations are achieved within 3 to 4 times the half-life, that is 3 to 5 days for digoxin and 1 to 2 days for digitoxin. Doubling the first dose results in the therapeutic concentration being reached more rapidly with minimal risk of toxic signs.

The use of digitoxin in the horse and the cat is not recommended.

Hypokalaemia resulting from prolonged diuretic therapy (see section 4.2) increases the animals' susceptibility to the toxic effects of cardiac glycosides. Signs of toxicity include arrhythmias, which may lead to sino-atrial block. Gastro-intestinal disturbances such as anorexia, vomiting, and diarrhoea may also be observed. Excessively slow heart-rates reduce cardiac output and cause renal dysfunction due to hypoperfusion.

DIGOXIN

Indications. Congestive heart failure; supraventricular arrhythmias
Contra-indications. Renal impairment; sinus or A-V node disease
Side-effects. Vomiting, diarrhoea; bradycardia, arrhythmias
Warnings. The higher rate of gastro-intestinal absorption of alcohol-based elixirs necessitates lower absolute doses. There is decreased absorption of digoxin with concurrent dosing of kaolin or pectin-based gastric protectants or antacid preparations
Dose. *Horses*: 40-70 micrograms/kg as a loading dose, followed by 15-35 micrograms/kg daily
Dogs: 10 micrograms/kg twice daily (maximum 750 micrograms daily). Reassess every other day until therapeutic effect is achieved
Cats: 7-15 micrograms/kg every other day

PoM **Digoxin** (Non-proprietary)
Tablets, digoxin 62.5 micrograms, 125 micrograms, 250 micrograms

PoM **Lanoxin-PG**™ (Wellcome)
Elixir, digoxin 50 micrograms/mL; 60 mL

DIGITOXIN

Indications. Congestive heart failure; supraventricular arrhythmias
Contra-indications. **Side-effects**. **Warnings**. See under Digoxin, see notes above
Dose. *Dogs*: 40-100 micrograms/kg daily in 3 divided doses

PoM **Digitoxin** (Animalcare)
Tablets, digitoxin 100 micrograms, for *dogs*; 250, 1000

4.1.2 Methylxanthines

The methylxanthines **aminophylline**, **diprophylline**, and **etamiphylline camsylate** (see section 5.1.1) are mainly used as bronchodilators but also have a mild diuretic action and positive chronotropic and inotropic activity.

They are used to relieve secondary bronchospasm. Aminophylline and diprophylline may cause tachycardia and vomiting.

4.2 Diuretics

4.2.1 Thiazides
4.2.2 Loop diuretics
4.2.3 Potassium-sparing diuretics
4.2.4 Osmotic diuretics

Diuretics are mainly used in veterinary medicine to reduce oedema in cases of cardiac failure, hepatic disease, cerebral oedema, hypoproteinaemia, inflammation, and trauma. They act by promoting sodium excretion, thus reducing the volume of the extracellular fluid (ECF). They also have vascular effects. Diuretics reduce hypertension and have been claimed to aid therapy of equine epistaxis.

Diuretics are rapidly absorbed and protein bound. They are secreted into the proximal tubule and reach their target site via the urine. Once an effective dose is reached, substantially higher doses are unlikely to achieve more than a slight prolongation of effect and a greater risk of side-effects. Increasing the frequency of dosing may increase the effectiveness of the drug. The requisite dose may be increased in renal failure due to reduced renal blood flow. Proteinuria also results in reduced drug efficacy as there is increased protein-binding of the diuretic.

With prolonged therapy, there may be excessive loss of potassium and magnesium in urine. Hypokalaemia increases the animal's susceptibility to toxicity from cardiac glycosides (see section 4.1.1) and to cardiac dysrhythmias and may impair carbohydrate metabolism. The risk of hypokalaemia is increased by anorexia

To avoid potassium depletion, dietary supplementation may be used or more potent diuretics may be combined with potassium-sparing diuretics (see section 4.2.3). Depletion of extracellular fluid volume without the loss of bicarbonate ions may lead to metabolic alkalosis. Excessive use of diuretics may also cause hypovolaemia leading to reduced renal blood flow and glomerular filtration-rate, thereby compromising renal function.

Attempts to mobilise oedema fluid with short periods of intensive diuresis will cause phases during which the animal is predisposed to acute hypovolaemia followed by extended phases when its kidneys negate the effect of the diuretic. On a 24-hour basis, therefore, a short-acting potent diuretic may have poorer efficacy than a less potent but longer-acting diuretic.

Diuretics are usually classified according to their site of action since this affects their likely side-effects. For example, loop diuretics are much more potent than diuretics acting distally because the loop is the site of greater sodium reabsorption. However, the animal responds to the induced sodium depletion by producing more aldosterone, thus the distal tubule becomes an important site of potassium loss. Some distally active potassium-sparing diuretics are used, therefore, to reduce this unwanted potassium loss, alongside a more powerful diuretic. Some preparations licensed for use in humans combine a potassium-sparing diuretic with more potent diuretics.

4.2.1 Thiazides

The thiazides inhibit sodium reabsorption in the early distal tubule. These drugs act proximal to the site of aldosterone-stimulated sodium and potassium exchange. The delivery of increased amounts of sodium to this area causes greater potassium loss and potassium supplementation may be necessary when using thiazides for diuresis. Thiazides reduce urinary calcium excretion.

Thiazides are used to treat cardiac or hypoproteinaemic oedema and may also be used as an adjunct to hormonal therapy in pseudopregnancy. Thiazides have also been used in the treatment of diabetes insipidus; they cause sodium, chloride, and water loss leading to hypovolaemia. This increases absorption of sodium and water from the proximal tubule. As a result, sodium delivery to the loop is reduced and formation of fully dilute urine is prevented; hence, the diuretic reduces the polyuria observed in diabetes insipidus.

Hydrochlorothiazide remains effective for up to 12 hours and is thus given in divided doses. **Bendrofluazide**, a more potent diuretic is effective for up to 24 hours and is usually administered in the morning.

BENDROFLUAZIDE

Indications. Oedema
Contra-indications. Side-effects. Warnings. See under Frusemide (4.2.2)
Dose. *Dogs, cats*: 125-250 micrograms/kg once daily in the morning

PoM **Bendrofluazide** (Non-proprietary)
Tablets, bendrofluazide 2.5 mg, 5 mg

HYDROCHLOROTHIAZIDE

Indications. Oedema; inhibition of lactation in pseudopregnancy in the bitch
Contra-indications. Side-effects. Warnings. See under Frusemide (4.2.2)
Dose. *Horses, cattle: by mouth*, initial dose 500 mg then 250 mg daily; *by intramuscular or slow intravenous injection*, 250 mg daily
Pigs: by intramuscular injection, 50-75 mg daily
Dogs, cats: by mouth, 1-2 mg/kg daily; *by intramuscular injection*, 12.5-25.0 mg daily

PoM **Vetidrex**™ (Ciba-Geigy)
Tablets, scored, hydrochlorothiazide 25 mg, for *dogs, cats*; 100, 500
Tablets, dispersible, hydrochlorothiazide 250 mg, for *horses, cattle*; 5
Injection, hydrochlorothiazide 50 mg/

mL, for *horses, cattle, pigs, dogs, cats*;
10 mL

4.2.2 Loop diuretics

Loop diuretics are the most potent group of diuretics, with a rapid onset of effect but a short duration of action. These drugs block sodium reabsorption in the loop of Henle. As loop diuretics are so potent, excessive doses can cause hypovolaemia and decompensate renal function. However, their potency allows them to remain effective even when urine delivery is poor, as in renal failure. Loop diuretics increase magnesium excretion and, as with thiazides, may cause severe potassium loss. Hypomagnesaemia potentiates the cardiac effects of hypokalaemia.

Frusemide is used to decrease oedema in conditions such as cardiovascular and pulmonary oedema, hepatic and renal dysfunction, hydrothorax, ascites, and non-specific oedema. Frusemide is detectable in milk for up to 30 hours after treatment.

FRUSEMIDE

Indications. Oedema
Contra-indications. Renal dysfunction with anuria
Side-effects. May cause hypokalaemia with prolonged administration and potassium supplementation may be necessary
Warnings. May potentiate the toxic effects of cardiac glycosides
Dose. *Horses*: *by intramuscular or intravenous injection*, 0.5-1.0 mg/kg 1-2 times daily
Cattle: *by mouth*, 2-5 mg/kg; *by intramuscular or intravenous injection*, 0.5-1.0 mg/kg
Pigs: *by intramuscular or intravenous injection*, 5 mg/kg
Dogs, cats: *by mouth*, 5 mg/kg 1-2 times daily. May be reduced to 1-2 mg/kg twice daily for maintenance; *by intravenous or intramuscular injection*, 2.5-5.0 mg/kg 1-2 times daily

PoM **Diuride**™ (BK)
Tablets, scored, frusemide 40 mg, for *dogs, cats*; 250, 1000

PoM **Frusidal**™ (Univet)
Tablets, scored, frusemide 40 mg, for *dogs, cats*; 500

PoM **Lasix**™ (Hoechst)
Tablets, scored, frusemide 40 mg, for *dogs, cats*; 250
Tablets, scored, frusemide 1 g, for *cattle*; 5
Injection, frusemide 50 mg/mL, for *horses, cattle, pigs, dogs, cats*; 10 mL

4.2.3 Potassium-sparing diuretics

These act in the late distal tubule and oppose the potassium secretion promoted by aldosterone. They can thus ameliorate the excessive potassium loss sometimes caused by more potent diuretics and are usually combined with them. **Spironolactone** acts by competitively antagonising aldosterone effects by blocking the same receptor. The action of spironolactone is self-limiting because any consequent hyperkalaemia will further increase aldosterone secretion allowing it to compete with the drug. **Amiloride** and **triamterene** produce effects on the distal nephron opposite to those of aldosterone. Potassium-sparing diuretics also reduce magnesium loss.

The use of potassium-sparing diuretics should be avoided in animals with conditions predisposing to hyperkalaemia such as renal failure, metabolic acidosis, and diabetes mellitus, or under therapy with beta-blockers which impair cellular uptake of potassium, or angiotensin-converting enzyme inhibitors, for example captopril, which may predispose to hyperkalaemia.

AMILORIDE HYDROCHLORIDE

Indications. Oedema
Contra-indications. Concurrent administration of potassium supplements and beta blockers (see Drug Interactions - Appendix 1); renal impairment; metabolic acidosis; diabetes mellitus

Dose. *Dogs, cats*: 1-2 mg/kg daily

PoM **Amiloride** (Non-proprietary)
Tablets, amiloride hydrochloride 5 mg

SPIRONOLACTONE

Indications. Oedema
Contra-indications. See under Amiloride hydrochloride
Dose. *Dogs, cats*: 1-2 mg/kg daily

PoM **Spironolactone** (Non-proprietary)
Tablets, spironolactone 25 mg, 50 mg, 100 mg

TRIAMTERENE

Indications. Oedema
Contra-indications. See under Amiloride hydrochloride
Dose. *Dogs, cats*: 0.5-3.0 mg/kg daily

PoM **Dytac**™ (Bridge)
Tablets, triamterene 50 mg; 30

4.2.4 Osmotic diuretics

Osmotic diuretics include hypertonic solutions of **mannitol**. Administration of mannitol causes water retention within the nephron, which dilutes urinary sodium and opposes its reabsorption especially in the proximal tubule and loop of Henle.

Mannitol is used to promote urine output, as in acute renal failure, or to reduce cellular oedema in cerebral oedema. It is not suitable for the mobilisation of general or local oedema as it may cause cardiac overload. Excessive administration of mannitol can produce severe hypovolaemia so maintenance of extracellular fluid volume may require administration of an electrolyte solution such as compound sodium lactate intravenous infusion (Hartmann's solution) (see section 16.1.2).

MANNITOL

Indications. Cerebral oedema; forced osmotic diuresis
Contra-indications. Congestive heart failure; pulmonary oedema
Warnings. Extravasation causes inflammation and thrombophlebitis

Dose. *Dogs*: *by intravenous injection*, 250-500 mg/kg test dose. Repeat as necessary if diuresis occurs

PoM **Mannitol** (Non-proprietary)
Intravenous infusion, mannitol 10%, 15%, 20%, 25%

4.3 Vasodilators

Vasodilators effectively decrease the myocardial workload and promote cardiac output by increasing the forward stroke volume. Venodilators reduce the preload and arteriodilators reduce afterload. Some drugs act on both veins and arteries. Vascular tone and intravascular pressure may be elevated in heart failure due to increased sympathetic tone, activation of angiotensin, release of vasopressin, or increased vascular wall stiffness due to salt and water retention. Afterload reduction is especially useful in conditions such as mitral insufficiency where the regurgitant fraction can be significantly reduced.

Captopril is an angiotensin-converting enzyme (ACE) inhibitor that blocks the production of aldosterone and reduces arteriole constriction.

Hydralazine is an arteriodilator causing relaxation of arteriole smooth muscle, probably by local mechanisms.

Prazosin blocks post-synaptic alpha receptors causing arterial and venous dilatation. Adequate monitoring must be provided as the initial dose may cause a precipitous fall in blood pressure.

Sodium nitroprusside is administered intravenously in severe congestive heart failure as it is a potent arterial and venous dilator. It is usually combined with a positive inotrope such as dobutamine (see section 4.5).

Glyceryl trinitrate and other nitrates relax venous smooth muscle and can be useful preload reducers especially in severe pulmonary congestion. Its use is limited in veterinary medicine since sublingual administration is impracticable. Topical ointment formulations may be used.

Isoxsuprine is an arterial dilator having its predominant effect on those vessels supplying skeletal muscles. It is also a positive inotrope.

CAPTOPRIL

Indications. Congestive heart failure
Contra-indications. Renal impairment

Side-effects. Hypotension; renal failure; gastro-intestinal disturbances; anorexia
Warnings. Low doses should be used initially and increased according to the patient's response. Doses should not exceed 2 mg/kg 3 times daily.
Dose. *Dogs*: 0.25-2.0 mg/kg 3 times daily
Cats: 12.5-18.75 mg daily in divided doses

PoM **Acepril**™ (DF)
Tablets, captopril 12.5 mg (scored), 25 mg, 50 mg (scored); 12.5-mg tablets 100; 25-mg, 50-mg tablets 56, 100

PoM **Capoten**™ (Squibb)
Tablets, captopril 12.5 mg (scored), 25 mg, 50 mg (scored); 12.5-mg tablets 100; 25-mg, 50-mg tablets 56, 90, 100

GLYCERYL TRINITRATE

Indications. Cardiogenic pulmonary oedema
Contra-indications. Cardiogenic shock
Side-effects. Hypotension; decreased cardiac output
Warnings. Always wear gloves during the application of ointment to patients
Dose. *Dogs, cats*: *by topical application*, 0.5-2.0 centimetres of a 2% ointment applied to inside of pinna or other area free of hair and inaccessible to the patient

P **Percutol**™ (Rorer)
Ointment, glyceryl trinitrate 2%; 30 g

HYDRALAZINE HYDROCHLORIDE

Indications. Mitral regurgitation and left-sided congestive heart failure
Side-effects. Reflex tachycardia; hypotension; gastro-intestinal disturbances; depression; anorexia

Dose. *Dogs*: 0.5-3.0 mg/kg twice daily
Cats. 2.5 mg twice daily, increasing to 10 mg twice daily if required

PoM **Hydralazine** (Non-proprietary)
Tablets, hydralazine hydrochloride 25 mg, 50 mg

ISOXSUPRINE HYDROCHLORIDE

Indications. Navicular disease
Contra-indications. Recent arterial haemorrhage; pregnant mares and mares up to two weeks post partum
Side-effects. Tachycardia
Dose. See preparation details

PoM **Duviculine**™ (Duphar)
Capsules, s/r, isoxsuprine hydrochloride 60 mg, for *horses*; 250
Withdrawal Periods. Should not be used in *horses* intended for human consumption
Dose. *Horses*: 900 micrograms/kg twice daily for 3 weeks, increasing to 1.2 mg/kg twice daily if required. Avoid sudden discontinuation of treatment. The dose should be reduced over a further 3-week period

PoM **Oralject Circulon**™ (Vetsearch; distributed by Millpledge)
Oral paste, isoxsuprine hydrochloride 40 mg/mL, for *horses*; 230 mL
Withdrawal Periods. Should not be used in *horses* intended for human consumption
Dose. *Horses*: 600 micrograms/kg twice daily for 3 weeks, increasing to 900 micrograms/kg twice daily if required. Avoid sudden discontinuation of treatment. The dose should be reduced over a further 3-week period

PRAZOSIN HYDROCHLORIDE

Indications. Congestive heart failure
Side-effects. Hypotension
Warnings. It is inadvisable to dose animals of less than 5 kg body-weight; efficacy is reduced with prolonged dosing
Dose. *Dogs*: (up to 15 kg body-weight) 1 mg 2-3 times daily; (more than 15 kg body-weight) 2 mg 2-3 times daily

PoM **Hypovase**™ (Invicta)
Tablets, prazosin hydrochloride 500 micrograms, 1 mg (scored), 2 mg (scored), 5 mg (scored); 56

SODIUM NITROPRUSSIDE

Indications. Life-threatening congestive heart failure
Side-effects. Hypotension
Warnings. Mean arterial blood pressure should be monitored
Dose. *By intravenous infusion*, 1 microgram/kg per minute increasing gradually, maintaining a mean arterial blood pressure above 70 mmHg

PoM **Sodium Nitroprusside** (Non-proprietary)
Intravenous infusion, for dilution, sodium nitroprusside 10 mg/mL; 5 mL. To be diluted before use

4.4 Anti-arrhythmics

4.4.1 Class I anti-arrhythmics
4.4.2 Class II anti-arrhythmics
4.4.3 Class III anti-arrhythmics
4.4.4 Class IV anti-arrhythmics
Abnormal heart rhythms may be controlled by anti-arrhythmic drugs. Permanent or progressive myocardial damage requires ongoing medication. However, if the cause is a focal or generalised inflammatory condition, which may itself resolve, the arrhythmia may cease and therapy can be discontinued. In dogs and cats atrial fibrillation is usually irreversible due to pathology of the atrial myocardium, whereas in the performance horse there is often no underlying cardiac abnormality and following treatment the animal returns to normal function.
Drugs used to control supraventricular and ventricular arrhythmias may be classified according to their mechanism of action. Many arrhythmias are secondary to an underlying cause such as trauma, gastric torsion, renal failure, central nervous disease, hypoxia, or electrolyte imbalance. It is important to address the primary cause where it can be determined.

4.4.1 Class I anti-arrhythmics

Drugs included in this class have a local anaesthetic action. They have a membrane-stabilising effect that results in a reduced rate of depolarisation. Although the subdivision of this class into A, B, and C is based on their varied effects on the action potential there is no clinical significance in these divisions. Only drugs in classes 1A (procainamide, quinidine) and 1B (lignocaine, phenytoin) are commonly used in veterinary medicine.
Quinidine is used mainly in cases of atrial fibrillation in the horse. It is less commonly used in the dog. **Procainamide** is rapidly absorbed after oral administration in the dog and has a plasma half-life of 2.5 to 4 hours. Most preparations are formulated as sustained-release dosage forms to overcome problems of frequent dosing. Procainamide is the drug of choice for ventricular arrhythmias in the dog. Disopyramide has a half-life of less than 2 hours and results in such significant myocardial depression as to preclude its routine use.
Lignocaine without adrenaline is given intravenously for severe acute ventricular arrhythmias of any cause. Efficient first-pass metabolism in the liver precludes oral dosing. **Phenytoin** (see section 6.9.1) has similar cardiovascular effects to lignocaine. It is used to treat cardiac glycoside toxicity♦ in dogs at a dose of 35 to 50 mg/kg by mouth 3 times daily. **Tocainide** is given by mouth and has a similar anti-arrhythmic action to lignocaine.

LIGNOCAINE HYDROCHLORIDE

Indications. Life-threatening ventricular arrhythmias
Contra-indications. Atrial fibrillation or flutter
Side-effects. Seizures; hypotension; central nervous system disturbances
Warnings. Not effective in the presence of hypokalaemia; doses should be

reduced in congestive heart failure or hepatic disease. See Drug Interactions – Appendix 1

Dose. *Dogs*: *by intravenous injection*, initial dose 2-4 mg/kg, followed by intravenous infusion at a rate of 25-75 micrograms/kg per minute

Cats: *by intravenous injection*, initial dose 250-500 micrograms, followed *by intravenous infusion* at a rate of 20 micrograms/kg per minute

PoM **Lignocaine** (Non-proprietary)
Intravenous infusion, lignocaine hydrochloride 1 mg/mL and 2 mg/mL in glucose intravenous infusion 5%; 500 mL, 1 litre

PoM **Min-I-Jet™ Lignocaine** (IMS)
Injection, lignocaine hydrochloride 10 mg/mL, 20 mg/mL; 10-mg/mL syringe 10 mL, 20-mg/mL syringe 5 mL

PoM **Select-A-Jet™ Lignocaine** (IMS)
Intravenous infusion, for dilution, lignocaine hydrochloride 200 mg/mL; 5 mL. To be diluted before use

PoM **Xylocard™** (Astra)
Injection, lignocaine hydrochloride (anhydrous) 20 mg/mL; 5 mL
Intravenous infusion, for dilution, lignocaine hydrochloride (anhydrous) 200 mg/mL; 5 mL, 10 mL. To be diluted before use

PROCAINAMIDE HYDROCHLORIDE

Indications. Supraventricular and ventricular arrhythmias such as ventricular premature depolarisations and ventricular tachycardia
Contra-indications. Untreated atrial fibrillation; renal impairment; conduction blocks
Side-effects. Gastro-intestinal disturbances
Dose. *Dogs*: *by mouth*, 8-20 mg/kg 4 times daily (tablets) or 3 times daily (sustained-release tablets); *by intramuscular injection*, 8-20 mg/kg 4 times daily; *by intravenous injection*, initial dose 2-15 mg/kg over 20 minutes, followed *by intravenous infusion* at a rate of 10-40 micrograms/kg per minute

PoM **Pronestyl™** (Squibb)
Tablets, scored, procainamide hydrochloride 250 mg; 100

Injection, procainamide hydrochloride 100 mg/mL; 10 mL

PoM **Procainamide Durules™** (Astra)
Tablets, s/r, procainamide hydrochloride 500 mg; 100

QUINIDINE SULPHATE

Indications. Supraventricular arrhythmias especially atrial fibrillation

Contra-indications. Hepatic impairment. See Drug Interactions – Appendix 1
Side-effects. Anorexia; vomiting, diarrhoea; tachycardia, ventricular fibrillation; allergic responses
Warnings. Increased toxicity in cases with hypoalbuminaemia
Dose. *Horses*: 20 mg/kg every 2 hours until arrhythmia is abolished (maximum 60 g daily)
Dogs: 6-16 mg/kg 3-4 times daily

PoM **Quinidine Sulphate** (Non-proprietary)
Tablets, quinidine sulphate 200 mg, 300 mg
Quinidine sulphate powder is available from Loveridge

TOCAINIDE HYDROCHLORIDE

Indications. Life-threatening ventricular arrhthymias
Contra-indications. Bradycardia, A-V block
Side-effects. Nausea, vomiting, anorexia; hypotension
Dose. *Dogs*: 10-20 mg/kg 3-4 times daily

PoM **Tonocard™** (Astra)
Tablets, tocainide hydrochloride 400 mg, 600 mg; 100

4.4.2 Class II anti-arrhythmics

Drugs included in this class are beta-adrenoceptor blocking drugs (beta blockers), which inhibit sympathetic activity. The heart-rate is decreased by a reduction in the sinus node rate and prolongation of atrio-ventricular (A-V) node conduction. These drugs prevent reflex tachycardia and decrease the occurrence of both atrial and ventricular premature depolarisations.

Propranolol is the most common beta blocker used in veterinary practice for atrial arrhythmias. It undergoes hepatic metabolism and has a plasma half-life of 1.5 hours. In cardiac failure, hepatic blood flow is reduced and propranolol metabolism is altered with prolonged administration, therefore the drug is given every 8 hours. Other compounds in this group include atenolol, pindolol, nadolol, metoprolol, and bisoprolol. Their properties are similar to propranolol. Dosages should be titrated on an individual patient basis.

PROPRANOLOL HYDROCHLORIDE

Indications. Supraventricular tachycardia; hypertrophic cardiomyopathy; thyrotoxicosis (7.1.2) especially in cats; atrial or ventricular premature depolarisations

Contra-indications. Concurrent administration of quinidine; hepatic impairment with decreased blood flow; asthma; small airway disease; sick sinus syndrome; A-V block

Side-effects. Bronchospasm; myocardial depression; bradycardia; hypotension

Warnings. Bronchospasm; negative inotropic properties may exacerbate congestive heart failure

Dose. *Dogs*: 100 micrograms/kg 3 times daily, increasing over 3-5 days to a maximum of 1 mg/kg 3 times daily as necessary

Cats: 2.5 mg 3 times daily, increasing over 3-5 days to up to 10 mg 3 times daily as necessary

PoM **Propranolol** (Non-proprietary)
Tablets, propranolol hydrochloride 10 mg, 40 mg, 80 mg, 160 mg

ATENOLOL

Indications. Supraventricular arrhythmias

Contra-indications. Side-effects. Warnings. See under Propranolol hydrochloride

Dose. *Dogs*: 20-100 mg 3 times daily

PoM **Atenolol** (Non-proprietary)
Tablets, atenolol 50 mg, 100 mg

METOPROLOL TARTRATE

Indications. Supraventricular arrhythmias

Contra-indications. Side-effects. Warnings. See under Propranolol hydrochloride

Dose. *Dogs*: 5-50 mg 3 times daily

PoM **Metoprolol Tartrate** (Non-proprietary)
Tablets, metoprolol tartrate 50 mg, 100 mg

NADOLOL

Indications. Supraventricular arrhythmias

Contra-indications. Side-effects. Warnings. See under Propranolol hydrochloride

Dose. *Dogs*: 5-40 mg 3 times daily

PoM **Corgard**™ (Squibb)
Tablets, nadolol 40 mg, 80 mg; 28

PINDOLOL

Indications. Supraventricular arrhythmias

Contra-indications. Side-effects. Warnings. See under Propranolol hydrochloride

Dose. *Dogs*: 1-3 mg 3 times daily

PoM **Visken**™ (Sandoz)
Tablets, scored, pindolol 5 mg, 15 mg; 5-mg tablets 100; 15-mg tablets 30

TIMOLOL MALEATE

Indications. Supraventricular arrhythmias

Contra-indications. Side-effects. Warnings. See under Propranolol hydrochloride

Dose. *Dogs*: 0.5-5.0 mg 3 times daily

PoM **Betim**™ (Leo)
Tablets, scored, timolol maleate 10 mg; 100

PoM **Blocadren**™ (MSD)
Tablets, scored, timolol maleate 10 mg; 100

4.4.3 Class III anti-arrhythymics

Drugs in this class prolong the action potential and hence the effective refractory period.

AMIODARONE HYDROCHLORIDE

Indications. Supraventricular and ventricular arrhythmias
Contra-indications.   Thyrotoxicosis; bradycardia
Side-effects. Pulmonary fibrosis; corneal deposits; thyroid disturbances
Dose. *Dogs*: 10 mg/kg twice daily

PoM **Cordarone**™ X (Sanofi)
Tablets, scored, amiodarone hydrochloride 100 mg, 200 mg; 28

BRETYLIUM TOSYLATE

Indications. Ventricular arrhythmias refractory to routine therapy
Side-effects. Rarely hypotension; ataxia; vomiting
Dose. *Dogs*: *by intravenous injection*, 2-6 mg/kg

PoM **Bretylate**™ (Wellcome)
Injection, bretylium tosylate 50 mg/mL; 2 mL

4.4.4 Class IV anti-arrhythmics

Drugs in this class inhibit slow calcium channels and cause arterial and venous dilatation. They have a profound depressant effect on A-V nodal conduction and are the drugs of choice for severe acute supraventricular tachycardias. In addition, they are potent coronary artery dilators and cause hypotension due to peripheral vasodilatation. A negative inotropic effect may exacerbate congestive heart failure.

DILTIAZEM HYDROCHLORIDE

Indications. Supraventricular tachyarrhythmias
Side-effects. Hypotension; bradycardia
Warnings. Care should be taken in case of sick sinus syndrome and untreated congestive heart failure
Dose. *Dogs*: 0.5-1.25 mg/kg 3-4 times daily

PoM **Diltiazem** (Non-proprietary)
Tablets, diltiazem hydrochloride 60 mg

VERAPAMIL HYDROCHLORIDE

Indications.   Supraventricular tachyarrhythmias; sustained and paroxysmal tachycardia
Side-effects. Hypotension; bradycardia; myocardial depression
Warnings. See under Diltiazem hydrochloride
Dose. *Dogs*: *by mouth*, 1-5 mg/kg 3 times daily; *by intravenous injection*, 50-150 micrograms/kg according to the patient's response

PoM **Verapamil** (Non-proprietary)
Tablets, verapamil hydrochloride 40 mg, 80 mg, 120 mg, 160 mg

PoM **Cordilox**™ (Abbott)
Injection, verapamil hydrochloride 2.5 mg/mL; 2 mL

PoM **Securon**™ (Knoll)
Injection, verapamil hydrochloride 2.5 mg/mL; 2 mL

4.5 Sympathomimetics

Sympathomimetic drugs are used for cardiovascular support in the management of critically ill patients. These are usually cases under anaesthesia or recovering from major surgery. Patients in shock, especially cardiogenic in origin may also benefit from this type of support.

The properties of sympathomimetics vary according to whether they act on alpha- or beta-adrenergic receptors.

Adverse effects of sympathomimetics include fear, anxiety, restlessness, vasoconstriction, and ventricular arrhythmias. All of the drugs discussed below have short plasma half-lives, but are useful for emergency care.

Adrenaline acts on both alpha- and beta-receptors and increases both heart-rate and contractility (beta$_1$ effects). It can cause peripheral vasodilatation (a beta effect) or vasoconstriction (an alpha effect). Adrenaline is used in the emergency treatment of acute allergic and anaphylactic reactions. Adrenaline may be administered by intracardiac injection in cases of cardiac arrest. **Adrenaline solutions should be diluted to at least 1 in 10 000 (100 micrograms/ mL) for all animal use.**

The cardiac stimulant **dobutamine** acts on beta$_1$ receptors in cardiac muscle, with minimal effect on heart-rate or blood pressure. It has a positive inotropic effect and is used for cardiogenic shock. **Isoprenaline** is less selective and increases both heart-rate and contractility.

The antimuscarinic drug, **atropine sulphate** (see section 6.6.1) is used for the treatment of bradycardia♦, incomplete A-V block♦, and sino-atrial arrest♦ in doses of 10 to 20 micrograms/ kg by intramuscular or intravenous injection or 30 to 40 micrograms/kg subcutaneously, in dogs and cats.

ADRENALINE

Indications. Anaphylaxis; cardiac arrest♦
Contra-indications. Manufacturer does not recommend administration by intravenous injection
Side-effects. Sweating in horses
Dose. *Dogs, cats*: *by intravenous injection*, 0.5-10.0 micrograms/kg; *by intracardiac injection*, 2-5 micrograms/kg (cardiac arrest)

PoM **Adrenaline Injection BP** (Non-proprietary)
Injection, adrenaline (as acid tartrate) 1 mg/ mL; 0.5 mL, 1.0 mL

Proprietary and non-proprietary medicines that are licensed for human use are printed in small type in The Veterinary Formulary

DOBUTAMINE

Indications. Cardiogenic shock; bradycardia; dilated cardiomyopathy with congestive heart failure
Side-effects. Tachyarrythmias; seizures in cats
Warnings. Monitor ECG
Dose. *Dogs*: *by intravenous infusion*, 2-7 micrograms/kg per minute (for up to 3 days in cases of cardiomyopathy)

Cats: *by intravenous infusion*, up to 4 micrograms/kg per minute

PoM **Dobutrex**™ (Lilly)
Intravenous infusion, for dilution, dobutamine (as hydrochloride) 12.5 mg/mL; 20 mL. To be diluted before use

ISOPRENALINE HYDROCHLORIDE

Indications. Heart block; bradycardia
Side-effects. Ventricular tachycardias
Warnings. Monitor ECG
Dose. *Dogs*: *by mouth*, 5-10 mg 3-4 times daily; *by intravenous infusion*, 10 nanograms/kg per minute

PoM **Saventrine**™ (Pharmax)
Tablets, isoprenaline hydrochloride 30 mg; 30, 250

PoM **Saventrine**™ iv (Pharmax)
Intravenous infusion, for dilution, isoprenaline hydrochloride 1 mg/mL; 2 mL. To be diluted before use

4.6 Anticoagulants

4.6.1 Parenteral anticoagulants
4.6.2 Oral anticoagulants

Anticoagulant drugs are much less frequently used in veterinary medicine than in human patients because atherosclerotic disease and prolonged postoperative recumbency are not common veterinary problems. Anticoagulants are part of the management of disseminated intravascular coagulation but are most commonly used to maintain patency of vascular catheters. There is evidence that warfarin can relieve the clinical signs of navicular disease in some horses. The main use of anticoagulants is to prevent thrombus formation or the extension of an existing thrombus. These agents act by affecting the clotting mechanisms. Heparin is rapidly effective, which makes it suitable for emergency situations. Coumarin derivatives, such as warfarin, act indirectly as vitamin K antagonists and are thus more suitable where prolonged therapy is required.

4.6.1 Parenteral anticoagulants

The action of **heparin** prevents thrombus formation but does not affect fibrin that is already present. It is metabolised in the liver and has a plasma half-life of 2 hours. For patients receiving treatment, the activated partial thromboplastin time and activated coagulation time should be maintained at 1.5 to 2.5 times normal. Practitioners are advised to use the normal values supplied by a local veterinary testing laboratory. Suggested normal values in the adult dog are:

Partial thromboplastin   15-25 seconds
time

Activated coagulation   60-125 seconds
time of whole blood
at room temperature

For maintaining catheter patency sodium chloride intravenous infusion 0.9% is as effective as heparin flushes for up to 48 hours and is therefore recommended for cannulas intended to be in place for 48 hours or less. Heparin flushes are recommended for cannulas intended to be in place longer than 48 hours. Heparin injection diluted to 5 units/mL in sodium chloride intravenous infusion 0.9% may be used.

HEPARIN SODIUM

Indications. Venous thrombosis; disseminated intravascular coagulation; pulmonary thrombo-embolism
Contra-indications. Hepatic impairment; haemorrhage. See Drug Interactions – Appendix 1
Side-effects. Haemorrhage
Dose. *Dogs*: *by subcutaneous injection*, 40-80 units/kg 3 times daily; *by intravenous injection*, initial dose 10-20 units/kg then 5 units/kg every 3 hours
Cats: *by subcutaneous injection*, 200 units/kg 3 times daily

PoM **Heparin** (Non-proprietary)
Injection, heparin sodium 1000 units/mL, 5000 units/mL, 10 000 units/mL, 25 000 units/mL; 1000-unit/mL, 5000-unit/mL vials, 1 mL, 5 mL; 10 000-unit/mL, 25 000-unit/mL vials 1 mL

4.6.2 Oral anticoagulants

Coumarin derivative anticoagulants inhibit the hepatic synthesis of vitamin K-dependent clotting factors. **Warfarin** is well absorbed from the intestine and is almost exclusively bound to plasma albumin. The onset of effect is 8 to 12 hours, with full benefit realised after 2 to 3 days.

Aspirin (see section 10.1) is used in cats with thrombo-embolism secondary to cardiomyopathy at a dose of up to 75 mg, by mouth, once every three days.

Many drugs are capable of displacing warfarin from plasma albumin, causing an increase in free warfarin and possible haemorrhage.

WARFARIN SODIUM

Indications. Venous thrombosis; navicular disease
Contra-indications. Purpura; malnutrition; haemorrhage. See Drug Interactions – Appendix 1
Side-effects. Haemorrhage
Warnings. Monitor effect using Quick test (one-stage prothrombin time) with samples taken at the same time each day for comparative purposes
Dose. *Horses*: 18 micrograms/kg increasing gradually to desired effect

PoM **Marevan**™ (DF)
Tablets, scored, warfarin sodium 1 mg, 3 mg, 5 mg; 100, 500

PoM **Warfarin WBP** (Boehringer Ingelheim)
Tablets, scored, warfarin sodium 1 mg, 3 mg, 5 mg; 100, 500

4.7 Fibrinolytics

Fibrinolytic drugs act as thrombolytics by activating plasminogens to form plasmin, which degrades fibrin, thereby breaking up the thrombus. **Streptokinase** has been used in the treatment of deep venous thrombosis. In such cases specialist advice should be sought.

4.8 Haemostatics

The use of **phytomenadione** (vitamin K_1) in the treatment of anticoagulant poisoning is described in Emergency treatment of poisoning. Preparation details are in section 16.5.6.

A mixture of **malonic and oxalic acids** has been given parenterally for certain haemorrhagic disorders. The efficacy of this preparation has not been confirmed. **Adrenaline** (see section 4.5) may be applied topically as a haemostatic. **Ferric chloride solution** has also been used topically to arrest bleeding from small wounds.

Dressings containing **calcium alginate** are available for control of wound haemorrhage during surgical procedures.

CALCIUM ALGINATE

Indications. Haemostasis

GSL **Hemovet**™ (Boehringer Ingelheim)
Fibrous wool swab, calcium alginate 400 mg
Fibrous wool pad, calcium alginate; 6 cm x 4 cm
Withdrawal Periods. Slaughter withdrawal period nil, milk withdrawal period nil

GSL **Kaltostat**™ (Hoechst)
Fibrous pad, calcium alginate, for *horses, cattle, sheep, pigs, dogs, cats, rabbits*; 7.5 cm x 12.0 cm, 10 cm x 20 cm

COMPOUND HAEMOSTATICS

PoM **Venagmin**™ (Willows Francis)
Injection, malonic acid 2.5 mg, oxalic acid 7.5 mg/mL for *horses, dogs*; 30 mL
Dose. Horses: *by intramuscular injection*, 10 mL in divided doses; *by intravenous injection*, 10 mL
Dogs: *by intramuscular or intravenous injection*, 0.08-0.16 mL/kg

5 Drugs used in the treatment of disorders of the
RESPIRATORY SYSTEM

5.1 Bronchodilators
5.2 Antihistamines and anti-inflammatory drugs
5.3 Mucolytics and expectorants
5.4 Antitussives
5.5 Respiratory stimulants
5.6 Nasal decongestants

Infection is one of the primary causes of respiratory distress. Wherever possible, the identity of the causative organism should be sought and appropriate treatment initiated before commencing symptomatic therapy. The use of anti-bacterial and antifungal drugs is described in Chapter 1 and the use of endoparasiticides is described in section 2.1. The use of vaccines to provide specific protection against pulmonary infection is described in Chapter 18.

5.1 Bronchodilators

5.1.1 Methylxanthines
5.1.2 Sympathomimetics

Bronchodilators are used where there is suspicion of bronchial narrowing due to bronchial secretion or broncho-constriction or where improved alveolar ventilation is required. In veterinary medicine these drugs are used for disorders including mild tracheo-bronchitis and severe chronic obstructive pulmonary disease (COPD) in horses, and bronchopneumonia and chronic pulmonary interstitial disease in all species.

The assessment of airway function, airway calibre, and bronchomotor tone is often subjective. The use and choice of a bronchodilator may be primarily on an empirical basis. The use of bronchodilators with or without con-current corticosteroid therapy is often used for the control of chronic bronchitis, and asthma syndrome in cats.

5.1.1 Methylxanthines

Methylxanthines including **aminophyl-line, diprophylline, etamiphylline,** and **theophylline** induce bronchodilation of the smaller airways by inhibition of phosphodiesterase, and have little effect on larger airways. These drugs may also increase tidal volume by stimulating the respiratory centre in the medulla oblongata.

Methylxanthines are more effective where there is reversible airway obstruction than in chronic respiratory disease. Their ability to induce bronchodilation is severely impaired by pathological changes both in the airway walls and pulmonary interstitium. This accounts for the wide variability of response seen with these drugs and individual animal treatment is often determined on a trial-and-error basis.

Methylxanthines are also central nervous and myocardial stimulants and diuretics. At therapeutic doses they cause increased alertness and activity. Signs of toxicity include restlessness, tachy-cardia, tachypnoea, and convulsions.

AMINOPHYLLINE

Indications. Respiratory disease where bronchodilation may be beneficial; myocardial stimulation (4.1.2)
Side-effects. Central nervous system and cardiovascular stimulation
Dose. *Dogs, cats: by mouth or by intramuscular or slow intravenous injection,* 10 mg/kg 2-3 times daily

Aminophylline (Non-proprietary)
P *Tablets,* aminophylline 100 mg

PoM *Injection*, aminophylline 25 mg/mL; 10 mL

PoM *Injection*, aminophylline 250 mg/mL; 2 mL

DIPROPHYLLINE

Indications. Respiratory disease where bronchodilation may be beneficial; myocardial stimulation (4.1.2)
Side-effects. See under Aminophylline
Dose. *Dogs, cats*: 200-400 mg 2 to 4 times daily

P **Theocardin™** (BK)
Tablets, diprophylline 200 mg, for *dogs, cats*; 100, 1000

ETAMIPHYLLINE CAMSYLATE

Indications. Respiratory disease where bronchodilation may be beneficial; respiratory stimulation of neonates (5.5); myocardial stimulation (4.1.2)
Side-effects. See under Aminophylline
Dose. *Horses, cattle*: *by addition to feed or as an oral solution*, 900 mg 3 times daily; *by subcutaneous or intramuscular injection*, 1.4 g repeated 3 times daily if required; *calves*: *by mouth*, 700 mg repeated after 3-4 hours if required; *by subcutaneous or intramuscular injection*, 0.7-1.05 g repeated 3 times daily if required
Sheep: *by subcutaneous or intramuscular injection*, 0.7-1.05 g repeated 3 times daily if required; *lambs*: *by mouth*, (less than 2.5 kg body-weight) 140 mg repeated after 3-4 hours if required; (more than 2.5 kg body-weight) up to 280 mg repeated after 3-4 hours if required
Dogs: *by mouth*, 100-300 mg 3 times daily; *by subcutaneous or intramuscular injection*, 140-700 mg repeated 3 times daily if required
Cats: *by mouth*, 100 mg 3 times daily; *by subcutaneous or intramuscular injection*, 140-280 mg repeated 3 times daily if required

PML **Dalophylline™** (Arnolds)
Oral gel, etamiphylline camsylate 140 mg/dose, for *calves, lambs*; 32-mL metered-dose applicator (1 dose = 3.2 mL)

Withdrawal Periods. *Calves, lambs*: slaughter 1 day

Millophyline-V™ (Arnolds)
P *Tablets*, etamiphylline camsylate 100 mg, for *dogs, cats*; 100, 500
P *Oral powder*, for addition to feed or to prepare an oral solution, etamiphylline camsylate 300 mg, for *horses, cattle, sheep*
PoM *Injection*, etamiphylline camsylate 140 mg/mL, for *horses, cattle, sheep, dogs, cats*; 50 mL

THEOPHYLLINE

Indications. Respiratory disease where bronchodilation may be beneficial
Contra-indications. Manufacturer does not recommend use in pregnant mares. Acute myocardial disease
Side-effects. See under Aminophylline

PoM **Euphyllin™ Retard** (Boehringer Ingelheim)
Pellets, for addition to feed, s/r, theophylline 817 mg/g, for *horses*; 3.67 g
Withdrawal Periods. Should not be used in *horses* intended for human consumption
Dose. *Horses*: initial dose 12 mg/kg of theophyline then 6 mg/kg daily

5.1.2 Sympathomimetics

Beta$_2$-adrenoceptor agonists are direct-acting sympathomimetic drugs and include **clenbuterol** and **terbutaline**. Clenbuterol has been shown to reduce transpulmonary pressure fluctuations in horses with COPD. Terbutaline may have a greater cardiac stimulant effect than clenbuterol. Aerosol adminis tration of these drugs reduces the cardiac effects but is impractical in most animals As well as bronchodilation these drugs increase ciliary beating of the respiratory mucosal cells and have a mucolytic action, which may contribute to their therapeutic effect.

CLENBUTEROL HYDROCHLORIDE

Indications. Bronchodilation in allergic respiratory disease, respiratory infection and inflammation, chronic obstructive pulmonary disease

Contra-indications. Concurrent administration of corticosteroids. Cardiac disease

Side-effects. Transient vasodilatation and tachycardia with sweating and muscle tremor

Warnings. May abolish uterine contractions

Dose. *Horses: by mouth or by slow intravenous injection*, 800 nanograms/kg twice daily

Cattle: by intramuscular or slow intravenous injection, 800 nanograms/kg twice daily; *calves*: 800 nanograms/kg twice daily

Dogs♦: by mouth or by slow intravenous injection, 800 nanograms/kg twice daily

PoM **Ventipulmin**™ (Boehringer Ingelheim)

Oral granules, for addition to feed, clenbuterol hydrochloride 16 micrograms/g, for *horses, calves*; 12.5 g, 500 g Withdrawal Periods. Should not be used in *horses* intended for human consumption. *Calves*: slaughter 12 days *Injection*, clenbuterol hydrochloride 30 micrograms/mL, for *horses, cattle*; 5 mL

Withdrawal Periods. Should not be used in *horses* intended for human consumption. *Cattle*: slaughter 12 days, milk 72 hours

---

TERBUTALINE SULPHATE

Indications. Respiratory disease where bronchodilation may be beneficial
Dose. *Dogs*: 1.25-5.0 mg 2-3 times daily
Cats: 1.25 mg 2-3 times daily

PoM **Bricanyl**™ (Astra)
Syrup, terbutaline sulphate 300 micrograms/mL; 300 mL, 1 litre

PoM **Monovent**™ (Lagap)
Syrup, terbutaline sulphate 300 micrograms/mL; 300 mL

5.2 Antihistamines and anti-inflammatory drugs

5.2.1 Antihistamines
5.2.2 Sodium cromoglycate
Allergic pulmonary disease may involve neutrophilic or eosinophilic migration into the lung parenchyma and airways, and mast-cell degranulation with release of inflammatory mediators such as histamine. Airway mucosal inflammatory mechanisms may be activated leading to the release of prostaglandins and leukotrienes. The symptoms of allergic pulmonary disease can vary from mild intractable coughing to severe respiratory distress and death.

Allergic respiratory diseases are a poorly defined group of conditions in animals, and include pulmonary infiltration with eosinophilia (PIE) in the dog, feline asthma syndrome, acute bovine allergic pneumonitis and alveolitis, and COPD in the horse. All are believed to involve an allergic reaction to either inhaled allergens or migrating pulmonary parasites. Human dander (epithelium) may be implicated in the cat disease.

Allergens causing reactions in horses include moulds from poor quality dusty hay and bedding. Control of COPD is achieved by avoiding allergens where possible, which involves keeping susceptible animals at pasture, using dust-free bedding, and feeding good quality mould-free hay. Treatment should always be directed at preventing further exposure to the allergen rather than the use of long-term therapy. In those horses where the symptoms are present, bronchodilators and corticosteroids may be used.

Corticosteroids (see section 7.2.1) are the drugs of choice in the treatment of canine and feline allergic respiratory disease and have also been used in cattle and horses.

Corticosteroids counteract the symptoms of respiratory disease in a variety of ways. They reduce airway inflammation due to histamine and prostaglandin release, prevent inflammatory mediator-induced bronchoconstriction, and may stabilise mast cell and lysosomal membranes. Reduction of inflammatory mediator release and mucus secretion improves mucociliary clearance of airway debris and reduces eosinophil migration into lung tissue. In emergency situations intravenous corticosteroids such as dexamethasone and betamethasone should be used, followed by oral prednisolone for long-term maintenance.

Flunixin meglumine (see section 10.1) is a non-steroidal anti-inflammatory drug (NSAID). It may be used in the treatment of acute bovine allergic pneumonitis and alveolitis, and may significantly reduce the mortality rate in this condition. It has also been used in calf pneumonias.

5.2.1 Antihistamines

Histamine is only one of many autacoids involved in hypersensitivity reactions and so antihistamines (H_1 antagonists) such as **promethazine**, **tripelennamine**, and **trimeprazine** have limited use in the treatment of allergic disorders in animals. These drugs are useful in the control of allergic rhinitis in the cat, but sedation often precludes long-term use. Nasal decongestants, such as pseudoephedrine (see section 5.6), are more effective therapy.

DIPHENHYDRAMINE HYDROCHLORIDE

Indications. Allergic respiratory disease; relief of coughing
Side-effects. CNS depression

P **Benylin™ Children's Cough Linctus** (Parke-Davis)
Linctus, diphenhydramine hydrochloride 1.4 mg, menthol 110 micrograms/mL; 125 mL
Warnings. May cause drowsiness
Dose. *Horses, cattle*: 60 mL as necessary; *foals, calves*: 10-20 mL 2-3 times daily
Dogs: 15-20 mL every 2-3 hours

PROMETHAZINE HYDROCHLORIDE

Indications. Allergic respiratory disease
Side-effects. CNS depression
Dose. *Dogs*: *by mouth or by subcutaneous injection*, 0.2-1.0 mg/kg 2-3 times daily

Phenergan™ (M&B)
P *Tablets*, promethazine hydrochloride 10 mg, 25 mg; 56
P *Elixir*, promethazine hydrochloride 1 mg/mL; 100 mL

PoM *Injection*, promethazine hydrochloride 25 mg/mL; 1 mL

TRIMEPRAZINE TARTRATE

Indications. Allergic respiratory disease
Dose. *Dogs*: 500-700 micrograms/kg daily

PoM **Vallergan™** (M&B)
Tablets, trimeprazine tartrate 10 mg; 28
Syrup, trimeprazine tartrate 1.5 mg/mL; 100 mL
Syrup forte, trimeprazine tartrate 6 mg/mL; 100 mL

TRIPELENNAMINE HYDROCHLORIDE

Indications. Allergic respiratory disease
Side-effects. CNS depression
Dose. *Horses, cattle, pigs*: *by intramuscular or intravenous injection*, 400-800 micrograms/kg
Dogs: *by intramuscular injection*, up to 20 mg
Cats: *by intramuscular injection*, up to 10 mg

PoM **Vetibenzamine™** (Ciba-Geigy)
Injection, tripelennamine hydrochloride 20 mg/mL, for *horses, cattle, pigs, dogs, cats*; 100 mL

5.2.2 Sodium cromoglycate

Sodium cromoglycate inhibits mast-cell degranulation on antigen challenge and may also have membrane-stabilising properties, but its precise mode of action is unclear. It is used for prophylaxis of COPD in the horse. Sodium cromoglycate should not be administered during an allergic attack, but may be delivered by inhalation, using a face mask, prior to expected exposure to an allergen. The length of protection is dependent on the number of consecutive days that the drug is administered. Four days of sodium cromoglycate administration will protect the horse for up to 20 days.

SODIUM CROMOGLYCATE

Indications. Prophylactic therapy of allergic respiratory disease

Contra-indications. Manufacturer does not recommend use during the first trimester of pregnancy in mares
Dose. *Horses*: *by inhalation*, 80 mg daily for 1-4 days. Protects for 3-20 days after exposure to allergen.

PoM **Cromovet™** (Fisons)
Nebuliser solution, sodium cromoglycate 20 mg/mL, for *horses*; 4 mL

5.3 Mucolytics and expectorants

5.3.1 Mucolytics
5.3.2 Expectorants

5.3.1 Mucolytics

Mucolytic agents such as **bromhexine** reduce mucus viscosity in the tracheobronchial tree and are often prescribed for chronic bronchitis in dogs, bronchopneumonia in cattle, and chronic coughing in the horse. The rationale for their use is that mucus of lower viscosity is more easily expectorated during coughing and is more easily carried up the tracheobronchial tree by the mucociliary clearance mechanism.
Dembrexine is used in the horse. In small animals inhalation of water vapour and chest physiotherapy are more effective methods of mucus removal.

BROMHEXINE

Indications. Respiratory disease where excess tenacious mucus is present
Dose. *Horses*: *by mouth or by intramuscular injection*, 100-250 micrograms/kg daily
Cattle, pigs: *by mouth or by intramuscular injection*, 200-500 micrograms/kg daily; *piglets*: *by mouth or by intramuscular injection*, 0.3-1.5 mg/kg daily
Dogs: *by mouth*, 1.6-2.5 mg/kg twice daily
Cats: *by mouth*, 1 mg/kg daily
Pigeons: *by addition to drinking water*, 192 mg for treatment of 10 birds

PoM **Bisolvon™** (Boehringer Ingelheim)
Oral powder, bromhexine hydrochloride 10 mg/g, for *horses, cattle, pigs, dogs, cats*; 5 g, 100 g, other sizes available

Injection, bromhexine hydrochloride 3 mg/mL, for *horses, cattle, pigs*; 100 mL
GSL **Broncholin™** (Harkers)
Oral powder, for addition to drinking water, bromhexine chloride 9.6 mg/g, for *pigeons*; 20 g

DEMBREXINE HYDROCHLORIDE

Indications. Respiratory disease where excess or tenacious mucus is present in the airways
Contra-indications. Manufacturers do not recommend use in pregnant animals
Dose. *Horses*: *by mouth*, 300 micrograms/kg twice daily

PoM **Sputolosin™** (Boehringer Ingelheim)
Oral powder, for addition to feed, dembrexine hydrochloride 5 mg/g, for *horses*; 420 g
Withdrawal Periods. *Horses*: slaughter 3 days

Injection, dembrexine hydrochloride 5 mg/mL, for *horses*; 100 mL
Note. Injection is only available directly from the manufacturers

5.3.2 Expectorants

Expectorants, such as ipecacuanha extract, are claimed to aid removal of mucus from the airways. These compounds are thought to act by mild irritation of the mucous membrane. They are included in compound preparations. Any therapeutic effect these preparations have is probably due to the inclusion of antihistamines, cough suppressants, and bronchodilators.

COMPOUND EXPECTORANT PREPARATIONS

PoM **Linct Morphinae Co** (Loveridge)
Linctus, camphor spirit 0.004 mL, ipecacuanha liquid extract 0.003 mL, morphine sulphate 600 micrograms, squill syrup 0.25 mL, tolu syrup 0.088 mL/mL, for *horses, dogs*; 2 litres
Contra-indications. Cats, see Prescribing for dogs and cats

Dose. *Horses*: 10-30 mL 2-3 times daily
Dogs: 0.5 mL/kg 2-3 times daily

5.4 Antitussives

Cough suppressants are only beneficial where coughing is persistent and unproductive, interferes with the animal's sleep and rest, or causes muscular fatigue and exhaustion. They should not be used where there are excess secretions in the tracheobronchial tree, as in chronic bronchitis or bronchopneumonia. In general, the use of antitussives is restricted to dogs.

Antitussive drugs are selected to exploit the cough suppressant effects of morphine-like drugs, while minimising the sedative and drug dependency characteristics of the opioids.

Butorphanol is the most effective antitussive and is also a potent analgesic. **Codeine phosphate** has little analgesic activity and can induce constipation. **Dextromethorphan** possesses some antitussive activity. All opioid drugs should be used with caution in cats.

BUTORPHANOL

Indications. Non-productive cough
Contra-indications. Chronic bronchitis, bronchiectasis, bronchopneumonia, or any other condition in which there is excess airway secretion. Conditions causing central nervous system depression. Hepatic impairment. Cats, see Prescribing for dogs and cats
Side-effects. Sedation, ataxia; respiratory depression; anorexia and diarrhoea
Dose. *Dogs*: *by mouth*, 500 micrograms/kg 2-4 times daily for up to 14 days; *by subcutaneous or intramuscular injection*, 50 micrograms/kg 2-4 times daily for up to 14 days

PoM **Torbutrol**™ (Willows Francis)
Tablets, butorphanol 1 mg, 5 mg, 10 mg, for *dogs*; 1-mg tablets 100; 5-mg tablets 50; 10-mg tablets 25
Injection, butorphanol 500 micrograms/mL, for *dogs*; 10 mL

CODEINE PHOSPHATE

Indications. Non-productive cough
Contra-indications. See under Butorphanol
Side-effects. Sedation, ataxia; respiratory depression; constipation
Dose. *Dogs*: 0.5-2.0 mg/kg twice daily

Codeine Phosphate (Non-proprietary)
PoM *Tablets*, codeine phosphate 15 mg, 30 mg, 60 mg

P **Codeine Linctus** (Non-proprietary)
Codeine phosphate 3 mg/mL; 100 mL

DEXTROMETHORPHAN HYDROBROMIDE

Indications. Non-productive cough
Contra-indications. See under Butorphanol
Side-effects. See under Codeine Phosphate
Dose. *Dogs*: up to 5 mg 3-4 times daily

P **Robitussin Cough Soother** (Wyeth)
Oral solution, dextromethorphan hydrobromide 7.5 mg/5 mL; 100 mL

P **Robitussin Junior Cough Soother** (Wyeth)
Oral solution, dextromethorphan hydrobromide 3.75 mg/5 mL; 100 mL

5.5 Respiratory stimulants

Respiratory stimulants are administered, at doses below the convulsive threshold, to stimulate respiration. Their main uses are to promote respiration in apnoeic newborn and preterm animals and to reverse respiratory depression associated with general anaesthetic, sedative, or hypnotic drugs (see Emergency treatment of poisoning).

These drugs should not be used as an alternative to patient management. In drug-induced respiratory depression maintenance of an adequate airway and airflow by intubation and positive-pressure ventilation are the recognised methods of treatment. While analeptic drugs will temporarily increase tidal and minute volume, the oxygen gain may be partly offset by increased brain oxygen consumption.

All analeptics are central nervous

stimulants and may induce convulsions. **Doxapram** is more selective as a respiratory stimulant and less likely to induce convulsions than **nikethamide** or the **cropropamide** and **crotethamide** combination. The principle mechanism of action of doxapram involves stimulation of the peripheral aortic and carotid body chemoreceptors rather than a central action.

The methylxanthines in addition to their bronchodilatory action are also non-specific central nervous stimulants. They increase respiratory drive by altering the respiratory centre's sensitivity to carbon dioxide. **Etamiphylline** (see section 5.1.1) is used as a respiratory stimulant in neonates.

DOXAPRAM HYDROCHLORIDE

Indications. Respiratory stimulation of neonates; reversal of respiratory depression associated with overdose of general anaesthetic, hypnotic, and sedative drugs

Contra-indications. Convulsions, renal or hepatic disease, hypocalcaemia

Side-effects. Hyperventilation leading to cerebral vasoconstriction and cerebral hypoxia, brain damage may occur with excessive doses; convulsions

Warnings. Airway should be patent; use with extreme caution in dogs that have been sedated with morphine; concurrent administration of cyclopropane or halogenated hydrocarbon anaesthetics may precipitate cardiac arrhythmias (see Drug Interactions – Appendix 1)

Dose. Neonatal use. *Calves*: by *subcutaneous, intramuscular or intravenous injection, or by sublingual application*, 40-100 mg

Lambs: by *subcutaneous or intravenous injection, or by sublingual application*, 5-10 mg

Puppies: by *subcutaneous or intravenous injection, or by sublingual application*, 1-5 mg

Kittens: by *subcutaneous or intravenous injection, or by sublingual application*, 1-2 mg

Post-anaesthetic use. *Horses*: by *intravenous injection*, 0.5-1.0 mg/kg

Dogs, cats: by *intravenous injection*, 1-2 mg/kg following inhalation anaesthetic; 5-10 mg/kg following intravenous anaesthetic

PoM **Dopram™-V** (Willows Francis)
Oral drops, doxapram hydrochloride 20 mg/mL, for *calves, lambs, puppies, kittens*; 5 mL
Withdrawal Periods. *Calves, lambs*: slaughter withdrawal period nil
Injection, doxapram hydrochloride 20 mg/mL, for *horses, calves, lambs, dogs, cats*; 20 mL
Withdrawal Periods. *Calves, lambs*: slaughter withdrawal period nil

CROPROPAMIDE AND CROTETHAMIDE

Indications. Respiratory stimulation of neonates; reversal of respiratory depression associated with overdose of general anaesthetic, hypnotic, and sedative drugs

Contra-indications. Side-effects. Warnings. See under Doxapram

PoM **Respirot™** (Ciba-Geigy)
Syrup, cropropamide 75 mg/mL, crotethamide 75 mg/mL, for *foals, calves, lambs, piglets, dogs, cats*; 15 mL
Dose. *Foals, calves*: up to 5 mL repeated at 30 second intervals if required. Repeat only twice
Lambs, piglets, dogs, cats: up to 0.06 mL/kg repeated at 30 second intervals if required. Repeat only twice

NIKETHAMIDE

Indications. Respiratory stimulation
Contra-indications. See under Doxapram
Warnings. Excessive dosage may cause convulsions followed by CNS depression
Dose. *Dogs*: by *subcutaneous, intramuscular, or intravenous injection*, 7-30 mg/kg

PoM **Nikethamide** (Non-proprietary)
Injection, nikethamide 250 mg/mL; 2 mL

5.6 Nasal decongestants

Nasal decongestants contain sympathomimetics and should be used with caution. **Pseudoephedrine** may be of use in cats with allergic rhinitis. Phenylephrine has been used in pigeons.

GSL **Nasal Drops** (Harkers)
Phenylephrine hydrochloride 0.25%, for *pigeons*; 14 mL

P **Sudafed**™ (Calmic)
Tablets, pseudoephedrine hydrochloride 60 mg; 12, 100
Elixir, pseudoephedrine hydrochloride 6 mg/mL; 100 mL
Dose. *Cats*: 2-4 mg/kg twice daily

6 Drugs acting on the

NERVOUS SYSTEM

6.1 Sedatives
6.2 Sedative antagonists
6.3 Opioid analgesics
6.4 Neuroleptanalgesics
6.5 Opioid antagonists
6.6 General anaesthetics
6.7 Drugs modifying neuromuscular transmission
6.8 Local anaesthetics
6.9 Antiepileptics
6.10 Drugs used for euthanasia

6.1 Sedatives

Sedatives produce calmness, drowsiness, and indifference to the surroundings. The division between sedatives and tranquillisers is indistinct but, in general, tranquillisers produce a state of calmness with less drowsiness.

Sedatives are commonly included in pre-anaesthetic medication, and used to facilitate handling and transport of animals, and to modify behaviour, for example to prevent fighting amongst pigs.

There is a continuous gradation of levels of sedation from light sedation to a depth approaching anaesthesia. The level of sedation is determined by the individual drug, dosage, route of administration, and the interacting effect of any other drugs that are being used to treat the animal at the time of administration. The doses given in each monograph below range from the lowest figure for light sedation to the highest amount appropriate for deep sedation. Deeply sedated animals require standards of monitoring equal to anaesthetised animals. Most sedatives have little or no analgesic activity and must be supplemented with opioid analgesics or local analgesia when painful procedures are carried out.

Acepromazine is widely used and produces mild to moderate sedation. Its effect is variable and unpredictable, and individual patients may fail to show an observable response. Absorption following oral administration is poor in dogs and cats, but good in horses. Subcutaneous absorption is variable and intravenous or intramuscular injection is preferred. Peak action is delayed for several minutes even after intravenous injection. Larger doses do not produce deeper sedation but lead to increased duration of action and side-effects, and many veterinary anaesthetists recommend limiting the parenteral dose of acepromazine to 50 micrograms/kg in dogs and cats. If deeper sedation is required then an opioid analgesic should be administered concomitantly or another drug selected. Acepromazine should not be used to treat status epilepticus as it lowers the seizure threshold. Chlorpromazine (see section 3.3.2) has been largely superseded by acepromazine for sedation but may still be used to prevent motion sickness.

Azaperone is used in pigs as a sedative to prevent fighting when mixing groups of animals and for pre-anaesthetic medication. Azaperone may cause violent reactions in horses and is not recommended in this species. The long duration of action of azaperone results in prolonged anaesthetic recovery when it is used as a premedicant.

Xylazine, medetomidine, and detomidine, are all alpha$_2$-adrenergic receptor agonists. **Xylazine** is a potent sedative with marked analgesic activity. It should be used with caution in dogs and cats as it produces deep and prolonged sedation with bradycardia and profound cardiovascular depression. When xylazine is used for pre-anaesthetic medication the amount of induction agent should be reduced considerably from that employed with other premedicants to avoid a fatal overdose. Vomiting occurs frequently when xylazine is administered to dogs and cats, which may be a disadvantage in its use, but an advantage if anaesthesia is to follow in an animal not starved during the previous 6 to 24 hours. Care should be exercised if xylazine is administered to elderly or debilitated patients.

Xylazine is a useful sedative in the horse. Approximately twice as much drug is required to achieve comparable sedation if given intramuscularly rather than intravenously. Xylazine may initially cause bradycardia and second degree heart block, which resolve after approximately 10 minutes. Arterial blood pressure will rise sharply after intravenous injection, then fall to a level slightly below normal. Peak sedation lasts for about 15 minutes and the total duration of effect is approximately one hour. Horses sedated with xylazine usually remain standing although they will sway if given high doses. Care must be exercised when using xylazine as an animal that appears deeply sedated can still kick accurately in response to a stimulus.

The depth and reliability of sedation can be increased by administering an opioid analgesic concomitantly, and drugs such as pethidine, morphine, methadone, or butorphanol have been used in combination with xylazine for standing sedation in horses. The duration of action of many opioid analgesics is longer than that of xylazine in the horse, and acepromazine is often included in combinations of xylazine and opioid analgesics, to provide continued sedation. This is particularly important when pure opioid agonists such as morphine or methadone are used.

Xylazine is also used for pre-anaesthetic medication in the horse. A dose of approximately 1 mg/kg, given by intravenous injection, may be followed by thiopentone, methohexitone, or ketamine. The induction agent should be given a few minutes after the xylazine when sedation has reached its peak level.

Cattle are more sensitive to xylazine than horses. Low doses of xylazine in cattle will produce sedation, while high doses will cause recumbency. Xylazine is useful for sedating animals before surgery under local analgesia. Before general anaesthesia, xylazine can be used to produce recumbency and permit endotracheal intubation with the laryngeal reflexes intact, therefore reducing the occurrence of inhalation of rumen contents.

Detomidine is used in horses. Deep sedation lasts for about 40 minutes after detomidine and its effects may persist for hours. Bradycardia, hypertension followed by hypotension, and second degree heart block are produced by detomidine as with xylazine. Fatal interactions have been reported when detomidine has been administered in conjunction with potentiated sulphonamides.

Detomidine is a good pre-anaesthetic medicant and can be followed by thiopentone, ketamine, or methohexitone. The induction agent should be given 5 minutes after intravenous detomidine to allow complete sedation to develop. Detomidine and xylazine increase the circulation time, and the loss of consciousness after intravenous injection of thiopentone or methohexitone will be longer than with other premedicants.

Detomidine has been used in combination with opioid analgesics to produce deeper and more reliable sedation in horses. Many opioid analgesics may be used but butorphanol has proved to be particularly useful. Ataxia is increased when opioid analgesics are used with detomidine in standing horses.

Medetomidine is structurally similar to xylazine and detomidine, and has similar side-effects when used in dogs and cats. The effects of medetomidine can be reversed by the specific antagonist atipamezole (see section 6.2) and the two drugs may be useful for procedures such as radiography in healthy animals.

ACEPROMAZINE

Indications. Pre-anaesthetic medication; sedation; motion sickness (3.3.2)
Contra-indications. Renal impairment. Should not be administered to male horses. Treatment of status epilepticus

Warnings. May cause syncope in canine brachycephalic breeds
Dose. *Horses*: *by mouth*, 130-260 micrograms/kg; *by intramuscular or slow intravenous injection*, 50-100 micrograms/kg.
Cattle, sheep, pigs: *by intramuscular or slow intravenous injection*, 50-100 micrograms/kg
Dogs, cats: *by mouth*, 1-3 mg/kg; *by intramuscular or slow intravenous injection*, 125-250 micrograms/kg

Oral preparations

PoM **ACP™** (C-Vet)
Tablets, acepromazine (as maleate) 10 mg, 25 mg, for *dogs, cats*; 250, 1000

PoM **BK-Ace™** (BK)
Tablets, acepromazine (as maleate) 10 mg, 25 mg, for *dogs, cats*; 500

Parenteral preparations

PoM **ACP™** (C-Vet)
Injection, acepromazine (as maleate) 2 mg/mL, for *dogs, cats*; 10 mL
Injection, acepromazine (as maleate) 10 mg/mL, for *horses, cattle, sheep, pigs*; 20 mL
Withdrawal Periods. *Cattle, sheep*: slaughter 7 days, milk 7 days. *Pigs*: slaughter 7 days

PoM **BK-Ace™** (BK)
Injection, acepromazine (as maleate) 2 mg/mL, for *dogs, cats*; 20 mL
Injection, acepromazine (as maleate) 10 mg/mL, for *horses, cattle, sheep, pigs*; 20 mL
Withdrawal Periods. *Cattle, sheep*: slaughter 7 days, milk 7 days. *Pigs*: slaughter 7 days

AZAPERONE

Indications. Behaviour modification; pre-anaesthetic medication; general anaesthesia in combination with Metomidate (6.6.2)
Side-effects. Transient salivation and panting with high doses
Dose. *Pigs*: *by intramuscular injection*, 1-4 mg/kg

PoM **Stresnil™** (Janssen)
Injection, azaperone 40 mg/mL, for *pigs*; 100 mL

Withdrawal Periods. *Pigs*: slaughter 3 days

DETOMIDINE HYDROCHLORIDE

Indications. Sedation; general anaesthesia in combination with Ketamine (6.6.2)
Contra-indications. Concurrent administration of sympathomimetics or potentiated sulphonamides (see Drug Interactions – Appendix 1). Manufacturer does not recommend use in last month of pregnancy in animals
Side-effects. Cardiac arrhythmias; sweating; incoordination; slight tremors
Dose. *Horses*: sedation, *by intramuscular or slow intravenous injection*, 10-80 micrograms/kg
Sedation, in combination with butorphanol, (200 kg body-weight or less) detomidine, *by intravenous injection*, 12 micrograms/kg, followed not more than 5 minutes later by butorphanol, *by intravenous injection*, 25 micrograms/kg; (more than 200 kg body-weight), detomidine, *by intravenous injection*, 5 mg, followed by butorphanol, *by intravenous injection*, 10 mg

PoM **Domosedan™** (SmithKline Beecham)
Injection, detomidine hydrochloride 10 mg/mL, for *horses*; 5 mL, 20 mL
Withdrawal Periods. Should not be used in *horses* intended for human consumption

MEDETOMIDINE HYDROCHLORIDE

Indications. Sedation; pre-anaesthetic medication
Contra-indications. Concurrent administration of sympathomimetics. Manufacturer does not recommend use in pregnant animals
Side-effects. Hyperthermia; occasional vomiting
Dose. Sedation. *Dogs*: *by subcutaneous, intramuscular, or intravenous injection*, 10-80 micrograms/kg
Cats: *by subcutaneous or intramuscular injection*, 50-150 micrograms/kg
Pre-anaesthetic medication. *Dogs*: *by*

subcutaneous, intramuscular, or intravenous injection, 10-20 micrograms/kg

PoM **Domitor**™ (SmithKline Beecham)
Injection, medetomidine hydrochloride
1 mg/mL, for *dogs, cats*; 10 mL

XYLAZINE

Indications. Sedation; pre-anaesthetic medication; general anaesthesia in combination with Ketamine (6.6.2)
Contra-indications. Latter stages of pregnancy in animals, except parturition; mechanical obstruction of the gastro-intestinal tract in dogs and cats
Side-effects. Vomiting in dogs and cats
Warnings. Caution when pulmonary disease is present or suspected; transient rise followed by fall in blood pressure in horses
Dose. *Horses*: *by intramuscular injection*, 2.2-3 mg/kg; *by slow intravenous injection*, 0.6-1.1 mg/kg
Cattle: *by intramuscular injection*, 50-300 micrograms/kg
Dogs: *by subcutaneous, intramuscular (preferred), or intravenous injection*, 1-3 mg/kg
Cats: *by intramuscular injection*, 3 mg/kg
Zoo animals: information on dose available from manufacturers

PoM **AnaSed**™ (BK)
Injection, xylazine 100 mg/mL, for *horses*; 10 mL
Withdrawal Periods. Should not be used for *horses* intended for human consumption

PoM **Rompun**™ (Bayer)
Injection, xylazine 20 mg/mL, for *horses, cattle, dogs, cats*; 25 mL
Injection, powder for reconstitution, xylazine 500 mg, for *horses, zoo animals*

6.2 Sedative antagonists

Atipamezole is an alpha$_2$-adrenergic receptor antagonist, which is used to reverse the sedative effects of medetomidine. The dose of atipamezole, in micrograms/kg, required, in dogs, is 5 times and, in cats, 2.5 times the previously administered medetomidine dose. Atipamezole is usually admin-

istered 15 minutes to one hour after the medetomidine.
Atipamezole will not reverse the sedative action of other classes of sedative or anaesthetic drugs. For example, care should be exercised if ketamine has also been previously administered to a dog as this drug is unsuitable as a sole anaesthetic agent in this species.

ATIPAMEZOLE HYDROCHLORIDE

Indications. Reversal of sedative effects of medetomidine
Contra-indications. Manufacturer does not recommend use in pregnant animals
Side-effects. Transient over-alertness and tachycardia with high dosage; transient hypotension; rarely vomiting and panting
Dose. *Dogs, cats*: *by intramuscular injection*, see notes above

PoM **Antisedan**™ (SmithKline Beecham)
Injection, atipamezole hydrochloride
5 mg/mL, for *dogs, cats*; 10 mL

6.3 Opioid analgesics

Opioid analgesics interact at opioid receptor sites in the central nervous system and other tissues. There are several distinct receptor types and the binding of opioid analgesics leads to their characteristic pharmacological actions.
Opioids may be agonists, antagonists, or a combination of both. Morphine, etorphine, and fentanyl are examples of potent agonists. Codeine and pethidine are less potent agonists. Pentazocine, buprenorphine, and butorphanol are regarded as mixed agonist-antagonists, capable of reversing the effects of an agonist and with selective opioid actions. Diprenorphine and nalorphine are also partial agonist-antagonists but closer to pure antagonists, reversing all of the effects of the agonist but retaining a degree of intrinsic activity that is expressed at higher doses. Naloxone is a pure antagonist having no sedative or analgesic action at recommended doses

Table 6.1. Relative analgesic potencies
of opioid analgesics

Drug	Equivalent analgesic potency
Buprenorphine†	1
Butorphanol	4–7
Etorphine	at least 1000
Fentanyl	80–100
Methadone	1
Morphine	1
Pentazocine	0.33–0.5
Pethidine	0.1

† In dogs

but capable of reversing the effects of
an agonist.

There are major species differences
in the responses elicited by opioid
analgesics. In the central nervous system,
opioid analgesics modify pain perception
and behavioural reaction to pain. They
also relieve anxiety and distress but may
induce drowsiness from which the animal
can usually be aroused. Cats, horses,
cattle, and pigs often become hyper-
excited at particularly high doses.
Excitement is less likely in animals in
pain than in pain-free animals. Spinal
cord reflexes may become exaggerated.
Due to their misuse potential, opioid
analgesics are subject to the Misuse of
Drugs Regulations, 1985 (see Legal
aspects of prescribing). It is recommended, therefore, that they should
only be used when there is no non-
opioid alternative, and that the newer,
less addictive drugs should be used
rather than morphine and methadone.

Morphine provides the standard against
which the analgesic potency of other
opioid analgesics are compared (see
Table 6.1). In addition to analgesia,
morphine depresses respiration and
induces sedation, which may lead to
coma according to dose.

Morphine remains the drug of choice
for severe pain as in injury sustained
in road traffic accidents. In such
circumstances, acepromazine should not
be given as it may cause fatal hypotension
in an already hypovolaemic animal.
Morphine is contra-indicated in patients

with head injuries. **Methadone** is a
synthetic opioid that has the same
analgesic potency as morphine, but less
sedative effect.

Pethidine is a synthetic opioid analgesic
that is structurally unlike morphine. It
produces a prompt but short-acting
analgesia. In cats, rapid detoxification
of pethidine results in unpredictable
effects. The recommended dose is 10 to
20 mg by intramuscular injection, which
produces satisfactory analgesia for more
than 2 hours. Doses of more than
6 mg/kg are unnecessarily high and may
result in excitation.

In dogs the maximum analgesic effect
of pethidine is reached about 45 minutes
after oral administration, or about 20
minutes after subcutaneous injection.
Pethidine also has an antispasmodic
action on the smooth muscle of the large
intestine and it is frequently used in the
treatment of equine colic.

Pentazocine has little sedative effect,
does not induce excitement, has little
action on the gastro-intestinal tract, and
does not cause vomiting. The respiratory
depression produced by pentazocine is
less than with morphine. Pentazocine is
a useful analgesic in the dog for both
musculoskeletal and visceral pain, and
it is helpful in the control of colic pain
in horses. It should not be used in cats.

Buprenorphine is mildly sedative and
this effect is potentiated by concurrent
administration of other sedatives. Buprenorphine does not cause excitement
and does not induce vomiting in animals.
Less respiratory depression is caused
than with morphine.

The analgesic effects of buprenorphine
are slow in onset, occurring after
approximately 15 minutes even when
administered intravenously. This,
together with the long duration of action,
may give rise to toxicity if repeated
doses are administered. The effects
of buprenorphine are only partially
reversed by naloxone, more of the latter
being needed than to reverse a pure
agonist.

Butorphanol is a synthetic opioid analgesic. It is particularly useful for the
relief of visceral pain in horses. It

may be combined with detomidine hydrochloride (see section 6.1).
Combinations of opioid analgesics and sedatives are used to provide neuroleptanalgesia (see section 6.4).

BUPRENORPHINE

Indications. Moderate to severe pain
Side-effects. Sedation; respiratory depression; sweating
Warnings. Repeated doses may cause overdosage, see notes above
Dose. *Dogs: by subcutaneous or intramuscular injection*, 10-20 micrograms/kg

CD **Temgesic**™ (Reckitt & Colman)
Injection, buprenorphine (as hydrochloride) 300 micrograms/mL; 1 mL, 2 mL

BUTORPHANOL

Indications. Moderate to severe pain; sedation; non-productive cough (5.4)
Contra-indications. Hepatic impairment; cats, see Prescribing for dogs and cats; horses with pre-existing cardiac dysrhythmias
Side-effects. Ataxia; respiratory depression
Dose. *Horses: analgesia, by intravenous injection*, 100 micrograms/kg
Sedation in combination with detomidine hydrochloride, see 6.1 for dosage details

PoM **Torbugesic**™ (C-Vet)
Injection, butorphanol (as tartrate) 10 mg/mL, for *horses*; 10 mL, 50 mL
Withdrawal Periods. Should not be used in *horses* intended for human consumption

METHADONE HYDROCHLORIDE

Indications. Severe pain
Side-effects. Respiratory depression; excitement at high doses
Dose. *Horses, dogs: by intramuscular injection*, 200 micrograms/kg; *by intravenous injection*, 100 micrograms/kg

CD **Physeptone**™ (Calmic)
Injection, methadone hydrochloride 10 mg/mL; 1 mL

MORPHINE SULPHATE

Indications. Severe pain
Side-effects. Respiratory depression, sedation; hyperexcitability in some species, see notes above
Dose. *Dogs: by subcutaneous or intramuscular injection*, 200 micrograms/kg

CD **Morphine Sulphate** (Non-proprietary)
Injection, morphine sulphate 10 mg/mL, 15 mg/mL, 30 mg/mL; 1 mL, 2 mL

PENTAZOCINE

Indications. Moderate to severe pain
Contra-indications. Should not be used in cats
Side-effects. Slight respiratory depression and mild sedation. Muscle tremors, ataxia and convulsions may occur at higher than recommended doses
Dose. *Horses: by intramuscular or slow intravenous injection*, 330 micrograms/kg, repeat after 15 minutes if required
Dogs: by intramuscular injection, 2 mg/kg

CD **Pentazocine** (Non-proprietary)
Injection, pentazocine (as lactate) 30 mg/mL; 1 mL, 2 mL

PETHIDINE HYDROCHLORIDE
(Meperidine hydrochloride)

Indications. Moderate to severe pain
Contra-indications. Renal impairment
Side-effects. Sedation; may cause emesis or constipation; occasional transient excitement
Warnings. Hyperexcitability in cats, see notes above
Dose. *Horses: by intramuscular injection*, 1-5 mg/kg
Dogs♦: *by intramuscular injection*, 1-2 mg/kg (maximum 10 mg/kg)
Cats♦: see notes above

CD **Pethidine** (Arnolds)
Injection, pethidine hydrochloride 50 mg/mL, for *horses*; 50 mL

COMPOUND ANALGESIC PREPARATIONS

CD **Budale-V**™ (Arnolds)
Tablets, scored, butobarbitone 60 mg, codeine phosphate 10 mg, paracetamol 250 mg, for *dogs*; 100, 500

Dose. *Dogs*: ½-3 tablets 3 times daily

PoM **Pardale-V™** (Arnolds)
Tablets, scored, caffeine hydrate 10 mg, codeine phsphate 9 mg, paracetamol 400 mg, for *dogs*; 100, 500
Dose. *Dogs*: ½-3 tablets 3 times daily

6.4 Neuroleptanalgesics

Neuroleptanalgesia is a state of sedation combined with analgesia. The animal no longer responds to surroundings or to pain but is not totally unconscious. Therefore, handling and minor surgical procedures may be carried out painlessly without having to resort to full anaesthesia.

Combinations of sedatives and opioid analgesics produce deeper and more reliable sedation than sedatives alone. In dogs and cats, acepromazine has been combined with a variety of opioid analgesics including pethidine and buprenorphine to produce deep sedation. Acepromazine, detomidine, and xylazine are often combined with opioid analgesics, especially butorphanol, in the horse to produce deep sedation.

Opioid antagonists may be used to reverse the sedation of neuroleptanalgesia, such that recovery is rapid and relatively safe.

Etorphine is a very potent derivative of thebaine and at least 1000 times more effective than morphine. In combination with a phenothiazine such as acepromazine or methotrimeprazine, neuroleptanalgesia is induced that is suitable for minor surgical procedures in horses, donkeys, cattle, sheep, pigs, and dogs. Some authorities suggest that the desired level of sedation, with less cardiovascular side-effects, may be achieved in dogs using approximately half the recommended manufacturer's dose. Only a small volume of the drug is required, therefore it is useful for darting, as in zoo practice and deer farming.

Fentanyl is a synthetic opioid analgesic similar in structure to pethidine. Its analgesic potency is at least 80 times that of morphine. Fentanyl is available in combination with the neuroleptic drug fluanisone. In the dog, the fentanyl and fluanisone combination can be used alone for minor surgical procedures or for pre-anaesthesia medication. For major surgery the dose of neuroleptanalgesic may be reduced to 25 to 30 percent of the usual dose and given in combination with barbiturates at 50 percent of the usual dose. This neuroleptanalgesic combination is also useful in the rabbit and guinea pig.

ETORPHINE HYDROCHLORIDE AND PHENOTHIAZINES

Indications. Reversible neuroleptanalgesia

Contra-indications. Horses with cardiac arrhythmias, endocarditis, or liver impairment; cats (see Prescribing for dogs and cats)

Side-effects. Tachycardia in horses, or bradycardia in dogs, hypertension or hypotension; mild sedation; priapism leading to paraphimosis in horses; respiratory depression; enterohepatic recirculation may cause excitement 6-8 hours after remobilisation

Warnings. Etorphine hydrochloride is a very potent neuroleptanalgesic, which is highly toxic to humans. In humans, it causes dizziness, nausea, and pinpoint pupils, followed by respiratory depression, lowered blood pressure, cyanosis, and in extreme cases, loss of consciousness and cardiac arrest.

Dose. See preparation details

> If there is any danger that a human may have absorbed or self-injected Immobilon™, the following steps should be taken IMMEDIATELY. Before calling medical assistance, inject reversing agent such as 0.8-1.2 mg naloxone (2-3 mL Narcan™) intravenously or intramuscularly (see section 6.5). Revivon™ may be used in humans in extreme emergencies. Repeat dose every 2 to 3 minutes until symptoms are reversed. Wash area with water. MAINTAIN RESPIRATION AND HEARTBEAT UNTIL MEDICAL ASSISTANCE ARRIVES. The data sheet or pack leaflet should be handed to the attending doctor.

CD **Large Animal Immobilon™** (C-Vet)
Injection, etorphine hydrochloride 2.45 mg, acepromazine maleate 10 mg/

mL, for *horses, cattle, sheep, pigs*;
10.5 mL
Withdrawal Periods. *Cattle*: slaughter
21 days, milk from treated animals
should not be used for human consumption. *Sheep, pigs*: slaughter 21 days
Dose. *Horses*: by intramuscular or
intravenous injection, 0.01 mL/kg
Donkeys♦: by intramuscular or intravenous injection, 0.005 mL/kg
Cattle: by intramuscular or intravenous
injection, 0.01 mL/kg
Sheep: by intramuscular injection,
0.005 mL/kg
Pigs: by intramuscular injection,
0.01 mL/kg
Notes. Reversal, see section 6.5
The Revivon™ component is an integral
part of the Immobilon™ product licence

co**Small Animal Immobilon**™ (C-Vet)
Injection, etorphine hydrochloride 74
micrograms, methotrimeprazine 18 mg/
mL, for *dogs*; 21 mL
Dose. *Dogs*: by intramuscular injection,
0.1 mL/kg; by intravenous injection,
0.05 mL/kg
Notes. Reversal, see section 6.5
The Revivon™ component is an integral
part of the Immobilon™ product licence

FENTANYL CITRATE AND FLUANISONE

Indications. Reversible neuroleptanalgesia
Contra-indications. Dogs in which respiration is significantly depressed; hepatic or renal impairment
Side-effects. Bradycardia; hypotension;
respiratory depression; salivation;
defaecation; hypersensitivity
Warnings. Involuntary movements
sometimes occur, especially in response
to stimulation
Dose. See preparation details

co**Hypnorm**™ (Janssen)
Injection, fentanyl citrate 315 micrograms, fluanisone 10 mg/mL, for *dogs,
rabbits, guinea pigs*; 10 mL
Dose. *Dogs, rabbits, guinea pigs*: by
subcutaneous injection, 0.55 mL/kg; by
intramuscular injection, 0.5 mL/kg

Note. Reversal, see section 6.5

6.5 Opioid antagonists

These drugs are used to reverse opioid-induced depression of the central
nervous system rapidly. They are
chemically related to the drugs that they
antagonise and are able to reverse the
analgesia and respiratory depression
induced by opioid analgesics.
Nalorphine was the first drug to be used
as an opioid antagonist but has now
been superseded by naloxone. **Naloxone**
is a pure antagonist so there is minimal
danger of overdose. However, the short
action in dogs means that the antagonistic
effect may cease before the action of
the opioid, previously administered, has
been eliminated, and sedation may reoccur. Naloxone is recommended in the
event of self-administration of etorphine
(see Warnings under Etorphine hydrochloride, section 6.4).
Diprenorphine is structurally similar to
etorphine and is used as an antagonist
to that drug.

DIPRENORPHINE

Indications. Reversing agent for etorphine in animals
Dose. See preparation details

PoM**Large Animal Revivon**™ (C-Vet)
Injection, diprenorphine (as hydrochloride) 3 mg/mL, methylene blue, for
horses, donkeys, cattle, sheep, pigs;
10.5 mL
Withdrawal Periods. *Cattle, sheep, pigs*:
slaughter 21 days
Dose. *Horses, donkeys, cattle, sheep, pigs*:
by intravenous injection, a volume
equal to the volume of Large Animal
Immobilon™ (Etorphine Hydrochloride, 6.4) previously administered

PoM**Small Animal Revivon**™ (C-Vet)
Injection, diprenorphine (as hydrochloride) 272 micrograms/mL, methylene blue, for *dogs*; 21 mL
Dose. *Dogs*: by intravenous injection, a
volume equal to the volume of Small

Animal Immobilon™ (Etorphine Hydro-chloride, 6.4) previously administered. Dogs can be left to recover spontaneously under supervision

NALOXONE HYDROCHLORIDE

Indications. Reversing agent for opioid agonist drugs in animals; reversal of accidental etorphine poisoning in humans (see Warnings under Etorphine Hydrochloride, 6.4)
Warnings. Short acting, possibility of relapse (see notes above)
Dose. *Dogs*: *by subcutaneous, intra-muscular, or intravenous injection*, 0.04-1.0 mg/kg

PoM **Naloxone** (Non-proprietary)
Injection, naloxone hydrochloride 400 micrograms/mL; 1 mL

PoM **Narcan™** (Du Pont)
Injection, naloxone hydrochloride 400 micrograms/mL; 1 mL, 10 mL

6.6 General anaesthetics

6.6.1 Antimuscarinic pre-anaesthetic medication
6.6.2 Injectable anaesthetics
6.6.3 Inhalational anaesthetics

The main aim of general anaesthesia is to produce unconsciousness so that surgical or other procedures may be carried out painlessly. Most anaesthetic drugs also cause profound alterations in the function of vital body systems, in particular the cardiovascular and respiratory systems. Careful technique with attention to basic principles such as airway management, constant patient monitoring, and the use of properly maintained equipment, all contribute to good anaesthetic recovery with minimal complications.

Most anaesthetic drugs have a narrow therapeutic index and careful attention to dose rates is required. A common source of error is inaccurate weight estimation and all patients should be weighed as part of their preparation for anaesthesia.

Anaesthetic drugs cause respiratory depression and, in general, during anaesthesia the inspired oxygen concentration should not be less than 30 percent, necessitating supplemental oxygen in all cases. This can be provided via a nasal tube or face mask but in most cases it is convenient to intubate the animal and connect it to a suitable circuit and anaesthetic machine, which also allows the use of inhalational drugs. In cats, intubation may be facilitated by the use of lignocaine spray (see section 6.8) to avoid laryngospasm.

The majority of patients undergo elective surgery or other treatment and can be prepared for general anaesthesia under optimal conditions. Cats, dogs, and horses should be starved for at least 6 hours so that the stomach is empty. Overnight starvation is convenient. Water should be allowed until 1 to 2 hours before anaesthesia. There is little point in starving ruminants as ruminal volume is maintained for several days. In general, very young and very small animals have high metabolic rates and food should be withheld for shorter periods. Sick and debilitated animals require individual pre-anaesthetic regimens. If possible, pre-existing disease should be treated and the animal stabilised before undergoing elective anaesthesia.

Pre-anaesthetic medication is appropriate in most patients. The main aims are to calm the patient, provide analgesia if needed, reduce the dose of anaesthetic agent, reduce or counteract the side-effects of anaesthetic drugs, and to provide a smooth anaesthetic induction and recovery. These aims are generally achieved by using sedatives, opioid analgesics, and antimuscarinic drugs either alone or in combination. The dose of barbiturate can be reduced by a third to a half, except in the horse, if a light pre-anaesthetic medication such as acepromazine is used. When heavier premedication is produced by drugs such as xylazine or medetomidine, the dose of barbiturate may need to be reduced further (or halved in the horse).

6.6.1 Antimuscarinic pre-anaesthetic medication

Antimuscarinic drugs are used to reduce salivation and bronchial secretion and to treat bradycardia. Their routine use in anaesthesia is declining as halogenated inhalation agents are less irritant to the airways than ether. Premedicants are indicated in cats and small dogs in which a small amount of saliva can block the airway but their routine use in larger dogs is controversial.

Atropine and **hyoscine** are not recommended for routine use in horses because the central excitation and mydriasis that these drugs produce can be unpleasant, and gastro-intestinal motility will be reduced. **Glycopyrronium** may be better for use in horses, if required, because it does not cross the blood-brain barrier. Administration of antimuscarinic drugs to ruminants does not inhibit salivation but results in production of a more viscid saliva and is therefore generally contra-indicated in these species.

Antimuscarinic drugs are still important for the treatment of bradycardia. Atropine (see section 4.5) is the most commonly used. It produces a more stable heart rate during anaesthesia than hyoscine. The latter also has greater central effects, which are generally undesirable.

ATROPINE SULPHATE

Indications. Drying secretions; adjunct in gastro-intestinal disorders characterised by smooth muscle spasm (3.6); antidote for organophosphorus compound poisoning (see Emergency treatment of poisoning); in combination with anticholinesterases to reverse competitive neuromuscular blockade
Contra-indications. Glaucoma
Side-effects. Tachycardia; constipation; urinary retention; dilation of pupils and photophobia
Dose. *By subcutaneous injection. Horses, cattle*: 30-60 micrograms/kg
Sheep: 80-160 micrograms/kg
Pigs: 20-40 micrograms/kg
Dogs, cats: 30-100 micrograms/kg

PoM **Atropine Sulphate** (Animalcare)
Injection, atropine sulphate 600 micrograms/mL, for *horses, cattle, sheep, pigs, dogs, cats*; 25 mL
PoM **Atropine Sulphate** (BK)
Injection, atropine sulphate 600 micrograms/mL, for *horses, cattle, sheep, pigs, dogs, cats*; 25 mL

GLYCOPYRRONIUM BROMIDE

Indications. Drying secretions; in combination with anticholinesterases to reverse competitive neuromuscular blockade
Side-effects. Tachycardia; reduced gastro-intestinal motility
Warnings. Concurrent administration of sympathomimetics may cause tachycardia and fatal dysrhythmias in horses
Dose. *Horses: by intravenous injection.* 1-3 micrograms/kg
Dogs: by intramuscular or intravenous injection, 2-8 micrograms/kg

PoM **Robinul**™ (Wyeth)
Injection, glycopyrronium bromide 200 micrograms/mL; 1 mL, 3 mL

HYOSCINE HYDROBROMIDE
(Scopolamine hydrobromide)

Indications. Drying secretions
Contra-indications. Glaucoma
Side-effects. Tachycardia
Dose. 10-20 micrograms/kg

PoM **Hyoscine Hydrobromide** (Non-proprietary)
Injection, hyoscine hydrobromide 400 micrograms/mL, 600 micrograms/mL; 1 mL

6.6.2 Injectable anaesthetics

Injectable anaesthetics have a rapid onset of action and are commonly used as induction agents to effect rapid passage through the light planes of anaesthesia during which the patient may struggle. These drugs are eliminated by metabolism and excretion and there is no way of increasing the rate of removal from the body to compensate for overdosage. Urinary pH may be altered to increase drug excretion by this is usually only employed for barbiturate poisoning.

Thiopentone is the standard drug for induction with which others are compared. It is administered as an aqueous solution of the sodium salt, which is alkaline and highly irritant. Perivascular injection may lead to tissue necrosis. Intra-arterial injection may lead to gangrene of an extremity and injection into the carotid artery may cause death. Solutions should be as dilute as possible, using a 1.25 percent solution for neonates and cats, and a 2.5 percent solution for dogs. Horses, ruminants, and pigs require more concentrated solutions, to minimise the volume required, and this should always be given via an intravenous catheter.

The initial dose of thiopentone reaches the brain, and is then redistributed to the viscera, muscles, and fat, and slowly metabolised in the liver. Therefore, recovery from a single dose of thiopentone is not dependent upon immediate excretion or metabolism. In general, when the animal recovers consciousness, the full dose of thiopentone is still present in its body. If repeated doses of thiopentone are given, the tissues may become saturated with thiopentone and recovery will be prolonged for many hours. Therefore, thiopentone is not generally suitable for maintenance of anaesthesia.

Greyhounds and other coursing hounds may take over 24 hours to recover from the effects of thiopentone. Methohexitone has been used for many years in these breeds but use of propofol is becoming popular due to the smoother induction and recovery observed with this drug.

Thiopentone should be used with a sedative pre-anaesthetic medicant in dogs and horses. If used alone the recovery may be violent in these species. When a phenothiazine premedicant is used in horses the dose of thiopentone should not be reduced.

Methohexitone is shorter acting than thiopentone, but causes greater respiratory depression. Induction and recovery are generally more excitable than with thiopentone. The solution is irritant and care should be taken to avoid perivascular injection. A one percent solution is suitable for use in dogs and cats. Methohexitone is more rapidly metabolised than thiopentone but recovery from a single dose is still mainly due to redistribution.

Alphadolone and **alphaxalone** in combination are insoluble in water and are solubilised in polyoxyl 35 castor oil. This vehicle may cause histamine release, which is usually mild in cats but can be severe in dogs. The drug combination is not irritant and may be given by intravenous or deep intramuscular injection. Recovery from alphaxalone and alphadolone anaesthesia is by metabolism and may be prolonged by repeated administration or continuous infusion.

Ketamine is a dissociative agent and interrupts the cerebral association between the limbic and cortical systems. The animal may appear to be in a light plane of anaesthesia but is insensitive to surgical stimulation. Muscle relaxation may be poor when ketamine is used alone and the addition of either an alpha$_2$-adrenergic agonist such as xylazine, or a benzodiazepine such as diazepam will increase muscle relaxation. Ketamine is only used alone in cats and primates. Cats' eyes remain open during ketamine anaesthesia and a bland eye ointment may be used to protect the cornea. Ketamine is a useful anaesthetic in many exotic species and can be given in a low dose to facilitate handling, followed by inhalational agents (see section 6.6.3) to deepen anaesthesia. Ketamine may be given intramuscularly or intravenously, although intramuscular injection is painful.

Ketamine should only be given to horses and donkeys after deep sedative premedication with xylazine or detomidine. Induction of anaesthesia in horses with ketamine is generally calm, but quiet surroundings and handling are important. There are a few reports of failure of ketamine to induce anaesthesia in horses and this potential problem should be remembered. Ketamine may produce convulsions in dogs when used as the sole anaesthetic agent.

Metomidate is only useful clinically in

the pig. The dose may be varied to give sedation or basal narcosis. The drug is not particularly good as a sole anaesthetic agent because analgesia is limited and the animal will respond to stimuli. Metomidate is usually administered in combination with azaperone, which increases recovery time. Metomidate may cause muscle tremors and pain on injection.

Pentobarbitone is now used only infrequently as a clinical anaesthetic drug as better alternatives such as thiopentone and propofol are available. Pentobarbitone is mainly used for status epilepticus (see section 6.9.2) or for long-term sedation (see Emergency treatment of poisoning) at a concentration of 60 mg/mL, and for euthanasia (see section 6.10) at a concentration of 200 mg/mL. The dose administered to animals convulsing due to poisoning depends upon the degree of CNS depression resulting from the toxin. Each animal should be treated according to individual response. Pentobarbitone is metabolised slowly and recovery from this drug is prolonged. Animals may vocalise and make repeated attempts to rise during recovery, resulting in injury.

Propofol produces anaesthesia after intravenous injection in a similar manner to thiopentone, although cardiovascular depression is slightly greater. The recovery from propofol is rapid and generally smooth, even when no sedative premedication has been given. Therefore, the drug is useful for minor out-patient procedures. Recovery from propofol is by metabolism rather than re-distribution so that repeated doses can be given with little increase in recovery time. Cats do not metabolise propofol as efficiently as dogs and the total anaesthetic time should not be prolonged in cats if this drug is used alone.

Propofol is not irritant to tissues and inadvertent perivascular injection does not cause problems, but pain on injection occurs in man and may be seen in some animals.

ALPHADOLONE ACETATE AND ALPHAXALONE

Indications. Induction and maintenance of general anaesthesia
Contra-indications. Dogs, see notes above
Side-effects. Transient unilateral or bilateral erythema and oedema of paws, pinnae, or both
Warnings. Rarely oedema of larynx; rarely necrotic lesions of the extremities
Dose. Expressed as alphadolone acetate + alphaxalone.
General anaesthesia (without pre-anaesthetic medication). *Cats*: *by intramuscular injection*, 18 mg/kg; *by intravenous injection*, initial dose 9 mg/kg, followed by 3 mg/kg increments if required
Monkeys: *by intramuscular injection*, 12-18 mg/kg; *by intravenous injection*, 6-9 mg/kg

PoM **Saffan**™ (Coopers Pitman-Moore)
Injection, alphadolone acetate 3 mg, alphaxalone 9 mg/mL, for *cats, monkeys*; 5 mL, 10 mL

KETAMINE

Indications. General anaesthesia, in combination with Xylazine or Detomidine (6.1)
Contra-indications. Sole anaesthetic in horses, donkeys, or dogs; hepatic or renal impairment; latter stages of pregnancy in animals
Side-effects. Hypersalivation in cats
Dose. General anaesthesia (without pre-anaesthesia medication). *Cats*: *by subcutaneous, intramuscular (preferred) or intravenous injection*, 11-33 mg/kg
Primates: information on dose available from manufacturers
General anaesthesia, in combination with detomidine hydrochloride (6.1)
Horses: detomidine hydrochloride, *by intravenous injection*, 20 micrograms/kg, followed 5 minutes later by ketamine *by intravenous injection*, 2.2 mg/kg
General anaesthesia, in combination with xylazine (6.1). *Horses, donkeys*: xylazine, *by slow intravenous injection*, 1.1 mg/kg, followed 2 minutes later by

ketamine, *by intravenous injection*, 2.2 mg/kg
Calves, sheep, goats: xylazine, *by intramuscular injection*, 200 micrograms/kg, followed 10-15 minutes later by ketamine, *by intramuscular injection*, 10 mg/kg
Dogs: (25 kg body-weight or less) xylazine, *by intramuscular injection*, 2 mg/kg, followed 10 minutes later by ketamine, *by intramuscular injection*, 10 mg/kg; (more than 25 kg body-weight) xylazine, *by intramuscular injection*, 1.3 mg/kg, followed 10 minutes later by ketamine, *by intramuscular injection*, 10 mg/kg
Cats: xylazine, *by intramuscular injection*, 1.1 mg/kg, followed by ketamine, *by intramuscular injection*, 22 mg/kg

PoM **Ketaset**™ (Willows Francis)
Injection, ketamine (as hydrochloride) 100 mg/mL, for **horses, donkeys, cats, primates**; 10 mL
Withdrawal Periods. Should not used in **horses** intended for human consumption

PoM **Vetaket**™ (C-Vet)
Injection, ketamine (as hydrochloride) 100 mg/mL, for **horses, donkeys, cats, primates**; 10 mL
Withdrawal Periods. Should not be used in **horses** intended for human consumption

PoM **Vetalar**™ (Parke-Davis)
Injection, ketamine (as hydrochloride) 100 mg/mL, for **horses, donkeys, calves, sheep, goats, dogs, cats, primates**; 5 mL, 10 mL, 20 mL

METHOHEXITONE SODIUM

Indications. Induction of general anaesthesia
Side-effects. Transient apnoea on induction
Dose. General anaesthetic induction (without pre-anaesthetic medication). **Dogs, cats**: *by intravenous injection*, 11 mg/kg

PoM **Brietal**™ **Sodium Veterinary** (Elanco)
Injection, powder for reconstitution, methohexitone sodium 500 mg, 2.5 g, for **dogs, cats**

METOMIDATE HYDROCHLORIDE

Indications. General anaesthesia in combination with azaperone (6.1)
Side-effects. Transient slight tremors
Dose. **Pigs**: general anaesthesia, in combination with azaperone, (less than 50 kg body-weight) azaperone, *by intramuscular injection*, 2 mg/kg, with metomidate, *by intraperitoneal injection*, 10 mg/kg; (more than 50 kg body-weight) azaperone, *by intramuscular injection*, 2 mg/kg, followed by metomidate 15 minutes later, *by intravenous injection*, 4 mg/kg
Caesarean section, azaperone, *by intramuscular injection*, 1 mg/kg, followed by metomidate 5-10 minutes later, *by intramuscular injection*, 2.5 mg/kg *or* azaperone, *by intravenous injection*, 400 micrograms/kg, with metomidate, *by intravenous injection*, 2.5 mg/kg *or* azaperone, *by intramuscular injection*, 1 mg/kg, followed by metomidate 15 minutes later, *by intraperitoneal injection*, 2.5 mg/kg

PoM **Hypnodil**™ (Janssen)
Injection, powder for reconstitution, metomidate hydrochloride 1 g, for **pigs**

PENTOBARBITONE SODIUM

Indications. General anaesthesia; long-term sedation in cases of poisoning; status epilepticus (6.9.2)
Contra-indications. Hepatic impairment
Warnings. Respiratory depression may be enhanced; perivascular injection may cause local irritation and slough
Dose. General anaesthesia (without pre-anaesthetic medication). **Dogs**: *by slow intravenous injection (preferred)*, 35 mg/kg; *by intraperitoneal injection*, 40 mg/kg
Cats: *by slow intravenous injection (preferred)*, 26 mg/kg; *by intraperitoneal injection*, 40 mg/kg
Rabbits, rodents: see Prescribing for rabbits and rodents
Long-term sedation after poisoning. **Dogs, cats**: from 10 mg/kg if there is only slight CNS or respiratory

depression. Adjust dose according to the individual patient's response

PoM **Sagatal**™ (RMB)
Injection, pentobarbitone sodium 60 mg/mL, for *dogs, cats, laboratory animals*; 100 mL

PROPOFOL

Indications. Induction and maintenance of general anaesthesia
Side-effects. During recovery phase vomiting and evidence of excitation may occur; if panting is evident before induction, this may continue through anaesthesia and recovery
Warnings. Caution in patients with cardiac, hepatic, respiratory, or renal impairment
Dose. General anaesthesia (without pre-anaesthetic medication). *Dogs: by intravenous injection*, 6.5 mg/kg
Cats: by intravenous injection, 8 mg/kg

PoM **Rapinovet**™ (Coopers Pitman-Moore)
Injection, propofol 10 mg/mL, for *dogs, cats*; 20 mL

THIOPENTONE SODIUM

Indications. Induction of general anaesthesia
Contra-indications. Animals less than 3 months of age
Warnings. Perivascular injection may cause local irritation and slough. Manufacturer advises that concomitant administration of chloramphenicol, streptomycin, and kanamycin may cause prolonged recovery
Dose. General anaesthetic induction (without pre-anaesthetic medication). *Horses, cattle, sheep, pigs: by intravenous injection*, 10 mg/kg; *calves: by intravenous injection*, 15 mg/kg of 5% solution
Dogs, cats: by intravenous injection, 25-30 mg/kg (maximum 1.25 g) of 1.25% or 2.5% solution; see notes above

PoM **Intraval**™ **Sodium** (RMB)
Injection, powder for reconstitution, thiopentone sodium 2.5 g, 5 g, for *horses, cattle, sheep, pigs, dogs, cats*

PoM **Thiovet**™ (C-Vet)
Injection, powder for reconstitution, thiopentone sodium 2.5 g, 5 g, for *horses, dogs, cats*
Withdrawal Periods. Should not be used in *horses* intended for human consumption

6.6.3 Inhalational anaesthetics

Inhalational drugs are for practical purposes absorbed and excreted unchanged via the lungs although some metabolism does occur for most agents. However, recovery does not depend upon drug metabolism and therefore these agents are useful in species for which there is little information on use of general anaesthetics, as their action will be similar in all mammals. Removal of an overdose of inhalational anaesthetic can be hastened by mechanical ventilation of the lungs. Humans should not be exposed to inhalational drugs for long periods, even in small doses, and some form of waste gas scavenging is needed when these agents are used.
Halothane is the most commonly used halogenated inhalational drug. Halothane, enflurane, and isoflurane are much less soluble than ether and the concentration in the brain and myocardium can rise quickly if high inspired concentrations are given, producing severe cardio-respiratory depression. These detrimental effects due to halothane are dose-dependent and the horse is particularly susceptible. The inhalation anaesthetics should always be administered using an appropriate precision vaporiser.
Enflurane produces more rapid induction and recovery than halothane because of its lower blood solubility. Cardiovascular depression is greater than that produced by halothane. Enflurane may produce seizure-like electroencephalogram activity and should be avoided in epileptic patients. Enflurane is not recommended for horses because cardiovascular depression is severe and recovery is rapid but violent.
Induction and recovery with **isoflurane** are more rapid than enflurane or halothane. Isoflurane may be used in

horses; it is not certain whether it offers any real advantages over halothane and there have been reports that recovery may be more violent than with halothane. **Methoxyflurane** produces good analgesia. Induction is slow because of its high blood solubility and low saturated vapour pressure. Recovery is also prolonged. It is used in dogs, cats, birds, and laboratory animals.

Nitrous oxide is a weak anaesthetic and is incapable of producing general anaesthesia when used alone in animals. It is used to supplement other drugs, especially inhalational anaesthetics, and provides analgesia and anaesthesia with relatively few detrimental effects. It is usually used at the highest inspired concentration possible, between 50 and 70 percent, with oxygen and an inhalational anaesthetic drug. Induction and recovery with nitrous oxide are rapid.

The main danger when using nitrous oxide is hypoxia. Modern anaesthetic machines have interlocks to shut off the nitrous oxide if the oxygen supply fails. If nitrous oxide is used in rebreathing circuits then an oxygen meter is needed to check that the inspired oxygen concentration does not fall below 30 percent. Diffusion hypoxia may occur at the end of nitrous oxide anaesthesia and the patient should be allowed to breath 100 percent oxygen for a few minutes before changing to room air.

Cyclopropane and **ether** are largely obsolete because they form explosive mixtures with oxygen and full anti-static precautions must be taken when they are used. Induction and recovery are rapid with cyclopropane but post-operative vomiting is a problem. Induction and recovery are slow with ether. It irritates the airways and antimuscarinic premedication is advisable. Cardiovascular function is well-maintained with ether because it causes sympathetic stimulation. Beta-adrenergic antagonists should never be used concurrently with ether.

Ether can be administered using relatively simple apparatus because the concentration in the body changes slowly even if high inspired levels are administered.

ENFLURANE

Indications. Inhalation anaesthesia
Contra-indications. Horses (see notes above); animals prone to seizures
Side-effects. Cardiovascular depression, seizures
Dose. Maintenance of anaesthesia, inspired concentration of 1.5-2.5%

ᴾ**Enflurane** (Abbott)
Enflurane; 250 mL

ETHER

Indications. Inhalation anaesthesia
Side-effects. Irritant locally causing nausea and vomiting
Warnings. Flammable and explosive. Concurrent use of beta-adrenoreceptor blocking drugs
Dose. Induction of anaesthesia, inspired concentration of up to 10%
Maintenance of anaesthesia, inspired concentration of 4-6%

Anaesthetic Ether BP

HALOTHANE

Indications. Inhalation anaesthesia
Contra-indications. Concurrent administration of adrenaline
Side-effects. Occasional malignant hyperpyrexia in pigs; cardiovascular depression
Dose. Induction of anaesthesia, inspired concentration of 2-3%
Maintenance of anaesthesia, inspired concentration of 0.5-1.8%

ᴾ**Fluothane**™ (Coopers Pitman-Moore)
Halothane, for *horses, cattle, sheep, pigs, dogs, cats, birds, reptiles*; 250 mL
ᴾ**Halothane** (RMB)
Halothane, for *horses, cattle, sheep, pigs, dogs, cats, non-domestic species including mammals, birds, reptiles*; 250 mL

ISOFLURANE

Indications. Inhalation anaesthesia
Side-effects. Cardiovascular depression

Dose. Maintenance of anaesthesia, inspired concentration of 1.0-2.5%

P **Isoflurane** (Abbott)
Isoflurane; 100 mL

METHOXYFLURANE

Indications. Inhalation anaesthesia
Contra-indications. Hepatic and renal impairment
Warnings. Renal toxicity with prolonged administration; absorbed by rubber and the inclusion of this material in anaesthetic circuits may result in prolonged induction and recovery times
Dose. Maintenance of anaesthesia, inspired concentration of 0.5-1.5%

PoM **Metofane**™ (C-Vet)
Methoxyflurane, for *horses, cattle, sheep, pigs, dogs, cats, birds*; 100 mL

NITROUS OXIDE

Indications. Inhalation anaesthesia in combination with other inhalational drugs
Warnings. The amount of oxygen used with nitrous oxide should not fall below 30%
Dose. Inspired concentration of 50-70%

Note. Cylinders are painted blue

6.7 Drugs modifying neuromuscular transmission

6.7.1 Non-depolarising muscle relaxants
6.7.2 Depolarising muscle relaxants
6.7.3 Muscle relaxant antagonists

Muscle relaxants are also known as neuromuscular blocking drugs or myoneural blocking drugs. These drugs interfere with transmission at the neuromuscular junction, thereby causing muscle paralysis or relaxation.
In veterinary anaesthesia muscle relaxants facilitate endotracheal intubation and endoscopy, and cause relaxation of skeletal muscle for easier surgical access and reduction of joint dislocation and bone fractures. They allow lighter levels of general anaesthesia to be employed, which facilitates artificial respiration.
Respiration should always be controlled in animals that have received a muscle relaxant until the drug has either been metabolised or antagonised. On humane grounds, muscle relaxants should only be used in unconscious animals.

6.7.1 Non-depolarising muscle relaxants

These drugs, also known as competitive muscle relaxants, block neuromuscular transmission by competing with acetylcholine for receptor sites on the motor end plate. The postsynaptic membrane is occupied but not depolarised. The action of non-depolarising muscle relaxants may be reversed (see section 6.7.3). In veterinary anaesthetic practice, these drugs are used mainly for orthopaedic or intrathoracic surgical procedures. Atracurium and vecuronium have been used in dogs suffering from myasthenia gravis, at one-fifth to one-tenth of the normal dosage to provide muscle relaxation during anaesthesia with adequate monitoring of neuromuscular transmission.
Tubocurarine is rarely used today in veterinary anaesthesia due to its histamine-releasing properties, particularly in the dog. It may also produce hypotension due to its ganglion-blocking properties. **Alcuronium** has a duration of action of about 70 minutes in the dog. It has minimal cardiovascular side-effects. It is excreted unchanged, mainly by the kidneys.
Atracurium has a duration of action of 30 to 40 minutes in horses, sheep, dogs, and cats, which may be prolonged by hypothermia. The drug has minimal vagolytic or sympatholytic properties. It can be administered to animals with hepatic or renal failure, and is non-cumulative after repeated doses.
Gallamine has a duration of action which varies between the species (see below). Gallamine causes an undesirable tachycardia due to its vagolytic action. The drug is excreted unchanged in urine.
Pancuronium has an initial duration of action of 30 to 45 minutes in horses,

cattle, sheep, goats, pigs, and cats. Although it does not cause histamine release or significant changes in blood pressure, pancuronium may produce tachycardia, especially in dogs and cats, due to its vagolytic properties. Pancuronium is excreted partly unchanged in urine.

Vecuronium has a duration of action of approximately 30 minutes in the dog and horse, and 15 minutes in sheep. It does not cause histamine release, sympathetic blockade, or vagolytic effects and therefore has minimal cardiovascular effects. The drug is relatively non-cumulative and is excreted mainly by the liver.

ALCURONIUM CHLORIDE

Indications. Non-depolarising muscle relaxant of long duration
Contra-indications. Renal impairment
Side-effects. See notes above
Warnings. Facilities for intermittent positive pressure ventilation should be present
Dose. *Horses*: *by intravenous injection*, initial dose 50 micrograms/kg then increments of 10 micrograms/kg
Dogs: *by intravenous injection*, initial dose 100 micrograms/kg then increments of 20 micrograms/kg

PoM **Alloferin**™ (Roche)
Injection, alcuronium chloride 5 mg/mL; 2 mL

ATRACURIUM BESYLATE

Indications. Non-depolarising muscle relaxant of medium duration
Side-effects. See notes above
Warnings. Facilities for intermittent positive pressure ventilation should be present. Inactivated by thiopentone and other alkaline solutions
Dose. *Horses*: *by intravenous injection*, initial dose 150 micrograms/kg then increments of 60 micrograms/kg
Sheep, dogs, cats: *by intravenous injection*, initial dose 500 micrograms/kg then increments of 200 micrograms/kg

PoM **Tracrium**™ (Calmic)
Injection, atracurium besylate 10 mg/mL; 2.5 mL, 5 mL, 25 mL

GALLAMINE TRIETHIODIDE

Indications. Non-depolarising muscle relaxant of medium duration
Contra-indications. Renal impairment
Side-effects. See notes above
Warnings. Facilities for intermittent positive pressure ventilation should be present
Dose. *By intravenous injection*. *Horses*: 1 mg/kg, which has an initial duration of action of 20-25 minutes, followed by increments of 200 micrograms/kg
Cattle: 500 micrograms/kg, which has an initial duration of action of 30-40 minutes, followed by increments of 100 micrograms/kg; *calves*: 400 micrograms/kg, which has an initial duration of 4 hours
Sheep: 400 micrograms/kg, which has an initial duration of action of more than 2 hours
Pigs: 1 mg/kg, which has an initial duration of action of 30 minutes, followed by increments of 200 micrograms/kg
Cats: 1 mg/kg, which has an initial duration of action of 15-20 minutes, followed by increments of 200 micrograms/kg

PoM **Flaxedil**™ (M&B)
Injection, gallamine triethiodide 40 mg/mL; 2 mL

PANCURONIUM BROMIDE

Indications. Non-depolarising muscle relaxant of medium duration
Contra-indications. Hepatic or renal impairment; obesity
Side-effects. See notes above
Warnings. Facilities for intermittent positive pressure ventilation must be present
Dose. *By intravenous injection*. *Horses*: initial dose 60 micrograms/kg then increments of 10 micrograms/kg
Cattle: initial dose 40 micrograms/kg then increments of 8 micrograms/kg
Sheep, goats: initial dose 25 micrograms/kg then increments of 5 micrograms/kg
Pigs: initial dose 100 micrograms/kg then increments of 20 micrograms/kg
Dogs: initial dose 60 micrograms/kg then increments of 10 micrograms/kg

Cats: initial dose 80 micrograms/kg then increments of 20 micrograms/kg

PoM **Pavulon**™ (Organon-Teknika)
Injection, pancuronium bromide 2 mg/mL; 2 mL

TUBOCURARINE CHLORIDE

Indications. Non-depolarising muscle relaxant of long duration
Contra-indications. Dogs and cats; hepatic or renal impairment
Side-effects. See notes above
Warnings. Facilities for intermittent positive pressure ventilation must be present
Dose. *By intravenous injection. Horses*: initial dose 300 micrograms/kg then increments of 50 micrograms/kg
Cattle: initial dose 60 micrograms/kg then increments of 10 micrograms/kg
Sheep: initial dose 40 micrograms/kg then increments of 10 micrograms/kg
Pigs: initial dose 400 micrograms/kg then increments of 80 micrograms/kg

PoM **Jexin**™ (DF)
Injection, tubocurarine chloride 10 mg/mL; 1.5 mL

PoM **Tubarine Miscible**™ (Calmic)
Injection, tubocurarine chloride 10 mg/mL; 1.5 mL

VECURONIUM BROMIDE

Indications. Non-depolarising muscle relaxant of medium duration
Contra-indications. Hepatic impairment
Side-effects. See notes above
Warnings. Facilities for intermittent positive pressure ventilation must be present
Dose. *By intravenous injection. Horses*: initial dose 100 micrograms/kg then increments of 20 micrograms/kg
Sheep: initial dose 40 micrograms/kg then increments of 10 micrograms/kg
Dogs, cats: initial dose 100 micrograms/kg then increments of 20 micrograms/kg

PoM **Norcuron**™ (Organon-Teknika)
Injection, powder for reconstitution, vecuronium bromide 10 mg

6.7.2 Depolarising muscle relaxants

The depolarising muscle relaxant **suxamethonium** produces a neuromuscular blockade by depolarising the motor end-plate similarly to the action of acetylcholine. Depolarisation is prolonged since disengagement from the receptor site and subsequent breakdown is slower than for acetylcholine. The initial depolarisation causes transient muscular spasm, which may be painful, and is followed by paralysis.
Paralysis is rapid, complete, and predictable, and recovery is spontaneous. Unlike non-depolarising muscle relaxants, the action of suxamethonium cannot be reversed.
In veterinary anaesthesia, suxamethonium is used to facilitate endotracheal intubation especially in pigs, cats, and primates. It may also be used by repeated injection for longer surgical procedures and is occasionally administered by infusion.
Suxamethonium is metabolised in the liver. It has a rapid onset and relatively short duration of action. The duration of action may be prolonged with concomitant administration of anticholinesterases (see section 6.7.3), or in animals which have received organophosphorus compounds within the preceding month.

SUXAMETHONIUM CHLORIDE

Indications. Depolarising muscle relaxant of short duration
Contra-indications. Hepatic impairment; administration of organophosphorus compounds within one month before administration of suxamethonium (see Drug Interactions—Appendix 1)
Side-effects. See notes above
Warnings. Facilities for intermittent positive pressure ventilation must be present
Dose. *By intravenous injection. Horses*: 100 micrograms/kg produces paralysis for up to 5 minutes
Cattle, sheep: 20 micrograms/kg produces paralysis for 6-8 minutes

Pigs: 2 mg/kg produces paralysis for 2-3 minutes
Dogs: 300 micrograms/kg produces paralysis for 25-30 minutes
Cats: 1.5 mg/kg produces paralysis for 5 minutes
Primates: 1 mg/kg produces paralysis for 5 minutes

PoM **Anectine**™ (Calmic)
Injection, suxamethonium chloride 50 mg/mL; 2 mL

PoM **Min-I-Mix**™ **Suxamethonium Chloride** (IMS)
Injection, powder for reconstitution, suxamethonium chloride 100 mg
Reconstitute to 20 mg/mL

PoM **Scoline**™ (DF)
Injection, suxamethonium chloride 50 mg/mL; 2 mL

6.7.3 Muscle relaxant antagonists

Muscle relaxant antagonists or anticholinesterases inhibit the hydrolysis of acetylcholine by cholinesterases. Consequently, acetylcholine accumulates and its action is prolonged. Anticholinesterase drugs reverse the effects of the non-depolarising muscle relaxant drugs, but they prolong the duration of action of the depolarising muscle relaxants.

These drugs are used to antagonise the neuromuscular block of non-depolarising muscle relaxants (see section 6.7.1), and are preferably adminstered on the return of muscular activity as determined by a nerve stimulator. Before administration of an anticholinesterase, an antimuscarinic drug such as atropine or glycopyrronium (see section 6.6.1) should be given to prevent excessive salivation, bradycardia, vomiting, and diarrhoea. If the initial dose of anticholinesterase is repeated, then the dose of atropine or glycopyrronium should also be repeated.

Neostigmine is commonly used for the reversal of non-depolarising neuromuscular block. It acts within 2 minutes of intravenous injection and has a duration of action of at least 30 minutes. **Edrophonium** has a rapid onset and a relatively short duration of action.

EDROPHONIUM CHLORIDE

Indications. Reversal of non-depolarising muscle relaxants
Side-effects. See notes above
Dose. *Horses, cattle, sheep, pigs, dogs, cats*: *by intravenous injection*, 0.5-1.0 mg/kg, repeat after 5 minutes if required

PoM **Tensilon**™ (Roche)
Injection, edrophonium chloride 10 mg/mL; 1 mL

NEOSTIGMINE METHYLSULPHATE

Indications. Reversal of non-depolarising neuromuscular block
Side-effects. See notes above
Dose. *Horses, cattle, sheep, pigs*: *by intravenous injection*, 50 micrograms/kg, repeat after 5 minutes if required
Dogs, cats: *by intravenous injection*, 100 micrograms/kg, repeat after 5 minutes if required

PoM **Prostigmin**™ (Roche)
Injection, neostigmine methylsulphate 500 micrograms/mL, 2.5 mg/mL; 1 mL

6.8 Local anaesthetics

Local anaesthetic drugs act by blocking conduction in nerve fibres. They will produce muscle paralysis, loss of sensation, or both depending on the type of fibre involved. Other effects such as vasodilatation may be seen if sympathetic autonomic fibres are blocked. Local anaesthetics are often used to block conduction in pain fibres, producing complete analgesia. This may be required for diagnostic purposes or to permit minor surgery. The use of local anaesthetics for the control of traumatic or postoperative pain is limited by anatomical considerations, but they are useful in certain circumstances, such as intercostal nerve blockade.

There are several ways in which local anaesthesic agents can be used to produce local analgesia.
Perineural injection is the technique used when the precise anatomical position of

the nerve supplying the area or region to be desensitised is known. A solution of a local anaesthetic is injected as closely as possible to the nerve and conduction in the nerve is blocked as the drug diffuses into the nerve trunk. For example, cornual anaesthesia or cornual nerve block, is produced when the drug is injected subcutaneously about 2.5 cm below the base of the horn or horn bud. In general, only small quantities of drug are needed for perineural blocks.

A *field block* occurs when a solution of a local anaesthetic is injected along a line, blocking conduction in the nerves which pass through the tissue. All regions supplied by the distal sections of these nerves will be desensitised. Much more local anaesthetic is required than for perineural injection.

Both perineural injection and field blocks may produce regional anaesthesia.

Epidural and *spinal injections* of local anaesthetics around the spinal cord will block conduction in spinal nerves or the entire spinal cord. Large areas of the body can be desensitised with small amounts of drug. Anterior epidural anaesthesia is used for surgery on the recumbent animal or extrusion of the penis in bulls. A caudal epidural injection is used mainly to desensitise the perineal region because of the problems of producing limb paralysis with higher blocks. It is useful for obstetric operations, surgery on the anal and peri-anal areas, and administering enemas to horses.

Intra-articular injection is mainly used as a diagnostic aid to confirm the presence of joint pain. Strict asepsis is essential. Excess joint fluid is aspirated before instilling the local anaesthetic and lameness is re-assessed after 15 to 45 minutes. The volume of the solution required depends on the joint size; the equine fetlock requires about 10 mL, the coffin joint 6 mL, and the stifle joint 50 mL.

Intravenous regional analgesia (IVRA) is produced when a local anaesthetic is injected intravenously distal to a tourniquet applied to isolate the blood supply to a limb. All sensation in the limb is lost until the tourniquet is released. Prilocaine is recommended for this technique because of its low toxicity.

Surface analgesia is application of local anaesthetics directly to the cornea or mucous membranes, producing desensitisation of the surface layer of tissue. Normal skin is too thick and impervious for most preparations of local anaesthetics to have much effect if applied topically. However, a cream containing lignocaine and prilocaine is available which will desensitise skin in about 60 minutes and allow painless venepuncture. An occlusive dressing should be applied over the cream. Lignocaine spray or gel are used on mucous membranes of the larynx and nasal passages.

The speed of onset of neuronal blockade produced by local anaesthetic drugs is determined by the drug, its concentration, the accuracy of injection, and the size of the nerve. Drugs that are more lipid soluble diffuse more readily through the tissues and nerve trunk. The duration of the block is determined by the type of drug, the amount used, the site of injection, and whether or not a vasoconstrictor has been added. The duration of action of local anaesthetics is increased by adding a vasoconstrictor, usually adrenaline, which decreases the rate of absorption of the drug into other tissues.

Vasoconstrictors such as adrenaline should not be added to solutions used for intra-articular, intravenous, epidural, or intradigital analgesia as tissue necrosis and cardiac arrhythmias may occur. Vasoconstrictors should be used with caution in horses because the coat colour at the site of injection may turn permanently white.

Local anaesthetics will cause systemic toxicity if excess amounts are used or if absorption is too rapid. The signs of toxicity seen in animals are convulsions followed by central nervous system depression.

Inadvertent intravenous injection of local anaesthetics may produce toxic plasma-drug concentrations and should be avoided. If intravenous regional analgesia is used the cuff should not be deflated, after the injection of the anaesthetic, until sufficient time has elapsed for the drug to become distributed in the tissues.

Bupivacaine has a long duration of action of up to 8 hours. It is therefore useful for spinal or epidural blocks where a prolonged action is required. It is also indicated when local anaesthetics are used for pain relief, for example in intercostal nerve blocks following rib trauma. Bupivacaine is more toxic than other local anaesthetics and the maximum dose should not exceed 2 mg/kg.

Lignocaine is widely used for most applications. It diffuses readily through the tissues and has a rapid onset of action. Duration of action is about 45 minutes without adrenaline and 90 minutes with adrenaline at a concentration of 1 in 200 000 (5 micrograms/mL). The use of adrenaline is limited as indicated previously.

Mepivacaine produces less tissue irritation than lignocaine and has been recommended when intra-articular analgesia is required. Its duration of action is similar to that of lignocaine.

Prilocaine is similar to lignocaine but of low toxicity and is preferred for intravenous regional anaesthesia. **Procaine** spreads through tissues less readily than lignocaine and is now rarely used.

Proxymetacaine is used for topical analgesia of the cornea. It produces less initial stinging than other agents (see section 12.7).

BUPIVACAINE HYDROCHLORIDE

Indications. Epidural, field block, and perineural anaesthesia

Contra-indications. Warnings. Should not be used for intravenous regional analgesia; care should be taken to avoid intravenous or intra-arterial injection; maximum dose should not exceed 2 mg/kg

Dose. *By perineural injection*, 1-2 mL/site of a 0.5% solution

PoM**Marcain**™ (Astra)
Injection, bupivacaine hydrochloride 5 mg/mL; 10 mL

BUTANILICAINE PHOSPHATE

Indications. Anterior and caudal epidural, field block, and perineural anaesthesia

PoM**Hostacain**™ **2%** (Hoechst)
This preparation is now discontinued

LIGNOCAINE HYDROCHLORIDE

Indications. Lignocaine without adrenaline. Epidural, field block, and perineural anaesthesia, see notes above; arrhythmias (see section 4.4.1)
Lignocaine with adrenaline. Field block and perineural anaesthesia, see notes above

Contra-indications. Lignocaine with adrenaline: intra-articular, intravenous, epidural, or intradigital administration

Dose. Expressed as Lignocaine.
Horses: by epidural, including caudal epidural injection, 0.26-1.67 g; by field block injection, 2-4 g/site
Cattle: by caudal epidural injection, 100-300 mg; by field block injection, 2-4 g/site; by perineural injection, 140 mg; by cornual injection, 40-120 mg
Sheep: by caudal epidural injection, 60-80 mg; by field block injection, 1.2-2.0 g/site
Pigs: by field block injection, 1.2-2.0 g/site
Dogs: by epidural injection, 74-260 mg; by field block injection, 0.4-1.0 g/site; by perineural injection, 20-40 mg/site
Cats: by epidural injection, 74-260 mg; by field block injection, 100-400 mg/site

Parenteral preparations of lignocaine

PML**Lignavet**™ (C-Vet)
Injection, lignocaine hydrochloride 20 mg/mL, for *cattle*; 100 mL
For cornual injection

PoM**Lignavet**™ **Epidural** (C-Vet)
Injection, lignocaine hydrochloride 20 mg/mL, for *horses, cattle, sheep, pigs, dogs, cats*; 10 mL

For caudal epidural and field block injection

Topical preparations of lignocaine

P **Xylocaine**™ (Astra)
Aerosol spray, lignocaine 10%, 10 mg/dose; 80-g dose applicator

PoM **Willotox**™ (Willows Francis)
See under Parenteral preparations of lignocaine with adrenaline below

Parenteral preparations of lignocaine with adrenaline

PML **Lignavet**™ **Plus** (C-Vet)
Injection, lignocaine hydrochloride 20 mg, adrenaline acid tartrate 20 micrograms/mL, for *horses, cattle, sheep, pigs, dogs, cats*; 100 mL
For field block and perineural injection, including cornual injection

PoM **Lignocaine-A** (Univet)
Injection, lignocaine hydrochloride 30 mg, adrenaline (as acid tartrate) 12.5 micrograms/mL, for *cattle*; 100 mL
For cornual injection

PML **Lignocaine Anaesthetic** (Battle Hayward & Bower)
Injection, lignocaine hydrochloride 20 mg, adrenaline acid tartrate 20 micrograms/mL, for *cattle*; 100 mL

PML **Lignocaine and Adrenaline** (Norbrook)
Injection, lignocaine hydrochloride 20 mg, adrenaline 12.5 micrograms/mL, for *cattle*; 100 mL
For cornual injection

PML **Lignodren**™ (Trilanco)
Injection, lignocaine hydrochloride 20 mg, adrenaline 12.5 micrograms/mL, for *cattle*; 100 mL
For cornual injection

PML **Lignodren**™**-TL** (Trilanco)
Injection, lignocaine hydrochloride 20 mg, adrenaline 20 micrograms/mL, for *cattle*; 100 mL
For field block and perineural injection, including cornual injection

PML **Lignol**™ (Arnolds)
Injection, lignocaine hydrochloride 20 mg, adrenaline 10 micrograms/mL, for *horses, cattle, sheep, pigs, dogs, cats*; 100 mL

For field block and perineural injection, including cornual injection

PoM **Locaine**™ (Animalcare)
Injection, lignocaine hydrochloride 20 mg, adrenaline acid tartrate 10 micrograms/mL, for *horses, cattle, sheep, pigs, dogs, cats*; 100 mL
For field block and cornual injection

PoM **Locovetic**™ (Bimeda)
Injection, lignocaine hydrochloride 30 mg, adrenaline (as acid tartrate) 12.5 micrograms/mL, for *cattle, sheep, pigs*; 100 mL
For field block and perineural injection, including cornual injection

PML **Local Anaesthetic** (Alfa-Laval)
Injection, lignocaine hydrochloride 20 mg, adrenaline acid tartrate 20 micrograms/mL, for *cattle*; 100 mL

PML **Nopaine**™ **Plus** (Crown)
Injection, lignocaine hydrochloride 20 mg, adrenaline acid tartrate 20 micrograms/mL, for *cattle*; 100 mL
For field block and perineural injection, including cornual injection

PML **Ruby Freezaject** (Spencer)
Injection, lignocaine hydrochloride 20 mg, adrenaline acid tartrate 20 micrograms/mL, for *cattle*; 100 mL
For cornual injection

PoM **Willotox**™ (Willows Francis)
Injection, lignocaine hydrochloride 37 mg, adrenaline 20 micrograms/mL, for *horses, cattle, dogs, cats*; 50 mL, 100 mL
For epidural, field block, and perineural injection, including cornual injection
Note. May also be used for topical application

MEPIVACAINE HYDROCHLORIDE

Indications. Epidural, field block, intra-articular, and perineural anaesthesia
Dose. *Horses*: *by epidural injection*, 80-200 mg; *by field block injection*, 40-100 mg; *by intra-articular injection*, 100 mg; *by perineural injection*, 40-200 mg

PoM **Intra-Epicaine**™ (Arnolds)
Injection, mepivacaine hydrochloride 20 mg/mL, for *horses*; 10 mL

Withdrawal Periods. Should not be used in *horses* intended for human consumption

PRILOCAINE HYDROCHLORIDE

Indications. Caudal epidural, field block, and intravenous regional analgesia
Dose. *Cattle*: *for intravenous regional analgesia*, 20-30 mL of a 0.5% solution; *by epidural and field block injection*, a suitable volume
Dogs: *for intravenous regional analgesia*, 2-3 mL of a 0.5% solution

PoM **Citanest™** (Astra)
Injection, prilocaine hydrochloride 5 mg/mL, 20 mL, 50 mL

PROCAINE HYDROCHLORIDE

Indications. Field block and perineural anaesthesia
Contra-indications. Intravenous administration
Dose. Expressed as Procaine. *Cattle*: *by field block or perineural injection*, 100-250 mg
Dogs, cats: *by field block or perineural injection*, 12.5-50.0 mg

PoM **Willcain™** (Arnolds)
Injection, procaine hydrochloride 50 mg, adrenaline 20 micrograms/mL, 100 mL
For field block and perineural injection, including cornual injection

COMPOUND LOCAL ANAESTHETICS

PoM **Corneocaine™** (Bimeda)
This preparation is now discontinued

PoM **Emla™** (Astra)
Cream, lignocaine 2.5%, prilocaine 2.5%; 5 g, 30 g

For topical anaesthesia, see notes above

> Proprietary and non-proprietary medicines that are licensed for human use are printed in small type in The Veterinary Formulary

6.9 Antiepileptics

6.9.1 Drugs used in control of epilepsy

Epilepsy may be defined as a condition of recurrent seizures. Therapy should not be commenced in any animal in which a single isolated seizure has occurred unless it develops into status epilepticus. In all cases, a thorough investigation should be carried out to determine any underlying cause. Therapy should be directed towards the disorder rather than routine use of antiepileptic drugs.

Epilepsy is most common in dogs, although cases do occur in cats, horses, and cattle. Some dogs, usually of the large breeds such as Golden Retrievers and German Shepherds suffer from cluster seizures, that is 3 to 15 seizures in close succession over 24 to 48 hours, followed by an interval of 1 to 3 weeks. In dogs it is often difficult to distinguish between generalised (grand mal) and partial (focal) seizures. Primary epilepsy is characterised by seizures that are generalised at the outset. Partial seizures may yield localising signs but often undergo rapid secondary generalisation. Epileptogenic foci within the temporal lobe of the cerebrum may result in psychomotor or behavioural seizures.

Partial seizures are more difficult to control than those that are generalised. There is no clear evidence that any of the antiepileptic drugs have a specific indication for a particular type of seizure in dogs.

The object of treatment is to suppress seizures by maintaining an effective concentration of the drug in plasma and brain tissue without producing side-effects. Therapy should be started in any dog having seizures at a frequency greater than once every 6 weeks, clusters of seizures more than once every 8 weeks, or recurrent seizures accompanied by aggression. Therapy should also be commenced in any dog suffering from epilepsy in which the seizures, although infrequent, are severe, generalised, and of concern to the owner. Successful control may not mean complete abolition of seizures. Partial control is being achieved if there is a significant increase in the time interval between fits.

The drug dose and the frequency of administration vary with the absorption, metabolism, and half-life of the drug and the species to which the drug is administered. Absorption is more rapid from an empty stomach. Antiepileptic drugs are mainly lipid soluble and are distributed readily to all tissues, including the nervous system, such that plasma-drug concentrations accurately reflect tissue levels.

Control is best achieved by the administration of a single drug. Multiple antiepileptic drug therapy does not necessarily give an additive therapeutic effect. Most antiepileptic drugs are potent liver enzyme inducers, enhancing their own metabolism and the metabolism of other drugs.

Sudden withdrawal of therapy may precipitate severe rebound seizures. In a dog that has not suffered a seizure for 3 to 4 months, a very gradual reduction in dosage may be attempted. Any change to another drug should be made with similar caution.

Patients should be monitored regularly during therapy to allow early detection of hepatotoxicity. The determination of plasma-drug concentrations is the only way to assess whether the dosing regimen is appropriate. Routine assays of some antiepileptics including phenobarbitone, primidone, and phenytoin are commercially available.

Apparent failure of therapy may be due to drug tolerance or concurrent disease affecting drug absorption. Alternatively, owner non-compliance or inadequate dosing may affect therapeutic efficacy. Incorrect diagnosis or the existence of refractory epilepsy will also lead to apparent failure of treatment.

Phenobarbitone is the drug of choice for the treatment of canine epilepsy and is also possibly the only drug that is both effective and safe to use in cats. The half-life of phenobarbitone in dogs varies from 47 to 74 hours so that therapy for 2 to 3 weeks is required to achieve a steady state plasma-drug concentration.

Primidone is commonly used in dogs. Approximately 85 percent of the anti-epileptic activity of primidone is due to its phenobarbitone metabolite, and it is therefore illogical to give primidone and phenobarbitone together. The half-life of primidone in dogs is between 5 and 10 hours. The rate of metabolic conversion increases after 14 days of treatment and results in lower plasma-drug concentrations. Initially, primidone therapy may cause temporary ataxia and depression. Thus it is recommended that therapy be commenced at low doses and then gradually increased over several weeks. Primidone is more hepatotoxic than phenobarbitone.

Phenytoin has a half-life of only 3 to 4 hours in the dog, but 24 to 100 hours in the cat and can cause toxicity in this species. In the horse the half-life is about 1.5 hours. Absorption and metabolism of phenytoin are variable, and it is difficult to achieve therapeutic plasma-drug concentrations in dogs because of its rapid metabolism.

Diazepam (see section 6.9.2) has anti-epileptic effects but its short half-life renders it unsuitable for maintenance therapy in canine epilepsy. Oral administration of diazepam leads to a bioavailability of only 2 to 3 percent.

Sodium valproate also has a short half-life in the dog. However, clinical trials have indicated that it may be effective in animals refractory to other medication, particularly when it is given in conjunction with another antiepileptic drug such as phenobarbitone.

PHENOBARBITONE

Indications. Epilepsy; see section 6.9.2 for use in status epilepticus
Contra-indications. Hepatic impairment
Side-effects. Transient ataxia, polyphagia, polydipsia, polyuria; weight gain
Warnings. Paradoxical hyperactivity may occur; abrupt cessation of therapy may precipitate seizures
Dose. *Dogs, cats*: 1.5-5.0 mg/kg twice daily
Note. For therapeutic purposes phenobarbitone and phenobarbitone sodium may be considered equivalent in effect

CD **Phenobarbitone** (Non-proprietary)
Tablets, phenobarbitone 15 mg, 30 mg, 60 mg, 100 mg
Elixir, phenobarbitone 3 mg/mL in a vehicle containing alcohol 38%; 100 mL

PHENYTOIN SODIUM

Indications. Epilepsy
Contra-indications. Cats, see notes above; hepatic impairment
Side-effects. Transient ataxia, gastric disturbance; hepatotoxicity and gingival hyperplasia have been reported
Warnings. Abrupt cessation of therapy may precipitate seizures
Dose. *Dogs*: initially 8-17 mg/kg daily in divided doses; adjust dose according to the patient's response. Doses of up to 35 mg/kg 3 times daily may be required for effective control

PoM **Epanutin**™ (Parke-Davis)
Capsules, phenytoin sodium 50 mg, 100 mg, for *dogs*; 500

PRIMIDONE

Indications. Epilepsy, aggressive behaviour
Contra-indications. Hepatic impairment
Side-effects. Transient ataxia, polydipsia
Warnings. Abrupt cessation of therapy may precipitate seizures
Dose. *Foals*: 25 mg/kg as a single dose
Sows: 1 g twice daily for 2-3 days. Gradual withdrawal over 7-10 days
Dogs, cats: 25 mg/kg twice daily

PoM **Mysoline**™ (Coopers Pitman-Moore)
Tablets, scored, primidone 250 mg, for *foals, pigs, dogs, cats*; 100, 1000

SODIUM VALPROATE

Indications. Epilepsy
Dose. *Dogs*: 60 mg/kg 3 times daily
When sodium valproate and phenobarbitone are used in combination, the dose of each drug should be reduced by 33-50% depending on plasma-drug concentrations and clinical signs

PoM **Epilim**™ (Sanofi)
Tablets, scored, sodium valproate 100 mg; 100
Tablets, e/c, sodium valproate 200 mg, 500 mg; 100
Oral liquid, sodium valproate 40 mg/mL; 300 mL

6.9.2 Drugs used in status epilepticus

The occurrence of repeated seizures without intervening periods of consciousness is called status epilepticus. Animals that suffer from cluster seizures are at particular risk from the development of status epilepticus. This is an emergency situation that requires prompt and appropriate therapy to avoid serious brain damage and death. Determination of the cause of status epilepticus will indicate the therapy to be instigated. Calcium, glucose, or thiamine, rather than treatment with antiepileptic drugs, may be required. Once the seizures are controlled, adequate ventilation must be maintained.
If other therapy is not necessary, the first priority is to administer an antiepileptic drug. **Diazepam**, given intravenously, is the drug of choice. When diazepam is given intravenously the risk of thrombophlebitis is minimised by using an emulsion formulation. Diazepam is only slightly soluble and it is important to avoid crystallisation in intravenous infusions.
If diazepam is not effective then **pentobarbitone sodium** (see section 6.6.2) should be given intravenously. Doses of up to 15 mg/kg may be administered to dogs. Overmedication should be avoided, only enough drug being given to suppress the seizures.
Phenobarbitone (see section 6.9.1) is slower in its action than pentobarbitone but has been used intravenously subsequent to the initial control.

DIAZEPAM

Indications. Status epilepticus; convulsions due to poisoning (see Emergency treatment of poisoning)

Side-effects. Respiratory depression at high doses

Dose. *Horses, cattle*: *by slow intravenous injection*, 25-100 mg doses according to the animal's response, followed by phenobarbitone, *by intravenous injection*, 5 mg/kg; *foals*: *by slow intravenous injection*, 5-10 mg doses according to the animal's response, followed by phenobarbitone, *by intravenous injection*, 9 mg/kg

Dogs, cats: *by intravenous injection*, 5-50 mg given in 5-10 mg doses, followed *by slow intravenous infusion* 2-5 mg/hour in glucose 5% intravenous infusion

PoM **Diazepam** (Non-proprietary)
Injection, diazepam 5 mg/mL; 2 mL

PoM **Diazemuls**™ (Dumex)
Injection (emulsion), diazepam 5 mg/mL; 2 mL
Note. For intravenous infusion, dilute to a maximum concentration of 200 mg in 500 mL of glucose 5% or 10% intravenous infusion. Allow not more than 6 hours between addition and completion of administration.

PoM **Valium**™ (Roche)
Injection, diazepam 5 mg/mL; 2 mL
Note. For intravenous infusion, dilute to a maximum concentration of 40 mg in 500 mL of glucose 5% intravenous infusion or sodium chloride 0.9% intravenous infusion. Allow not more than 6 hours between addition and completion of administration.

6.10 Drugs used for euthanasia

Euthanasia of animals is carried out in veterinary practice to prevent suffering from incurable or painful conditions. Other reasons for euthanasia requested by clients may include unacceptable behaviour, aggression, unwanted litters of puppies or kittens, relocation of the owner, or poor performance in racing. Whatever the reason, once the veterinary surgeon is satisfied that euthanasia is the only option, and that the client fully understands the situation and gives written consent, an agent for euthanasia is chosen to satisfy several criteria. Euthanasia should be as painless as possible and the procedure should not cause undue anxiety or fear.

Barbiturates are the most suitable drugs to comply with the criteria for acceptable agents. Intravenous injection of **pentobarbitone sodium 200 mg/mL** produces a smooth and rapid loss of consciousness. Overdosage of barbiturates causes death by depression of medullary respiratory and vasomotor centres. A compound preparation for euthanasia is also available.

Other methods of euthanasia of animals are described in *Humane Killing of Animals*. 4th ed. England: UFAW, 1988.

PENTOBARBITONE SODIUM 200 mg/mL

Indications. Euthanasia only
Dose. *By intravenous (preferred), intraperitoneal, or intracardiac injection*, 140-200 mg/kg as necessary

> Animals given pentobarbitone sodium 200 mg/mL should not be used for animal or human consumption

CD **Euthanasia Injection** (Univet)
Pentobarbitone sodium 200 mg/mL, for *cattle, dogs, cats*; 100 mL

CD **Euthatal**™ (RMB)
Injection, pentobarbitone sodium 200 mg/mL, for *dogs, cats*; 100 mL

CD **Euthesate**™ (Willows Francis)
Injection, pentobarbitone sodium 200 mg/mL, for *dogs, cats*; 100 mL

CD **Expiral**™ (Sanofi)
Injection, pentobarbitone sodium 200 mg/mL, 100 mL

CD **Lethobarb**™ (Duphar)
Injection, pentobarbitone sodium 200 mg/mL, for *small farm animals, dogs, cats*; 100 mL

CD **Pentobarbitone** (Loveridge)
Injection, pentobarbitone sodium 200 mg/mL, for *small farm animals, dogs, cats*; 100 mL

CD **Pentobarbitone Forte** (Animalcare)
Injection, pentobarbitone sodium 200 mg/mL, for *dogs, cats, mink*; 100 mL (for dogs, cats), 500 mL (for mink)

COMPOUND PREPARATIONS FOR EUTHANASIA

CD**Somulose**™ (Arnolds)
Injection,   cinchocaine   hydrochloride 25 mg, quinalbarbitone sodium 400 mg/ mL, for *dogs, cats*; 25 mL
Dose. *Dogs, cats*: *by intravenous injection*, 0.25 mL/kg

7 Drugs used in the treatment of disorders of the
ENDOCRINE SYSTEM

7.1 Thyroid and antithyroid drugs
7.2 Corticosteroids
7.3 Anabolic steroids
7.4 Drugs used in diabetes mellitus
7.5 Pituitary and hypothalamic hormones
7.6 Other endocrine drugs

7.1 Thyroid and antithyroid drugs

7.1.1 Thyroid drugs
7.1.2 Antithyroid drugs

Hypothyroidism is one of the most common endocrine disorders of the dog, but is uncommonly diagnosed in other domestic animals. In the dog, the most common causes of hypothyroidism are related to impaired production and secretion of the thyroid hormones, thyroxine (T_4) and tri-iodothyronine (T_3), which usually result from destruction of the thyroid gland (primary hypothyroidism). However, hypothyroidism may also result from pituitary disorders (secondary hypothyroidism) or hypothalamic dysfunction (tertiary hypothyroidism).

Hyperthyroidism is recognised most commonly in the older cat, but has been reported rarely in dogs. Feline hyperthyroidism is associated with increased circulating levels of T_4 and T_3 and is usually caused by nodular hyperplasia of the thyroid or thyroid adenomas.

Thyrotrophin (thyroid-stimulating hormone, TSH) or thyrotrophin-releasing hormone (TRH) may be used in the assessment of thyroid function (see sections 7.5.1 and 7.5.3).

7.1.1 Thyroid drugs

Thyroid hormones are used in the treatment of hypothyroidism regardless of the cause. Congenital hypothyroidism requires prompt treatment if normal development is to be attained.

Thyroxine sodium is commonly used for maintenance therapy since thyroxine is the main secretory product of the thyroid gland. Part of the absorbed dose of thyroxine is de-iodinated in peripheral tissues, to the more active tri-iodothyronine (T_3). The clinical effects of thyroxine sodium may not be apparent for several days. Although rare, signs of thyrotoxicosis may develop while receiving thyroxine treatment. These signs include polyuria, polydipsia, nervousness, panting, tachycardia, weight loss, diarrhoea, and increase in appetite.

Liothyronine sodium (T_3) has a similar action to thyroxine, but is more rapidly metabolised and thus has a shorter duration of activity. Although T_3 is the active intracellular hormone, liothyronine is only indicated when thyroxine therapy has failed to achieve a response in a dog with confirmed hypothyroidism. The dog is relatively resistant to thyrotoxicosis from over-supplementation with thyroid drugs, due to efficient metabolism and excretion of thyroid hormone. However, patients with pre-existing cardiac disorders should receive lower doses of thyroid drug initially.

Dried thyroid gland preparations should not be used as their potency varies and their effects are unpredictable.

THYROXINE SODIUM

Indications. Hypothyroidism
Side-effects. See notes above
Dose. *Dogs, cats*: initially 20-40 micrograms/kg daily in divided doses. Adjust dose for each individual animal after approximately 8 weeks of therapy. Once-daily administration is usually adequate for maintenance and treatment should be continued for life.

PoM **Thyroxine** (Non-proprietary)
Tablets, thyroxine sodium 25 micrograms, 50 micrograms, 100 micrograms

LIOTHYRONINE SODIUM

Indications. Hypothyroidism
Side-effects. See notes above
Dose. *Dogs*: initially 2-3 micrograms/kg 3 times daily, increasing to 4-6 micrograms/kg if required. Adjust dose for each individual animal

PoM **Tertroxin**™ (Coopers Pitman-Moore)
Tablets, scored, liothyronine sodium 20 micrograms, for *dogs*; 100

7.1.2 Antithyroid drugs

Antithyroid drugs are used in the pre-operative preparation of hyperthyroid patients for thyroidectomy or for long-term management of hyperthyroidism. **Carbimazole** is the drug of choice and should be used in preference to **propylthiouracil**, which has a much higher incidence of side-effects. Methimazole is the active metabolite of carbimazole. These antithyroid drugs act primarily by interfering with the synthesis of thyroid hormones.

Iodine and **iodide** are used prior to thyroidectomy to block the release of T_4 and T_3 and to reduce the vascularity of the thyroid gland. Iodine should not be used for long-term treatment since its antithyroid action tends to diminish and it may not even achieve the euthyroid state.

Propranolol (see section 4.4.2) is used to prevent many of the cardiovascular and neuromuscular effects of excess thyroid hormones and controls the tachycardia, tachyarrhythmias, and hyperexcitability associated with hyperthyroidism. It is generally considered to have no effect on serum concentrations of thyroid hormones and has been used with antithyroid drugs in the pre-operative management of hyperthyroid patients.

CARBIMAZOLE

Indications. Hyperthyroidism
Side-effects. Anorexia, vomiting; lethargy; pruritus; bleeding diatheses; jaundice
Dose. *Cats*: 10-15 mg daily in divided doses for 1 to 3 weeks will produce a euthyroid state in most patients. Then adjust dose for each individual animal to the lowest effective dosage. At least once-daily administration is required to control thyroid hormone synthesis.

PoM **Neo-Mercazole**™ (Nicholas)
Tablets, carbimazole 5 mg (scored), 20 mg; 5-mg tablets 100, 500; 20-mg tablets 100

IODINE AND IODIDE

Indications. Hyperthyroidism (pre-operative management)
Side-effects. Hypersalivation; anorexia, vomiting
Dose. *Cats*: Aqueous Iodine Oral Solution, 3 to 5 drops daily for 7-14 days before surgery

Aqueous Iodine Oral Solution (Lugol's Solution)
Iodine 5 g, potassium iodide 10 g, water to 100 mL, containing free iodine 50 mg, total iodine (free and combined) 130 mg/mL

PROPYLTHIOURACIL

Indications. Hyperthyroidism
Side-effects. See under Carbimazole; immune-mediated haemolytic anaemia; development of serum antinuclear antibodies; lupus-like syndrome
Dose. *Cats*: 50 mg 3 times daily. Adjust dose as described under Carbimazole

PoM **Propylthiouracil** (Non-proprietary)
Tablets, propylthiouracil 50 mg

7.2 Corticosteroids

7.2.1 Glucocorticoids
7.2.2 Treatment of hypoadrenocorticism

The corticosteroids secreted by the adrenal cortex constitute the glucocorticoids that alter glucose, protein, and calcium metabolism and possess anti-inflammatory activity; and the mineralocorticoids that affect water and electrolyte balance.

Corticosteroids are used in pharmacological doses primarily for their anti-inflammatory and immunosuppressive properties and for the treatment of shock. They are also used in physiological doses for replacement therapy in adrenal insufficiency (see section 7.2.2).

7.2.1 Glucocorticoids

The action of glucocorticoids in suppressing inflammatory reactions may be useful in a wide variety of conditions. Many conditions may benefit from corticosteroid therapy including respiratory disease such as chronic obstructive pulmonary disease and feline asthma syndrome (section 5.2), gastro-intestinal disease including colitis in the dog (section 3.1.3), inflammatory lesions of the eye (section 12.3), ear (section 13.1), and a variety of skin disorders (section 14.4). The use of glucocorticoids in the treatment of mastitis is described in section 11.1.1. Glucocorticoids are capable of producing symptomatic improvement in many conditions, but without treating the underlying disease. In musculoskeletal disorders (section 10.2) the benefits of suppression of the disease process are weighed against the protective effects of reduced activity if therapy is withheld. Glucocorticoids are not indicated where only mild analgesia is required.

Clinical signs of hypersensitivity disorders including allergic dermatitis and urticaria, and auto-immune diseases such as haemolytic anaemia, thrombocytopenia, systemic lupus erythematosus, and pemphigus variants may be improved by glucocorticoid administration.

Glucocorticoids may also be used as adjunctive therapy in the management of mast cell and lymphoid neoplasia (see section 9.5).

Early administration of large doses of intravenous corticosteroids such as betamethasone, dexamethasone, hydrocortisone, or methylprednisolone may

Table 7.1. Relative anti-inflammatory potencies of glucocorticoids

Drug	Equivalent anti-inflammatory potency
Hydrocortisone	1
Prednisolone	4
Methylprednisolone	5
Triamcinolone	5
Betamethasone	30
Dexamethasone	30
Flumethasone	40

be of benefit in acute circulatory failure or shock irrespective of the cause.

Glucocorticoids are used for the induction of parturition in cattle and sheep. Induction of parturition in late pregnancy may be effected by administration of soluble esters of betamethasone, and dexamethasone. These drugs are recommended in cases of possible fetal oversize and periparturient oedema of the udder in cattle, and in sheep when it is necessary to compress or shorten the lambing season or to aid in the treatment of pregnancy toxaemia. Glucocorticoids should be given after day 260 of gestation in cattle and after day 138 in sheep to minimise the adverse effects of prematurity in the offspring. Glucocorticoids are commonly used in the treatment of ketosis (see section 16.3) in cattle and goats and also for pregnancy toxaemia in sheep and goats.

Administration of glucocorticoids. Acceptable doses of glucocorticoids vary widely depending upon the potency of the drug employed, its formulation, rate and route of administration; the nature and severity of the condition being managed; and the goals of therapy. **Betamethasone, dexamethasone, methylprednisolone, prednisolone**, and **triamcinolone** are commonly used for their anti-inflammatory activity. The anti-inflammatory effect of a corticosteroid parallels its gluconeogenic potency.

Sodium phosphate salts and succinate esters are soluble, readily absorbed, and eliminated within 8 to 24 hours. They can be administered intravenously and are used when high plasma or tissue concentrations are required rapidly such as in cases of shock or allergic reactions. Despite the rapid elimination of some of these corticosteroid formulations, suppression of the hypothalamic-pituitary-adrenal (HPA) axis may be prolonged. Other esters including acetate, adamantoate, dipropionate, isonicotinate, phenylpropionate, pivalate, and trioxa-undecanoate are insoluble and should not be given intravenously. They are less rapidly absorbed and metabolised. Insoluble esters of dexamethasone are usually intermediate-acting and effective for 8 to 14 days.

Depot or long-acting corticosteroids such as insoluble esters of methylprednisolone or triamcinolone may be effective for 3 to 6 weeks. These preparations are used for sustained therapy including intra-articular (see section 10.2) and intra-lesional injections. Where necessary, continued treatment may be effected by oral administration of prednisolone. In courses of therapy lasting longer than 2 weeks, the dose of prednisolone should be tapered to the lowest clinically acceptable maintenance level with a gradual transition to administration of twice this maintenance dose on alternate days. This regimen, combined with morning medication in the dog and evening medication in the cat may minimise HPA axis suppression.

Compound preparations usually contain a potent corticosteroid such as betamethasone or dexamethasone. A soluble, short-acting ester may be combined with an insoluble prolonged acting ester. In addition, preparations may include a corticosteroid in combination with an antimicrobial drug although their use is thought not to be generally justified.

Side-effects of glucocorticoids. Prolonged corticosteroid treatment with both rapidly eliminated formulations and depot preparations may have suppressive effects on the HPA axis and lead to adrenal atrophy.

Unnecessarily prolonged therapy should be avoided in order to minimise the possibility of precipitating signs of adrenal insufficiency during superimposed stress or when glucocorticoid treatment is finally withdrawn.

Corticosteroids should be used with caution in pregnancy as they may cause abortion. The use of glucocorticoids to induce parturition is associated with an increased incidence of retained placenta in cattle, although subsequent fertility is unaffected. Fetal abnormalities have been observed in laboratory animals, particularly when the drug is given during the first third of pregnancy. Corticosteroids may induce a temporary fall in milk yield when given to lactating animals.

Catabolic effects of glucocorticoids include muscle wasting, cutaneous atrophy, telogen arrest of hair follicles, and delayed wound healing. In cases of corneal ulceration, repair of corneal stroma and epithelium is suppressed. Chronic use of exogenous glucocorticoids may lead to iatrogenic hyperadrenocorticism.

Diabetes mellitus may be unmasked by glucocorticoid therapy and alteration of insulin requirements in established diabetics may occur. Gastric and colonic ulceration, sometimes with perforation, may occur.

Immunosuppressive effects and modification of inflammatory reactions by glucocorticoids may facilitate the spread of concurrent infectious disease. In pre-existing infections, an appropriate antimicrobial drug should be administered concurrently if glucocorticoids are used. Corticosteroids should not be administered concurrently with a vaccination.

BETAMETHASONE

Indications. Shock; inflammatory and allergic disorders; acetonaemia; induction of parturition in cattle

Contra-indications. Side-effects. Warnings. See notes above

Dose. *Horses*: *by intramuscular or intravenous injection*, 20-200 micrograms/kg

Cattle: *by intramuscular or intravenous injection*, 20-200 micrograms/kg

Induction of parturition, *by intramuscular or intravenous injection*, 20-30 mg and repeat after 3 days if required
Sheep, goats, pigs: *by intramuscular or intravenous injection*, 20-200 micrograms/kg
Dogs, cats: *by mouth*, 25 micrograms/kg; *by intramuscular or intravenous injection*, 40-80 micrograms/kg

PoM **Betsolan**™ (Coopers Pitman-Moore)
Tablets, scored, betamethasone 250 micrograms, for **dogs, cats**; 1000
Injection, betamethasone 2 mg/mL, for **horses, cattle, sheep, goats, pigs, dogs**; 20 mL, 50 mL
For intramuscular injection

PoM **Betsolan**™ **Soluble** (Coopers Pitman-Moore)
Injection, betamethasone (as sodium phosphate) 2 mg/mL, for **horses, cattle, sheep, goats, pigs, dogs, cats**; 20 mL, 50 mL
For intramuscular or intravenous injection

Compound betamethasone preparations

PoM **Canisone**™ (Schering-Plough)
Injection, betamethasone (as dipropionate) 5 mg, betamethasone (as sodium phosphate) 2 mg/mL, for **dogs**; 5 mL
Dose. Dogs: *by intramuscular injection*, 0.03-0.06 mL/kg (maximum 1 mL), repeat as necessary (maximum of 4 doses)

DEXAMETHASONE

Indications. Shock; inflammatory and allergic disorders; acetonaemia; induction of parturition in cattle and sheep; hypoadrenocorticism (7.2.2)
Contra-indications. Side-effects. Warnings. See notes above
Dose. Horses: *by mouth*, 10-30 mg, repeat after 48 hours if required; *by intramuscular or intravenous injection*, 20-200 micrograms/kg
Shock, *by intravenous injection*, 3 mg/kg, repeat after 3-6 hours if required
Cattle: *by mouth*, 10-30 mg, repeat after 24-48 hours if required; *by intramuscular or intravenous injection*, 20-200 micrograms/kg

Induction of parturition, *by intramuscular or intravenous injection*, 20-30 mg and repeat in 3 days if necessary
Shock, *by intravenous injection*, 3 mg/kg, repeat after 3-6 hours if required
Sheep: *by intramuscular or intravenous injection*, 20-200 micrograms/kg
Induction of parturition, *by intramuscular or intravenous injection*, 8-16 mg and repeat in 3 days if necessary
Shock, *by intravenous injection*, 3 mg/kg, repeat after 3-6 hours if required
Pigs: *by intramuscular or intravenous injection* 20-200 micrograms/kg
Shock, *by intravenous injection*, 3 mg/kg, repeat after 3-6 hours if required
Dogs, cats: *by mouth*, 50 micrograms/kg in divided doses; *by subcutaneous, intramuscular, or intravenous injection*, 20-200 micrograms/kg
Shock, *by intravenous injection*, 3 mg/kg, repeat after 3-6 hours if required

Note. Dexamethasone 1 mg $\equiv$ dexamethasone acetate 1.1 mg $\equiv$ dexamethasone isonicotinate 1.3 mg $\equiv$ dexamethasone sodium phosphate 1.3 mg $\equiv$ dexamethasone trioxa-undecanoate 1.4 mg (approximately)

Oral preparations

PoM **Opticorten**™ (Ciba-Geigy)
Tablets, scored, dexamethasone 250 micrograms, for **dogs, cats**; 1000, 5000
Tablets, dispersible, scored, dexamethasone 5 mg, for **horses, cattle**; 20

Parenteral preparations

PoM **Azium**™ (Schering-Plough)
Injection, dexamethasone (as dexamethasone alcohol) 2 mg/mL, for **horses, cattle, dogs, cats**; 50 mL
Withdrawal Periods. **Cattle**: slaughter 21 days, milk 36 hours
For intramuscular or intravenous injection

PoM **Colvasone**™ (Norbrook)
Injection, dexamethasone sodium phosphate 2 mg/mL, for **horses, cattle, sheep, goats, pigs, dogs, cats**; 50 mL
For intramuscular or intravenous injection

PoM **Dectan**™ (Hoechst)
Injection, dexamethasone trioxa-undecanoate 2.5 mg/mL, for *horses, cattle, sheep, pigs, dogs, cats*; 50 mL
For subcutaneous or intramuscular injection
Note. May also be administered by intra-articular, intrasynovial, or peritendinous injection (see section 10.2)

PoM **Dexadreson**™ (Intervet)
Injection, dexamethasone (as sodium phosphate) 2 mg/mL, for *horses, cattle, sheep, goats, pigs, dogs, cats*; 50 mL
For subcutaneous, intramuscular, or intravenous injection
Note. May also be administered by intra- or peri-articular injection (see section 10.2)

PoM **Dexazone**™ (Bimeda)
Injection, dexamethasone (as sodium phosphate) 2 mg/mL, for *cattle*; 50 mL
For intramuscular or intravenous injection
Note. May also be administered by intra-articular injection (see section 10.2)

PoM **Duphacort**™ **Q** (Duphar)
Injection, dexamethasone sodium phosphate 2 mg/mL, for *horses, cattle, sheep, goats, pigs, dogs, cats*; 50 mL
For intramuscular or intravenous injection

PoM **Soludex**™ (Mycofarm)
Injection, dexamethasone (as dexamethasone alcohol) 2 mg/mL, for *horses, cattle, dogs, cats*; 50 mL
Withdrawal Periods. *Cattle*: slaughter 21 days, milk 36 hours
For intramuscular or intravenous injection

PoM **Voren**™ (Boehringer Ingelheim)
Injection, dexamethasone isonicotinate 1 mg/mL, for *horses, cattle, pigs, dogs, cats*; 50 mL
For subcutaneous, intramuscular, or intravenous injection

PoM **Voren**™ **14** (Boehringer Ingelheim)
Injection, dexamethasone isonicotinate 3 mg/mL, for *horses, dogs, cats*; 50 mL
Withdrawal Periods. Should not be used in *horses* intended for human consumption
For intramuscular injection

Compound dexamethasone preparations

PoM **Dexafort**™ (Intervet)
Injection, dexamethasone (as phenylpropionate) 2 mg, dexamethasone (as sodium phosphate) 1 mg/mL, for *horses, cattle, sheep, goats, pigs, dogs, cats*; 50 mL
Dose. *By subcutaneous or intramuscular injection*. *Horses, cattle*: 10 mL
Foals, calves, sheep, goats, pigs: 1-3 mL
Dogs: 0.5-1.0 mL
Cats: 0.25-0.5 mL

ISOFLUPREDONE ACETATE

Indications. Shock; inflammatory and allergic disorders; acetonaemia
Contra-indications. Side-effects. Warnings. See notes above
Dose. *By intramuscular injection*. *Horses*: 5-20 mg, repeat as necessary
Cattle: 10-20 mg, repeat after 12-24 hours as necessary
Pigs: 37 micrograms/kg

PoM **Predef**™ **2X** (Upjohn)
Injection, isoflupredone acetate 2 mg/mL, for *horses, cattle, pigs*; 100 mL
For intramuscular injection
Note. May also be administered by intrasynovial or intratendinous injection (see section 10.2)

METHYLPREDNISOLONE

Indications. Shock; inflammatory and allergic disorders
Contra-indications. Side-effects. Warnings. See notes above
Dose. *Horses*: *by depot intramuscular injection*, 200 mg, repeat as necessary
Dogs, cats: *by intramuscular, slow intravenous injection or intravenous infusion*, 20-30 mg/kg 4-6 times daily for 1-2 days as necessary; *by depot intramuscular injection*, 1-2 mg/kg

PoM **Depo-Medrone**™ **V** (Upjohn)
Depot injection, methylprednisolone acetate 40 mg/mL, *horses, dogs, cats*; 5 mL
For intramuscular injection
Note. May be administered by intrasynovial or intratendinous injection or subcutaneous infiltration for periostitis (see section 10.2)

PoM **Solu-Medrone™** V (Upjohn)
Injection, powder for reconstitution, methylprednisolone (as sodium succinate) 125 mg, 500 mg, for *dogs*
For intramuscular or intravenous injection

PREDNISOLONE

Indications. Shock; suppression of inflammatory and allergic disorders; acetonaemia; adrenocortical insufficiency
Contra-indications. Side-effects. Warnings. See notes above
Dose. *Horses, cattle, sheep, pigs: by intramuscular injection*, 0.5-3.0 mg/kg
Dogs, cats: by mouth or by intramuscular injection, 0.5-3.0 mg/kg

PoM **Prednisolone** (Animalcare)
Tablets, prednisolone 1 mg, 5 mg, for *dogs, cats*; 500, 1000

> **Proprietary and non-proprietary medicines that are licensed for human use are printed in small type in The Veterinary Formulary**

TRIAMCINOLONE ACETONIDE

Indications. Inflammatory and allergic disorders; acetonaemia
Contra-indications. Side-effects. Warnings. See notes above
Dose. *Horses: by subcutaneous or intramuscular injection*, up to 40 micrograms/kg
Cattle: by intramuscular injection, up to 40 micrograms/kg
Dogs, cats: by subcutaneous or intramuscular injection, 100-200 micrograms/kg

PoM **Vetalog™ Long-Acting** (Ciba-Geigy)
Injection, triamcinolone acetonide 6 mg/mL, for *horses, cattle, dogs, cats*; 5 mL
For subcutaneous or intramuscular injection
Note. May be administered by intra-articular or intrasynovial injection (see section 10.2)

COMPOUND GLUCOCORTICOID PREPARATIONS

PoM **Opticortenol™** S (Ciba-Geigy)
Injection, dexamethasone pivalate 2.5 mg, prednisolone 7.5 mg/mL, for *horses, cattle, sheep, pigs, dogs, cats*; 20 mL
Dose. *by intraperitoneal, subcutaneous, intramuscular, or intravenous injection*.
Horses: 6-10 mL, repeat every 2-5 days as necessary
Cattle: 4-8 mL, repeat every 2-5 days as necessary
Sheep: 2-3 mL, repeat every 2-5 days as necessary
Pregnancy toxaemia, up to 10 mL, repeat after 2-5 days as necessary
Pigs: 4-8 mL, repeat every 2-5 days as necessary
Dogs, cats: 0.04 mL/kg, repeat every 2-5 days as necessary
Note. May also be administered by intra-articular injection (see section 10.2)

7.2.2 Treatment of hypoadrenocorticism

Hypoadrenocorticism is a syndrome that results from a deficiency of both glucocorticoid and mineralocorticoid secretion from the adrenal cortices. Destruction of both adrenal cortices is termed primary hypoadrenocorticism (Addison's disease). Secondary hypoadrenocorticism is caused by a deficiency of ACTH that leads to atrophy of the zona fasciculata of the adrenal cortices and impaired secretion of glucocorticoids. The production of mineralocorticoids from the zona glomerulosa, however, usually remains adequate. Primary hypoadrenocorticism is seen in the dog, cat, and horse.
In acute primary hypoadrenocorticism, sodium chloride 0.9% intravenous infusion and glucocorticoid therapy should be given. **Hydrocortisone sodium succinate** and **dexamethasone sodium phosphate** are suitable for intravenous glucocorticoid therapy. However, if plasma-cortisol concentrations are to be

measured for diagnosis, then dexamethasone should be used to avoid interference with the assay. Dexamethasone 0.5 to 1.0 mg/kg twice daily by intravenous injection should be administered until oral therapy can be tolerated. Once the animal has improved, maintenance therapy with mineralocorticoids can be instigated.

Chronic primary hypoadrenocorticism requires supplementation with **fludrocortisone acetate**, an oral synthetic adrenocortical steroid with mineralocorticoid activity. The dose should be adjusted until the plasma-sodium concentration and plasma-potassium concentration are within the normal range. The majority of cases do not require continuous daily glucocorticoid supplementation after initial stabilisation. However, owners should be given a supply of **prednisolone** or **hydrocortisone** tablets and clear instructions for their appropriate use in animals requiring additional glucocorticoid treatment. Either prednisolone at a dose of 100 to 200 micrograms/kg daily or hydrocortisone at a dose of 500 micrograms/kg twice daily can be used for replacement therapy.

Salt supplementation is required initially to correct hyponatraemia but is not usually required long term. Dogs requiring unusually high doses of fludrocortisone may respond to lower doses with salt supplementation.

It is advisable to administer hydrocortisone to patients with adrenocortical insufficiency before situations that may be stressful to an animal such as general anaesthesia and surgery.

FLUDROCORTISONE ACETATE

Indications. Mineralocorticoid replacement in adrenocortical insufficiency
Dose. *Dogs*: 100-500 micrograms daily. The dose may need to be increased during the first 6 to 18 months of therapy and may be required twice daily in a few cases.

PoM **Florinef**™ (Squibb)
Tablets, scored, fludrocortisone acetate 100 micrograms; 100

HYDROCORTISONE

Indications. Glucocorticoid replacement in adrenocortical insufficiency; shock
Contra-indications. Side-effects. Warnings. See section 7.2.1
Dose. *Dogs*: *by mouth*, 500 micrograms/kg twice daily; *by intramuscular injection*, 5-10 mg/kg; *by intravenous injection*, 1-10 mg/kg
Shock, *by intravenous injection*, 50 mg/kg, repeat after 3-6 hours if required

Oral preparations

PoM **Hydrocortistab**™ (Boots)
Tablets, scored, hydrocortisone 20 mg; 100

PoM **Hydrocortone**™ (MSD)
Tablets, scored, hydrocortisone 10 mg, 20 mg; 100

Parenteral preparations

PoM **Hydrocortisone Sodium Succinate** (Organon)
Injection, powder for reconstitution, hydrocortisone (as sodium succinate) 100 mg, 500 mg

PoM **Efcortelan Soluble**™ (Glaxo)
Injection, powder for reconstitution, hydrocortisone (as sodium succinate) 100 mg

PoM **Solu-Cortef**™ (Upjohn)
Injection, powder for reconstitution, hydrocortisone (as sodium succinate) 100 mg

7.3 Anabolic steroids

Anabolic steroids are synthetic derivatives of testosterone. They have some androgenic activity but less virilising effects. The use of anabolic steroids in animals intended for human consumption and in animals used in competitions is prohibited.

Anabolic steroids are indicated to promote nitrogen retention in animals with catabolic diseases. They also cause retention of sodium, calcium, potassium, chloride, sulphate, and phosphate.

The effects of anabolic steroids are to stimulate appetite, increase muscle mass, retain intracellular water, increase skin thickness, increase skeletal mass, close growth plates prematurely, and to increase production of erythrocytes.

Despite potential benefits, the clinical efficacy of anabolic steroids is unproven. Anabolic steroids are recommended as an adjunct to the treatment of chronic renal failure, in debilitating diseases and convalescence, and to promote tissue repair.

Anabolic steroids are also indicated in the management of hypoplastic anaemia and anaemia due to uraemia and neoplasia. The erythropoietic effects result partly from increased erythropoietin production and partly from direct stimulatory effect on bone marrow stem cells. Nandrolone decanoate may be used to treat anaemia, although treatment for 3 to 6 months may be required before a response is observed.

Oral and injectable preparations are available. The injectable products contain esters in oil to prolong absorption. Phenylpropionate esters slow absorption for about one week, whereas laurate and undecenoate esters prolong absorption for 3 to 4 weeks.

Anabolic steroids, particularly the alkylated compounds, including ethyloestrenol, oxymetholone, and methyltestosterone (see section 8.2.3) must be administered with care because of potential hepatotoxicity.

ETHYLOESTRENOL

Indications. Aid in convalescence, debility; wound healing, fracture repair
Contra-indications. Androgen-dependent neoplasia
Side-effects. Virilism with high doses; hepatopathy
Warnings. Caution in hepatic impairment
Dose. *Dogs, cats*: 50 micrograms/kg daily in divided doses if possible

PoM **Nandoral**™ (Intervet)
Tablets, scored, ethyloestrenol 500 micrograms, for *dogs, cats*; 500

BOLDENONE UNDECENOATE

Indications. See under Ethyloestrenol
Contra-indications. Androgen-dependent neoplasia; pregnant animals
Side-effects. Warnings. See under Ethyloestrenol

Dose. *Horses*: *by intramuscular injection*, 500-600 micrograms/kg every 2-4 weeks
Dogs, cats: *by subcutaneous or intramuscular (preferred) injection*, 2.5 mg/kg every 2-4 weeks

PoM **Vebonol**™ (Ciba-Geigy)
Depot injection (oily), boldenone undecenoate 25 mg/mL, for *horses, dogs, cats*; 10 mL
Withdrawal Periods. Should not be used in *horses* intended for human consumption

NANDROLONE

Indications. See under Ethyloestrenol; anaemia (nandrolone decanoate)
Contra-indications. Androgen-dependent neoplasia
Side-effects. Warnings. See under Ethyloestrenol. Prolonged treatment may cause symptoms of androgenic activity to occur
Dose. See preparation details

PoM **Deca-Durabolin 100**™ (Organon)
Depot injection (oily), nandrolone decanoate 25 mg/mL, 50 mg/mL, 100 mg/mL; 1 mL
Dose. Anaemia. *Dogs, cats*: *by intramuscular injection*, 1-3 mg/kg weekly

PoM **Laurabolin**™ (Intervet)
Depot injection (oily), nandrolone laurate 25 mg/mL, 50 mg/mL, for *dogs, cats*; 10 mL
Dose. *Dogs*: *by subcutaneous or intramuscular injection*, 1 mg/kg (maximum 40 mg) every 3 weeks
Cats: *by subcutaneous or intramuscular injection*, 1 mg/kg (maximum 20 mg) every 3 weeks

PoM **Nandrolin**™ (Intervet)
Depot injection (oily), nandrolone phenylpropionate 25 mg/mL, 50 mg/mL, for *dogs, cats*; 25-mg/mL vial 10 mL; 50-mg/mL vial 25 mL
Dose. *Dogs*: *by subcutaneous or intramuscular injection*, up to 50 mg weekly
Cats: *by subcutaneous or intramuscular injection*, up to 25 mg weekly

OXYMETHOLONE

Indications. See under Ethyloestrenol
Contra-indications. Side-effects. Warnings. See under Ethyloestrenol

Dose. *Dogs, cats*: 2 mg/kg twice daily

PoM **Anapolon™ 50** (Syntex)
Tablets, scored, oxymetholone 50 mg; 100

7.4 Drugs used in diabetes mellitus

7.4.1 Insulin
7.4.2 Oral antidiabetic drugs
7.4.3 Treatment of diabetic ketoacidosis
7.4.4 Treatment of hypoglycaemia

Diabetes mellitus results from an absolute or relative deficiency of insulin and is recognised particularly in the dog, cat, and horse. Although insulin and oral antidiabetic drugs are available for treatment, the majority of spontaneous cases are insulin dependent.

7.4.1 Insulin

7.4.1.1 Short-acting insulin
7.4.1.2 Intermediate- and long-acting insulins
Insulin plays a key role in the regulation of carbohydrate, fat, and protein metabolism. A relative or absolute deficiency in insulin results in a decreased utilisation of glucose, amino acids, and fatty acids by peripheral tissues, including the liver, muscle, and adipose cells. The majority of animals with diabetes mellitus require exogenous insulin to maintain satisfactory control.
Insulin is a polypeptide hormone of complex structure. It is extracted mainly from beef or pork pancreas and purified by crystallisation. Human insulins can be made biosynthetically by recombinant DNA technology using *Escherichia coli* (prb or crb depending on the precise technique) or yeast (pyr). They may also be prepared semisynthetically by enzymatic modification of porcine insulin and are termed emp. All insulin preparations are likely to be immunogenic in animals to a greater or lesser extent, but resistance to exogenous insulin action is uncommon.
Insulin is inactivated by gastro-intestinal enzymes and therefore must be given by injection. The subcutaneous route is ideal for most circumstances. However, when treating diabetic ketoacidosis (see section 7.4.3), insulin should be given by the intravenous or intramuscular route, since absorption from subcutaneous depots may be slow and erratic. Insulin is usually administered using a specific 0.5 mL or 1 mL syringe calibrated in units (100 units/mL). Insulin preparations should be stored in a refrigerator at 2°C to 8°C as they are adversely affected by heat or freezing. They should be shaken well before use.
Management of diabetes mellitus. The aim of the treatment is to achieve the best possible control of plasma-glucose concentration throughout the day in order to maintain the patient's ideal body-weight with normal water consumption and urine output while avoiding periods of hypoglycaemia. Intermediate- or long-acting insulins are usually used in doses of 0.5 to 1.0 unit/kg body-weight when initiating treatment. The dose is then tailored to the individual requirements of the patient.
Stabilisation requires understanding on behalf of the owner and a regular fixed daily routine for the patient. Intermediate-acting insulin is usually given subcutaneously once daily followed by 2 or more small meals of a constant and measured diet to minimise postprandial hyperglycaemia. The meals should be timed to coincide with the activity of the insulin preparation used. Increased dietary fibre intake is believed to improve control of blood glucose. A regular and constant pattern of exercise is also essential, since the amount of exercise will affect the daily insulin requirement. An animal will usually require 3 to 4 days to equilibrate to changes in insulin dosage or preparation. The dose should be gradually increased until optimal control of blood glucose is reached without periods of hypoglycaemia.
Insulin requirements will be increased by infection, oestrus, pregnancy, glucocorticoid therapy, and ketoacidosis. Obesity must be avoided as this will increase insulin resistance.
The duration of action of different insulin preparations varies considerably

from one patient to another and needs to be assessed for each individual. The times indicated below are only approximations.

7.4.1.1 SHORT-ACTING INSULIN

Soluble Insulin is a short-acting form of insulin. It is the only appropriate form of insulin for use in diabetic emergencies (see section 7.4.3) and may be used at the time of surgical operations. It has the great advantage that it can be given intravenously and intramuscularly as well as subcutaneously.

When injected subcutaneously or intramuscularly, soluble insulin has a rapid onset of action of 15 to 30 minutes, peak activity between 2 and 4 hours, and a duration of action of up to 8 hours. When injected intravenously, soluble insulin has a very short half-life and its effect disappears within 2 to 4 hours.

SOLUBLE INSULIN
(Insulin Injection; Neutral Insulin)

A sterile solution of insulin (i.e. bovine or porcine) or of human insulin; pH 6.6-8.0

Indications. Diabetes mellitus; diabetic ketoacidosis (7.4.3)
Side-effects. See notes above; overdosage causes hypoglycaemia
Dose. *Dogs, cats*: *by subcutaneous, intramuscular, or intravenous injection, or intravenous infusion*, according to patient's requirements; see notes above

Highly purified animal insulins

PoM **Neutral Insulin Injection** (Evans)
Injection, soluble insulin (bovine, highly purified) 100 units/mL; 10 mL

PoM **Hypurin Neutral**™ (CP)
Injection, soluble insulin (bovine, highly purified) 100 units/mL; 10 mL

PoM **Velosulin**™ (Novo Nordisk)
Injection, soluble insulin (porcine, highly purified) 100 units/mL; 10 mL

Human sequence insulins

PoM **Human Actrapid**™ (Novo Nordisk)
Injection, soluble insulin (human, pyr) 100 units/mL; 10 mL

PoM **Human Velosulin**™ (Novo Nordisk)
Injection, soluble insulin (human, emp) 100 units/mL; 10 mL

PoM **Humulin S**™ (Lilly)
Injection, soluble insulin (human, prb) 100 units/mL; 10 mL

7.4.1.2 INTERMEDIATE- AND LONG-ACTING INSULINS

When given by subcutaneous injection, intermediate-acting insulin has an onset of activity of approximately 1 to 2 hours, a peak activity at 6 to 12 hours, and a duration of action of 18 to 26 hours in the dog. The times for peak activity and duration of action are often shorter in the cat. Intermediate-acting insulins are usually administered once daily.

Insulin Zinc Suspension (30% amorphous, 70% crystalline) is a mixture of **Insulin Zinc Suspension (Amorphous)**, which has an intermediate duration of action and **Insulin Zinc Suspension (Crystalline)**, which has a more prolonged duration of action. It has proved a useful preparation in the long-term management of diabetes mellitus in the dog and cat. **Isophane Insulin** is a suspension of insulin with protamine but is shorter acting and needs to be administered twice daily in most patients to achieve blood glucose control. **Biphasic Insulins** are ready-mixed combinations of an intermediate-acting insulin with soluble insulin and may require twice daily injection.

Protamine Zinc Insulin and Insulin Zinc Suspension (Crystalline) are long-acting insulins. When injected subcutaneously they have an onset of activity of 4 to 6 hours, peak action around 14 to 24 hours and duration of activity 32 to 36 hours. All types of insulin are used in veterinary practice, although Insulin Zinc Suspension, Isophane Insulin, and Protamine Zinc Insulins are used most commonly.

INSULIN ZINC SUSPENSION
(Insulin Zinc Suspension (Mixed); I.Z.S.)

A sterile neutral suspension of bovine and/or porcine insulin or of human insulin in the form of a complex obtained by the addition of a suitable zinc salt

Indications. Diabetes mellitus
Side-effects. See notes above; over-dosage causes hypoglycaemia
Dose. *Dogs, cats: by subcutaneous injection*, according to patient's requirements; see notes above

Highly purified animal insulin

PoM **Insulin Zinc Suspension Lente** (Evans)
Injection, insulin zinc suspension (bovine, highly purified) 100 units/mL; 10 mL

PoM **Hypurin Lente™** (CP)
Injection, insulin zinc suspension (bovine, highly purified) 100 units/mL; 10 mL

PoM **Lentard MC™** (Novo Nordisk)
Injection, insulin zinc suspension (bovine and porcine, highly purified) 100 units/mL; 10 mL

Human sequence insulin

PoM **Human Monotard™** (Novo Nordisk)
Injection, insulin zinc suspension (human, pyr) 100 units/mL; 10 mL

PoM **Humulin Lente™** (Lilly)
Injection, insulin zinc suspension (human, prb) 100 units/mL; 10 mL

INSULIN ZINC SUSPENSION (AMORPHOUS)
(Amorph. I.Z.S.)

A sterile neutral suspension of bovine or porcine insulin in the form of a complex obtained by the addition of a suitable zinc salt

Indications. Diabetes mellitus
Side-effects. See under Insulin Zinc Suspension
Dose. *Dogs, cats: by subcutaneous injection*, according to patient's requirements; see notes above

PoM **Semitard™ MC** (Novo Nordisk)
Injection, insulin zinc suspension, amorphous (porcine, highly purified) 100 units/mL; 10 mL

INSULIN ZINC SUSPENSION (CRYSTALLINE)
(Cryst. I.Z.S.)

A sterile neutral suspension of bovine insulin or of human insulin in the form

of a complex obtained by the addition of a suitable zinc salt

Indications. Diabetes mellitus
Side-effects. See under Insulin Zinc Suspension
Dose. *Dogs, cats: by subcutaneous injection*, according to patient's requirements; see notes above

PoM **Human Ultratard™** (Novo Nordisk)
Injection, insulin zinc suspension, crystalline (human, pyr) 100 units/mL; 10 mL

PoM **Humulin Zn™** (Lilly)
Injection, insulin zinc suspension, crystalline (human, prb) 100 units/mL; 10 mL

ISOPHANE INSULIN
(Isophane Insulin Injection; Isophane Protamine Insulin Injection; Isophane Insulin (NPH))

A sterile suspension of bovine or porcine insulin or of human insulin in the form of a complex obtained by the addition of protamine sulphate or another suitable protamine

Indications. Diabetes mellitus
Side-effects. See under Insulin Zinc Suspension
Dose. *Dogs, cats: by subcutaneous injection*, according to patient's requirements; see notes above

Highly purified animal insulin

PoM **Isophane Insulin Injection** (Evans)
Injection, isophane insulin (bovine, highly purified) 100 units/mL; 10 mL

PoM **Hypurin Isophane™** (CP)
Injection, isophane insulin (bovine, highly purified) 100 units/mL; 10 mL

PoM **Insulatard™** (Novo Nordisk)
Injection, isophane insulin (porcine, highly purified) 100 units/mL; 10 mL

Human sequence insulin

PoM **Human Insulatard™** (Novo Nordisk)
Injection, isophane insulin (human, emp) 100 units/mL; 10 mL

PoM **Human Protaphane™** (Novo Nordisk)
Injection, isophane insulin (human, pyr) 100 units/mL; 10 mL

PoM **Humulin I™** (Lilly)
Injection, isophane insulin (human, prb)
100 units/mL; 10 mL

PROTAMINE ZINC INSULIN
(Protamine Zinc Insulin Injection)

A sterile suspension of insulin in the form of a complex obtained by the addition of a suitable protamine and zinc chloride

Indications. Diabetes mellitus
Side-effects. See under Insulin Zinc Suspension
Dose. *Dogs, cats*: *by subcutaneous injection*, according to patient's requirements; see notes above

PoM **Hypurin Protamine Zinc™** (CP)
Injection, protamine zinc insulin (bovine, highly purified) 100 units/mL; 10 mL

BIPHASIC INSULIN
(Biphasic Insulin Injection)

A sterile suspension of crystals containing bovine insulin in a solution of porcine insulin

Indications. Diabetes mellitus
Side-effects. See under Insulin Zinc Suspension
Dose. *Dogs, cats*: *by subcutaneous injection*, according to patient's requirements; see notes above

PoM **Rapitard MC™** (Novo Nordisk)
Injection, biphasic insulin (highly purified) 100 units/mL; 10 mL

BIPHASIC ISOPHANE INSULIN
(Biphasic Isophane Insulin Injection)

A sterile buffered suspension of porcine insulin complexed with protamine sulphate (or another suitable protamine) in a solution of porcine insulin *or* a sterile buffered suspension of human insulin complexed with protamine sulphate (or another suitable protamine) in a solution of human insulin

Indications. Diabetes mellitus
Side-effects. See under Insulin Zinc Suspension
Dose. *Dogs, cats*: *by subcutaneous*

injection, according to patient's requirements; see notes above

Highly purified animal insulin

PoM **Initard 50/50™** (Novo Nordisk)
Injection, biphasic isophane insulin (porcine, highly purified), 50% soluble, 50% isophane, 100 units/mL; 10 mL

PoM **Mixtard 30/70™** (Novo Nordisk)
Injection, biphasic isophane insulin (porcine, highly purified), 30% soluble, 70% isophane, 100 units/mL; 10 mL

Human sequence insulin

PoM **Human Actraphane 30/70™** (Novo Nordisk)
Injection, biphasic isophane insulin (human, pyr), 30% soluble, 70% isophane, 100 units/mL; 10 mL

PoM **Human Initard 50/50™** (Novo Nordisk)
Injection, biphasic isophane insulin (human, emp), 50% soluble, 50% isophane, 100 units/mL; 10 mL

PoM **Human Mixtard 30/70™** (Novo Nordisk)
Injection, biphasic isophane insulin (human, emp), 30% soluble, 70% isophane, 100 units/mL; 10 mL

PoM **Humulin M1™** (Lilly)
Injection, biphasic isophane insulin (human, prb), 10% soluble, 90% isophane, 100 units/mL; 10 mL

PoM **Humulin M2™** (Lilly)
Injection, biphasic isophane insulin (human, prb), 20% soluble, 80% isophane, 100 units/mL; 10 mL

PoM **Humulin M3™** (Lilly)
Injection, biphasic isophane insulin (human, prb), 30% soluble, 70% isophane, 100 units/mL; 10 mL

PoM **Humulin M4™** (Lilly)
Injection, biphasic isophane insulin (human, prb), 40% soluble, 60% isophane, 100 units/mL; 10 mL

7.4.2 Oral antidiabetic drugs

Oral antidiabetic drugs are rarely successful in controlling non-insulin dependent diabetes mellitus in animals. The two major groups of oral antidiabetic drugs are the sulphonylureas and the biguanides. The sulphonylureas act mainly by augmenting insulin secretion and consequently are only effective when some residual pancreatic beta-cell activity is present. The biguanides act mainly by decreasing gluconeogenesis and increasing peripheral utilisation of glucose and are again only effective with some residual functioning pancreatic islet cells.

The sulphonylureas, which include **chlorpropamide, tolbutamide, glipizide**, and **glibenclamide** have been used very occasionally in dogs. Chlorpropamide may also enhance the effect of anti-diuretic hormone and has been used in the treatment of partial cranial diabetes insipidus (see section 7.5.2).

The biguanide, **metformin** has also been used for the treatment of non-insulin dependent diabetes mellitus.

CHLORPROPAMIDE

Indications. Non-insulin dependent diabetes mellitus, diabetes insipidus (7.5.2)
Side-effects. Overdosage causes hypoglycaemia
Dose. *Dogs*: 10-40 mg/kg daily in divided doses. Adjust dose as necessary to produce normoglycaemia

PoM **Chlorpropamide** (Non-proprietary)
Tablets, chlorpropamide 100 mg, 250 mg

GLIBENCLAMIDE

Indications. Non-insulin dependent diabetes mellitus
Side-effects. Overdosage causes hypoglycaemia
Dose. *Dogs*: 200 micrograms/kg daily. Adjust dose as necessary to produce normoglycaemia

PoM **Glibenclamide** (Non-proprietary)
Tablets, glibenclamide 2.5 mg, 5 mg

GLIPIZIDE

Indications. Non-insulin dependent diabetes mellitus
Side-effects. Overdosage causes hypoglycaemia
Dose. *Dogs*: 250-500 micrograms/kg twice daily. Adjust dose as necessary to produce normoglycaemia

PoM **Glibenese**™ (Pfizer)
Tablets, scored, glipizide 5 mg; 56

PoM **Minodiab**™ (Farmitalia Carlo Erba)
Tablets, glipizide 2.5 mg, 5 mg (scored); 60

METFORMIN HYDROCHLORIDE

Indications. Non-insulin dependent diabetes mellitus
Side-effects. Overdosage causes hypoglycaemia
Dose. *Dogs*: 250-500 mg twice daily with food. Adjust dose as necessary to produce normoglycaemia

PoM **Metformin** (Non-proprietary)
Tablets, metformin hydrochloride 500 mg, 850 mg

TOLBUTAMIDE

Indications. Non-insulin dependent diabetes mellitus
Side-effects. Hepatopathy, overdosage causes hypoglycaemia
Dose. *Dogs*: 20-100 mg/kg daily. Adjust dose as necessary to produce normoglycaemia

PoM **Tolbutamide** (Non-proprietary)
Tablets, tolbutamide 500 mg

7.4.3 Treatment of diabetic ketoacidosis

Signs of diabetic ketoacidosis include anorexia, vomiting, diarrhoea, lethargy weakness, and increased depth and rate of respiration.

Soluble insulin may be used in the management of diabetic ketoacidosis and hyperosmolar non-ketotic coma in dogs and cats. It is the only form of insulin that may be given intravenously It is necessary to achieve and maintain an adequate plasma-insulin concentration until the metabolic disturbance is brought under control.

Soluble insulin is best given by intravenous infusion since a single bolus dose will only achieve an adequate concentration for a short period of time Plasma concentrations are effectively maintained with infusion rates of 0.1 unit/kg per hour. Insulin is diluted in the replacement fluids taking care to ensure the insulin is not injected into the 'dead space' of the injection port of the infusion bag and is thoroughly mixed with the replacement fluid. The infusion should be continued until the blood-glucose concentration has fallen to 10 mmol/litre and the patient is willing to eat. Subcutaneous administration of an intermediate- or long-acting preparation can then be started.

If facilities for administering insulin by continuous infusion are inadequate, 0.25 unit/kg of soluble insulin may be given intravenously and 0.75 unit/kg intramuscularly. The dose should be repeated every 4 to 6 hours until the blood-glucose concentration reaches 10 mmol/litre. Some clinicians consider this is more likely to result in hypokalaemia than the infusion technique.

Intravenous replacement of fluid and electrolytes with sodium chloride 0.9% infusion is an essential part of the management of ketoacidosis. Potassium chloride should be included in the infusion as appropriate to prevent hypokalaemia induced by the insulin. The rate of potassium administration should not exceed 0.5 mmol/kg bodyweight per hour. Sodium bicarbonate 2.74% infusion is only used in life-threatening acidosis, since the acid-base disturbance is normally corrected by insulin and fluid therapy.

7.4.4 Treatment of hypoglycaemia

Signs of hypoglycaemia include disorientation, weakness, hunger, shaking, ataxia, convulsions and coma. The occurrence of clinical signs is thought to be dependent on the rate of decline of plasma-glucose concentration as well as on the severity of hypoglycaemia.

Acute hypoglycaemia occurs most commonly when a diabetic animal is given too much insulin or exercises too strenuously. If mild signs of hypoglycaemia are seen, the animal should be fed its normal food. Alternatively, glucose or sugar dissolved in a little water may be given and repeated, if necessary, after 10 to 15 minutes. If severe signs are observed, **glucose** (see section 16.1.2) should be given intravenously. A dose of 1 mL/kg of 50% glucose intravenous infusion should be adequate to correct the hypoglycaemia. The dose of insulin should be adjusted to prevent further episodes.

Chronic hypoglycaemia usually results from excess endogenous insulin secretion from an islet cell tumour (insulinoma). Islet cell tumours in dogs are generally malignant, but slow growing. Surgical excision is the treatment of choice, although virtually all islet cell tumours recur after excision. The mean survival-time following excision is about one year. If surgical treatment is not possible or not successful, or if hypoglycaemic episodes return after surgery, medical therapy is indicated.

Initial medical management for chronic hypoglycaemia should include giving small frequent meals high in proteins, fats, and complex carbohydrates. Glucocorticoids are also recommended. **Prednisolone** (see section 7.2.1) at a dose of 0.5 to 1.0 mg/kg daily in divided doses is used most frequently.

Diazoxide is a non-diuretic benzothiadiazine antihypertensive drug, which acts primarily by suppressing insulin secretion by the pancreas. It is useful in treating hypoglycaemia due to islet cell tumours, but is of no value in the management of acute hypoglycaemia.

DIAZOXIDE

Indications. Chronic hypoglycaemia
Side-effects. Anorexia, vomiting; cataract formation
Dose. *Dogs*: 10 mg/kg daily in divided doses increasing up to 60 mg/kg daily if necessary. Usually used in combination with frequent feeding and prednisolone (see notes above).

PoM **Eudemine**™ (A&H)
Tablets, diazoxide 50 mg; 100

7.5 Pituitary and hypothalamic hormones

7.5.1 Anterior pituitary hormones
7.5.2 Posterior pituitary hormones
7.5.3 Hypothalamic hormones

7.5.1 Anterior pituitary hormones

The anterior lobe of the pituitary gland produces and releases a number of trophic hormones of which thyrotrophin (TSH), corticotrophin (ACTH), growth hormone (GH), follicle-stimulating hormone (FSH), luteinising hormone (LH), and prolactin are the most important.

Protirelin (thyrotrophin-releasing hormone, TRH) (see section 7.5.3) is used as a diagnostic agent to confirm the presence of hypothyroidism and to distinguish between primary and secondary forms of the disease.

Corticotrophin and **tetracosactrin** are used mainly as diagnostic agents to assess adrenocortical function. Failure of the plasma-cortisol concentration to increase after administration of corticotrophin or tetracosactrin indicates adrenocortical insufficiency due to either hypoadrenocorticism (Addison's disease) or the exogenous administration of glucocorticoids. An excessive elevation of plasma-cortisol concentration following administration of corticotrophin or tetracosactrin indicates hyperadrenocorticism (Cushing's syndrome). An exaggerated response may also result from uncontrolled diabetes mellitus, pyometra, or chronic renal disease.

GH has been used in the treatment of panhypopituitarism (pituitary dwarfism) and in growth hormone-responsive alopecia. The use of GH preparations in food animals is illegal. Potential side-effects to GH therapy include hypersensitivity reactions and diabetes mellitus.

In theory, prolactin secretion may be increased with the use of dopamine antagonists such as metoclopramide, although this drug is used clinically to inhibit the side-effects of bromocriptine treatment. Prolactin secretion may be decreased with the use of dopamine agonists such as bromocriptine (see section 7.6.1).

CORTICOTROPHIN
(ACTH)

Indications. Diagnostic use; see notes above

Side-effects. See under Glucocorticoids (see section 7.2.1)

Dose. *Dogs: by intramuscular injection*, 2.2 units/kg

PoM **Acthar Gel™** (Rorer)
Injection, corticotrophin (with gelatin) 20 units/mL, 40 units/mL, 80 units/mL; 20-unit vial 5 mL, 40-unit vial 2 mL and 5 mL, 80-unit vial 5 mL
Note. Preparations of corticotrophin are not generally available. A written order, stating case details, should be sent to the manufacturer to obtain a supply of the preparation.

TETRACOSACTRIN

Indications. Diagnostic use; see notes above

Side-effects. See under Glucocorticoids (see section 7.2.1)

Dose. *Horses: by intravenous injection*, 1 mg

Dogs: by intramuscular or intravenous injection, (less than 5 kg body-weight) 125 micrograms; (more than 5 kg body-weight) 250 micrograms

PoM **Synacthen™** (Ciba)
Injection, tetracosactrin (as acetate) 250 micrograms/mL; 1 mL

7.5.2 Posterior pituitary hormones

The posterior lobe of the pituitary gland releases stored vasopressin (antidiuretic hormone, ADH) and oxytocin, which are synthesised in the hypothalamus. Oxytocin (see section 8.4) is used mainly in obstetrics. The domestic species, like man, store arginine-vasopressin (argipressin) except for the pig, which has lysine-vasopressin (lypressin).

Diabetes insipidus is a syndrome caused by an absolute or relative deficiency of ADH. It may result from a partial or total failure to synthesise or release ADH (cranial diabetes insipidus) or from a failure of the kidney to respond to ADH (nephrogenic diabetes insipidus). **Desmopressin** has been used in the treatment of cranial diabetes insipidus and is particularly indicated when the disease is severe. The dose must be adjusted to the requirements of the individual patient.

Desmopressin is considered to have a longer duration of action than vasopressin and does not possess its vascoconstrictor activity. The intranasal solution is effective if placed in the conjunctival sac. This route of administration is preferred since repeated intranasal use may prove difficult. The maximal effect of the drug occurs from 2 to 8 hours after administration and its duration of action varies from 8 to 24 hours.

Desmopressin injection is used in the differential diagnosis of diabetes insipidus to distinguish the cranial form of the disease from the nephrogenic form. This test is performed after a water-deprivation test has confirmed that the animal cannot concentrate its urine. Restoration of the ability to concentrate urine confirms a diagnosis of cranial diabetes insipidus. Failure to respond is indicative of nephrogenic diabetes insipidus.

Excessive desmopressin medication can lead to hyponatraemia and water intoxication. Clinical signs may include depression, salivation, vomiting, ataxia, muscle tremors, convulsions, and coma. Desmopressin is almost devoid of pressor activity.

Aqueous **vasopressin** is not suitable for long-term management of cranial diabetes insipidus since its duration of action is only a few hours. However, it is a suitable agent for an ADH test. In dogs or cats with nephrogenic or partial cranial diabetes insipidus, thiazides (see section 4.2.1) may have a paradoxical effect in reducing urinary output. **Hydrochlorothiazide** at a dose of 2 to 4 mg/kg twice daily by mouth and **chlorothiazide** 20 to 40 mg/kg twice daily by mouth have been used in conjunction with low-sodium diets. Plasma-electrolyte concentrations should be checked periodically so that disturbances, particularly hypokalaemia, can be corrected.

Chlorpropamide (see section 7.4.2) has also been used in the treatment of partial cranial diabetes insipidus and is thought to act by potentiating the renal tubular effects of remaining endogenous ADH. A suggested dose for the dog is 10 to 40 mg/kg daily and the cat 50 mg per day. Results are inconsistent and it may take 1 to 2 weeks of trial medication to obtain an effect. Hypoglycaemia is a potential side-effect.

Desmopressin injection is also used to boost von Willebrand factor antigen concentrations and thus reduce the bleeding time in von Willebrand's disease.

DESMOPRESSIN

Indications. Cranial diabetes insipidus; von Willebrand's disease; see notes above
Side-effects. See notes above
Dose. *Dogs, cats*: cranial diabetes insipidus, *by instillation into the conjunctival sac*, 2-4 drops (of the intranasal solution) 1-2 times daily; *by intramuscular injection*, 1-4 micrograms 1-2 times daily

ADH test, *by intramuscular injection*, (less than 15 kg body-weight) 2 micrograms; (dogs more than 15 kg body-weight) 4 micrograms. Urine samples should be collected 2-hourly following the injection until maximum concentration is achieved

Von Willebrand's disease, *by intravenous injection*, 1 microgram/kg if the patient is bleeding

PoM **DDAVP**™ (Ferring)
Injection, desmopressin 4 micrograms/mL; 1 mL
Intranasal solution, desmopressin 100 micrograms/mL; 2.5 mL

VASOPRESSIN

Indications. See notes above
Side-effects. Vasoconstriction and hypersensitivity reactions; see notes above
Dose. *Dogs, cats*: ADH test, *by intramuscular injection*, 0.5 unit/kg (maximum 5 units). Urine samples should be

collected 2-hourly following the injection until maximum concentration is achieved.

PoM **Pitressin™** (Parke-Davis)
Injection, argipressin 20 units/mL; 1 mL
Note. Preparations of argipressin are not generally available. A written order, stating case details, should be sent to the manufacturer to obtain a supply of the preparation.

7.5.3 Hypothalamic hormones

Protirelin (thyrotrophin-releasing hormone, TRH) is used mainly for diagnostic purposes in the evaluation of hypothyroidism. Thyroid hormone concentrations are measured before and after intravenous administration of protirelin. Failure to respond adequately suggests primary or secondary hypothyroidism. Post-stimulation levels tend to be lower than following thyrotrophin (TSH) stimulation.

Doses of protirelin greater than 100 micrograms/kg may produce salivation, vomiting, miosis, tachycardia, and tachypnoea.

PROTIRELIN

Indications. Diagnostic use in hypothyroidism
Side-effects. See notes above
Dose. *Dogs, cats*: *by intravenous injection*, 200 mg *or* 100 micrograms/kg according to the protocol used. Blood samples should be taken for thyroid hormone estimations before and at 4 or 6 hours after injection.

PoM **TRH** (Roche)
Injection, protirelin 100 micrograms/mL; 2 mL
Note. Preparations of protirelin are not generally available. A written order, stating case details, should be sent to the manufacturer to obtain a supply of the preparation.

7.6 Other endocrine drugs

7.6.1 Bromocriptine
7.6.2 Drugs used in hyperadrenocorticism

7.6.1 Bromocriptine

Bromocriptine is a potent dopamine receptor agonist. It also inhibits prolactin release from the anterior pituitary gland. Bromocriptine is used in the treatment of pseudopregnancy in the bitch. It should be reserved for cases where other methods fail because side-effects of bromocriptine are common and may be severe.

Metoclopramide (see section 3.3.1) can be used concurrently as an anti-emetic even though it has dopamine receptor blocking properties.

Bromocriptine may decrease the secretion of ACTH in some animals with pituitary-dependent hyperadrenocorticism (Cushing's syndrome). Its use is limited because of the small percentage of cases that do respond and the frequency with which relapses occur.

BROMOCRIPTINE

Indications. Pseudopregnancy, pituitary-dependent hyperadrenocorticism
Side-effects. Vomiting, anorexia, depression, and behavioural changes; see notes above
Dose. *Dogs*: pseudopregnancy, 10 micrograms/kg twice daily for 10 days *or* 30 micrograms/kg once daily for 16 days
Pituitary-dependent hyperadrenocorticism, up to 100 micrograms/kg daily in divided doses given in gradually increasing amounts

PoM **Bromocriptine** (Non-proprietary)
Tablets, bromocriptine (as mesylate) 2.5 mg

PoM **Parlodel™** (Sandoz)
Tablets, scored, bromocriptine (as mesylate) 1 mg, 2.5 mg; 1-mg tablets 100; 2.5-mg tablets 30, 100, 500
Capsules, bromocriptine (as mesylate) 5 mg, 10 mg; 100

7.6.2 Drugs used in hyperadrenocorticism

Hyperadrenocorticism (Cushing's syndrome) is associated with excessive production or administration of glucocorticoids and is one of the most commonly diagnosed endocrinopathies affecting dogs. It is seen rarely in cats and horses.

Hyperadrenocorticism can be spontaneous or iatrogenic. Spontaneously occurring hyperadrenocorticism may be associated with inappropriate secretion of ACTH by the pituitary gland (pituitary-dependent hyperadrenocorticism) or associated with an adrenal tumour (adrenal-dependent hyperadrenocorticism). Pituitary-dependent hyperadrenocorticism accounts for over 80 percent of dogs with naturally occurring hyperadrenocorticism.

Although pituitary-dependent hyperadrenocorticism has been managed surgically by hypophysectomy or bilateral adrenalectomy, medical management using mitotane is the treatment of choice. **Mitotane** is a cytotoxic drug that selectively destroys the zona fasciculata and zona reticularis of the adrenal cortex while tending to preserve the zona glomerulosa. Although considerable care is required in its use, many cases have been successfully managed long term with this drug. Some clinicians recommend routine replacement of glucocorticoids at the start of mitotane therapy. However, most patients do not exhibit signs of glucocorticoid deficiency and do not require replacement therapy.

Ketoconazole (see section 1.2), an imidazole derivative used primarily for its antifungal properties, is a promising alternative to mitotane. It has a reversible inhibitory effect on glucocorticoid synthesis whilst having negligible effects on mineralocorticoid production. Hepatoxicity may occur in some patients.

Cyproheptadine and **bromocriptine** (see section 7.6.1) may decrease the secretion of ACTH in some animals with pituitary-dependent hyperadrenocorticism. However, both appear to have limited usefulness because of the small percentage of cases that do respond and the frequency with which relapses occur. Surgical adrenalectomy is considered the treatment of choice for adrenal-dependent hyperadrenocorticism, although mitotane therapy is also recommended. Presurgical treatment with ketoconazole may reduce the relatively high morbidity and mortality associated with surgical extirpation of the adrenal glands.

CYPROHEPTADINE HYDROCHLORIDE

Indications. Pituitary-dependent hyperadrenocorticism
Side-effects. Polyphagia
Dose. *Horses*: 0.6 mg/kg increasing to 1.2 mg/kg daily
Dogs: 0.3 mg/kg increasing to 3.0 mg/kg daily

P **Periactin**™ (MSD)
Tablets, scored, cyproheptadine hydrochloride 4 mg; 100
Syrup, cyproheptadine hydrochloride 400 micrograms/mL; 200 mL

KETOCONAZOLE

Indications. Pituitary-dependent hyperadrenocorticism, adrenal-dependent hyperadrenocorticism (presurgery)
Side-effects. Anorexia, vomiting, diarrhoea, hepatopathy, and jaundice
Dose. *Dogs*: 5 mg/kg twice daily for 7 days increasing to 10 mg/kg twice daily for 7 to 14 days, then 15 mg/kg twice daily

PoM **Nizoral**™ (Janssen)
See section 1.2 for preparation details

MITOTANE

Indications. Pituitary-dependent hyperadrenocorticism, adrenal-dependent hyperadrenocorticism
Side-effects. Lethargy, anorexia, vomiting, weakness, diarrhoea, and neurological signs such as ataxia, incoordination, circling, blindness, facial paralysis, and seizures
Dose. *Dogs*: 50 mg/kg daily until thirst returns to normal, usually 7 to 10 days. Then 50 mg/kg every 1-2 weeks to prevent recurrence of clinical signs. Mitotane should be given with food to improve absorption.

Mitotane preparations are not generally available in the UK.

Supplies of mitotane tablets and mitotane powder are available from Idis Ltd who import the preparations from the US.

8 Drugs acting on the

REPRODUCTIVE SYSTEM and URINARY TRACT

8.1 Drugs used to promote gonadal function
8.2 Sex hormones
8.3 Prostaglandins
8.4 Myometrial stimulants
8.5 Myometrial relaxants
8.6 Drugs for uterine infections
8.7 Drugs used for disorders of the urinary tract

8.1 Drugs used to promote gonadal function

8.1.1 Gonadotrophins
8.1.2 Gonadotrophin-releasing hormones
8.1.3 Immunogens

8.1.1 Gonadotrophins

Chorionic gonadotrophin is a complex glycoprotein that has a similar effect to luteinising hormone (LH) secreted by the anterior pituitary gland in both males and females.

In veterinary practice, it is used to supplement or replace luteinising hormone in cases of ovulation failure or delay and to induce lactation post partum. In males, chorionic gonadotrophin stimulates the secretion of testosterone by interstitial testicular cells. It is used to treat genital hypoplasia and reduced libido.

Serum gonadotrophin is also a complex glycoprotein. It is extracted from mares' serum during a well-defined stage of pregnancy and is more accurately referred to as pregnant mare serum gonadotrophin (PMSG, or equine chorionic gonadotrophin). The effects of serum gonadotrophin in animals are similar to both luteinising hormone and, more predominantly, follicle-stimulating hormone (FSH) secreted by the anterior pituitary gland.

Serum gonadotrophin is commonly used to induce follicular growth and ovulation during anoestrus or following the application of progestogen-impregnated vaginal sponges in sheep (see section 8.2.2). It is used routinely to induce superovulation in cattle, sheep, and goats for use as donors in embryo transfer programmes. In males, serum gonadotrophin promotes spermatogenesis. Individuals may show a variable response to serum gonadotrophin.

Before hormonal treatment the status of the reproductive tract should be ascertained by rectal palpation or milk-progesterone assays. The efficacy of therapy will depend on both the presence and responsiveness of the target organ. Both chorionic gonadotrophin and serum gonadotrophin may become ineffective after repeated doses due to antibody formation. Occasionally, treatment may cause an anaphylactic reaction in some animals.

CHORIONIC GONADOTROPHIN

Indications. See notes above and under Dose

Side-effects. Immune-mediated reduced effect after repeated doses; occasional anaphylactic reactions

Dose. *Horses. Females*: suboestrus with follicles greater than 2 cm in diameter, *by subcutaneous or intramuscular injection*, 1500-3000 units, repeat after 2-3 days if required

Postpartum agalactia, *by subcutaneous or intramuscular injection*, 1500-3000 units, repeat after 1 day if required

Nymphomania, *by intravenous injection*, 1500-5000 units, repeat after 4 weeks if required

Anoestrus, see Serum Gonadotrophin below

Males: deficient libido, *by intramuscular injection*, 1500 units twice weekly for 4-6 weeks

Genital hypoplasia, *by intramuscular injection*, 1500-5000 units twice weekly for 4-6 weeks

Cryptorchidism (before castration), *by intramuscular injection*, 1500-15 000 units twice weekly for 4-6 weeks

Cattle. Females: ovulatory failure or delay, prolonged oestrus, *by intravenous injection*, 1500-3000 units on day of insemination. Repeat dose *by subcutaneous or intramuscular injection*, 8-10 days later if required

Suboestrus, true anoestrus in heifers, *by subcutaneous or intramuscular injection*, 1500-3000 units

Cystic ovaries, *by intravenous injection*, 1500-3000 units after expression or drainage of cysts

Males: deficient libido, *by intramuscular injection*, 1500 units twice weekly for 4-6 weeks

Genital hypoplasia, *by intramuscular injection*, 1500-5000 units twice weekly for 4-6 weeks

Cryptorchidism (before castration), *by intramuscular injection*, 1500-15 000 units twice weekly for 4-6 weeks

Sheep. Males: deficient libido, genital hypoplasia, *by intramuscular injection*, 500 units twice weekly for 4-6 weeks

Goats. Females: repeated failure to hold to service, fetal resorption, *by intramuscular injection*, 100-500 units on day of insemination

Nymphomania, *by intramuscular injection*, 1000 units

Males: deficient libido, genital hypoplasia, *by intramuscular injection*, 500 units twice weekly for 4-6 weeks

Cryptorchidism (before castration), *by intramuscular injection*, 500-1500 units twice weekly for 4-6 weeks

Pigs. Females: repeated failure to hold to service, fetal resorption, *by intramuscular injection*, 500-1000 units on day of insemination

Postpartum agalactia, *by subcutaneous or intramuscular injection*, 500-1000 units, repeat after 1 day if required

Males: deficient libido, genital hypoplasia, *by intramuscular injection*, 500 units twice weekly for 4-6 weeks

Cryptorchidism (before castration), *by intramuscular injection*, 500-1500 units twice weekly for 4-6 weeks

Dogs. Females: repeated failure to hold to service, fetal resorption, *by intramuscular injection*, 200-500 units on day of insemination

Postpartum agalactia, *by intramuscular injection*, 100-500 units, repeat after 1 day if required

Nymphomania, *by intramuscular injection*, 100-500 units

Males: deficient libido, genital hypoplasia, feminisation at puberty, *by intramuscular injection*, 100-500 units twice weekly for 4-6 weeks

Cryptorchidism (before castration), *by intramuscular injection*, 100-1500 units twice weekly for 4-6 weeks

Cats. Females: suppression of oestrus, *by intramuscular injection*, 100-500 units as a single dose

PoM **Chorionic Gonadotrophin** (Univet)
Injection, powder for reconstitution, chorionic gonadotrophin 1500 units, for **horses, cattle**

PoM **Chorulon**™ (Intervet)
Injection, powder for reconstitution, chorionic gonadotrophin 1500 units, for **horses, cattle, pigs, sheep, goats, dogs, cats**

PoM **LH 1500**™ (Paines & Byrne)
Injection, powder for reconstitution, chorionic gonadotrophin 1500 units, for **horses, cattle**
Withdrawal Periods. *Cattle*: slaughter withdrawal period nil, milk withdrawal period nil

See also section 8.2.5

SERUM GONADOTROPHIN

Indications. See notes above and under Dose

Side-effects. Immune-mediated decreased effect after repeated doses; occasional anaphylactic reactions

Dose. Horses. Females: anoestrus, *by subcutaneous or intramuscular injection*, 3000-6000 units, followed by chorionic gonadotrophin 1500-3000 units at time of insemination

Males: impaired spermatogenesis, *by intramuscular injection*, 1000-3000 units twice weekly for 4-6 weeks

Cattle. Females: anoestrus, *by subcutaneous or intramuscular injection*, 1500-3000 units, repeat after 10-14 days if required

Males: impaired spermatogenesis, *by intramuscular injection*, 1000-3000 units twice weekly for 4-6 weeks

Sheep, goats. Females: anoestrus, to induce superovulation, *by subcutaneous or intramuscular injection*, 1000 units, followed by 750 units after 1 day if required

Males: impaired spermatogenesis, *by intramuscular injection*, 500-750 units twice weekly for 4-6 weeks

Pigs. Females: anoestrus, *by subcutaneous or intramuscular injection*, 1000 units

Males: impaired spermatogenesis, *by intramuscular injection*, 500-750 units twice weekly for 4-6 weeks

Dogs. Females: to induce oestrus, *by subcutaneous injection*, 50-200 units daily for up to 3 weeks (usually 8-10 days)

Males: impaired spermatogenesis, *by intramuscular injection*, 400-800 units twice weekly for 4-6 weeks

PoM **Folligon**™ (Intervet)
Injection, powder for reconstitution, serum gonadotrophin 1000 units, for *horses, cattle, sheep, goats, pigs, dogs*

PoM **Fostim**™ (Paines & Byrne)
Injection, powder for reconstitution, serum gonadotrophin 6000 units, for *cattle, sheep, goats, pigs, dogs*

See also section 8.2.5

8.1.2 Gonadotrophin-releasing hormones

Endogenous gonadotrophin-releasing hormone (GnRH) is a decapeptide secreted by the hypothalamus. Gonadotrophin releasing-hormone causes release of both LH and FSH from the anterior pituitary gland. **Buserelin**, **fertirelin**, and **gonadorelin** are synthetic analogues of GnRH.

The increase in LH concentration that follows treatment with GnRH can be used to induce ovulation in horses, cattle, and rabbits in cases of anoestrus or delayed oestrus, in cattle with follicular cysts, or in mares with prolonged oestrus. Administration at the time of service or insemination may improve conception rates in mares, cows, and does. Buserelin is also used in the fish farming industry.

BUSERELIN

Indications. See notes above and under Dose

Warnings. Avoid contamination of product with traces of disinfectant or alcohol

Dose. *Horses*: *by subcutaneous, intramuscular (preferred), or intravenous injection*.

Anovulation with prolonged oestrus and a well developed follicle, 40 micrograms 6 hours before insemination, repeat after 1 day if required

Improvement of conception rate, 40 micrograms, 6 hours before insemination

Cattle: *by subcutaneous, intramuscular (preferred), or intravenous injection*.

Anoestrus, 20 micrograms, repeat after 8-22 days if required

Ovulatory delay, follicle atresia, improvement of conception rate, 10 micrograms 6-8 hours before or at time of insemination

Cystic ovaries, 20 micrograms, repeat after 10-14 days if required

Rabbits: *by subcutaneous injection*.

Induction of ovulation post partum, 800 nanograms 24 hours after parturition and followed by insemination

Improvement of conception rate, 800 nanograms at time of insemination

Rainbow trout: to facilitate stripping and to reduce mortality due to egg binding, *by intramuscular injection*, 3-4 micrograms/kg

PoM **Receptal**™ (Hoechst)
Injection, buserelin 4 micrograms/mL, for *horses, cattle, rabbits, rainbow trout*; 10 mL

Withdrawal Periods. *Cattle, rabbits*: slaughter withdrawal period nil. Should not be used in *fish* intended for human consumption

FERTIRELIN ACETATE

Indications. See notes above and under Dose

Dose. *Cattle*: cystic ovaries, *by intramuscular injection*, 100 micrograms

PoM **Ovalyse™** (Upjohn)
Injection, fertirelin acetate 50 micrograms/mL, for *cattle*; 2 mL
Withdrawal Periods. *Cattle*: slaughter 0.5 days, milk 12 hours

GONADORELIN

Indications. See notes above and under Dose
Warnings. See under Buserelin
Dose. *Cattle*: *by intramuscular injection.*
Delayed ovulation, 500 micrograms on day of insemination
Cystic ovaries, 500 micrograms, repeat after 14 days if required
Improvement of conception rate, 500 micrograms 5-6 weeks post partum
Rabbits: *by intramuscular injection*, induction of ovulation post partum, 20 micrograms 48 hours after parturition and followed by insemination

PoM **Fertagyl™** (Intervet)
Injection, gonadorelin 100 micrograms/mL, for *cattle, rabbits*; 5 mL

PoM **Fertilin™** (Mycofarm)
Injection, gonadorelin 100 micrograms/mL, for *cattle, rabbits*; 5 mL

8.1.3 Immunogens

Ovandrotone albumin is a protein-bound steroid preparation used to immunise sheep against their own androstenedione. Active immunity of this type results in a variable increase in ovulation rate and is maintained by annual re-administration.
Under the correct conditions of management, a 25 percent increase in live births can be expected. The increase occurs indiscriminately and not simply as an increase in the number of twins.

Therefore, conditions should be suitable to manage an increase in multiple births.

OVANDROTONE ALBUMIN

Indications. See notes above
Side-effects. Occasional anaphylactic or local hypersensitivity reactions
Warnings. Conditions should be suitable to cope with an increase in multiple births
Dose. *Sheep*: *by subcutaneous injection*, 1.2 mg at 8 weeks before insemination, repeat dose 4 weeks before insemination. Immunity can be maintained thereafter with a single annual dose 4 weeks before insemination.

PML **Fecundin™** (Coopers Pitman-Moore)
Injection, ovandrotone albumin 600 micrograms/mL, for *sheep*; 100 mL
Withdrawal Periods. *Sheep*: slaughter withdrawal period nil

8.2 Sex hormones

8.2.1 Oestrogens
8.2.2 Progestogens
8.2.3 Androgens
8.2.4 Anti-androgens
8.2.5 Compound hormonal preparations

8.2.1 Oestrogens

Oestrogens are responsible physiologically for initiating behavioural signs of heat, preparing the female reproductive tract for fertilisation and developing the secretory tissue of the mammary gland. They also have anabolic activity.
In veterinary practice, they are used to induce oestrus during suboestrus and anoestrus, and also to induce ovulation to aid removal of detritus following retained placenta, pyometra, or mummified fetus. The status of the reproductive tract should be ascertained before treatment. Oestrogens are used in the treatment of misalliance in the bitch. They act by inhibiting the movement of the fertilised ova down the oviducts as well as causing hypertrophy

of the uterine mucosa. Urinary incontinence in the bitch may also be controlled with oestrogens (see section 8.7.2).

In males, oestrogens are used in the treatment of excess libido, anal adenoma, and prostate hyperplasia. All oestrogenic effects are dose sensitive. The use of stilbenes, such as stilboestrol, is banned in food animals as they have been found to be carcinogenic in humans under some circumstances. Oestrogens may cause aplastic anaemia in dogs and overdosage can cause severe inhibition of pituitary function.

ETHINYLOESTRADIOL

Indications. See notes above and under Dose
Side-effects. Feminisation
Dose. *Dogs*: prostatic hyperplasia, anal adenoma, 50-100 micrograms/kg daily. If feminisation occurs, cease treatment. Recommence therapy at half original dose

PoM **Ethinyloestradiol** (Non-proprietary)
Tablets, ethinyloestradiol 10 micrograms, 20 micrograms, 50 micrograms, 1 mg

See also section 8.2.5

OESTRADIOL BENZOATE

Indications. See notes above and under Dose; urinary incontinence (8.7.2)
Contra-indications. Misalliance in cats
Warnings. Overdosage may cause severe inhibition of pituitary function; aplastic anaemia in dogs
Dose. *By subcutaneous or intramuscular injection*. *Horses*: suboestrus, 5-15 mg as a single dose
Cattle: removal of detritus, 15 mg immediately post partum
Retained placenta, 10-20 mg, repeat after 3 days if required
Metritis, pyometra, 20-25 mg weekly for 2-3 weeks
Mummified fetus, 20-25 mg, repeat with concomitant dose of oxytocin (see section 8.4) if required
Sheep, goats: anoestrus, 250 micrograms daily for 4 days
Pigs: anoestrus, 5-10 mg at least 40 days after farrowing

Dogs. *Females*: misalliance, 5-10 mg as a single dose and within 4 days of insemination
Males: anal adenoma, 5-10 mg weekly as a single dose
Prostatic hyperplasia, 5 mg weekly
Excess libido, 0.5-1.0 mg daily

PoM **Oestradiol Benzoate** (Intervet)
Injection (oily), oestradiol benzoate 5 mg/mL, for *horses, cattle, sheep, goats, pigs, dogs*; 10 mL

See also section 8.2.5

STILBOESTROL

Indications. See notes above and under Dose
Contra-indications. See notes above
Dose. *Dogs*: prostatic hyperplasia, anal adenoma, up to 1 mg daily, reducing to maintenance dose

PoM **Stilboestrol** (Non-proprietary)
Tablets, stilboestrol 1 mg, 5 mg

8.2.2 Progestogens

Progestogens are steroids that mimic the effects of progesterone and thus prepare and maintain the female reproductive tract for implantation and pregnancy. They cause development of the mammary glands to the point of lactation. Progestogens inhibit oestrus and ovulation by depressing the production of hormones from the anterior pituitary gland, and consequently, the development of ovarian follicles. In male animals, progestogens cause reduced testosterone production.

In mares, cows, ewes, and sows, progestogens are used to synchronise oestrus in groups of animals. Administration of a progestogen for 10 to 14 days will suppress heat. On removal of the progestogen source, oestrus is initiated. This facilitates the use of artificial insemination and stud males. This treatment may also be used in individual animals. **Altrenogest** is administered in the feed to mares and sows. **Fluorogestone** and **medroxyprogesterone** are administered as intravaginal sponges in ewes. Daily injections of **progesterone** are administered to cattle. Animals are usually mated at synchronised oestrus, although ewes may be mated at the second oestrus after removal of a progestogen-impregnated sponge.

Altrenogest may reduce habitual abortion, thought to be due to progesterone deficiency, in mares.

In dogs and cats, **medroxyprogesterone**, **megestrol**, **progesterone** and **proligestone** are used to postpone or suppress oestrus. They are used for the treatment of pseudopregnancy, oestrogen-dependent mammary tumours in bitches, and prostatic hyperplasia in dogs. Progesterone is also used for habitual abortion in bitches. In cats, eosinophilic granuloma and miliary dermatitis are responsive to progestogens. These drugs may be given for behavioural problems in dogs and cats.

Progestogens should be used with caution. All synthetic progestogens differ in their pharmacological profile and their capacity to produce side-effects in different animal species. For example, although some progestogens may be used to inhibit or retard the growth of certain oestrogen-dependent mammary tumours and treat pseudopregnancy in bitches, it is known that other progestogens can cause or aggravate these conditions.

Progestogens stimulate the proliferative and secretory activity of the uterine endometrium leading to cystic endometrial hyperplasia, mucometra, or pyometra. Therefore, progestogens should not be administered to animals with a history of vaginal discharge or reproductive abnormalities, sexually immature animals, or dogs and cats intended for breeding. When used for suppression of oestrus in dogs and cats, animals should be allowed to have a normal cycle every 18 to 24 months.

Progestogens antagonise the hypoglycaemic effects of antidiabetic drugs and therefore should not be given to diabetic animals. They may induce acromegaly in entire bitches. Subcutaneous injection of progestogens may cause hair discoloration and localised alopecia.

ALTRENOGEST

Indications. See notes above and under Dose

Contra-indications. Male animals, see notes above

Side-effects. See notes above

Warnings. Partly consumed feed should be safely destroyed and not given to any other animal. Care must be taken to avoid contact between the product and women of child bearing age.

Dose. *Horses*: anoestrus, suppression of oestrus in prolonged oestrus, 44 micrograms/kg daily for 10 days
Suppression of oestrus in cycling mares, 44 micrograms/kg daily for 15 days
Pigs: oestrus synchronisation, 20 mg daily for 18 days

PoM **Regumate™ Equine** (Hoechst)
Oral solution, for addition to feed, altrenogest 2.2 mg/mL, for *horses*; 250 mL
Withdrawal Periods. Should not be used in *horses* intended for human consumption

PoM **Regumate™ Porcine** (Hoechst)
Oral suspension, for addition to feed, altrenogest 20 mg/dose, for *pigs*; 360-mL metered-dose applicator (1 dose = 5 mL)
Withdrawal Periods. *Pigs*: slaughter 15 days

FLUOROGESTONE ACETATE

Indications. See notes above and under Dose

Contra-indications. Side-effects. See notes above; use of alcohols, cresols, phenols, or sheep-dip disinfectants to cleanse applicator

Dose. *Sheep*: *by intravaginal administration*, one 30-mg sponge. Remove after 12-14 days

PoM **Chronogest™** (Intervet)
Vaginal sponge, fluorogestone acetate 30 mg, for *sheep*; 25, 50, 100
Withdrawal Periods. *Sheep*: slaughter 14 days after removal of sponge

MEDROXYPROGESTERONE ACETATE

Indications. See notes above and under Dose

Contra-indications. Side-effects. See notes above

Dose. Sheep: *by intravaginal administration*, one 60-mg sponge. Remove after 13 days

Dogs. Females: prevention of oestrus, *by subcutaneous injection*, (up to 15 kg body-weight) 50 mg; (more than 15 kg body-weight) 3 mg/kg, given 6-8 weeks before oestrus. Repeat after 5-6 months

Postponement of oestrus, *by mouth*, (less than 25 kg body-weight) 5 mg daily as necessary; (more than 25 kg body-weight) 10 mg daily as necessary, given in anoestrus and 5 days before postponement is required

Suppression of oestrus, *by mouth*, (less than 25 kg body-weight) 10 mg daily for 4 days then 5 mg daily for 12 days; (more than 25 kg body-weight) 20 mg daily for 4 days then 10 mg daily for 12 days, given at pro-oestrus

Behavioural problems, *by subcutaneous injection*, 10 mg/kg every 4-6 months as necessary

Males: prostatic hypertrophy, *by subcutaneous injection*, 50-100 mg every 3-4 months

Behavioural problems, *by subcutaneous injection*, 10 mg/kg every 4-6 months as necessary

Cats. Females: postponement and suppression of oestrus, *by mouth*, 2.5 mg daily, given in pro-oestrus

Behavioural problems, *by subcutaneous injection*, 10 mg/kg every 3-6 months

Males: behavioural problems, *by subcutaneous injection*, 10 mg/kg every 3-6 months

PoM **Perlutex**™ (Leo)
Tablets, scored, medroxyprogesterone acetate 5 mg, for *dogs, cats*; 20
Injection, medroxyprogesterone acetate 5 mg/mL, for *dogs, cats*; 10 mL

PoM **Promone**™**-E** (Upjohn)
Injection, medroxyprogesterone acetate 50 mg/mL, for *dogs*; 5 mL

PoM **Veramix**™ **Sheep Sponge** (Upjohn)
Vaginal sponge, medroxyprogesterone acetate 60 mg, for *sheep*; 20, 100

MEGESTROL ACETATE

Indications. See notes above and under Dose

Contra-indications. Side-effects. See notes above

Dose. Dogs. Females: prevention of oestrus, 2 mg/kg daily for 8 days *or* 2 mg/kg daily for 4 days then 500 micrograms/kg daily for 16 days, given at pro-oestrus

Postponement of oestrus, 500 micrograms/kg daily for up to 40 days given in anoestrus and 7-14 days before postponement is required *or* 500 micrograms daily for 40 days then 100-200 micrograms/kg twice weekly for up to 4 months

Pseudopregnancy, 2 mg/kg daily for 5-8 days given at onset of clinical signs

Oestrogen-dependent mammary tumour, 2 mg/kg daily for 10 days *or* 2 mg/kg daily for 5 days then 0.5-1.0 mg/kg daily for 10 days

Males: behavioural problems, 2 mg/kg daily for 7 days then 4 mg/kg for 7 days if no improvement, followed by 1 mg/kg daily for 14 days if some improvement *or* 2 mg/kg daily for 7 days then 1 mg/kg daily for 14 days if some improvement

Cats. Miliary dermatitis, eosinophilic granuloma, 2.5-5.0 mg every 2-3 days until lesions regress then 2.5 mg every 7-14 days as necessary

Females: prevention of oestrus, 5 mg daily for 3 days given in pro-oestrus

Postponement of oestrus, 2.5 mg daily for up to 8 weeks and given in dioestrus *or* 2.5 mg once weekly for up to 18 months and given in anoestrus

PoM **Ovarid**™ (Coopers Pitman-Moore)
Tablets, scored, megestrol acetate 5 mg, 20 mg, for *dogs, cats*; 200

PROGESTERONE

Indications. See notes above and under Dose

Contra-indications. Side-effects. See notes above

Dose. *By subcutaneous or intramuscular*

injection. **Cattle**: postponement of oestrus, 100 mg daily beginning before day 15 of the oestrus cycle
Dogs: habitual abortion, 2-3 mg/kg daily
Cats: postponement of oestrus, 2.5-5.0 mg every 3 days and given in anoestrus

PoM**Progesterone Injection** (Intervet)
Progesterone 25 mg/mL, for *cattle, dogs, cats*; 50 mL

See also section 8.2.5

PROLIGESTONE

Indications. See notes above and under Dose
Contra-indications. See notes above
Side-effects. Occasional anaphylactic reactions; see notes above
Dose. *By subcutaneous injection. Dogs*: postponement of oestrus, 33 mg/kg, repeat after 3, 4, and 5 months
Suppression of oestrus, pseudopregnancy, 33 mg/kg as a single dose
Cats: postponement and suppression of oestrus, 100 mg
Miliary dermatitis, 100 mg, repeat every 4 months

PoM**Covinan**™ (Intervet)
Injection, proligestone 100 mg/mL, for *dogs, cats*; 20 mL

PoM**Delvosteron**™ (Mycofarm)
Injection, proligestone 100 mg/mL, for *dogs, cats*; 20 mL

8.2.3 Androgens

Testosterone esters promote and maintain primary and secondary anatomical, physical, and psychological male sexual characteristics. In the female, their anti-oestrogenic properties are useful.
Androgens are used in the treatment of hypogonadism and deficient libido in males. They are administered for the treatment of hormonal alopecia in dogs and cats and mammary tumours and pseudopregnancy with lactation in bitches.
Care should be taken to avoid inducing excess virilism. Androgen therapy should not be given to animals suffering from conditions known to be aggravated by testosterone such as prostatic hypertrophy in dogs.
The duration of action of testosterone esters varies. The effects of **methyltestosterone** last for 1 to 3 days, while oily injections of **testosterone phenylpropionate** are effective for 14 days.

METHYLTESTOSTERONE

Indications. See notes above and under Dose
Contra-indications. Dogs with prostatic hypertrophy
Side-effects. Virilisation with overdosage
Warnings. Reduce dose in male castrated cats
Dose. *Dogs. Females*: pseudopregnancy, 5-30 mg daily in divided doses for 5-7 days
Males: hormonal alopecia, feminisation, 5-30 mg daily, reducing to 2-3 times weekly
Cats. Males, castrated: hormonal alopecia, feline urolithiasis syndrome, up to 5 mg daily, reducing to 2-3 times weekly

PoM**Orandrone**™ (Intervet)
Tablets, methyltestosterone 5 mg, for *dogs, cats*; 500

See also section 8.2.5

TESTOSTERONE ESTERS

Indications. See notes above and under Dose
Contra-indications. **Side-effects**. See under Methyltestosterone
Dose. See preparation details

PoM**Androject**™ (Intervet)
Injection (oily), testosterone phenyl propionate 10 mg/mL, for *horses, cattle sheep, goats, pigs, dogs, cats*; 10 mL
Dose. *By subcutaneous or intramuscular injection.*
Horses, cattle: deficient libido, 25-50 mg every 7-10 days
Hypogonadism, 20 mg every 7 days
Sheep, goats, pigs: deficient libido, 10 mg every 10-14 days
Hypogonadism, 10-20 mg every 10-14 days
Dogs. Females: pseudopregnancy, 5-10 mg every 7 days

Mammary neoplasia, 10 mg every 7 days
Oestrus suppression, 10 mg every 10-14 days
Males: cryptorchidism (before castration), deficient libido, feminisation, hormonal alopecia, hypogonadism, 5-10 mg every 7-14 days
Cats. Females: suppression of oestrus, 10 mg every 10-14 days
Males, castrated: hormonal alopecia, 5 mg every 14 days

PoM **Durateston**™ (Intervet)
Injection (oily), testosterone decanoate 20 mg, testosterone isocaproate 12 mg, testosterone phenylpropionate 12 mg, testosterone propionate 6 mg/mL, for *horses, cattle, sheep, pigs, dogs, cats*; 10 mL
Dose. *By intramuscular injection.*
Horses, cattle: 5-10 mL every 4 weeks
Sheep: 2-4 mL every 4 weeks
Pigs: 5 mL every 4 weeks
Dogs: 0.5-3.0 mL every 4 weeks
Cats: 0.25-0.5 mL every 4 weeks

8.2.4 Anti-androgens

Anti-androgens compete with androgens for receptor sites. They are used to treat conditions aggravated by excessive androgenic activity in male dogs and cats.
Delmadinone is used in the treatment of prostatic hypertrophy, prostatic carcinoma, and perianal tumours. It improves behaviour in some forms of aggression, nervousness, and hypersexuality.

DELMADINONE ACETATE

Indications. See notes above
Warnings. Avoid use in animals intended for breeding
Dose. *Dogs, cats*: *by subcutaneous or intramuscular injection*, 1-2 mg/kg depending on the severity of the condition, repeat dose after 8 days if no improvement. Repeat dose every 3-4 weeks in animals showing improvement

PoM **Tardak**™ (SmithKline Beecham)
Injection, delmadinone acetate 10 mg/mL, for *dogs, cats*; 10 mL

8.2.5 Compound hormonal preparations

A combination of hormones is used to induce preseasonal ovulation or synchronise oestrus in a group of animals. These preparations are also used in the treatment of ovarian cysts. These preparations are unlikely to produce satisfactory results in animals in deep anoestrus, immature animals, animals with genital-tract abnormalities, or when breeding problems have resulted from severe nutritional deficiency or other stresses.

PoM **Crestar**™ (Intervet)
Injection, oestradiol valerate 2.5 mg, norgestomet 1.5 mg/mL, for *cattle*; 2 mL
Implant, norgestomet 3 mg, for *cattle*
Withdrawal Periods. *Cattle:* slaughter 4 days after removal of implant
Note. Not for use in *cattle* producing milk for human consumption
Dose. *Cattle*: oestrus synchronisation, *by subcutaneous implantation*, 1 implant, then *by intramuscular injection*, 2 mL. Remove implant after at least 9 days, followed by insemination

PoM **Nymfalon**™ (Intervet)
Injection, powder for reconstitution, chorionic gonadotrophin 3000 units, progesterone 125 mg, for *horses, cattle*
Dose. *Horses*: oestrus synchronisation, *by slow intravenous injection*, 1 vial of reconstituted solution. Repeat after 10-14 days if required
Cattle: oestrus regulation, *by slow intravenous injection*, 1 vial of reconstituted solution. Repeat after 7 days if required

PoM **PG 600**™ (Intervet)
Injection, powder for reconstitution, chorionic gonadotrophin 200 units, serum gonadotrophin 400 units, for *pigs*; 5 mL when reconstituted
Dose. *Pigs*: oestrus induction, *by subcutaneous injection*, 5 mL of reconstituted solution

PoM **Prid**™ (Sanofi)
Intravaginal device, progesterone 1.55 g, oestradiol benzoate 10 mg, for *cattle*; 6
Withdrawal Periods. *Cattle*: milk withdrawal period nil

Contra-indications. Pregnant animals; see notes above
Note. Intravaginal device should be removed before slaughter
Dose. *Cattle*: cystic ovaries, oestrus induction, *by intravaginal administration*, one device. Remove after 12 days, followed by insemination

PoM **Sesoral**™ (Intervet)
Tablets, scored, ethinyloestradiol 5 micrograms, methyltestosterone 4 mg, for *dogs*; 500
Dose. *Dogs*: pseudopregnancy, initial dose, up to 8 tablets then 6-8 tablets daily in divided doses for 5 days

8.3 Prostaglandins

Alfaprostol, cloprostenol, dinoprost, fenprostalene, luprostiol, and **tiaprost** are synthetic prostaglandins available for veterinary use.

Prostaglandins cause functional and morphological regression of the corpus luteum, associated with either the oestrus cycle or pregnancy.

In veterinary practice, they may be used to terminate pregnancy. Prostaglandins are effective in causing abortion from early pregnancy until around day 150 of gestation in cattle. They are used to advance parturition if used within one week of full term in cattle or 3 days in pigs. A knowledge of the distribution of gestation lengths in individual pig herds is necessary in order to exploit this property to maximum advantage.

Prostaglandins cause luteolysis of a persistent corpus luteum associated with retained mummified fetus, pyometra, and luteinised cystic ovaries in cattle or pseudopregnancy in horses.

Prostaglandins are also used to induce ovulation and synchronise oestrus in groups of animals. In cycling mares and cows there is a refractory period of 3 to 5 days after ovulation when the corpus luteum is not fully formed and is not sensitive to the luteolytic effects of prostaglandins. In horses, administration of a prostaglandin after day 5 of the oestrus cycle will cause oestrus within 2 to 4 days and ovulation 6 to 8 days after injection. In cows, injection

between days 5 and 17 of the oestrus cycle will cause oestrus and ovulation in 2 to 4 days. Although luteolysis may occur consistently, oestrus and ovulation will only follow if the ovary is capable of responding to normal gonadotrophin stimulation.

Side-effects such as transient sweating and mild colic with or without diarrhoea frequently follow the use of prostaglandins in mares. Some prostaglandins are potent thromboxane agonists and may produce severe reactions at the site of intramuscular injections.

Prostaglandins can be absorbed through the skin and care should be taken when handling these compounds, especially by asthma sufferers and women of childbearing age. All accidental spillage on skin should be washed off immediately. Prostaglandins should not be dispensed for use by lay persons except under very carefully controlled circumstances (BVA. Code of practice for using prostaglandins in cattle and pigs. *The Veterinary Record* 1987; **120**: 511-12). Prostaglandins should always be administered to cattle by a veterinarian. Prostaglandins may be dispensed to a pig farmer and administered to pigs by a lay person only to synchronise farrowings and under the strict guidelines outlined in the BVA code.

ALFAPROSTOL

Indications. See notes above
Contra-indications. Concurrent treatment with non-steroidal anti-inflammatory drugs; pregnant animals unless termination required
Side-effects. See notes above
Warnings. Operators should wear protective clothing and wash hands after use. Prostaglandins should be handled with care by women of child-bearing age and by asthmatics
Dose. *Horses*: *by intramuscular injection* 3 mg
Cattle: *by intramuscular injection* 15 micrograms/kg (maximum dose 8 mg)
Pigs: *by intramuscular injection*, 2 mg

PoM **Alphacept**™ (SmithKline Beecham)
Injection, alfaprostol 2 mg/mL, for *horses, cattle, pigs*; 40 mL
Withdrawal Periods. *Cattle*: slaughter 1 day, milk withdrawal period nil. *Pigs*: slaughter 1 day

CLOPROSTENOL

Indications. See notes above
Contra-indications. **Side-effects**. See under Alfaprostol and notes above
Warnings. Operators should wear protective clothing and wash hands after use. Prostaglandins should be handled with care by women of child-bearing age and by asthmatics
Dose. *By intramuscular injection. Horses*: 125-500 micrograms
Donkeys: 125-250 micrograms
Cattle: 500 micrograms
Pigs: 175 micrograms

PML **Estrumate**™ (Coopers Pitman-Moore)
Injection, cloprostenol (as sodium salt) 250 micrograms/mL, for *horses, donkeys, cattle*; 10 mL, 20 mL
Withdrawal Periods. Should not be used in *horses* intended for human consumption. *Cattle*: slaughter 1 day, milk withdrawal period nil

PoM **Planate**™ (Coopers Pitman-Moore)
Injection, cloprostenol (as sodium salt) 87.5 micrograms/mL, for *pigs*; 10 mL, 20 mL
Withdrawal Periods. *Pigs*: slaughter 1 day

DINOPROST

Indications. See notes above
Contra-indications. See under Alfaprostol
Side-effects. Transient sweating and decreased rectal temperature in horses; transient abdominal pain in pigs; overdosage may cause increased rectal temperature in cattle
Warnings. Operators should wear protective clothing and wash hands after use. Prostaglandins should be handled with care by women of child-bearing age and by asthmatics
Dose. *By intramuscular injection. Horses*: 5 mg

Cattle: 25-35 mg
Pigs: 10 mg

PoM **Lutalyse**™ (Upjohn)
Injection, dinoprost (as tromethamine salt) 5 mg/mL, for *horses, cattle, pigs*; 10 mL, 30 mL
Withdrawal Periods. *Cattle*: slaughter 1 day, milk withdrawal period nil. *Pigs*: slaughter 1 day

FENPROSTALENE

Indications. See notes above
Contra-indications. See under Alfaprostol
Side-effects. Overdosage may cause increased rectal temperature in cattle
Warnings. Operators should wear protective clothing and wash hands after use. Prostaglandins should be handled with care by women of child-bearing age and by asthmatics
Dose. *Cattle*: by subcutaneous injection, 1 mg, repeat dose if required
Pigs: by subcutaneous injection, 500 micrograms

PoM **Synchrocept**™ **B** (Syntex)
Injection, fenprostalene 500 micrograms/mL, for *cattle, pigs*; 20 mL
Withdrawal Periods. *Cattle*: slaughter 1 day, milk withdrawal period nil. *Pigs*: slaughter 2 days

LUPROSTIOL

Indications. See notes above
Contra-indications. See under Alfaprostol
Side-effects. Transient sweating and diarrhoea in horses; abdominal discomfort in cattle
Warnings. Operators should wear protective clothing and wash hands after use. Prostaglandins should be handled with care by women of child-bearing age and by asthmatics
Dose. *By intramuscular injection. Horses*: 7.5 mg, repeat dose if required
Cattle: 7.5-15.0 mg, repeat dose if required
Pigs: 7.5 mg

PoM **Prosolvin**™ (Intervet)
Injection, luprostiol 7.5 mg/mL, for *horses, cattle, pigs*; 10 mL, 20 mL

Withdrawal Periods. *Cattle, pigs*: slaughter 1 day

PoM **Prostamate**™ (Mycofarm)
Injection, luprostiol 7.5 mg/mL, for *horses, cattle, pigs*; 10 mL, 20 mL
Withdrawal Periods. *Cattle, pigs*: slaughter 1 day

TIAPROST

Indications. See notes above
Contra-indications. **Side-effects**. See under Alfaprostol and notes above
Warnings. Operators should wear protective clothing and wash hands after use. Prostaglandins should be handled with care by women of child-bearing age and by asthmatics
Dose. *Pigs: by intramuscular injection*, 300-600 micrograms

PoM **Iliren**™ (Hoechst)
Injection, tiaprost (as trometamol salt) 150 micrograms/mL, for *pigs*; 10 mL
Withdrawal Periods. *Pigs*: slaughter 1 day

8.4 Myometrial stimulants

This group includes extracts of mammalian **posterior pituitary gland** and preparations of **oxytocin**. They stimulate contraction of the oestrogen-sensitised uterine myometrium and mammary myoepithelial cells. This activity may be of benefit in dystocia due to primary uterine inertia. Myometrial stimulants should not be used when dystocia is due to malpresentation or obstruction.
Myometrial stimulants are also used in the control of postpartum haemorrhage in all species and to remove retained placenta in mares, sows, bitches, and queens. Oxytocics are also used to reduce the size of a uterine prolapse before replacement in cattle and occasionally mares. In mares, oxytocin may be administered by intravenous infusion in sodium chloride 0.9% intravenous infusion or sodium chloride 0.18% and glucose 4% intravenous infusion. In other species single injections suffice.

Myometrial stimulants may lead to milk 'let down' in all species.

OXYTOCIN

Indications. See notes above and under Dose
Contra-indications. Dystocia due to obstruction
Side-effects. Occasionally swelling and sloughing at the site of injection
Dose. *Horses, cattle*: uterine inertia, *by subcutaneous or intramuscular injection*, 10-40 units; *by slow intravenous injection*, 2.5-10.0 units of diluted solution
Agalactia, *by subcutaneous or intramuscular injection*, 20-80 units; *by slow intravenous injection*, 5-20 units of diluted solution
Sheep, goats, pigs, dogs: uterine inertia, *by subcutaneous or intramuscular injection*, 2-10 units; *by slow intravenous injection*, 0.5-2.5 units of diluted solution
Agalactia, *by subcutaneous or intramuscular injection*, 4-20 units; *by slow intravenous injection*, 1-5 units of diluted solution
Cats: uterine inertia, *by subcutaneous or intramuscular injection*, 2-5 units; *by slow intravenous injection*, 0.5-1.25 units of diluted solution
Agalactia, *by subcutaneous or intramuscular injection*, 4-10 units; *by slow intravenous injection*, 1.0-2.5 units of diluted solution

PoM **Oxytocin** (Leo)
Injection, oxytocin 10 units/mL, for *horses, cattle, sheep, pigs*; 20 mL

PoM **Oxytocin-S** (Intervet)
Injection, oxytocin 10 units/mL, for *horses, cattle, sheep, goats, pigs, dogs, cats*; 25 mL
For intravenous injection dilute 1 volume with 9 volumes water for injections

PITUITARY (POSTERIOR LOBE) INJECTION

Indications. Uterine inertia; agalactia; see notes above
Contra-indications. **Side-effects**. See under Oxytocin
Dose. Expressed as units of oxytocic activity

Horses, cattle: *by subcutaneous or intramuscular injection*, 30-100 units; *by slow intravenous injection*, 10-50 units
Sheep, goats: *by subcutaneous or intramuscular injection*, 20-50 units; *by slow intravenous injection*, 6-25 units
Pigs: *by subcutaneous or intramuscular injection*, 10-30 units; *by slow intravenous injection*, 3-15 units
Dogs: *by subcutaneous or intramuscular injection*, 2.5-20.0 units; *by slow intravenous injection*, 1-10 units
Cats: *by subcutaneous or intramuscular injection*, 2.5-5.0 units; *by slow intravenous injection*, 1.0-2.5 units

PoM **Hyposton**™ (Paines & Byrne)
Injection, oxytocic activity 10 units/mL, for *horses, cattle, sheep, goats, pigs, dogs, cats*; 50 mL

PoM **Pituitary Extract Injection** (Animalcare)
Oxytocic activity 10 units/mL, for *horses, cattle, sheep, pigs, dogs, cats*; 50 mL
Note. For subcutaneous and intramuscular injection only

PoM **Pituitary (Posterior Lobe) Injection** (Univet)
Oxytocic activity 10 units/mL, for *horses, cattle, sheep, goats, pigs, dogs, cats*; 50 mL

8.5 Myometrial relaxants

These preparations cause relaxation of the uterus and are used to aid obstetrical manoeuvres during dystocias and to facilitate handling of the uterus during caesarean section. They help to minimise uterine trauma during embryo transfer and to facilitate replacement of a prolapsed uterus.
Clenbuterol is a beta-adrenoceptor stimulant and therefore is antagonistic to the effects of oxytocin and prostaglandins. **Dimophebumine** is not as effective as clenbuterol but can be used for ringwomb in sheep. **Proquamezine** is a smooth muscle relaxant. It has similar indications to clenbuterol but may also be used for the treatment of oesophageal obstruction, relief of urolithiasis in cattle and dogs, and relief of flatulent colic in horses.

CLENBUTEROL HYDROCHLORIDE

Indications. Facilitate obstetrical manoeuvres
Contra-indications. Concurrent administration of atropine, corticosteroids, sympathomimetics, vasodilators, or general anaesthetics
Side-effects. Transient vasodilatation and tachycardia with sweating and muscle tremors with high dosage
Dose. *Cattle*: *by intramuscular or slow intravenous injection*, initial dose 300 micrograms then 200-300 micrograms given after 4 hours if required

PoM **Planipart**™ (Boehringer Ingelheim)
Injection, clenbuterol hydrochloride 30 micrograms/mL, for *cattle*; 10 mL
Withdrawal Periods. *Cattle*: slaughter 3 days, milk 72 hours

DIMOPHEBUMINE HYDROCHLORIDE

Indications. Facilitate obstetrical manoeuvres
Contra-indications. Should not be used in cats
Dose. *By intramuscular injection.*
Horses, cattle: 1.0-1.5 g
Sheep: 150-250 mg
Pigs: 200-400 mg
Dogs: 25-100 mg

PoM **Monzaldon**™ (Boehringer Ingelheim)
Injection, dimophebumine hydrochloride 100 mg/mL, for *horses, cattle, sheep, pigs, dogs*; 50 mL

PROQUAMEZINE FUMARATE

Indications. See under Dose
Contra-indications. Concurrent administration of other phenothiazines; repeated treatment on the same day
Side-effects. Mild sedation
Dose. *Horses*: flatulent or impaction colic, *by slow intravenous injection*, 300-900 mg

Cattle: mummified fetus, retained placenta, *by intramuscular or slow intravenous injection*, 240-750 mg
Obstetrical manoeuvres, prolapsed uterus, oesophageal obstruction, urolithiasis, *by slow intravenous injection*, 240-750 mg; *calves*: *by slow intravenous injection*, 30-240 mg
Sheep: mummified fetus, retained placenta, *by intramuscular or slow intravenous injection*, 150-240 mg
Obstetrical manoeuvres, prolapsed uterus, *by slow intravenous injection*, 150-240 mg
Dogs: obstetrical manoeuvres, urolithiasis, *by slow intravenous injection*, 3 mg/kg
Cats: urolithiasis, *by slow intravenous injection*, 3 mg/kg

PoM **Myspasmol™** (RMB)
Injection, proquamezine fumarate 30 mg/mL, for *horses, cattle, sheep, dogs, cats*; 50 mL

8.6 Drugs for uterine infections

Endometritis and metritis may be treated with intra-uterine antimicrobials in the form of pessaries, pastes, or instillations. The quantity of antibacterial in the formulation is rarely sufficient to have much effect on acute or extensive infections, which should be treated with parenteral antibacterials (see section 1.1). There is evidence to show that intra-uterine antibacterials can, particularly in cattle, interfere with the animal's own response to infection.
Prostaglandins (see section 8.3) may be given concurrently with antimicrobials to cause regression of persistent luteal cysts. Oestrogens (see section 8.2.1) may also aid in the expulsion of detritus by sensitising the uterus to endogenous oxytocin.

PoM **Aureomycin™ Soluble Oblets** (Cyanamid)
Tablets, used as pessaries, chlortetracycline hydrochloride 500 mg, for *horses, cattle, sheep, pigs*; 48
Dose. *Horses, cattle*: *by intra-uterine administration*, 1-2 pessaries

Sheep, pigs: *by intra-uterine administration*, ½-1 pessary
Note. May also be used for oral administration (see section 1.1.2)

PoM **Duphatrim™** (Duphar)
Tablets, used as pessaries, co-trimazine 200/1000 [trimethoprim 200 mg, sulphadiazine 1 g], for *horses, cattle, sheep, pigs*; 10
Withdrawal Periods. *Cattle, sheep*: slaughter 5 days, milk 48 hours. *Pigs*: slaughter 5 days
Dose. *Horses, cattle*: *by intra-uterine administration*, 2-4 pessaries, repeat if required
Sheep, pigs: *by intra-uterine administration*, 1-2 pessaries, repeat if required
Note. May also be used for oral administration (see section 1.1.6.2)

GSL **Pevidine™ Antiseptic Solution** (BK)
Solution, available iodine (as povidone-iodine) 1%; 500 mL, 5 litres. May be diluted before use
Dilute 1 volume with 5 volumes water for uterine instillation
Note. May also be used undiluted for wound cleansing
Dose. *By intra-uterine instillation*.
Low-grade endometritis, 20 mL of diluted solution 1-2 days after insemination
Postpartum endometritis, 100 mL of diluted solution 1-3 weeks post partum then 50 mL 3 weeks later

Compound preparations for uterine infections

PoM **Metrijet™** (Intervet)
Suspension, clioquinol 500 mg, ethinyloestradiol 500 micrograms, furazolidone 500 mg, oxytetracycline hydrochloride 500 mg, for *cattle*; 19-g intra-uterine applicator
Withdrawal Periods. *Cattle*: slaughter 2 days, milk 48 hours
Dose: *by intra-uterine administration*, the contents of 1 applicator, repeat after 4-7 days if required

PoM **Utocyl™** (Ciba-Geigy)
Pessaries, benzylpenicillin 100 mg, ethinyloestradiol 500 micrograms, formo-

sulphathiazole 1.75 g, streptomycin (as sulphate) 50 mg, for *cattle*; 20
Withdrawal Periods. *Cattle*: slaughter 2 days, milk 48 hours
Dose. *Cattle*: *by intra-uterine administration*, 6 pessaries for prophylaxis only

8.7 Drugs used for disorders of the urinary tract

8.7.1 Drugs for cystitis
8.7.2 Drugs for urinary retention and incontinence
8.7.3 Drugs for urolithiasis

8.7.1 Drugs for cystitis

Cystitis is commonly caused by organisms that include *Escherichia coli* and other coliforms, *Proteus*, *Pseudomonas aeruginosa*, staphylococci, and streptococci. Chronic cystitis may be complicated by urinary calculi or neoplasia. Treatment for acute cystitis usually requires a 7 to 10 day course of a systemic antibacterial (see section 1.1) that is excreted unchanged by the kidneys. Chronic cystitis may require therapy for up to 3 weeks. Effective drugs include amoxicillin, cephalexin, co-amoxiclav, co-trimazine, nitrofurantoin, and penicillin.
The urinary pH may affect the efficacy of antibacterials. Erythromycin, streptomycin, and co-trimazine are more effective at pH 8, whereas penicillin, tetracycline, and nitrofurantoin are more active at pH 5.5. The antimicrobial action of hexamine is due to formaldehyde, which is liberated during acid hydrolysis.
Ethylenediamine hydrochloride acidifies the urine, which is useful in the treatment of cystitis. In cases of infection appropriate antimicrobials should be given. Urine alkalisation may be attempted with **sodium bicarbonate**.

GSL **Chelidon™ Compound** (Animalcare)
Tablets, extract of chelidonium 65 mg, extract of buchu 32.5 mg, sodium tauroglycocholate 11 mg, hexamine 22 mg, for *dogs, cats*; 500, 1000

Dose. *Dogs*: (10 kg body-weight) 1 tablet 3 times daily
Cats: 1 tablet twice daily

P **Chelidon™** (Duphar)
Tablets, berberis 30 mg, extract of chelidonium 45 mg, extract of kava 30 mg, hexamine 20 mg, sodium tauroglycocholate 10 mg, for *dogs, cats*; 500
Dose. *Dogs*: 1-2 tablets 3 times daily
Cats: 1 tablet twice daily

P **Chelix™** (Arnolds)
Elixir, extract of chelidonium 0.15 mL, extract of kava 0.025 mL, glycerol 0.2 mL/mL, for *dogs, cats*; 2 litres
Dose. *Horses*♦: 60 mL twice daily
Cattle♦: 90 mL twice daily
Dogs, cats: 5-15 mL

PoM **Chlorethamine™** (Intervet)
Tablets, ethylenediamine dihydrochloride 90 mg, for *dogs, cats*; 500
Dose. *Dogs, cats*: 1 tablet 3 times daily. Adjust dose according to urinary pH

Sodium Bicarbonate Powder available from wholesalers
Dose. *Dogs, cats:* 325 mg 3 times daily

> In The Veterinary formulary, the ♦ symbol denotes an unlicensed indication for a preparation that is licensed for use in animals in the UK

8.7.2 Drugs for urinary retention and incontinence

Urinary retention and incontinence may affect animals of all ages. Non-neurogenic causes include inherited lesions or acquired conditions such as cystitis, neoplasia, or urinary calculi. Neurological deficits may follow spinal trauma.
Bladder wall irritability leading to frequent micturition may be caused by cystitis and antibacterial therapy should be instigated (see section 8.7.1). **Propantheline** is an antimuscarinic drug, which increases bladder capacity by diminishing unstable muscle contractions.
Incontinence may be caused by flaccidity of the urethral sphincter. This condition commonly affects ovariohysterectomised bitches and may be responsive to

oestrogen therapy (see section 8.2.1). Drugs used for treatment include **stilboestrol** at doses of 0.1 to 1.0 mg daily for 3 to 5 days, followed by weekly treatment.

Excessive urinary retention that may lead to incontinence is caused by detrusor muscle paralysis or excessive urethral sphincter contraction. Paralysis of the bladder wall may occur following spinal trauma or overdistention of the bladder due to obstruction. **Bethanechol** has cholinergic activity causing an increase in the tone and contractions of the detrusor muscle.

Phenoxybenzamine acts by blocking alpha-adrenergic receptors of the bladder neck and proximal urethra allowing relaxation of the urethral sphincter. **Acepromazine** (see section 6.1) or **diazepam** (see section 6.9.2) may also help by causing relaxation and reduction of urethral resistance.

BETHANECHOL CHLORIDE

Indications. Urinary retention
Contra-indications. Urinary obstruction
Side-effects.   Salivation,   vomiting, diarrhoea
Dose. *Dogs*: 5-25 mg 3 times daily

PoM **Myotonine**™ (Glenwood)
Tablets, scored, bethanechol chloride 10 mg, 25 mg; 100

PHENOXYBENZAMINE HYDROCHLORIDE

Indications. Urinary retention
Contra-indications. Urinary obstruction
Side-effects. Hypotension
Dose. *Dogs*: 0.25-0.5 mg/kg 3 times daily

PoM **Dibenyline**™ (SK&F)
Capsules, phenoxybenzamine hydrochloride 10 mg; 30

PROPANTHELINE BROMIDE

Indications. Urinary incontinence
Contra-indications. Urinary obstruction

Side-effects. Dry mouth, constipation
Dose. *Dogs*: 7.5-15.0 mg 3 times daily

PoM **Pro-Banthine**™ (Gold Cross)
Tablets, propantheline bromide 15 mg; 100, 1000

8.7.3 Drugs for urolithiasis

The management and treatment of urolithiasis will depend on the type of calculus present and may include surgery, dietary control, antibacterial therapy, urinary acidifiers and alkalinisers as well as specific drug therapy. Struvite calculi may form when urease-positive staphylococci or *Proteus* bacteria and high concentrations of magnesium or phosphate salts are present in the bladder. Medical therapy includes appropriate antibacterials to eliminate bacteria, dietary control to reduce protein intake and induce polyuria, and urinary acidifiers (see section 8.7.1). **Walpole's solution** may be used to irrigate the bladder in cats with feline urological syndrome (FUS).

Urate uroliths are more soluble in alkaline urine. Dietary control to reduce protein intake and urine alkalinisers (see section 8.7.1) are used as preventive treatment. **Allopurinol** reduces the formation of uric acid from purines by inhibiting xanthine oxidase.

Penicillamine reacts with cystine to form a more soluble sulphide compound that is more readily excreted. It is used as an adjunct to dietary management and urinary alkalinisation in the management of cystinuria.

ALLOPURINOL

Indications. Urate calculi
Side-effects. Erythema, hypersensitivity
Warnings. Reduce dosage for patients with renal impairment
Dose. *Dogs*: 10 mg/kg 3 times daily for 4 weeks then 10 mg/kg twice daily

PoM **Allopurinol** (Non-proprietary)
Tablets, allopurinol 100 mg, 300 mg

PENICILLAMINE

Indications. Cystine calculi; copper and lead poisoning (see Emergency treatment of poisoning)
Side-effects. Anorexia, vomiting; pyrexia; nephrotic syndrome
Dose. *Dogs*: cystine calculi, 15 mg/kg twice daily preferably on an empty stomach

PoM **Distamine**™ (Dista)
Tablets, penicillamine 50 mg (scored), 125 mg, 250 mg; 100

PoM **Penicillamine** (Non-proprietary)
Tablets, penicillamine 125 mg, 250 mg

COMPOUND PREPARATIONS FOR UROLITHIASIS

PoM **Walpole's Buffer Solution** (Arnolds)
Glacial acetic acid 0.685%, sodium acetate 1.17%, for struvite calculi in *cats*; 25 mL
Use undiluted to irrigate bladder

9 Drugs used in the treatment of
MALIGNANT DISEASE

9.1 Alkylating drugs
9.2 Antimetabolites
9.3 Antitumour antibiotics
9.4 Vinca alkaloids
9.5 Other cytotoxic drugs

The use of cytotoxic drugs to treat cancer is increasing in veterinary medicine with chemotherapy becoming the treatment of choice in certain neoplastic diseases of companion animals.

Cytotoxic drugs are classified according to their characteristic sites or modes of action. Most cytotoxic drugs act upon the processes of cell growth and division. These drugs are potent and potentially dangerous and extreme care is required in their use. Careful consideration must be given to the pharmacology and toxicity of the drug, the spectrum of drug activity, and the condition of the patient.

> In veterinary medicine, the prescribing and administration of these drugs is usually confined to specialists in the field and empirical use is to be discouraged.

The main indications for cytotoxic drugs in veterinary medicine are management of lymphoproliferative and myeloproliferative disorders including lymphosarcoma, leukaemia, and multiple myeloma. These drugs are of little value in the treatment of large solid tumours, although they may have a palliative role as adjuncts to surgery or radiation therapy in the prevention or management of metastatic disease. The value of cytotoxic drugs in this role has yet to be proven and this use must therefore be regarded as experimental. Generally, the use of cytotoxic drugs in combination protocols is favoured as the most effective approach, for example, the combination of cyclophosphamide, vincristine, cytarabine, and prednisolone (COAP) as used in the treatment of lymphoma.

Toxicity is the major treatment-limiting factor in cancer chemotherapy. Commonly used dosages and protocols are a compromise between efficacy and toxicity, due to the low therapeutic index of these drugs. The intensive medical support often necessary for human patients to manage the severe toxicity resulting from chemotherapy is not routinely available or feasible in veterinary practice. Rapidly dividing cells such as bone marrow are most susceptible to toxic effects and myelosuppression occurs commonly with administration of cytotoxic drugs. Bone marrow suppression may lead to leukopenia, resulting in an increased risk of infection and sepsis; anaemia; or thrombocytopenia. Peripheral blood cell counts should be regularly monitored and drug dosage reduced or therapy withheld if critical blood cell counts are reached.

Toxic effects may also manifest in the gastro-intestinal tract and the skin. Poor hair growth or alopecia may occur, particularly in fine or curly-coated breeds such as poodles. Several drugs, for example vincristine and doxorubicin, are extremely irritant and will cause severe local tissue necrosis if injected perivascularly.

Dosage. In this chapter, only approximate guidelines are given regarding doses and indications. Doses of cytotoxic drugs are calculated as a function of body surface area (m^2) rather than body-weight because the blood supply to the organs responsible for detoxification, that is the kidney and liver, is more closely related to surface area than body-weight. Body surface area in square

Table 9.1 Weight to surface area in square metres for dogs†

kg	m^2	kg	m^2	kg	m^2
0.5	0.06	18	0.69	36	1.09
1	0.1	19	0.71	37	1.11
2	0.15	20	0.74	38	1.13
3	0.2	21	0.76	39	1.15
4	0.25	22	0.78	40	1.17
5	0.29	23	0.81	41	1.19
6	0.33	24	0.83	42	1.21
7	0.36	25	0.85	43	1.23
8	0.4	26	0.88	44	1.25
9	0.43	27	0.9	45	1.26
10	0.46	28	0.92	46	1.28
11	0.49	29	0.94	47	1.3
12	0.52	30	0.96	48	1.32
13	0.55	31	0.99	49	1.34
14	0.58	32	1.01	50	1.36
15	0.6	33	1.03		
16	0.63	34	1.05		
17	0.66	35	1.07		

† Adapted from Ettinger, SJ, ed. *Textbook of Veterinary Internal Medicine*. Philadelphia: WB Saunders Company, 1975: vol 1

metres for dogs and cats may be obtained from the following formula:

$$BSA = \frac{K \times W^{2/3}}{10^4}$$

K = constant (10.1 for dogs; 10.0 for cats)
W = weight in grams
BSA = body surface area in square metres
Table 9.1 gives the weight to surface area for dogs up to 50 kg.
The mode of drug metabolism and excretion should be known, as drug dosage may need to be reduced in patients with hepatic or renal impairment.

Extreme care is required in handling and using cytotoxic drugs. Administration should preferably be limited to veterinarians with the necessary expertise. Many cytotoxic substances are irritant to skin and mucous membranes and are suspected of having mutagenic, teratogenic, or carcinogenic potential. Thus even low dose exposure may be hazardous.

9.1 Alkylating drugs

In veterinary medicine, alkylating drugs are the most widely used in cancer chemotherapy. They act by interfering with DNA replication. Myelosuppression is the major side-effect of these drugs. Alkylating drugs may also severely affect gametogenesis and the gastro-intestinal tract, and cause alopecia.

Cyclophosphamide is widely used in the treatment of lymphoproliferative diseases, especially lymphosarcoma in cats and dogs. Use in the treatment of myeloma has been reported. Cyclophosphamide may also have a palliative role as an adjunct in the treatment of certain solid carcinomas and sarcomas. It is converted to active alkylating metabolites by the liver and primarily excreted by the kidney.

One of the metabolites, acrolein, may cause a sterile necrotising haemorrhagic cystitis. This is a serious complication which precludes further use of the drug. An increased water intake may help to avoid this complication. Prolonged therapy may also result in insidious fibrosis of the bladder.

Chlorambucil is the slowest acting and least toxic of the alkylating drugs. It is primarily used for maintenance therapy in lymphosarcoma, in the treatment of chronic lymphocytic leukaemia and multiple myeloma. The use of chlorambucil in the treatment of polycythaemia vera has been described. Myelosuppression is reversible on discontinuation of the drug.

Melphalan is primarily indicated in the treatment of multiple myeloma, but is also useful in lymphoproliferative disorders. It has been included in combined protocols to treat osteogenic sarcoma and mammary carcinoma. Myelosuppression is the major side-effect and may be delayed in onset. Anorexia and vomiting may also occur.

Busulphan has a selective action against granulocytes and is almost exclusively used in the treatment of chronic granulocytic leukaemia. Use in the treatment of polycythemia has been described. Myelosuppression is the main side-effect although pulmonary fibrosis may occur rarely.

Thiotepa may be administered by instillation in the treatment of superficial transitional cell carcinoma of the bladder. It has been used experimentally in the management of malignant pleural or ascitic effusions.

BUSULPHAN

Indications. Side-effects. See notes above
Dose. *Dogs, cats*: initial dose, 3-6 mg/m² daily until white blood cell count approaches normal values
Maintenance dose. 2 mg/m² daily, repeat as necessary to maintain the white blood cell count at 20000-25000 x 10⁹/litre

PoM **Myleran**™ (Calmic)
Tablets, busulphan 500 micrograms, 2 mg; 25

CHLORAMBUCIL

Indications. Side-effects. See notes above
Dose. *Dogs, cats*: 2 mg/m² every 24 or 48 hours

PoM **Leukeran**™ (Calmic)
Tablets, chlorambucil 2 mg, 5 mg; 25

CYCLOPHOSPHAMIDE

Indications. Side-effects. See notes above
Dose. *Dogs, cats*: *by mouth*, 50 mg/m² every other day or 50 mg/m² for the first 4 days of each week *or* 100-300 mg/m² every 3 weeks; *by intravenous injection*, 100-300 mg/m² every 3 weeks (maximum recommended dose for *dogs*, 250 mg/m²)

Oral preparations

PoM **Cyclophosphamide** (Farmitalia Carlo Erba)
Tablets, cyclophosphamide (as hydrate) 50 mg; 100, 250

PoM **Endoxana**™ (Degussa)
Tablets, cyclophosphamide 50 mg; 100

Parenteral preparations

PoM **Cyclophosphamide** (Farmitalia Carlo Erba)
Injection, powder for reconstitution, cyclophosphamide (as hydrate) 100 mg, 200 mg, other sizes available

PoM **Endoxana**™ (Degussa)
Injection, powder for reconstitution, cyclophosphamide (as hydrate) 100 mg, 200 mg, other sizes available

MELPHALAN

Indications. Side-effects. See notes above
Dose. *Dogs, cats*: multiple myeloma, 1-2 mg/m² every other day until plasma-protein concentrations approach normal values *or* 1-2 mg/m² daily for 7-14 days with repeat cycles at intervals of 2-4 weeks
Lymphoproliferative disorders, up to 5 mg/m² every other day

PoM **Alkeran**™ (Calmic)
Tablets, melphalan 2 mg, 5 mg; 25

THIOTEPA

Indications. Side-effects. See notes above
Dose. *Dogs, cats*: *by instillation into the bladder*, up to 60 mg in 60-100 mL water, instilled and retained for 30 minutes every 7 days; *by intravenous injection*, 9 mg/m² as a single dose *or* 9 mg/m² in 2-4 divided doses on successive days. Repeat dose every 7-28 days

PoM **Thiotepa** (Lederle)
Injection, powder for reconstitution, thiotepa 15 mg

9.2 Antimetabolites

Antimetabolites interfere with DNA and RNA synthesis by interaction with enzymes.
Cytarabine acts by interfering with pyrimidine synthesis. It is primarily used to induce remission in lympho-proliferative or myeloproliferative diseases and has been used intrathecally for the treatment of CNS lymphoma in dogs. The drug is rapidly degraded after

injection and is therefore more effective but also more toxic, if given by slow intravenous infusion. Cytarabine is a potent myelosuppressant leading to leukopenia, which is more severe with prolonged infusions.

Fluorouracil has been used in the treatment of carcinomas of the mammary gland, gastro-intestinal tract, liver, and lung in dogs, but is at best palliative. In addition to myelosuppression, fluorouracil causes neurotoxicity, manifest as cerebellar ataxia and seizures. These effects are transitory in dogs but fatal in cats. It is usually administered intravenously, but a preparation is also available for topical use for the treatment of superficial squamous cell or basal cell carcinoma.

Methotrexate competitively inhibits the enzyme dihydrofolate reductase, which is essential for the synthesis of purines and pyrimidines. Methotrexate may be used in the treatment of lympho-proliferative and myeloproliferative disorders. Its use has also been described in transmissible venereal tumours, Sertoli cell tumours, osteosarcoma and other sarcomas.

The 'high-dose' regimen described for human use of methotrexate is not generally advisable in veterinary medicine due to the toxic effects. Even at low doses, some dogs will show side-effects. Methotrexate is primarily excreted unchanged by the kidney and renal tubular necrosis may occur with high-dose regimens. Myelosuppression and gastro-intestinal ulceration are common side-effects.

Mercaptopurine is a purine analogue. It is used in the treatment of lympho-proliferative disorders including acute lymphocytic and granulocytic leukaemia. It may cause myelo-suppression, particularly leukopenia.

CYTARABINE

Indications. Side-effects. See notes above
Dose. *Dogs, cats*: *by subcutaneous or intravenous injection*, 100 mg/m^2 daily for 2-4 days; *by intravenous infusion*, 100 mg/m^2 given over 24 hours; *by*

intrathecal injection, 20 mg/m^2 every 1-5 days

PoM **Cytarabine** (Non-proprietary)
Injection, powder for reconstitution, cytarabine 100 mg, 500 mg, 1 g
For subcutaneous, intramuscular, or intravenous injection

PoM **Alexan**™ (Pfizer)
Injection, cytarabine 20 mg/mL; 2 mL, 5 mL
For subcutaneous, intramuscular, intravenous, or intrathecal injection

FLUOROURACIL

Indications. Side-effects. See notes above
Contra-indications. Cats, see notes above
Dose. *Dogs*: *by intravenous injection*, 150-200 mg/m^2 every 7 days

Parenteral preparations

PoM **Fluorouracil** (Non-proprietary)
Injection, fluorouracil (as sodium salt) 25 mg/mL; 10 mL, 20 mL, 100 mL

Topical preparations

PoM **Efudix**™ (Roche)
Cream, fluorouracil 5%; 20 g

MERCAPTOPURINE

Indications. Side-effects. See notes above
Dose. *Dogs, cats*: 50 mg/m^2 daily to effect then 50 mg/m^2 every other day or as necessary

PoM **Puri-Nethol**™ (Calmic)
Tablets, scored, mercaptopurine 50 mg; 25

METHOTREXATE

Indications. See notes above
Contra-indications. Side-effects. Renal impairment. See notes above
Dose. *Dogs, cats*: *by mouth or by intravenous injection*, 2.5 mg/m^2 daily. Dose frequency should be adjusted according to toxicity (see notes above)

Oral preparations

PoM **Methotrexate** (Lederle)
Tablets, scored, methotrexate 2.5 mg, 10 mg; 2.5-mg tablets 100; 10-mg tablets 50

Parenteral preparations

PoM **Methotrexate** (Lederle)
Injection, methotrexate (as sodium salt)
2.5 mg/mL; 1 mL, 2 mL
Injection, methotrexate (as sodium salt)
25 mg/mL; 1 mL, 2 mL, other sizes available
Injection, powder for reconstitution, methotrexate (as sodium salt) 500 mg

9.3 Antitumour antibiotics

These drugs act by forming complexes with DNA thus inhibiting synthesis.
Doxorubicin is an anthracycline antibiotic, and is one of the most effective of the cytotoxic drugs. In veterinary therapy, doxorubicin is used to treat lymphoproliferative and myeloproliferative disorders. It is also a palliative in soft tissue and osteogenic sarcomas and in carcinomas of mammary, thyroid, and prostatic origin. Doxorubicin is administered by intravenous injection and is severely irritant if injected perivascularly. It is myelosuppressive with the lowest leukocyte count occurring 10 to 14 days after treatment. Doxorubicin also causes myocardial damage leading to a dose-dependent congestive cardiomyopathy, and cardiac monitoring is advisable. Doxorubicin is excreted in the biliary tract.

Tachyarrhythmias, cutaneous anaphylaxis, and collapse may occur during infusion; premedication with an antihistamine is advisable (see section 5.2.1). Treatment with this drug should be supervised by specialists familiar with its use.

Bleomycin is used in the treatment of lymphoproliferative disorders and has shown some efficacy against squamous cell carcinoma in cats and dogs. Bleomycin causes minimal myelosuppression but hypersensitivity reactions may occur. Lung changes including interstitial pneumonia, pleural scarring, and pulmonary fibrosis have been reported with high doses in the dog.

Actinomycin D has not been widely used in veterinary chemotherapy. There is limited investigational experience in the treatment of canine lymphoproliferative

disorders, carcinomas, and sarcomas. Toxicities include leukopenia, anorexia, vomiting, diarrhoea, and weight loss, due to selective damage of the haemopoietic and intestinal tissues.

ACTINOMYCIN D
(Dactinomycin)

Indications. Side-effects. See notes above
Dose. *Dogs, cats*: *by intravenous injection*, 1.5 mg/m^2 every 7 days

PoM **Cosmegen Lyovac**™ (MSD)
Injection, powder for reconstitution, actinomycin D (with mannitol) 500 micrograms

BLEOMYCIN

Indications. Side-effects. See notes above
Dose. *Dogs, cats*: *by intravenous injection*, 10-15 units/m^2 weekly to a maximum dose of 250 units/m^2

PoM **Bleomycin** (Lundbeck)
Injection, powder for reconstitution, bleomycin (as sulphate) 15 units

DOXORUBICIN HYDROCHLORIDE

Indications. See notes above
Contra-indications. Side-effects. Hepatic impairment, see notes above
Dose. *Dogs, cats*: *by intravenous injection*, 30 mg/m^2 every 21 days to a maximum cumulative dose of 240 mg/m^2

PoM **Doxorubicin Rapid Dissolution**™ (Farmitalia Carlo Erba)
Injection, powder for reconstitution, doxorubicin hydrochloride 10 mg, 50 mg

PoM **Doxorubicin**™ **Solution for Injection** (Farmitalia Carlo Erba)
Doxorubicin hydrochloride 2 mg/mL; 5 mL, 25 mL

9.4 Vinca alkaloids

These drugs are plant alkaloids. They bind to microtubular proteins, causing metaphase arrest. They may also cause enzyme inhibition.
Vincristine is the most widely used vinca alkaloid in veterinary medicine. The

main indications are in the treatment of lymphoproliferative disorders and transmissible venereal tumour. The latter is extremely sensitive to vincristine. The experimental use of vincristine in the treatment of soft tissue sarcomas and carcinomas has also been reported. Vincristine is also of value in the management of thrombocytopenia by virtue of its stimulation of platelet release from megakaryocytes.

Vincristine causes virtually no myelosuppression but is severely vesicant if injected perivascularly. Peripheral and autonomic neuropathies rarely occur in dogs and cats. Constipation may result from long term therapy.

Vinblastine is less frequently used than vincristine. Its uses include treatment of lymphoproliferative disorders and solid carcinomas but efficacy in the latter case is limited. Unlike vincristine, vinblastine causes myelosuppression, and will also cause severe perivascular reactions.

VINBLASTINE SULPHATE

Indications. Side-effects. See notes above
Dose. *Dogs, cats*: *by intravenous injection*, 2.0-2.5 mg/m^2 every 7 or 14 days

PoM **Vinblastine** (Non-proprietary)
Injection, powder for reconstitution, vinblastine sulphate 10 mg

VINCRISTINE SULPHATE

Indications. Side-effects. See notes above
Dose. *Dogs, cats*: *by intravenous injection*, 500-750 micrograms/m^2 every 7 or 14 days

PoM **Vincristine** (Non-proprietary)
Injection, vincristine sulphate 1 mg/mL; 1 mL, 2 mL
Injection, powder for reconstitution, vincristine sulphate 1 mg, 2 mg, 5 mg

9.5 Other cytotoxic drugs

Prednisolone is widely used in cancer therapy. Corticosteroids have antimitotic and cytolytic effects on lymphoid tissues and are therefore used in the treatment of lymphoproliferative disorders. They are also useful in the treatment of mast cell tumours and may be indicated in brain tumours as these drugs are able to cross the blood-brain barrier. Corticosteroids may also be used in the management of secondary complications of neoplasia and palliation of advanced disease. They are also potent immunosuppressants.

Toxic effects include pancreatitis and diarrhoea. Hyperadrenocorticism may result from chronic, long-term therapy. Corticosteroids cause little or no myelosuppression.

PREDNISOLONE

Indications. Side-effects. See notes above
Dose. *Dogs, cats*: 10-60 mg/m^2 daily or every other day

See section 7.2.1 for preparation details

Cisplatin inhibits protein synthesis by cross-linking strands of DNA. The drug is severely toxic, which limits its veterinary use. Cisplatin has been used in the treatment of osteosarcoma, soft tissue sarcoma and various carcinomas. Cisplatin is nephrotoxic, causing acute proximal tubular necrosis. Vomiting and myelosuppression also occur. Pretreatment hydration and diuresis are recommended and toxicity frequently necessitates dose reduction. It is preferable that treatment with this drug be supervised by specialists familiar with its use.

CISPLATIN

Indications. See notes above
Contra-indications. Side-effects. Renal impairment, see notes above
Dose. *Dogs, cats*: *by intravenous infusion* 50-70 mg/m^2, combined with hydration and diuresis

PoM **Cisplatin** (Non-proprietary)
Injection, cisplatin 1 mg/mL; 10 mL, 50 mL 100 mL
Injection, powder for reconstitution, cisplatin 10 mg, 50 mg, other sizes available

Crisantaspase is the enzyme asparaginase produced by *Erwinia chrysanthemi*. It hydrolyses asparagine, an essential amino acid, and is used i the treatment of lymphoproliferative disorders. It has also been used in the treatment of canine melanoma and mast cell tumours. Crisantaspase may be administered by the intravenous, intramuscular, or intraperitoneal routes but anaphylaxis may follow administration and the intramuscular route appears to be the safest and most effective. Premedication with antihistamine (see section 5.2.1) is necessary if used by other routes. Haemorrhagic pancreatitis has been reported in dogs.

CRISANTASPASE

Indications. Side-effects. See notes above
Dose. *Dogs, cats: by intramuscular (preferred), intravenous, or intraperitoneal injection*, 10 000-40 000 units/m^2 every 7 days or more

PoM **Erwinase**™ (Porton)
Injection, powder for reconstitution, crisantaspase 10 000 units

Dacarbazine has alkylating actions but also inhibits DNA and protein synthesis. It is not commonly used in veterinary medicine due to its toxic effects but it has been included in some combination protocols for the treatment of lymphoproliferative disorders. In addition to myelosuppression, gastro-intestinal toxicity has been reported. Dacarbazine can cause pain on injection and severe perivascular reactions.

DACARBAZINE

Indications. Side-effects. See notes above
Dose. *Dogs, cats: by intravenous injection*, 200-250 mg/m^2 daily on days 1-5, repeat cycle every 21-28 days

PoM **DTIC-Dome**™ (Bayer)
Injection, powder for reconstitution, dacarbazine 100 mg, 200 mg

Hydroxyurea inhibits the enzyme ribonucleotide reductase. It is administered orally and is excreted by the kidney. It is used in the treatment of polycythaemia vera and chronic granulocytic leukaemia. Myelosuppression is the main toxic effect.

HYDROXYUREA

Indications. See notes above
Contra-indications. Side-effects. Renal impairment, see notes above
Dose. *Dogs, cats*: 50 mg/kg daily *or* 80 mg/kg every 3 days

PoM **Hydrea**™ (Squibb)
Capsules, hydroxyurea 500 mg; 100

10 Drugs used in the treatment of disorders of the
MUSCULOSKELETAL SYSTEM and JOINTS

Many classes of drugs are used to suppress or abolish one or more of the cardinal signs of acute inflammation. The principal value of these drugs is to relieve pain and reduce swelling. In addition to the drug classes discussed in this chapter, **corticosteroids** (see section 7.2) are used extensively for the treatment of inflammatory conditions.

Not all of the drugs considered in this chapter are, strictly, anti-inflammatory. Chondroprotective agents, for example polysulphated glycosaminoglycan (see section 10.2), retard the degradation and promote the synthesis of cartilage components in non-inflamed joints.

Drugs used in the management of musculoskeletal and joint disorders interfere with the action, release, or synthesis of mediators and modulators of inflammation and cartilage degradation. These mediators and modulators include histamine, bradykinin, prostaglandins, leukotrienes, platelet-activating factor, complement components, and oxygen-derived free radicals. The many mediators that are implicated in acute and chronic inflammation may interact either synergistically or antagonistically. Anti-inflammatory drugs that antagonise the action or release of a single mediator or group of mediators often suppress, but usually do not abolish, inflammatory or arthritic changes.

10.1 Non-steroidal anti-inflammatory drugs

Almost all non-steroidal anti-inflammatory drugs (NSAIDs) are weak carboxylic or enolic acids. They are analgesics, antipyretics, and have peripheral anti-inflammatory activity. They act mainly by inhibiting cyclo-oxygenase leading to reduced synthesis of prostaglandins and related compounds. This mechanism probably underlies their principal therapeutic and toxic activity. Toxicity varies with the species and the individual drug and is therefore not readily predictable.

The principal side-effect of NSAIDs is gastro-intestinal irritation and ulceration. Lesions may occur throughout the gastro-intestinal tract and may lead to a life-threatening plasma protein-losing enteropathy in the horse. Lesions may occur after parenteral as well as oral dosing. Other side-effects include vomiting, blood dyscrasias, hepatotoxicity due to cholestatic and parenchymal cell damage, renal papillary necrosis, and occasionally skin rashes. Some NSAIDs, such as aspirin, have been shown to be teratogenic in animal studies.

Paracetamol is an analgesic but with relatively weak anti-inflammatory activity. It should not be administered to cats. Cats have a reduced capacity for glucuronide conjugation and the drug is converted to a reactive electrophilic metabolite in this species. Clinical signs of toxicity include anaemia, methaemoglobinaemia, and liver failure.

The pharmacokinetics of NSAIDs vary between species, which leads to marked inter-species differences in dosage requirements. Variations in naproxen

Table 10.1 Species difference in elimination half-life of NSAIDs in hours

Species	Flunixin	Indomethacin	Naproxen	Phenylbutazone	Salicylate
Horse	1.6–2.1	—	5	4.5–8.0†	1.0–3.0
Cattle	8	—	—	36–55	0.5 (i.v.) 3.7 (by mouth)
Pig	—	—	5	4	5.9
Dog	3.7	0.3	35–74‡	2.5–6.0†	8.6
Cat	—	—	—	—	22–45
Monkey	—	0.3	1.9	7	—
Man	—	2	14	72	3.0 (by mouth)

† dose-dependent kinetics: half-life increases with administered dose
‡ breed dependent

half-life have been reported for different breeds of dog. Table 10.1 indicates the half-life of NSAIDs in domestic species, monkey, and man.

Most NSAIDs are well absorbed following administration by mouth, although drug-induced gastric irritation in monogastric species may lead to persistent vomiting, for example, with ibuprofen. Parenteral formulations of flunixin and compound analgesic preparations may be given by both intravenous and intramuscular injection but phenylbutazone is too irritant for injection by non-vascular routes. With the exception of salicylate, NSAIDs are highly bound to plasma proteins, commonly in excess of 99 percent, which limits extravascular penetration of NSAIDs. However, penetration into acute inflammatory exudate is generally good since exudate is rich in extravasated plasma protein.

NSAIDs have been used for their analgesic and anti-oedematous action in acute inflammatory conditions including the control of pain following surgery. They have also been used to control joint pain in various arthritides, particularly osteoarthritis and they may ameliorate symptoms of endotoxaemic shock, for example, in peracute mastitis. Flunixin has been used to reduce morbidity and mortality in calf pneumonias by suppressing pulmonary oedema. Flunixin is also used to reduce pain in equine colic. Aspirin, unlike other NSAIDs, combines with cyclo-oxygenase covalently to produce irreversible enzyme blockade. This action has been utilised to prevent clotting in thrombo-embolic disorders.

ASPIRIN

Indications. Inflammation and pain; thrombo-embolic disorders (see section 4.6.2)
Contra-indications. Pregnant animals
Side-effects. Prolonged use may cause gastro-intestinal lesions, see notes above
Warnings. Should not be administered to animals with gastric ulceration
Dose. *Dogs*: 25 mg/kg 3 times daily
Cats: 25 mg/kg once daily

PAspirin (Non-proprietary)
Tablets, aspirin 300 mg; pack sizes greater than 25
Tablets, dispersible, aspirin 75 mg, 300 mg; pack sizes greater than 25

FLUNIXIN

Indications. Inflammation and pain; endotoxic shock
Contra-indications. Racehorses within 8 days prior to racing (see Prescribing for animals used in competitions). Manufacturer does not recommend use

in pregnant animals or treatment in conjunction with methoxyflurane anaesthesia
Side-effects. Warnings. See under Aspirin
Dose. *Horses*: *by mouth or by intramuscular or intravenous injection*, 1.1 mg/kg once daily for up to 5 days
Cattle: *by intravenous injection*, 2.2 mg/kg once daily for up to 5 days
Dogs: *by mouth or by subcutaneous injection*, 1 mg/kg daily for up to 3 days; *by slow intravenous injection*, 1 mg/kg up to twice daily for a maximum of 3 doses if required

PoM **Finadyne™** (Schering-Plough)
Tablets, scored, flunixin (as meglumine) 5 mg, 20 mg, for *dogs*; 100
Oral paste, flunixin (as meglumine) 110 mg/division, for *horses*; 30-g metered-dose applicator
Withdrawal Periods. Should not be used in *horses* intended for human consumption
Oral granules, for addition to feed, flunixin (as meglumine) 25 mg/g, for *horses*; 10 g
Withdrawal Periods. *Horses*: slaughter 7 days
Injection, flunixin (as meglumine) 10 mg/mL, for *dogs*; 20 mL
Injection, flunixin (as meglumine) 50 mg/mL, for *horses, cattle*; 50 mL
Withdrawal Periods. *Horses*: slaughter 7 days. *Cattle*: slaughter 7 days, milk 36 hours

MECLOFENAMIC ACID

Indications. Inflammation and pain
Contra-indications. Gastro-intestinal, hepatic, or renal impairment. Discontinue administration 5 days prior to administration of prostaglandins for breeding purposes. Racehorses 8 days prior to racing (see Prescribing for animals used in competitions)
Side-effects. Warnings. See under Aspirin
Dose. *Horses*: 2.2 mg/kg once daily for 5-7 days, then adjust dose frequency to suit each individual patient if further treatment is necessary

PoM **Arquel™** (Parke-Davis)
Oral granules, for addition to feed, meclofenamic acid 50 mg/g, for *horses*; 10 g
Withdrawal Periods. *Horses*: slaughter 5 days

PoM **Equafen™** (Duphar)
Oral granules, for addition to feed, meclofenamic acid 50 mg/g, for *horses*; 10 g
Withdrawal Periods. *Horses*: slaughter 5 days

NAPROXEN

Indications. Inflammation and pain
Contra-indications. Racehorses 8 days prior to racing (see Prescribing for animals used in competitions)
Side-effects. Warnings. See under Aspirin
Dose. *Horses*: 10 mg/kg twice daily for up to 14 days
Dogs: initial dose 5 mg/kg then 2 mg/kg once daily

PoM **Naproxen** (Non-proprietary)
Tablets, naproxen 250 mg, 500 mg

PHENYLBUTAZONE

Indications. Inflammation and pain
Contra-indications. Cardiac, hepatic, or renal impairment; anaemia. Racehorses 8 days prior to racing (see Prescribing for animals used in competitions)
Side-effects. Warnings. See under Aspirin; occasional oedema of limbs
Dose. *Horses*: *by mouth*, 4.4 mg/kg twice daily on day one then 4.4 mg/kg once daily for 4 days, followed by 4.4 mg/kg every other day for 4 days; *by slow intravenous injection*, 2.2-4.4 mg/kg for up to 5 days
Dogs: *by mouth or by slow intravenous injection*, 2-20 mg/kg daily (maximum 800 mg). Parenteral treatment should only be given for up to 3 days.

Oral preparations

PoM **Equipalazone™** (Arnolds)
Oral paste, phenylbutazone 1 g/division, for *horses*; 35-mL metered-dose applicator

Oral powder, for addition to feed, phenylbutazone 1 g/sachet, for *horses*

PoM **Flexazone**™ (BK)
Tablets, phenylbutazone 100 mg, 200 mg, for *dogs*; 1000

PoM **Phenogel**™ (Duphar)
Tablets, phenylbutazone 100 mg, 200 mg, for *dogs*; 1000

PoM **Phenylbutazone** (Animalcare)
Tablets, phenylbutazone 100 mg, 200 mg, for *horses, dogs*; 250, 500, 1000

PoM **Phenylbutazone** (Loveridge)
Tablets, phenylbutazone 100 mg, 200 mg, for *dogs*; 250, 500, 1000

PoM **Phenyzene**™ (C-Vet)
Oral paste, phenylbutazone 200 mg/division, for *horses*; 25-g metered-dose applicator
Withdrawal Periods. Should not be used in *horses* intended for human consumption

PoM **Pro-Dynam**™ (Leo)
Oral powder, for addition to feed, phenylbutazone 1 g/sachet, for *horses*

Parenteral preparations

PoM **Equipalazone**™ (Arnolds)
Injection, phenylbutazone 200 mg/mL, for *horses*; 50 mL

PoM **Phenyzene**™ (C-Vet)
Injection, phenylbutazone 200 mg/mL, for *horses, dogs*; 50 mL

PIROXICAM

Indications. Inflammation and pain
Side-effects. **Warnings**. See under Aspirin
Dose. *Dogs*: 300 micrograms/kg every other day

PoM **Piroxicam** (Non-proprietary)
Capsules, piroxicam 10 mg, 20 mg

10.2 Other anti-inflammatory drugs

Several classes of drugs are used to treat arthritis by intra-articular injection in horses and in dogs. Some of these are also recommended for intramuscular administration. Some **corticosteroids** (see section 7.2), sodium hyaluronate, and the chondroprotective drug, poly-sulphated glycosaminoglycan (PSGAG) may be given by intra-articular injection.
Sodium hyaluronate is a high molecular-weight mucopolysaccharide, which is a constituent of the higher molecular-weight cartilage matrix molecules, aggregated proteoglycans, and is also present in synovial fluid. This accounts for the high viscosity of synovial fluid. In some forms of joint disease depolymerisation of hyaluronate occurs, which affects the thixotropic properties of synovial fluid. Sodium hyaluronate is administered by intra-articular injection for the therapy of joint diseases in the horse, especially in cases associated with synovitis. The mechanism of action may be partially attributable to restoration of normal viscosity of synovial fluid and partially due to its anti-inflammatory properties, although sodium hyaluronate is probably not chondroprotective.
Pentosan polysulphate sodium is a semi-synthetic polymer with molecular-weight of 2000. **Polysulphated glycosamino-glycan** (PSGAG) is based on hexosamine and hexuronic acid and has a molecular weight of 10000. These high molecular-weight polymers bind to damaged cartilage matrix consisting of aggregated proteoglycans, and stimulate the synthesis of new aggregated glycosaminoglycan molecules. Several possible modes of action have been identified. The ability of these compounds to inhibit a range of proteolytic enzymes may be of particular importance.

PENTOSAN POLYSULPHATE SODIUM

Indications. Osteoarthritis and non immune arthritides
Contra-indications. Septic arthritis; haemorrhage; hepatic impairment; renal impairment; malignant disease
Dose. *Horses*♦: *by intra-articular injection*, 250 mg/joint, repeat after 7-10 days
Dogs: *by subcutaneous injection*, 3 mg/kg. Repeat 3 times at 5-7 day intervals
by intra-articular injection,♦ 10-20 mg

PoM **Cartrophen Vet**™ (Univet)
Injection, pentosan polysulphate sodium 100 mg/mL, for *dogs*; 10 mL

POLYSULPHATED GLYCOSAMINOGLYCAN

Indications. Non-infectious and non-immune arthritides
Contra-indications. Hepatic or renal impairment. Manufacturer does not recommend use in pregnant animals
Side-effects. Increased oedema at joint site
Dose. *Horses*: *by intramuscular injection*, 500 mg twice weekly for 7 doses; *by intra-articular injection*, 250 mg/joint weekly for 5 doses

PoM **Adequan**™ (Panpharma)
Injection, polysulphated glycosaminoglycan 100 mg/mL, for *horses*; 5 mL
For intramuscular injection
Withdrawal Periods. Should not be used in *horses* intended for human consumption
Injection, polysulphated glycosaminoglycan 250 mg/mL, for *horses*; 1 mL
For intra-articular injection
Withdrawal Periods. Should not be used in *horses* intended for human consumption

SODIUM HYALURONATE

Indications. Arthritides associated with synovitis
Side-effects. Transitory local reactions
Dose. *Horses*: *by intra-articular injection*, 10-40 mg/joint, repeat if required

Note. For therapeutic purposes sodium hyaluronate and hyaluronic acid may be considered equivalent in effect.

PoM **Equron**™ (Duphar)
Injection, sodium hyaluronate 5 mg/mL, for *horses*; 2-mL syringe
Withdrawal Periods. *Horses*: slaughter withdrawal period nil
PoM **Hyalovet**™ **20** (C-Vet)
Injection, hyaluronic acid (as sodium salt) 10 mg/mL, for *horses*; 2-mL syringe
Withdrawal Periods. *Horses*: slaughter withdrawal period nil

PoM **Hylartil**™ **Vet** (Fisons)
Injection, sodium hyaluronate 10 mg/mL, for *horses*; 2-mL syringe

10.3 Compound preparations of anti-inflammatory analgesic drugs

A number of preparations containing combinations of NSAIDs and opioid drugs or two NSAIDs are licensed for veterinary use. These latter preparations should only be used at the recommended dose rates since the 2 drugs may be additive in their toxic as well as their therapeutic effects. Other, less rational, drug combinations are also available.

Oral preparations

PoM **Buta-Leucotropin**™ (BK)
Oral powder, for addition to feed, cinchophen 1 g, phenylbutazone 500 mg/sachet, for *horses*
Dose. *Horses*: (450 kg body-weight) 4 sachets daily in divided doses for 4 days, then 2 sachets daily in divided doses for 4 days, then 1 sachet on alternate days for 12 days

PoM **Leucotropin**™ (BK)
Tablets, cinchophen 280 mg, hexamine 100 mg, quinine hydrochloride 70 mg, for *dogs, cats*; 100, 1000
Dose. *Dogs*: (less than 7 kg body-weight) ½ tablet twice daily; (7-20 kg body-weight) 1 tablet twice daily; (20-30 kg body-weight) 1 tablet 3 times daily; (more than 30 kg body-weight) 2 tablets twice daily
Cats: ½ tablet twice daily

PoM **Predno-Leucotropin**™ (BK)
Tablets, cinchophen 200 mg, hexamine 100 mg, prednisolone 1 mg, for *dogs, cats*; 100, 1000
Dose. *Dogs*: given with food, (less than 7 kg body-weight) ½ tablet twice daily; (7-20 kg body-weight) 1 tablet twice daily; (20-30 kg body-weight) 1 tablet 3 times daily; (more than 30 kg body-weight) 2 tablets twice daily
Cats: ½ tablet twice daily

Parenteral preparations

PoM **Adzoid™** (Arnolds)
Injection, phenylbutazone 200 mg, prednisolone sodium phosphate 2 mg/mL,
for *horses*; 50 mL
Dose. *Horses*: *by slow intravenous
injection*, up to 0.02 mL/kg

PoM **Buscopan™ Compositum** (Boehringer
Ingelheim)
Injection, dipyrone 500 mg, hyoscine
butylbromide 4 mg/mL, for *horses,
cattle, pigs, dogs*; 100 mL
Dose. *Horses*: *by intravenous injection*,
0.05 mL/kg
Cattle, pigs: *by intramuscular or intravenous (preferred) injection*, 0.1 mL/kg
Dogs: *by intramuscular or intravenous
(preferred) injection*, 0.05 mL/kg

PoM **Tomanol™** (Intervet)
Injection, phenylbutazone (as sodium
salt) 120 mg, ramifenazone 240 mg/mL,
for *horses, cattle, pigs, dogs, cats*; 100
mL
Dose. Repeat daily for 2-3 days if
required. *Horses*: *by slow intravenous
injection*, 0.04 mL/kg
Cattle: *by intramuscular or slow intravenous injection*, 0.04 mL/kg
Pigs: *by subcutaneous or intramuscular
injection*, 0.07 mL/kg
Dogs: *by intramuscular or slow intravenous injection*, 0.5-4.0 mL
Cats: *by intramuscular or slow intravenous injection*, 0.5-1.0 mL

10.4 Topical anti-inflammatory preparations

The topical drugs used most extensively
for their anti-inflammatory properties
are the corticosteroids (see section 7.2,
section 14.4. Skin, section 12.3 Eye, and
section 13.1 Ear). Topical drugs that
may also be applied include dimethyl
sulphoxide (DMSO) and certain non-
steroidal anti-inflammatory drugs, such
as methyl salicylate. Preparations containing copper in combination with
NSAIDs and formulated in a DMSO
basis have been evaluated and found to
be more effective than NSAIDs dissolved
in DMSO but without the copper
component.
DMSO is a solvent that readily dissolves
both water-soluble and lipid-soluble
drugs and can be used to transport drugs
through skin. It also possesses some
anti-inflammatory activity and causes
dissolution of collagen. The mode of
action as an anti-inflammatory drug is
unknown but it may act through
scavenging free radicals.
Copper and copper-containing compounds may also act by the same
mechanism. They possess superoxide
dismutase activity. However, the therapeutic value of copper-containing compounds in joint disease remains to be
established.
Combination preparations are available,
which are used for tendonitis and
synovitis mainly in horses.

COMPOUND TOPICAL ANTI-INFLAMMATORY OR ANALGESIC PREPARATIONS

PML **Tensolvet™** (C-Vet)
Gel, glycol salicylate 50 mg, menthol 5
mg, heparin sodium 50 units/g, for
horses; 300 g
Withdrawal Periods. Should not be
used on *horses* intended for human
consumption
Contra-indications. Racehorses 48 hours
prior to racing

PML **Trisolgel™** (Crown)
Gel, glycol salicylate 50 mg, menthol
5 mg, heparin sodium 50 units/g, for
horses; 300 g
Withdrawal Periods. Should not be
used on *horses* intended for human
consumption
Contra-indications. Racehorses 48 hours
prior to racing

GSL **Veterinary Embrocation** (Battle Hayward & Bower)
Liniment, acetic acid 3.3%, strong
ammonia solution 7.2%, turpentine oil

11.1%, for *horses*, *cattle*; 300 mL, 500 mL

10.5 Cytotoxic immunosuppressants

Cytotoxic drugs with immunosuppressant properties such as methotrexate, cyclophosphamide, chlorambucil, and mercaptopurine have been used in the treatment of immune-based arthritides principally in the dog. These drugs are usually given in combination with a corticosteroid such as prednisolone.

Cyclophosphamide (see section 9.1) is administered to dogs at a dose of 25 mg/m^2 for dogs weighing less than 10 kg, 20 mg/m^2 for dogs weighing 10 to 35 kg, and 15 mg/m^2 for dogs weighing more than 35 kg. Doses of up to 50 mg/m^2 have been used. Cyclophosphamide is given for 4 consecutive days every week, in combination with decreasing doses of prednisolone (see section 7.2.1) 3-4 mg/kg daily.

After 4 months, treatment should be changed to **mercaptopurine** (see section 9.2) given at a dose of 20 mg/m^2 on alternate days.

10.6 Disease-modifying drugs

Drugs in this class include the gold salts sodium aurothiomalate and auranofin, penicillamine, and levamisole, an anthelmintic drug that also possesses immunomodulatory properties.

These drugs are used in man to suppress symptoms and retard degenerative changes in rheumatoid and other immune-based arthritides. The mechanism of action has not been fully elucidated. Some of the drugs have been used to treat immune-based arthritides but the slow onset of action, difficulty in assessing efficacy, and potential toxicity to the haematopoietic system have limited their veterinary usage.

Sodium aurothiomalate treatment regimens consist of progressively increasing doses over a period of 13 weeks although it is possible to modify such courses according to the severity of the condition and the size and breed of the animal treated.

SODIUM AUROTHIOMALATE

Indications. Immune-based arthritides
Warnings. See notes above
Dose. *By intramuscular injection. Horses, cattle*: 10 mg, then 20 mg, then 2 injections of 50 mg, and then 9 injections of 100 mg, at weekly intervals over 13 weeks
Dogs: 10 mg, then 6 injections of 20 mg, and then 6 injections of 50 mg, at weekly intervals over 13 weeks

PoM **Myocrisin**™ (M&B)
Injection, sodium aurothiomalate 20 mg/mL, 40 mg/mL, 100 mg/mL; 0.5 mL

11 Drugs used in the treatment of
MASTITIS

11.1 Intramammary preparations
11.2 Preparations for the care of teats and udders

Mastitis is of economic importance in dairy herds because it causes decreased milk production often leading to early culling. Peracute mastitis may result in death. Other species affected include ewes, sows, does, and mares.

Generally, infecting organisms enter the udder via the teat canal during milking. Contamination may arise from the udders of infected cows, teat abrasions, soiled environment, inadequate milking machines, and in the case of summer mastitis, the head fly *Hydrotoea irritans*. The main pathogens causing inflammation of the udder and teat canal are *Streptococcus agalactiae*, *Strep. dysgalactiae*, *Strep. uberis*, *Staphylococcus* species; *Actinomyces pyogenes* (summer mastitis); *Escherichia coli*, *Klebsiella* species, *Enterobacter aerogenes* (coliform mastitis); *Mycoplasma* species; various other bacteria, some fungi, and yeasts.

These pathogens enter the teat canal and cause infection and inflammation of the mammary gland. A systemic reaction may also occur in some cases.

In peracute clinical mastitis, there is acute inflammation of the mammary gland with toxaemia. The causal bacteria may include *Staph. aureus*, *A. pyogenes*, *Pseudomonas*, or coliforms. Treatment should include intravenous fluids, antibiotics, and supportive therapy. Fluids (see section 16.1.2) such as sodium chloride 0.9% intravenous infusion should be administered rapidly at a rate of 10 litres over 30 minutes and repeated as necessary. Concurrently 25 litres of fluid can be administered into the rumen via a stomach tube. Flunixin meglumine (see section 10.1) is indicated in the treatment of toxaemia at a dose of 2 mg/kg body-weight by intravenous injection. Parenteral antibiotics (see section 1.1) such as penicillin and streptomycin in combination, cephalosporins, and oxytetracycline should be given as well as intramammary preparations. Multivitamin preparations (see section 16.5.7) containing B vitamins may also aid recovery.

In acute mastitis there is swelling and inflammation of the mammary gland with little systemic reaction. The milk is found to be abnormal. Treatment consists of thorough stripping of the udder to remove milk clots before applying intramammary preparations for lactating cows (see section 11.1.1). Oxytocin (see section 8.4) may also be used to cause emptying of the udder.

In cases of subclinical mastitis the main evidence of disease is an abnormality of the milk cell count. These cases are usually treated when the animal is no longer lactating by using long-acting intramammary preparations (see section 11.1.2). Preparations for non-lactating animals are also used to prevent cases of summer mastitis due to *A. pyogenes*. Mastitis may cause a significant loss of production and prevention and control of the disease is practised. Guidelines have been set by MAFF/MMB which include hygiene standards in the dairy and housing areas, equipment maintenance, monitoring of herd status using bulk and individual milk cell counts, culling policy, and judicious use of antibiotic and disinfectant preparations.

11.1 Intramammary preparations

11.1.1 Intramammary preparations for lactating animals
11.1.2 Intramammary preparations for non-lactating animals

11.1.1 Intramammary preparations for lactating animals

These preparations are used to treat clinical mastitis (see notes above). Initial treatment is usually empirical and chosen to provide the widest possible cover. A sample of the infected secretion may be collected and refrigerated or deep frozen for future examination should treatment be unsuccessful.

Antibacterials included in intra-mammary preparations give either narrow or broad spectrum protection against mastitic pathogens. Details of antibacterial spectra of activity may be found in section 1.1. Procaine penicillin, erythromycin, novobiocin in combination with procaine penicillin, and cloxacillin are effective against Gram-positive bacteria including streptococci and staphylococci although procaine penicillin is ineffective against beta-lactamase-producing staphylococci.

Broad-spectrum antibiotic activity is achieved with co-amoxiclav, oxytetra-cycline, cephalosporins such as cephace-trile, cefoperazone, and cefuroxime, and compound intramammary preparations. Some compound preparations also contain corticosteroids to help reduce inflammation within the udder.

For the treatment of bovine mastitis, one dose of antibiotic preparation per infected quarter is infused into the teat orifice immediately after milking, ensuring that the teat does not become contaminated. Disinfectant teat dips, sprays, and creams (see section 11.2) may then be applied.

> When using antibacterial intramammary preparations, operators should avoid contact of the product with the skin as occasional allergic reactions may occur.

CEFOPERAZONE

Indications. Mastitis, see notes above
Dose. See preparation details

PoM **Pathocef™** (Pfizer)
Intramammary suspension (oily), cefoperazone (as sodium salt) 250 mg/dose, for *cattle*; 10-mL dose applicator
Withdrawal Periods. *Cattle*: slaughter 2 days, milk 3.5 days
Dose. *Cattle*: *by intramammary infusion*, one dose per infected quarter. One dose is usually sufficient for treatment

CEFUROXIME

Indications. Mastitis, see notes above
Dose. See preparation details

PoM **Spectrazol™ Milking Cow** (Coopers Pitman-Moore)
Intramammary paste (oily), cefuroxime (as sodium salt) 250 mg/dose, for *cattle*; single-dose applicator
Withdrawal Periods. *Cattle*: slaughter 1 day, milk 60 hours
Dose. *Cattle*: *by intramammary infusion*, one dose per infected quarter. Repeat twice at 12-hour intervals

CEPHACETRILE SODIUM

Indications. Mastitis, see notes above
Dose. See preparation details

PoM **Vetimast™** (Ciba-Geigy)
Intramammary suspension, cephacetrile sodium 250 mg/dose, for *cattle*; 10-g dose applicator
Withdrawal Periods. *Cattle*: slaughter 7 days, milk 4 days
Dose. *Cattle*: *by intramammary infusion*, one dose per infected quarter. One dose is usually sufficient for treatment

CLOXACILLIN

Indications. Mastitis, see notes above
Dose. See preparation details

PoM **Kloxerate™ QR** (Duphar)
Intramammary suspension, cloxacillin (as sodium salt) 200 mg/dose, for *cattle* 5-g dose applicator
Withdrawal Periods. *Cattle*: slaughter ' days, milk 60 hours
Dose. *Cattle*: *by intramammary infusion* one dose per infected quarter. Repeat twice at 12-hour intervals

PoM **Noroclox™ QR** (Norbrook)
Intramammary suspension, cloxacillin (as sodium salt) 200 mg/dose, for *cattle*; 5-g dose applicator
Withdrawal Periods. *Cattle*: slaughter 7 days, milk 60 hours
Dose. *Cattle*: *by intramammary infusion*, one dose per infected quarter. Repeat twice at 12-hour intervals

PoM **Orbenin™ LA** (SmithKline Beecham)
Intramammary suspension, cloxacillin (as sodium salt) 200 mg/dose, for *cattle, sheep*; 3-g dose applicator
Withdrawal Periods. *Cattle*: slaughter 7 days, milk 3.5 days
Dose. *Cattle*: *by intramammary infusion*, one dose per infected quarter. Repeat twice at 48-hour intervals
Sheep: *by intramammary infusion*, one dose per teat at weaning

PoM **Orbenin™ QR** (SmithKline Beecham)
Intramammary suspension, cloxacillin (as sodium salt) 200 mg/dose, for *cattle*; 3-g dose applicator
Withdrawal Periods. *Cattle*: slaughter 7 days, milk 60 hours
Dose. *Cattle*: *by intramammary infusion*, one dose per infected quarter. Repeat twice at 12-hour intervals

ERYTHROMYCIN

Indications. Mastitis, see notes above
Dose. See preparation details

PoM **Erythrocin™ Intramammary** (Sanofi)
Intramammary solution, erythromycin 300 mg/dose, for *cattle*; 6-mL dose applicator
Withdrawal Periods. *Cattle*: slaughter 7 days, milk 36 hours
Dose. *Cattle*: *by intramammary infusion*, one dose per infected quarter. Repeat twice at 12-hour intervals

OXYTETRACYCLINE HYDROCHLORIDE

Indications. Mastitis, see notes above
Dose. See preparation details

PoM **Oxymast™** (Bimeda)
Intramammary suspension (oily), oxytetracycline hydrochloride 500 mg/dose, for *cattle*; single-dose applicator

Withdrawal Periods. *Cattle*: slaughter 7 days, milk 72 hours
Dose. *Cattle*: *by intramammary infusion*, one dose per infected quarter every 12 hours as necessary after milking

PoM **Terramycin™** (Pfizer)
Intramammary solution, oxytetracycline hydrochloride (as magnesium complex) 426 mg/dose, for *cattle*; 14.2-g dose applicator
Withdrawal Periods. *Cattle*: slaughter 7 days, milk 72 hours
Dose. *Cattle*: *by intramammary infusion*, one dose per infected quarter daily for 3 days

PROCAINE PENICILLIN

Indications. Mastitis, see notes above
Dose. See preparation details

PoM **Mylipen™ QR** (Coopers Pitman-Moore)
Intramammary paste (oily), procaine penicillin 300 mg/dose, for *cattle*; single-dose applicator
Withdrawal Periods. *Cattle*: slaughter 4 days, milk 3.5 days
Dose. *Cattle*: *by intramammary infusion*, one dose per infected quarter. Repeat once after 48 hours

PoM **Pen-3-Mast™** (Bimeda)
Intramammary suspension (oily), procaine penicillin 300 mg/dose, for *cattle*; single-dose applicator
Withdrawal Periods. *Cattle*: slaughter 7 days, milk 72 hours
Dose. *Cattle*: *by intramammary infusion*, one dose per infected quarter every 12 hours as necessary after milking

COMPOUND ANTIBACTERIAL PREPARATIONS FOR LACTATING ANIMALS

PoM **Albacillin™** (Upjohn)
Intramammary suspension (oily), novobiocin (as sodium salt) 150 mg, procaine penicillin 100 mg/dose, for *cattle*; 10-mL dose applicator
Withdrawal Periods. *Cattle*: slaughter 7 days, milk 72 hours
Dose. *Cattle*: *by intramammary infusion*,

one dose per infected quarter daily for 2 days

PoM **Ampiclox™ Lactating Cow** (Smith-Kline Beecham)
Intramammary suspension, ampicillin (as sodium salt) 75 mg, cloxacillin (as sodium salt) 200 mg/dose, for *cattle*; 3-g dose applicator
Withdrawal Periods. *Cattle*: slaughter 7 days, milk 60 hours
Dose. *Cattle*: *by intramammary infusion*, one dose per infected quarter. Repeat twice at 12-hour intervals

PoM **Cloxamast™** (Bimeda)
Intramammary suspension, ampicillin (as sodium salt) 75 mg, cloxacillin (as sodium salt) 200 mg/dose, for *cattle*; 4.5-g dose applicator
Withdrawal Periods. *Cattle*: slaughter 7 days, milk 72 hours
Dose. *Cattle*: *by intramammary infusion*, one dose per infected quarter. Repeat twice at 12-hour intervals

PoM **Embacillin™ C** (RMB)
Intramammary suspension, ampicillin sodium 75 mg, cloxacillin sodium 200 mg/dose, for *cattle*; 5-g dose applicator
Withdrawal Periods. *Cattle*: slaughter 7 days, milk 60 hours
Dose. *Cattle*: *by intramammary infusion*, one dose per infected quarter. Repeat twice at 12-hour intervals

PoM **Kloxerate Plus™** (Duphar)
Intramammary suspension, ampicillin (as sodium salt) 75 mg, cloxacillin (as sodium salt) 200 mg/dose, for *cattle*; 5-g dose applicator
Withdrawal Periods. *Cattle*: slaughter 7 days, milk 60 hours
Dose. *Cattle*: *by intramammary infusion*, one dose per infected quarter. Repeat twice at 12-hour intervals

PoM **Lactaclox™** (Norbrook)
Intramammary suspension, ampicillin (as sodium salt) 75 mg, cloxacillin (as sodium salt) 200 mg/dose, for *cattle*; 5-g dose applicator
Withdrawal Periods. *Cattle*: slaughter 7 days, milk 60 hours
Dose. *Cattle*: *by intramammary infusion*, one dose per infected quarter. Repeat twice at 12-hour intervals

PoM **Lamoxin™** (Univet)
Intramammary suspension, ampicillin (as sodium salt) 75 mg, cloxacillin (as sodium salt) 200 mg/dose, for *cattle*; 5-g dose applicator
Withdrawal Periods. *Cattle*: slaughter 7 days, milk 60 hours
Dose. *Cattle*: *by intramammary infusion*, one dose per infected quarter. Repeat twice at 12-hour intervals

PoM **Nafpenzal™ MC** (Mycofarm)
Intramammary suspension, benzylpenicillin sodium 180 mg, dihydrostreptomycin (as sulphate) 100 mg, nafcillin (as sodium salt) 100 mg/dose, for *cattle*; 3-g dose applicator
Withdrawal Periods. *Cattle*: slaughter 7 days, milk 3.5 days
Dose. *Cattle*: *by intramammary infusion*, one dose per infected quarter daily for 3-4 days

PoM **Penstreptomast™** (Bimeda)
Intramammary suspension (oily), procaine penicillin 100 mg, streptomycin (as sulphate) 250 mg/dose, for *cattle*; single-dose applicator
Withdrawal Periods. *Cattle*: slaughter 7 days, milk 72 hours
Dose. *Cattle*: *by intramammary infusion*, one dose per infected quarter. Repeat at 12-hour intervals as necessary

PoM **Streptopen™ Milking Cow** (Coopers Pitman-Moore)
Intramammary suspension, dihydrostreptomycin (as sulphate) 500 mg, procaine penicillin 1 g/dose, for *cattle*; single-dose applicator
Withdrawal Periods. *Cattle*: slaughter 7 days, milk 4.5 days
Dose. *Cattle*: *by intramammary infusion*, one dose per infected quarter. Repeat twice at 12-hour intervals

PoM **Streptopen™ QR** (Coopers Pitman-Moore)
Intramammary paste (oily), dihydrostreptomycin (as sulphate) 100 mg, procaine penicillin 100 mg/dose, for *cattle*; single-dose applicator
Withdrawal Periods. *Cattle*: slaughter 7 days, milk 72 hours
Dose. *Cattle*: *by intramammary infusion*, one dose per infected quarter daily after milking for 3 days

PoM**Strypen™ Forte Rapid** (RMB)
Intramammary suspension, dihydro-streptomycin (as sulphate) 250 mg, procaine penicillin 300 mg/dose, for *cattle*; 5-mL dose applicator
Withdrawal Periods. *Cattle*: slaughter 7 days, milk 72 hours
Dose. *Cattle*: *by intramammary infusion*, one dose per infected quarter daily after milking for 3 days

PoM**Synermast™ Lactating Cow** (Virbac)
Intramammary suspension, ampicillin (as trihydrate) 200 mg, cloxacillin (as sodium salt) 200 mg/dose, for *cattle*; 10-mL dose applicator
Withdrawal Periods. *Cattle*: slaughter 2 days, milk 48 hours
Dose. *Cattle*: *by intramammary infusion*, one dose per infected quarter. Repeat twice at 12-hour intervals

PoM**Targot™** (Cyanamid)
Intramammary suspension (oily), chlortetracycline hydrochloride 200 mg, dihydrostreptomycin (as sulphate) 100 mg, neomycin (as sulphate) 100 mg/dose, for *cattle, sheep, goats*; 6-mL dose applicator
Withdrawal Periods. *Cattle*: slaughter 7 days, milk 4 days. *Sheep, goats*: slaughter 7 days
Dose. *Cattle, sheep, goats*: *by intramammary infusion*, one dose per infected quarter daily as necessary

PoM**Vonapen™ Milking Cow** (Intervet)
Intramammary paste, neomycin (as sulphate) 300 mg, procaine penicillin 500 mg/dose, for *cattle*; 6-g dose applicator
Withdrawal Periods. *Cattle*: slaughter 7 days, milk 72 hours
Dose. *Cattle*: *by intramammary infusion*, one dose per infected quarter daily for 3 days

Compound antibacterial preparations with corticosteroids for lactating animals

PoM**Aureomycin™ Mastitis Suspension** (Cyanamid)
Intramammary suspension, chlortetracycline hydrochloride 426 mg, hydrocortisone 2 mg/dose, for *cattle, sheep, goats*; 6-mL dose applicator

Withdrawal Periods. *Cattle*: slaughter 7 days, milk 4.5 days. *Sheep, goats*: slaughter 7 days
Dose. *Cattle, sheep, goats*: *by intramammary infusion*, one dose per infected quarter daily as necessary

PoM**Duphacerate™ Co** (Duphar)
Intramammary paste (oily), neomycin sulphate 100 mg, prednisolone 10 mg, procaine penicillin 100 mg, streptomycin sulphate 100 mg/dose, for *cattle*; 5-g dose applicator
Withdrawal Periods. *Cattle*: slaughter 7 days, milk 72 hours
Dose. *Cattle*: *by intramammary infusion*, one dose per infected quarter daily for 3 days

PoM**Leo Yellow Milking Cow™** (Leo)
Intramammary paste, dihydrostreptomycin (as sulphate) 150 mg, framycetin sulphate 50 mg, penethamate hydriodide 150 mg, prednisolone 5 mg/dose, for *cattle*; single-dose applicator
Withdrawal Periods. *Cattle*: slaughter 7 days, milk 3.5 days
Dose. *Cattle*: *by intramammary infusion*, one dose per infected quarter daily for 3 days

PoM**Multiject™ IMM** (Norbrook)
Intramammary paste (oily), neomycin sulphate 100 mg, prednisolone 10 mg, procaine penicillin 100 mg, streptomycin sulphate 100 mg/dose, for *cattle*; 5-g dose applicator
Withdrawal Periods. *Cattle*: slaughter 7 days, milk 72 hours
Dose. *Cattle*: *by intramammary infusion*, one dose per infected quarter daily for 3 days

PoM**Synulox™ Lactating Cow** (SmithKline Beecham)
Intramammary suspension (oily), co-amoxiclav 200/50 [amoxycillin (as trihydrate) 200 mg, clavulanic acid (as potassium salt) 50 mg] prednisolone 10 mg/dose, for *cattle*; 3-g dose applicator
Withdrawal Periods. *Cattle*: slaughter 7 days, milk 48 hours
Dose. *Cattle*: *by intramammary infusion*, one dose per infected quarter. Repeat twice at 12-hour intervals

PoM **Tetra-Delta**™ (Upjohn)
Intramammary suspension (oily), dihydrostreptomycin sulphate 125 mg, neomycin sulphate 150 mg, novobiocin (as sodium salt) 100 mg, prednisolone 10 mg, procaine penicillin 100 mg/dose, for *cattle*; 10-mL dose applicator
Withdrawal Periods. *Cattle*: slaughter 7 days, milk 72 hours
Dose. *Cattle*: *by intramammary infusion*, one dose per infected quarter. Repeat after 24 or 48 hours if required

11.1.2 Intramammary preparations for non-lactating animals

In non-lactating animals, therapy is used to eliminate subclinical infection present at the end of lactation, prevent summer mastitis, and treat other causes of mastitis.

Herd management plays a major part in the control of mastitis during the dry period. Non-lactating animals should be examined frequently. It is preferable to run these animals through the milking parlour twice a day so that the udders can be handled to ascertain that they are normal. An early case of mastitis detected at this time will respond to intramammary treatment. The head fly, *Hydrotoea irritans* may contribute to the spread of bacteria. This insect frequents shady areas, not flying more than 35 metres from these areas. Fly repellents (see section 2.2) will help to protect cows from fly bites.

Cloxacillin, erythromycin, novobiocin, and procaine penicillin are effective against mastitis caused by Gram-positive bacteria. Broad-spectrum antibacterial activity is achieved by preparations containing cephalosporins such as cefuroxime and cephalonium, and compound preparations. Details of antibacterial spectra of activity may be found in section 1.1.

The preparations are formulated with aluminium monostearate or in an oily basis, which may prolong effective tissue-antibacterial concentrations for up to several weeks. Therefore, these preparations should not be used in animals with a dry period of less than the duration of action of the preparation or in animals intended to calve within the effective drug duration. If calving does occur within the effective drug duration, milk should not be used for human consumption for this period and, in addition, for a specified time after calving. Milk should be withheld from the bulk supply until testing shows it to be free from antibacterial residues.

One dose is infused into each quarter immediately after the last milking before drying off. Teat dips or sprays containing disinfectants (see section 11.2) are then applied.

CEFUROXIME

Indications. Mastitis, see notes above
Contra-indications. Lactating animals, see notes above
Dose. *Cattle*: *by intramammary infusion*, one dose per quarter after the last milking before drying off

PoM **Spectrazol**™ **Dry Cow** (Coopers Pitman-Moore)
Intramammary paste, cefuroxime (as sodium salt) 375 mg/dose, for *cattle*; 3-g dose applicator
Withdrawal Periods. *Cattle*: slaughter 7 days, milk not less than 21 days after administration and 4 days after calving

CEPHALONIUM

Indications. Mastitis, see notes above
Contra-indications. Lactating animals, see notes above
Dose. *Cattle*: *by intramammary infusion*, one dose per quarter after the last milking before drying off

PoM **Cepravin**™ **Dry Cow** (Coopers Pitman-Moore)
Intramammary paste, cephalonium 250 mg/dose, for *cattle*; 3-g dose applicator
Withdrawal Periods. *Cattle*: slaughter 21 days, milk not less than 51 days after administration and 4 days after calving

CLOXACILLIN

Indications. Mastitis, see notes above
Contra-indications. Lactating animals, see notes above
Dose. *Cattle*: *by intramammary infusion*, one dose per quarter after the last milking before drying off

PoM **Cloxacillin 1000DC**™ (Virbac)
Intramammary suspension, cloxacillin (as benzathine salt) 1 g/dose with aluminium monostearate, for *cattle*; 10-mL dose applicator
Withdrawal Periods. *Cattle*: slaughter 30 days, milk not less 28 days after administration and 4 days after calving

PoM **Embaclox**™ **Dry Cow** (RMB)
Intramammary suspension, cloxacillin (as benzathine salt) 500 mg/dose with aluminium monostearate, for *cattle*; 4.5-g dose applicator
Withdrawal Periods. *Cattle*: slaughter 28days, milk not less than 28 days after administration and 60 hours after calving

PoM **Kloxerate**™ **DC** (Duphar)
Intramammary suspension, cloxacillin (as benzathine salt) 500 mg/dose with aluminium monostearate, for *cattle*; 4.5-g dose applicator
Withdrawal Periods. *Cattle*: slaughter 28 days, milk not less than 28 days after administration and 60 hours after calving

PoM **Noroclox**™ **DC** (Norbrook)
Intramammary suspension, cloxacillin (as benzathine salt) 500 mg/dose with aluminium monostearate, for *cattle*; 4.5-g dose applicator
Withdrawal Periods. *Cattle*: slaughter 28 days, milk not less than 28 days after administration and 60 hours after calving

PoM **Orbenin**™ **Dry Cow** (SmithKline Beecham)
Intramammary suspension, cloxacillin (as benzathine salt) 500 mg/dose with aluminium monostearate, for *cattle*; 3-g dose applicator
Withdrawal Periods. *Cattle*: slaughter 28 days, milk not less than 28 days after administration and 4 days after calving

PoM **Orbenin**™ **Extra Dry Cow** (Smith-Kline Beecham)
Intramammary suspension (oily), cloxacillin (as benzathine salt) 600 mg/dose, for *cattle*; 3.6-g dose applicator
Withdrawal Periods. *Cattle*: slaughter 28 days, milk not less than 42 days after administration and 4 days after calving

ERYTHROMYCIN

Indications. Mastitis, during the dry and lactating period

PoM **Erythrocin**™ **Intramammary** (Sanofi)
See section 11.1.1 for preparation details
Dose. *Cattle*: *by intramammary infusion*, one dose per infected quarter every 12 hours for 3 consecutive infusions

NOVOBIOCIN

Indications. Mastitis, see notes above
Contra-indications. Lactating animals, see notes above
Dose. *Cattle*: *by intramammary infusion*, one dose per quarter after the last milking before drying off

PoM **Albadry**™ (Upjohn)
Intramammary suspension (oily), novobiocin (as sodium salt) 400 mg/dose, for *cattle*; 10-mL dose applicator
Withdrawal Periods. *Cattle*: slaughter 10 days, milk not less than 14 days after administration

PROCAINE PENICILLIN

Indications. Mastitis, see notes above
Contra-indications. Lactating animals, see notes above
Dose. *Cattle*: *by intramammary infusion*, one dose per quarter after the last milking before drying off

PoM **Mylipen**™ **Dry Cow** (Coopers Pitman-Moore)
Intramammary paste (oily), procaine penicillin 300 mg/dose, for *cattle*; single-dose applicator
Withdrawal Periods. *Cattle*: slaughter 10

days, milk not less than 28 days after administration and 4 days after calving

COMPOUND ANTIBACTERIAL PREPARATIONS FOR NON-LACTATING ANIMALS

PoM **Ampiclox™ Dry Cow** (SmithKline Beecham)
Intramammary suspension (oily), ampicillin (as trihydrate) 250 mg, cloxacillin (as benzathine salt) 500 mg/dose, for *cattle*; 3-g dose applicator
Withdrawal Periods. *Cattle*: slaughter 28 days, milk not less than 7 days after administration and 4 days after calving
Dose. *Cattle*: prophylaxis, *by intramammary infusion*, one dose per quarter after the last milking before drying off
Summer mastitis, repeat dose every 3 weeks during the dry period

PoM **Bovaclox™ DC (Dry Cow)** (Norbrook)
Intramammary suspension, ampicillin (as trihydrate) 250 mg, cloxacillin (as benzathine salt) 500 mg/dose with aluminium monostearate, for *cattle*; 4.5-g dose applicator
Withdrawal Periods. *Cattle*: slaughter 28 days, milk not less than 30 days after administration and 4 days after calving
Dose. *Cattle*: prophylaxis, *by intramammary infusion*, one dose per quarter after the last milking before drying off
Summer mastitis, repeat dose every 3 weeks during the dry period

PoM **Depomycin™ Dry Cow** (Mycofarm)
Intramammary suspension, dihydro-streptomycin (as sulphate) 100 mg, procaine penicillin 300 mg/dose, for *cattle*; 3-g dose applicator
Withdrawal Periods. *Cattle*: slaughter 28 days, milk not less than 28 days after administration and 4.5 days after calving
Dose. *Cattle*: *by intramammary infusion*, one dose per quarter after the last milking before drying off, repeat after 3-4 weeks

PoM **Embacillin™ C Dry Cow** (RMB)
Intramammary suspension, ampicillin (as trihydrate) 250 mg, cloxacillin (as benzathine salt) 500 mg/dose with aluminium monostearate, for *cattle*; 4.5-g dose applicator

Withdrawal Periods. *Cattle*: slaughter 28 days, milk not less than 30 days after administration and 4 days after calving
Dose. *Cattle*: prophylaxis, *by intramammary infusion*, one dose per quarter after the last milking before drying off
Summer mastitis, repeat dose every 3 weeks during the dry period

PoM **Ilcocillin™ Dry Cow** (Ciba-Geigy)
Intramammary suspension, dihydro-streptomycin (as sulphate) 1 g, procaine penicillin 1 g/dose, for *cattle*; 10-mL dose applicator
Withdrawal Periods. *Cattle*: slaughter 28 days, milk not less than 28 days after administration and 4.5 days after calving
Dose. *Cattle*: *by intramammary infusion*, one dose per quarter after the last milking before drying off

PoM **Kloxerate Plus DC™ (Dry Cow)** (Duphar)
Intramammary suspension, ampicillin (as trihydrate) 250 mg, cloxacillin (as benzathine salt) 500 mg/dose with aluminium monostearate, for *cattle*; 4.5-g dose applicator
Withdrawal Periods. *Cattle*: slaughter 28 days, milk not less than 30 days after administration and 4 days after calving
Dose. *Cattle*: prophylaxis, *by intramammary infusion*, one dose per quarter after the last milking before drying off
Summer mastitis, repeat dose every 3 weeks during the dry period

PoM **Lamoxin™ (Dry Cow)** (Univet)
Intramammary suspension, ampicillin (as trihydrate) 250 mg, cloxacillin (as benzathine salt) 500 mg/dose with aluminium monostearate, for *cattle*; 4.5-g single-dose applicator
Withdrawal Periods. *Cattle*: slaughter 28 days, milk not less than 7 days after administration and 4 days after calving
Dose. *Cattle*: prophylaxis, *by intramammary infusion*, one dose per quarter after the last milking before drying off
Summer mastitis, repeat dose every 3 weeks during the dry period

PoM **Leo Red Dry Cow™** (Leo)
Intramammary paste, framycetin sulphate 100 mg, penethamate hydriodide 100 mg, procaine penicillin

300 mg/dose, for *cattle*; single-dose applicator
Withdrawal Periods. *Cattle*: slaughter 28 days, milk not less than 28 days after administration and 3.5 days after calving
Dose. *Cattle*: *by intramammary infusion*, one dose per quarter after the last milking before drying off

PoM **Nafpenzal**™ **Dry Cow** (Mycofarm)
Intramammary suspension, dihydro-streptomycin (as sulphate) 100 mg, nafcillin (as sodium salt) 100 mg, procaine penicillin 300 mg/dose, for *cattle*; 3-g dose applicator
Withdrawal Periods. *Cattle*: slaughter 28 days, milk not less than 28 days after administration and 4.5 days after calving
Dose. *Cattle*: *by intramammary infusion*, one dose per quarter after the last milking before drying off

PoM **Novomast DC**™ (Bimeda)
Intramammary suspension (oily), novo-biocin (as sodium salt) 250 mg, procaine penicillin 300 mg/dose, for *cattle*; single-dose applicator
Withdrawal Periods. *Cattle*: slaughter 28 days, milk not less than 28 days after administration and 96 hours after calving
Dose. *Cattle*: *by intramammary infusion*, one dose per quarter after the last milking before drying off, repeat in the second half of the dry period

PoM **Streptopen**™ **Dry Cow** (Coopers Pitman-Moore)
Intramammary paste (oily), dihydro-streptomycin (as sulphate) 500 mg, procaine penicillin 1 g/dose, for *cattle, sheep*; single-dose applicator
Withdrawal Periods. *Cattle*: slaughter 10 days, milk not less than 32 days after administration and 4 days after calving.
Sheep: slaughter 10 days
Dose. *Cattle*: *by intramammary infusion*, one dose per quarter after the last milking before drying off, repeat after 3-4 weeks
Sheep: *by intramammary infusion*, ½ dose per udder half not more than 2 weeks after weaning

PoM **Tetra-Delta**™ **Dry Cow** (Upjohn)
Intramammary suspension (oily), novo-biocin (as sodium salt) 400 mg, procaine

penicillin 200 mg/dose, for *cattle*; 10-mL dose applicator
Withdrawal Periods. *Cattle*: slaughter 30 days, milk not less than 30 days after administration and 3.5 days after calving
Dose. *Cattle*: *by intramammary infusion*, one dose per quarter after the last milking before drying off

PoM **Vonapen**™ **Dry Cow** (Intervet)
Intramammary suspension, benzylpenicillin potassium 314 mg, neomycin 500 mg, procaine penicillin 1 g/dose, for *cattle*; 9-g dose applicator
Withdrawal Periods. *Cattle*: slaughter 28 days, milk not less than 35 days after administration
Dose. *Cattle*: *by intramammary infusion*, one dose per quarter after the last milking before drying off

Compound antibacterial preparations with corticosteroids for non-lactating animals

PoM **Neobiotic**™ **Dry Cow** (Upjohn)
Intramammary suspension (oily), hydrocortisone acetate 20 mg, hydrocortisone sodium succinate 12.5 mg, neomycin sulphate 500 mg/dose, for *cattle*; 10-mL dose applicator
Withdrawal Periods. *Cattle*: slaughter 28 days, milk not less than 28 days after administration and 4 days after calving
Dose. *Cattle*: *by intramammary infusion*, one dose per quarter after the last milking before drying off, repeat after 2 days if required

11.2 Preparations for the care of teats and udders

The care and hygiene of udders and teats are important factors in mastitis control. Proper maintenance of the milking machine to avoid pressure variations which may lead to teat damage, and disinfection of the machine to reduce contamination from cow to cow are essential. Hygiene in the milking parlour and housing cubicles as well as the use of skin disinfectants will reduce the population of pathogenic micro-organisms.
Before milking, udders should be

cleaned with individual dry paper tissues or disinfectant-impregnated towels to remove excess contamination. Only in cases where the udders are obviously contaminated with mud or faeces is it necessary to wash the teats with a disinfectant diluted to be used as an udderwash. The udder and teats should be dried thoroughly before applying teat cups. Post-milking disinfectants help to reduce the bacterial population on the teats and assist abrasions to heal. They are applied after every milking during lactation and after the final milking before drying off.

Cetrimide, chlorhexidine, and **polyhexanide** are effective against Gram-positive and Gram-negative bacteria. These disinfectants are inactivated by soaps and anionic substances. **Glutaraldehyde** is effective against Gram-positive and Gram-negative bacteria, although concentrated solutions may cause dermatitis. **Iodophores** have broad-spectrum antibacterial activity.

Preparations for udder and teat hygiene are formulated as dips, sprays, or udderwashes, which may require dilution before use. Glycerol, hydrous wool fat (lanolin), white and yellow soft paraffin, and sorbitol are added to preparations to promote skin hydration, to soften skin, and allow lesions to heal. Emollients (see section 14.2) may be applied to dry teats immediately after milking. In the case of suckler cows, the calf should be kept away from the cow for at least an hour after application. Other preparations used for skin sores and wounds may also be applied to teats and udders (see section 14.2).

CETRIMIDE

Indications. Cleaning and disinfection of udder and teats
Contra-indications. Concurrent use of soaps and anionic substances
Warnings. Do not contaminate ponds, waterways, ditches with disinfectants. Avoid contact of product with eyes and do not use internally

GSL **Capritect**™ (Goat Nutrition)
Cream, cetrimide 1%; 454 g

GSL **Cetrex**™ (Univet)
Cream, cetrimide 2%, 450 g

GSL **Cetriad**™ (Duphar)
Cream, cetrimide 2%, 450 g

GSL **Strepolene**™ (Crown)
Cream, cetrimide 0.5%, for *cattle*; 500 g, 2 kg

GSL **Udder Cream** (Alfa Laval)
Cetrimide 0.5%; 1.2 kg, 3.5 kg

GSL **Udder Cream** (Battle Hayward & Bower)
Cetrimide 0.5%, for *cattle, goats*; 250 g, 400 g, other sizes available

GSL **Vanodine**™ **Udder Cream** (Evans Vanodine)
Cetrimide 2%, 4 kg
Withdrawal Periods. *Cattle*: slaughter withdrawal period nil, milk withdrawal period nil

CHLORHEXIDINE

Indications. Contra-indications. Warnings. See under Cetrimide

GSL **Alfa Blue Plus** (Alfa Laval)
Teat dip or spray, chlorhexidine gluconate 0.425%, glycerol 2%, isopropyl alcohol 3.16%, sorbitol 5.6%; 25 litres

GSL **Alfa Red +** (Alfa Laval)
Teat dip or spray, chlorhexidine gluconate 0.425%, glycerol 2%, isopropyl alcohol 3.16%, sorbitol 5.6%; 25 litres

GSL **Blue**™ **Dip** (Deosan)
Teat dip, spray, or udderwash, Chlorhexidine Gluconate Solution BP 10.5% (=chlorhexidine gluconate 2.1%), glycerol 35%; 5 litres
Teat dip or spray. Dilute 1 volume with 4 volumes water
Udderwash. Dilute 3 mL in 1 litre water

GSL **C-Dip**™ (Kilco)
Teat dip or spray, chlorhexidine gluconate 0.5%, glycerol, hydrous wool fat, for *cattle*; 25 litres, 200 litres

GSL **Elite Chlorhexidine Teat Dip** (Dalgety)
Teat dip, spray, or udderwash, chlorhexidine 0.5%, glycerol, for *cattle*
Teat dip or spray. Use undiluted
Udderwash. Dilute 1 volume in 80 volumes water

GSL **Hibitex**™ (Coopers Pitman-Moore)
Teat dip or spray, Chlorhexidine Gluconate Solution BP 3.75% (=chlorhexidine gluconate 0.75%), for *cattle*; 5 litres (N. Ireland only), 25 litres

GSL **Summer Teatcare Plus**™ (Deosan)
Teat dip or spray, chlorhexidine gluconate 0.425%, glycerol, fly repellents, for *cattle*; 25 litres

GSL **Superspray**™ (Ciba-Geigy)
Teat dip or spray, chlorhexidine gluconate 0.425%, glycerol 7%, for *cattle*; 25 litres, 200 litres

GSL **Teatcare**™ (Deosan)
Teat dip or spray, chlorhexidine gluconate 0.425%, glycerol, sorbitol, hydrous wool fat, for *cattle*; 25 litres, 200 litres

GSL **Teatcare Plus**™ (Deosan)
Teat dip or spray, chlorhexidine gluconate 0.425%, glycerol, for *cattle*; 25 litres, 200 litres

GSL **Teat-Ex**™ (Deosan)
Teat dip or spray, chlorhexidine gluconate 0.425%, glycerol, sorbitol, for *cattle*; 25 litres

GSL **Uddercare**™ (Deosan)
Udderwash, Chlorhexidine Gluconate Solution BP 4% (=chlorhexidine gluconate 0.8%), sorbitol; 25 litres
Dilute 6 mL in 1 litre water

GSL **Uddercream** (Deosan)
Chlorhexidine 2%, hydrous wool fat; 250 g, 2 kg

GLUTARALDEHYDE

Indications. Cleaning and disinfection of teats and udders
Side-effects. Concentrated solutions may cause dermatitis
Warnings. See under Cetrimide

GSL **Leo Yellow Super Dip** (Leo)
Teat dip or spray, glutaraldehyde 1.5%, glycerol, hydrous wool fat, for *cattle, sheep, goats*; 200 mL, 5 litres
Dilute 1 volume with 4 volumes water

IODINE COMPOUNDS

Indications. Cleaning and disinfection of teats and udders

GSL **Coopercare**™ **1** (Coopers Pitman-Moore)
Teat dip, spray, or udderwash, available iodine 2%, glycerol, sorbitol, for *cattle*; 25 litres
Teat dip or spray. Dilute 1 volume with 3 volumes water
Udderwash. Dilute 2 mL in 1 litre water

GSL **Coopercare**™ **3** (Coopers Pitman-Moore)
Teat dip or spray, available iodine 1.5%, glycerol, sorbitol, for *cattle*; 8.33 litres
Dilute 1 volume with 2 volumes water

GSL **Dipal Concentrate** (Alfa Laval)
Teat dip, spray, or udderwash, available iodine 1.5%, glycerol; 10 litres, 25 litres

GSL **Elite Iodine Teat Dip: Concentrate** (Dalgety)
Teat dip, spray, or udderwash, available iodine 1.5%, glycerol, for *cattle*; 5 litres
Teat dip or spray. Dilute 1 volume with 3 volumes water
Udderwash. Dilute 1 volume in 500 volumes water

GSL **Elite Iodine Teat Dip: Ready to use** (Dalgety)
Teat dip, spray, or udderwash, available iodine 0.5%, sorbitol, for *cattle*; 25 litres
Teat dip or spray. Use undiluted
Udderwash. Dilute 1 volume with 80 volumes water

GSL **Elite Udder Salve** (Dalgety)
Ointment, available iodine 0.2%; 2 kg

GSL **Iodo-Care Concentrate**™ (Deosan)
Teat dip, spray, or udderwash, available iodine 2%, glycerol, sorbitol, for *cattle*; 25 litres
Teat dip or spray. Dilute 1 volume with 3 volumes water
Udder wash. Dilute 2 mL in 1 litre water

GSL **Iodophor Udderwash**™ (Deosan)
Available iodine 1.6%; 25 litres
Dilute 3.3 mL in 1 litre water

GSL **Iosan**™ **CCT** (Ciba-Geigy)
Teat dip, spray, or udderwash, available iodine 1.6%, for *cattle*; 10 litres, 25 litres
Teat dip or spray. Dilute 1 volume with 2 volumes water
Udderwash. Dilute 6.25 mL in 1 litre water

GSL **Iosan™ Superdip** (Ciba-Geigy)
Teat dip, spray, or udderwash, available iodine 0.5%, glycerol, for *cattle*; 25 litres, 200 litres
Teat dip or spray. Use undiluted
Udderwash. Dilute 18.75 mL in 1 litre water

GSL **Iosan™ Teat Dip** (Ciba-Geigy)
Teat dip, spray, or udderwash, available iodine 1.55%, glycerol, for *cattle*; 5 litres, 25 litres, 200 litres
Teat dip or spray. Dilute 1 volume with 2 volumes water
Udderwash. Dilute 6.25 mL in 1 litre water

GSL **Lanodip Readymix™** (Kilco)
Teat dip, spray, or udderwash, available iodine 0.53%, hydrous wool fat, for *cattle*; 25 litres, 200 litres

GSL **Lanodip Readymix Gold™** (Kilco)
Teat dip, spray, or udderwash, available iodine 0.5%, hydrous wool fat, for *cattle*; 25 litres, 200 litres

GSL **Lanodip Super Concentrate** (Kilco)
Teat dip, spray, or udderwash, available iodine 2%, hydrous wool fat, for *cattle*; 5 litres, 25 litres
Dilute 1 volume with 3 volumes water

GSL **Masocare™** (Evans Vanodine)
Teat dip or spray, available iodine 0.5%, glycerol, sorbitol, for *cattle*; 25 litres, 200 litres
Withdrawal Periods. *Cattle*: slaughter withdrawal period nil, milk withdrawal period nil

GSL **Masodine™ 1:3** (Evans Vanodine)
Teat dip or spray, available iodine 2%, glycerol, sorbitol, for *cattle*; 5 litres, 25 litres, other sizes available
Withdrawal Periods. *Cattle*: slaughter withdrawal period nil, milk withdrawal period nil
Dilute 1 volume with 3 volumes water

GSL **Masodine™ RTU** (Evans Vanodine)
Teat dip or spray, iodine 0.5%, sorbitol, glycerol, for *cattle*; 25 litres, 60 litres, 200 litres
Withdrawal Periods. *Cattle*: slaughter withdrawal period nil, milk withdrawal period nil

GSL **Masodine™ Udder Wash** (Evans Vanodine)
Glycerol, iodophore, sorbitol, for *cattle*; 5 litres, 25 litres, 200 litres
Withdrawal Periods. *Cattle*: slaughter withdrawal period nil, milk withdrawal period nil
Dilute 1 volume in 500 volumes water

GSL **Novatex™** (IndChemNI)
Teat dip, iodophore, for *cattle*; 5 litres, 25 litres
Dilute 1 volume with 3 volumes water

GSL **Orbisan™ Forte** (SmithKline Beecham)
This preparation is now discontinued

GSL **Ready-Dip™** (Deosan)
Teat dip or spray, available iodine 0.5%, glycerol, sorbitol, for *cattle*; 25 litres

GSL **Super Ex-Cel™** (Deosan)
Teat dip or spray, available iodine 0.5%, glycerol, sorbitol, for *cattle*; 25 litres, 200 litres

GSL **Super Iodip™** (Deosan)
Teat dip, spray, or udderwash, available iodine 2%, glycerol, sorbitol, for *cattle*; 5 litres, 25 litres
Teat dip. Dilute 1 volume with 3 volumes water
Teat spray. Dilute 1 volume with 4 volumes water
Udderwash. Dilute 3.5 mL in 1 litre water

GSL **T-Dip** (Alfa Laval)
Teat dip, spray, or udderwash, available iodine 0.5%, glycerol, for *cattle*; 25 litres
Teat dip or spray. Use undiluted
Udderwash. Dilute 18.75 mL in 1 litre water

GSL **T-Spray** (Alfa Laval)
Teat spray, available iodine 0.5%, glycerol, for *cattle*; 25 litres

GSL **Theratec (surge)** (Babson)
Teat dip or spray, available iodine 0.5%, 25 litres

GSL **Vanodine™ Uddersalve** (Evans Vanodine)
Ointment, iodine 0.2%, for *cattle*; 4 kg
Withdrawal Periods. *Cattle*: slaughter

withdrawal period nil, milk withdrawal period nil

POLYHEXANIDE

Indications. Contra-indications. Warnings. See under Cetrimide

GSL **Sapphire**™ (Evans Vanodine)
Teat dip or spray, polyhexanide 0.5%, glycerol, for *cattle*; 25 litres
Withdrawal Periods. *Cattle*: slaughter withdrawal period nil, milk withdrawal period nil

SODIUM HYPOCHLORITE

Indications. Warnings. See under Cetrimide

GSL **Uddersan** (Alfa Laval)
Udderwash, available chlorine (as sodium hypochlorite) 4.2%; 10 litres
Dilute 16 mL in 1 litre water

OTHER PREPARATIONS FOR THE CARE OF TEATS AND UDDERS

GSL **Antiseptic Teat Ointment** (Arnolds)
Phenol 0.5%, wool fat 8.5%, zinc oxide 7%; 500 g, 4 kg

GSL **Blu-Gard** (Ecolab)
Teat dip or spray, dodecylbenzene-sulphonic acid 1-2%, for *cattle*; 5 litres, 20 litres

GSL **Blu-Gard Towels** (Ecolab)
Non-woven fibre, impregnated with benzalkonium chloride 7.7%, polyhexanide 3.3%, for *cattle*; 24 towels

GSL **Coopercare**™ **2** (Coopers Pitman-Moore)
Teat dip or spray, chlorhexidine 1.7%, quaternary ammonium compound 0.45%, sorbitol, for *cattle*; 2.5 litres
Dilute 1 volume with 9 volumes water

Cow Salve (Battle Hayward & Bower)
Ointment, boric acid 11%, yellow soft paraffin 87.5%; 200 g, 450 g, other sizes available

GSL **Fectan**™ (Ciba-Geigy)
Teat dip or spray, powder for reconstitution, benzalkonium chloride complex 1.52%, polyhexanide 3.82%, for *cattle*; 3.3 kg
Reconstitute 3.3 kg powder in 25 litres water (=benzalkonium chloride complex 0.2%, polyhexanide 0.5%)

GSL **Golden Udder** (Shep-Fair)
Ointment, salicylic acid 1.5%, sulphur 10%, for *cattle*, *sheep*, *goats*; 360 g, 1 kg

GSL **Leo Yellow Teat Ointment** (Leo)
Colophony, industrial methylated spirit, wool fat, yellow beeswax, yellow soft paraffin, zinc oleostearate, for *cattle*; 400 g, 2.75 kg

GSL **Masodip**™ (Evans Vanodine)
Teat dip or spray, benzalkonium chloride, chlorhexidine, glycerol, sorbitol, for *cattle*; 25 litres, 200 litres
Withdrawal Periods. *Cattle*: slaughter withdrawal period nil, milk withdrawal period nil

PML **Variola**™ **Salve** (Bimeda)
Ointment, diacetylaminoazotoluene 2%, lignocaine 1%, yellow soft paraffin 97%, for *cattle*; 200 g

12 Drugs acting on the

EYE

12.1 Administration of drugs to the eye

Many owners have difficulty in administering eye drops and eye ointments to animals and therefore the procedure should always be demonstrated to them. Eye drops should be instilled into the lower conjunctival sac. Eye ointment should be applied into the conjunctival fornix inside the lower lid by everting the lid with the index finger or thumb. The softer eye ointments may be put onto the cornea but owners may be afraid of injuring the eye. Eye drops are easy to use in dogs and cats, but eye ointments are probably easier to use in larger species such as horses. Some antibacterial drugs are formulated as topical powders for use in eye disorders including New Forest Disease in cattle. Eye drops generally require frequent application in order to achieve acceptable ocular and intra-ocular concentrations, as rapid elimination of solutions will occur from the conjunctival sac after dilution with tears. When 2 different eye drop formulations are to be administered, there should be an interval of at least 5 minutes between applications to avoid dilution and overflow. Eye ointments have a longer contact time resulting in higher ocular and intra-ocular drug concentrations and thereby necessitating less frequent application. Eye ointments may be preferred for night-time treatment.

The frequency of administration of eye drops or eye ointment depends on the type and severity of the disease. The absorption and effect of a drug used topically may be dependent upon the inflamed or diseased state of the conjunctival and corneal epithelium.

Preparations for the eye contain suitable preservatives and provided that contamination is avoided they may be used for about one month, after which a new container should be opened, if treatment is to be continued, and the old one discarded.

Subconjunctival injections may be carried out in all species following the topical administration of 1 or 2 drops of a local anaesthetic. The drug should be placed under the bulbar conjunctiva rather than the palpebral conjunctiva. Volumes of injectable solutions used are approximately 0.5 mL for dogs and cats, and up to 1 mL for horses and cattle.

Subpalpebral lavage systems, ocular inserts, and contact lenses have all been used with success in veterinary ophthalmology.

Systemic therapy may be undertaken in conjunction with topical therapy in cases of severe intra-ocular infection.

12.2 Anti-infective eye preparations

12.2.1 Antibacterial preparations
12.2.2 Antifungal preparations
12.2.3 Antiviral preparations

Care should be taken to distinguish superficial ocular disease caused by infections from other conditions that may result in a red or inflamed eye. A stained smear preparation may be useful. Where possible the causative organism should be identified and any initial choice of a broad-spectrum antibiotic, or combination of antibiotics, modified according to sensitivity data. The severity of an infection may determine the choice of drug and frequency of application. Where possible, antibiotics likely to be useful systemically should be avoided. Primary bacterial conjunctivitis is usually acute and corticosteroids are unnecessary. The normal conjunctival flora of the dog consists of a number of species whereas the cat conjunctiva is relatively sterile.

Where only one eye is involved, it may be appropriate to apply the chosen preparation to the other eye, before treating the infected side, to minimise the possibility of cross-infection.

12.2.1 Antibacterial preparations

Bacterial infections of the eye in animals are generally due to *Staphylococcus*, *Streptococcus*, *Bacillus*, *Actinobacillus*, *Chlamydia*, *Moraxella*, *Micrococcus*, or *Clostridium* species. Ocular infections usually present as conjunctivitis, blepharitis, keratitis, or keratoconjunctivitis. **Neomycin** has a broad spectrum of activity, which includes *Proteus*, but its corneal penetration is poor. **Cloxacillin** has been shown to persist in the eye for many hours and is appropriate for the treatment of New Forest Disease in cattle and contagious ophthalmia in sheep. **Chloramphenicol** combines a broad spectrum of activity with lipid solubility and hence is particularly useful for intra-ocular infections. **Gentamicin sulphate** is often used together with **acetylcysteine** (see section 12.6) and **atropine sulphate** (see section 12.4) in the treatment of collagenase ulcers. The **sulphonamides** are bacteriostatic and may also be active against *Toxoplasma*. The use of compound preparations containing an antibiotic and a corticosteroid requires careful judgement and the potential deleterious effects of corticosteroids (see section 12.3) should always be taken into account.

Subconjunctival injections may be advantageous. Chloramphenicol sodium succinate has been given by this route.

CEPHALONIUM

Indications. Bacterial eye infections
Dose. *Cattle*: apply as a single dose, repeat after 2-3 days as necessary
Dogs: apply as a single dose, repeat daily as necessary

PoM **Cepravin**™ (Coopers Pitman-Moore)
Eye ointment, cephalonium 8%, for *cattle*, *dogs*; 2 g
Withdrawal Periods. *Cattle*: slaughter withdrawal period nil, milk withdrawal period nil

CHLORAMPHENICOL

Indications. Bacterial eye infections, see notes above
Dose. *Eye drops or ointment*, apply up to 8 times daily for at least 2 days
By subconjunctival injection, 100-200 mg (0.5-1.0 mL) of a 20% solution into bulbar subconjuntival tissue

PoM **Chloromycetin**™ **Succinate Injection** (Parke-Davis)
See section 1.1.5 for preparation details
PoM **Chloromycetin**™ **Ophthalmic Ointment** (Parke-Davis)
Eye ointment, chloramphenicol 1%; 4 g
Withdrawal Periods. Slaughter withdrawal period nil, milk from treated animals should not be used for human consumption

PoM **Chloromycetin**™ **Redidrops** (Parke-Davis)
Eye drops, chloramphenicol 0.5%, for *dogs*, *cats*; 5 mL, 10 mL

CHLORTETRACYCLINE HYDROCHLORIDE

Indications. Bacterial eye infections

PoM **Aureomycin**™ **Ophthalmic Ointment** (Cyanamid)
Eye ointment, chlortetracycline hydrochloride 1%; 3.5 g
Dose. Apply every 2 hours or more frequently according to severity of condition

PoM **Aureomycin™ Topical Powder** (Cyanamid)
See section 14.2.1 for preparation details

PoM **PEP™** (Intervet)
See section 14.2.1 for preparation details

CLOXACILLIN

Indications. Bacterial eye infections, see notes above

PoM **Orbenin™** (SmithKline Beecham)
Eye ointment, cloxacillin (as benzathine salt) 16.7% with aluminium monostearate, for *horses*, *cattle*, *sheep*, *dogs*, *cats*; 3 g
Dose. *Horses*: apply as a single dose, repeat daily as necessary
Cattle, *sheep*: apply as a single dose, repeat after 2-3 days as necessary
Dogs, *cats*: apply as a single dose, repeat daily as necessary

PoM **Opticlox™** (Norbrook)
Eye ointment, cloxacillin (as benzathine salt) 16.7%, for *horses*, *cattle*, *sheep*, *dogs*, *cats*; 5 g
Withdrawal Periods. *Cattle*, *sheep*: slaughter withdrawal period nil, milk withdrawal period nil
Dose. *Horses*, *cattle*, *sheep*, *dogs*, *cats*: apply as a single dose, repeat after 2-3 days as necessary

FRAMYCETIN SULPHATE

Indications. Bacterial eye infections
Dose. *Eye drops*, apply 3 times daily
Eye ointment, apply 3 times daily

PoM **Framycetin Sulphate** (Non-proprietary)
Eye drops, framycetin sulphate 0.5%; 5 mL
Eye ointment, framycetin sulphate 0.5%; 3.5 g

GENTAMICIN SULPHATE

Indications. Bacterial eye infections, see notes above
Dose: *Eye drops*, apply 3-4 times daily
Eye ointment, apply 3-4 times daily

PoM **Cidomycin™** (Roussel)
Drops (eye drops or ear drops), gentamicin (as sulphate) 0.3%; 8 mL
Eye ointment, gentamicin (as sulphate) 0.3%; 3 g

PoM **Garamycin™** (Schering-Plough)
Drops (eye drops or ear drops), gentamicin (as sulphate) 0.3%; 10 mL

PoM **Genticin™** (Nicholas)
Eye drops, gentamicin (as sulphate) 0.3%; 10 mL
Eye ointment, gentamicin (as sulphate) 0.3%; 3 g

PoM **Minims™ Gentamicin** (S&N Pharm.)
Eye drops, gentamicin (as sulphate) 0.3%; 0.5 mL

NEOMYCIN SULPHATE

Indications. Bacterial eye infections, see notes above
Dose. Apply 2-4 times daily

PoM **Neobiotic™** (Upjohn)
Eye ointment, neomycin sulphate 0.5%; 3.9 g

SULPHACETAMIDE SODIUM

Indications. Bacterial eye infections, see notes above
Dose. *Dogs*, *cats*: apply 3-4 times daily

PoM **Albucid™** (Nicholas)
Eye drops, sulphacetamide sodium 10%; 10 mL

PoM **Minims™ Sulphacetamide Sodium** (S&N Pharm.)
Eye drops, sulphacetamide sodium 10%; 0.5 mL

TOBRAMYCIN

Indications. Bacterial eye infections
Dose. Apply 3-6 times daily

PoM **Tobralex™** (Alcon)
Eye drops, tobramycin 0.3%; 5 mL

COMPOUND ANTIBACTERIAL PREPARATIONS

PoM **Biophth™ LA** (Mycofarm)
Eye ointment, dihydrostreptomycin (as sulphate) 3.3%, procaine penicillin 10%, for *cattle*, *sheep*; 3 g
Withdrawal Periods. *Cattle*, *sheep*: slaughter withdrawal period nil, milk withdrawal period nil
Dose. *Cattle*, *sheep*: apply as a single

dose, repeat at 2-3 day intervals as necessary

12.2.2 Antifungal preparations

Ocular fungal infections may be superficial such as mycotic keratitis, or endogenous such as mycotic endophthalmitis. Mycotic keratitis is common in the horse. Endogenous ocular manifestations of systemic mycotic infections in dogs and cats, such as blastomycosis, cryptococcosis, geotrichosis, and histoplasmosis, usually present as a focal granulomatous posterior uveitis, often involving the retina and other tissues of the eye. Most topical antifungal drugs have poor corneal penetration. Thiomersal and povidone-iodine have some antifungal activity. Antifungal drugs are usually formulated in combination with corticosteroids and an antibacterial (see section 12.3).

12.2.3 Antiviral preparations

Conjunctivitis in the cat caused by feline herpes virus, a potential respiratory pathogen, has been treated with topical **idoxuridine.**

IDOXURIDINE

Indications. See notes above
Dose. *Cats*: *eye drops*, apply every 1-2 hours
Eye ointment, apply 5-6 times daily

PoM **Idoxene**™ (Spodefell)
Eye ointment, idoxuridine 0.5%; 3 g

PoM **Kerecid**™ (Allergan)
Eye drops, idoxuridine 0.1%, polyvinyl alcohol 1.4%; 15 mL

12.3 Corticosteroids and other anti-inflammatory preparations

The anti-inflammatory effects of corticosteroids are based upon their ability to suppress capillary dilatation, vascular exudation, and leucocyte migration regardless of the causative agent. In chronic conditions they inhibit neovascularisation and fibroblastic activity in the eye. This may be useful in preventing scarring and pigment deposition in the cornea but disadvantageous by retarding healing. In general, topical preparations readily penetrate the cornea. Topical corticosteroids are particularly useful in the treatment of uveitis, various specific and non-specific inflammatory disorders of the cornea, such as pannus in the German Shepherd dog, and in reducing post-surgical inflammation, such as that following cataract or lens extraction.

Following administration, therapeutic levels remain in the eye for only about 3 hours and this may necessitate frequent application to prevent treatment failure. Topical corticosteroids should not be used in the presence of corneal ulceration; non-steroidal anti-inflammatory drugs (NSAIDs) should be considered. Corticosteroids may be used in the presence of glaucoma in animals but care should obviously be taken in the differential diagnosis of a 'red eye'.

Subconjunctival injections may augment, or replace, topical instillation. Preparations of methylprednisolone acetate or triamcinolone acetonide may be effective for up to 3 weeks. Their use may sometimes be effective for owners experiencing difficulty in applying drops. The use of systemic corticosteroids for ocular therapy is limited because lower concentrations are achieved than with topical application. However, systemic therapy may be useful for idiopathic partial serous retinal detachments, posterior uveitis, and optic neuritis. There is an association between cataractogenesis and steroid therapy in man but this has not been described in animals. The adverse effects of prolonged administration of systemic corticosteroids may be minimised by alternate day therapy. Systemic NSAIDs may be useful when corticosteroids are contra-indicated. They are administered pre-operatively to reduce inflammation during intraocular surgery.

Antihistamines may have a limited use in reducing inflammation associated with immunoglobulin (IgE)-mediated immediate hypersensitivity reactions

Antihistamine therapy has been largely replaced by the use of corticosteroids.

DEXAMETHASONE

Indications. See notes above
Dose. Apply every 2-3 hours

PoM **Maxidex™** (Alcon)
Eye drops, dexamethasone 0.1%, hypromellose 0.5%; 5 mL, 10 mL

COMPOUND CORTICOSTEROID AND ANTIBIOTIC OPHTHALMIC PREPARATIONS

PoM **Betsolan™ Eye and Ear Drops** (Coopers Pitman-Moore)
Drops, betamethasone sodium phosphate 0.1%, neomycin sulphate 0.5%; 5 mL
Dose. Apply every 2-3 hours

PoM **Chloromycetin™ Hydrocortisone** (Parke-Davis)
Eye ointment, chloramphenicol 1%, hydrocortisone acetate 0.5%; 4 g
Withdrawal Periods. Slaughter withdrawal period nil, milk from treated animals should not be used for human consumption
Dose. Apply up to 8 times daily for at least 2 days

PoM **Maxitrol™** (Alcon)
Eye drops, dexamethasone 0.1%, hypromellose 0.5%, neomycin (as sulphate) 0.35%, polymyxin B sulphate 6000 units/mL; 5 mL
Eye ointment, dexamethasone 0.1%, neomycin (as sulphate) 0.35%, polymyxin B sulphate 6000 units/g; 3.5 g

PoM **Neobiotic™ HC** (Upjohn)
Drops (eye drops or ear drops), hydrocortisone acetate 0.5%, neomycin sulphate 0.5%; 5 mL
Dose. Apply 3-6 times daily, reducing to 2-4 times daily after improvement

PoM **Vetsovate™ Eye and Ear Drops** (Coopers Pitman-Moore)
Drops, betamethasone valerate 0.05%, neomycin sulphate 0.5%, for *dogs*, *cats*; 5 mL

Dose. *Dogs*, *cats*: apply 4 times daily

12.4 Mydriatics and cycloplegics

Sympathomimetic drugs such as adrenaline and phenylephrine dilate the pupil by stimulating the dilator muscle of the iris. Antimuscarinic drugs including atropine, cyclopentolate, homatropine, and tropicamide paralyse the iris sphincter muscle and the ciliary muscle.

Atropine is frequently used to relieve muscle spasm, and therefore pain, associated with anterior uveitis (iridocyclitis). It is also useful in maintaining a patent pupil in the presence of exudation and to prevent the formation or break down of anterior and posterior synechiae. The duration of action, several days in the normal eye, is greatly reduced in uveitis and 3 to 4 applications per day may be necessary. Atropine is contra-indicated in glaucoma and keratoconjunctivitis sicca.

Homatropine is less potent than atropine and has been used in combination with phenylephrine for subconjunctival injection to maintain mydriasis during cataract surgery. **Tropicamide**, a poor cycloplegic, has the most rapid action and is the mydriatic of choice for intraocular examination and funduscopy. The effect is maximal within 30 minutes and persists for several hours. **Cyclopentolate** has a longer action and is more effective when combined with 10% solution of phenylephrine. **Phenylephrine** alone, usually as a 10% solution, is effective as a mydriatic in dogs but not in cats, unless used in combination with homatropine. Phenylephrine is useful in the diagnosis and investigation of Horner's syndrome. The affected pupil responds more rapidly to phenylephrine, due to denervation hypersensitivity.

ATROPINE SULPHATE

Indications. See notes above
Contra-indications. Keratoconjunctivitis sicca, glaucoma

Dose. Apply up to 3-4 times daily

PoM **Atropine** (Non-proprietary)
Eye drops, atropine sulphate 1%; 10 mL

PoM **Atropine** (Non-proprietary)
Eye ointment, atropine sulphate 1%; 3 g

PoM **Minims™ Atropine Sulphate** (S&N Pharm.)
Eye drops, atropine sulphate 1%; 0.5 mL

PoM **Opulets™ Atropine Sulphate** (Alcon)
Eye drops, atropine sulphate 1%; 0.5 mL

CYCLOPENTOLATE HYDROCHLORIDE

Indications. See notes above

PoM **Minims™ Cyclopentolate** (S&N Pharm.)
Eye drops, cyclopentolate hydrochloride 0.5%, 1%; 0.5 mL

PoM **Mydrilate™** (Boehringer Ingelheim)
Eye drops, cyclopentolate hydrochloride 0.5%, 1%; 5 mL

PoM **Opulets™ Cyclopentolate** (Alcon)
Eye drops, cyclopentolate hydrochloride 1%; 0.5 mL

HOMATROPINE HYDROBROMIDE

Indications. See notes above

PoM **Homatropine** (Non-proprietary)
Eye drops, homatropine hydrobromide 1%, 2%; 10 mL

PoM **Minims™ Homatropine Hydrobromide** (S&N Pharm.)
Eye drops, homatropine hydrobromide 2%; 0.5 mL

PHENYLEPHRINE HYDROCHLORIDE

Indications. See notes above

PoM **Phenylephrine** (Non-proprietary)
Eye drops, phenylephrine hydrochloride 10%; 10 mL

PoM **Minims™ Phenylephrine Hydrochloride** (S&N Pharm.)
Eye drops, phenylephrine hydrochloride 2.5%, 10%; 0.5 mL

TROPICAMIDE

Indications. See notes above
Dose. *Dogs*: tropicamide 1%

Cats: tropicamide 0.5%

PoM **Minims™ Tropicamide** (S&N Pharm.)
Eye drops, tropicamide 0.5%, 1%; 0.5 mL

PoM **Mydriacyl™** (Alcon)
Eye drops, tropicamide 0.5%, 1%; 5 mL

12.5 Drugs used in glaucoma

12.5.1 Miotics
12.5.2 Carbonic anhydrase inhibitors

Glaucoma is a common condition in dogs and occurs, to a lesser extent, in other species. It almost invariably arises through impairment of aqueous drainage. The causes are many and include acquired or inherited ocular disease, uveitis, cataract, lens luxation, neoplasia and intra-ocular haemorrhage. In some breeds of dog, glaucoma is inherited as a primary condition. Chronic simple glaucoma, as seen in man, is not recognised as a significant problem in animals. As subjective signs of glaucoma are difficult to assess, many cases present at a late stage of the disease when medical therapy alone is unlikely to succeed. In such cases, surgical intervention to facilitate aqueous drainage is the only practical alternative. The clinical history, presenting signs, intra-ocular pressure, and gonioscopic findings will influence the choice of treatment. Medical therapy will not succeed in a globe which has become enlarged, such as in hydrophthalmos or buphthalmos. Medical therapy usually comprises a combination of a miotic to increase aqueous humour outflow and a carbonic anhydrase inhibitor to inhibit aqueous humour production. Sympathomimetics are infrequently used and topical beta-adrenoceptor blockers, such as timolol maleate appear not to be particularly effective in dogs. In emergencies, hyperosmotic agents, such as oral **glycerol** (see section 16.3) 1 to 2 mL/kg or intravenous **mannitol** (see section 4.2.4) 1 to 2 g/kg as a 20% solution over 10 to 15 minutes are used in combination with a carbonic anhydrase inhibitor, such as intravenous **acetazolamide**, and frequent applications of topical **pilo-carpine**.

12.5.1 Miotics

The most useful drugs are **pilocarpine**, a parasympathomimetic miotic and **demecarium bromide**, a cholinesterase inhibitor. Pilocarpine penetrates the cornea, produces miosis within 15 minutes and is effective for 6 to 8 hours. Initially, frequent applications are required, thereafter it is instilled 3 to 4 times daily. Pilocarpine may produce local irritation. Cats appear to be more susceptible to side-effects of pilocarpine. Demecarium bromide has a longer action than pilocarpine and is usually less irritant. **Carbachol** also has longer action than pilocarpine. Other anticholinesterases, such as **physostigmine sulphate** and **ecothiopate iodide** have been used in the dog.

CARBACHOL

Indications. Glaucoma, see notes above
Dose. *Dogs*: apply 2-3 times daily

PoM **Isopto Carbachol**™ (Alcon)
Eye drops, carbachol 3%, hypromellose 1%; 10 mL

DEMECARIUM BROMIDE

Indications. Glaucoma, see notes above
Dose. *Dogs*: apply 1-2 times daily

PoM **Tosmilen**™ (Sinclair)
Eye drops, demecarium bromide 0.25%; 5 mL
Note. No longer on the UK market but available on a named-patient basis for use under expert supervision

ECOTHIOPATE IODIDE

Indications. Glaucoma, see notes above
Dose. *Dogs*: apply 1-2 times daily

PoM **Phospholine Iodide**™ (Wyeth)
Eye drops, ecothiopate iodide 0.03%, 0.06%, 0.125%, 0.25%; 5 mL
Note. No longer on the UK market but available on a named-patient basis for use under expert supervision

PHYSOSTIGMINE SULPHATE

Indications. Glaucoma, see notes above
Dose. *Dogs*: apply 3-4 times daily

PoM **Physostigmine** (Non-proprietary)
Eye drops, physostigmine sulphate 0.25%, 0.5%; 10 mL

PILOCARPINE

Indications. Glaucoma, see notes above; improvement of tear secretion (12.6)
Side-effects. Local irritation
Dose. Apply 1 or 2% solution 3-4 times daily

PoM **Pilocarpine** (Non-proprietary)
Eye drops, pilocarpine hydrochloride 0.5%, 1%, 2%; 10 mL

PoM **Minims**™ **Pilocarpine Nitrate** (S&N Pharm.)
Eye drops, pilocarpine nitrate 1%, 2%; 0.5 mL

PoM **Opulets**™ **Pilocarpine** (Alcon)
Eye drops, pilocarpine hydrochloride 1%, 2%; 0.5 mL

12.5.2 Carbonic anhydrase inhibitors

These substances act by inhibiting the carbonic anhydrase enzyme present in the ciliary epithelium, which catalyses the reversible hydration of carbon dioxide and leads to aqueous humour production. **Acetazolamide** administered orally results in a lowering of intraocular pressure within an hour and the effect may persist for at least 8 hours. Acetazolamide may be administered intravenously in emergencies. **Dichlorphenamide**, which may only be administered orally, has a similar duration of action but has the advantage of fewer side-effects. Administering the drug in divided doses may minimise the side-effects.

ACETAZOLAMIDE

Indications. Glaucoma, see notes above
Side-effects. Vomiting, diarrhoea, polydipsia, polyuria

Dose. *Dogs*: *by mouth*, 5-10 mg/kg 2-4 times daily; *by intravenous injection*, 50 mg/kg

PoM **Acetazolamide** (Non-proprietary)
Tablets, acetazolamide 250 mg

PoM **Diamox™** (Lederle)
Injection, powder for reconstitution, acetazolamide (as sodium salt) 500 mg

DICHLORPHENAMIDE

Indications. Glaucoma, see notes above
Dose. *Dogs*: 2-4 mg/kg 3 times daily

PoM **Daranide™** (MSD)
Tablets, scored, dichlorphenamide 50 mg; 100

12.6 Drugs used in keratoconjunctivitis sicca

Keratoconjunctivitis sicca (KCS) occurs in the dog but it is rare in other species. Treatment consists of the replacement of tear secretions, or the improvement of tear secretion. Management of the condition by surgical procedures may be necessary.

Successful replacement therapy with artificial or false tears is dependent on frequent application. Treatment should be given 8 to 10 times daily. It may be necessary to try a number of different preparations to find that most satisfactory for each individual patient.

Hypromellose eye drops are the most commonly used tear substitute and are particularly useful where the deficiency is in the aqueous phase of the precorneal tear film, as is almost invariably the case in the dog.

A mucolytic, such as **acetylcysteine**, may be beneficial where tears are particularly mucoid and viscous.

Pilocarpine (see section 12.5.1) has been used to improve tear secretion in patients that have some residual lachrymal gland function. One to two drops of a 1% solution are administered by mouth,

once or twice daily, for an initial trial period of 4 to 6 weeks.

ACETYLCYSTEINE

Indications. Tear deficiency; collagenous ulcers
Dose. See notes above

PoM **Ilube™** (DF)
Eye drops, acetylcysteine 5%, hypromellose 0.35%; 15 mL

HYPROMELLOSE

Indications. Tear deficiency
Dose. See notes above

P **Hypromellose** (Non-proprietary)
Eye drops, hypromellose '4000' (or '4500' or '5000') 0.3%; 10 mL

P **BJ6** (Martindale; Thornton & Ross)
Eye drops, hypromellose 0.25%; 10 mL

P **Isopto Alkaline™** (Alcon)
Eye drops, hypromellose 1%; 10 mL

P **Isopto Plain™** (Alcon)
Eye drops, hypromellose, 0.5%; 10 mL

P **Tears Naturale™** (Alcon)
Eye drops, hypromellose 0.3%, dextran '70' 0.1%; 15 mL

LIQUID PARAFFIN

Indications. Tear deficiency
Dose. See notes above

P **Lacri-Lube™** (Allergan)
Eye ointment, liquid paraffin; 3.5 g

POLYVINYL ALCOHOL

Indications. Tear deficiency
Dose. See notes above

P **Hypotears™** (CooperVision)
Eye drops, macrogol '8000' 2%, polyvinyl alcohol 1%; 10 mL

P **Liquifilm Tears™** (Allergan)
Eye drops, polyvinyl alcohol 1.4%; 15 mL

P **Sno Tears™** (S&N Pharm.)
Eye drops, polyvinyl alcohol 1.4%; 10 mL

12.7 Local anaesthetics

Proxymetacaine hydrochloride is the most widely used topical local anaesthetic in veterinary ophthalmology for both diagnostic and minor surgical procedures. Proxymetacaine has a rapid action and the effect persists for 15 to 20 minutes. **Amethocaine** has a more prolonged effect.

Amethocaine hydrochloride and lignocaine hydrochloride are sometimes included in combination preparations in an ointment basis for their topical anaesthetic properties.

AMETHOCAINE HYDROCHLORIDE

Indications. See notes above

PoM **Amethocaine** (Non-proprietary)
Eye drops, amethocaine hydrochloride 0.5%, 1%; 10 mL

PoM **Minims™ Amethocaine Hydrochloride** (S&N Pharm.)
Eye drops, amethocaine hydrochloride 0.5%, 1%; 0.5 mL

PROXYMETACAINE HYDROCHLORIDE

Indications. See notes above

PoM **Ophthaine™** (Ciba-Geigy)
Drops (for ear, eye, or nose), proxymetacaine hydrochloride 0.5%; 15 mL

12.8 Diagnostic stains

The ophthalmic stains **fluorescein sodium** and **rose bengal** are used for the diagnosis of disorders of the cornea and conjunctiva. Following instillation excess stain should be washed out of the eye with sodium chloride solution 0.9%. The main use of fluorescein sodium is in the diagnosis of corneal epithelial defects, in which areas of denuded epithelium are stained bright fluorescent green. It is also used to prove the patency, or otherwise, of the nasolachrymal duct system and in fluorescein angiography of both anterior and posterior segments of the eye. Rose bengal stains devitalised epithelial cells an intense dark red. It also stains mucus and is used in the diagnosis of keratoconjunctivitis sicca.

FLUORESCEIN SODIUM

Indications. See notes above

P **Fluorets** (S&N Pharm.)
Paper strips, impregnated with fluorescein sodium 1 mg; 100

P **Minims™ Fluorescein Sodium** (S&N Pharm.)
Eye drops, fluorescein sodium 1%, 2%; 0.5 mL

P **Opulets™ Fluorescein Sodium** (Alcon)
Eye drops, fluorescein sodium 1%; 0.5 mL

ROSE BENGAL

Indications. See notes above

P **Minims™ Rose Bengal** (S&N Pharm.)
Eye drops, rose bengal 1%; 0.5 mL

13 Drugs acting on the

EAR

13.1 Anti-infective ear preparations
13.2 Cleansers and sebolytics

Diseases of the pinna and external ear canal more commonly affect the smaller species of domestic animals.

In all species the pinna may be affected by inflammation caused by either bites from insects such as the stable fly, *Stomoxys calcitrans*, or self-inflicted trauma secondary to otitis.

The principal disorder of the ear canal is otitis externa. Inflammation may also involve the pinna and in chronic cases result in perforation of the tympanic membrane leading to middle-ear disease. Otitis externa commonly affects the dog, especially breeds with pendulous ears such as spaniels, or breeds that have a lot of hair in the ear canal, for example poodles. The highest incidence is usually in dogs 5 to 8 years of age. The disease is less common in the cat because the pinna is erect and well drained, and even less common in livestock.

Micro-organisms commonly involved in cases of otitis externa are yeasts, mainly *Pityrosporum*, and bacteria including *Actinomyces*, *Proteus*, *Pseudomonas*, staphylococci, and streptococci. The ear mite *Otodectes cynotis* commonly causes otitis externa in dogs and cats, while *Psoroptes cuniculi* similarly affects rabbits.

13.1 Anti-infective ear preparations

Prevention of insect attacks requires use of fly repellents, fly sprays, or flea sprays, (see section 2.2.2.6) to minimise repeated bites. If possible the affected animal should be housed indoors away from flies while lesions heal.

For otitis externa, a suitable antibiotic is used to control infections by micro-organisms and many preparations are available. **Neomycin** is the most frequently used antibacterial, but others such as **polymyxin B sulphate** and **fusidic acid** may also be used. **Nystatin**, **natamycin**, and **miconazole** are used for fungal infections and mites are controlled with ectoparasiticides such as **monosulfiram**. Some preparations incorporate a corticosteroid or a local anaesthetic such as amethocaine or benzocaine to help relieve pain and inflammation. Treatment of severe otitis may include systemic therapy. In chronic cases, other measures may be needed such as microbial sensitivity testing before medication or surgery. Due to the varied aetiology of otitis externa, available preparations are usually combinations of the above groups of drugs. Liquid formulations are commonly used for ease of administration.

Before examination and treatment can be carried out, restraint or general anaesthesia may be required. In most cases, a few drops of the preparation are instilled into the ear canal twice daily. To eliminate *Otodectes cynotis*, treatment should be continued for the duration of the life-cycle of the parasite, namely 3 weeks. Any other susceptible species likely to be in contact with the infected carrier should also be treated. Ensure that the tympanum is not perforated before administering these preparations.

PoM **Auroto**™ (Arnolds)
Ear drops, amethocaine hydrochloride 1%, neomycin sulphate 0.5%, thiabendazole 4%, for *dogs, cats*; 10 mL

PoM **Betsolan**™ **Cream** (Coopers Pitman-Moore)
See section 14.4 for preparation details

PoM **Betsolan**™ **Eye and Ear Drops** (Coopers Pitman-Moore)
See section 12.3 for preparation details

PoM **Canaural**™ (Leo)
Ear drops (oily), diethanolamine fusidate 0.5%, framycetin 0.5%, nystatin 100 000 units/g, prednisolone 0.15%, for *dogs, cats*; 7.5 mL, 15 mL, other sizes available

PoM **Fucidin**™ **Ointment** (Leo)
See section 14.2.1 for preparation details

PoM **Fucidin**™ **H Ointment** (Leo)
See section 14.4 for preparation details

PoM **GAC**™ (Arnolds)
Ear drops, amethocaine hydrochloride 1%, lindane 0.1%, neomycin undecenoate 0.5%, for *dogs, cats*; 10 mL

PoM **Neobiotic**™ **HC Drops** (Upjohn)
See section 12.3 for preparation details

PoM **Oterna**™ (Coopers Pitman-Moore)
Ear drops (oily), betamethasone 0.1%, monosulfiram 5%, neomycin sulphate 0.5%, for *dogs, cats*; 20 mL

PoM **Panolog**™ **Ointment** (Ciba-Geigy)
Liquid (oily), neomycin (as sulphate) 0.25%, nystatin 100 000 units/mL, thiostrepton 2500 units/mL, triamcinolone acetonide 0.1%, for *dogs, cats*; 7.5 mL, 100 mL

PoM **Pimavecort**™ (Mycofarm)
Ear drops, hydrocortisone 0.5%, natamycin 1%, neomycin (as sulphate) 0.175%, for *dogs, cats*; 20 mL

P **Polynoxylin Gel** (BK)
See section 14.2.1 for preparation details

PoM **Surolan**™ (Janssen)
Suspension, miconazole nitrate 2.3%, polymyxin B sulphate 5000 units/mL, prednisolone acetate 0.5%, for *dogs, cats*; 15 mL

PoM **Vetsovate**™ **Cream** (Coopers Pitman-Moore)
See section 14.4 for preparation details

PoM **Vetsovate**™ **Eye and Ear Drops** (Coopers Pitman-Moore)
See section 12.3 for preparation details

13.2 Cleansers and sebolytics

A significant proportion of otic disorders in animals will improve with flushing and cleansing of the ear canal to remove wax and debris. Preparations are available using solvents such as propylene glycol, squalane, or xylene, and incorporating benzoic acid and salicylic acid.

There are many preparations available. This is not a comprehensive list.

Auroclens™ (Arnolds)
Liquid, vegetable oil emulsion, for *dogs, cats*; 30 mL

P **Dermisol**™ (SmithKline Beecham)
Cream, benzoic acid 0.02%, malic acid 0.4%, propylene glycol 1.7%, salicylic acid 0.006%; 30 g, 100 g

P **Dermisol**™ **Multicleanse** (SmithKline Beecham)
Solution, benzoic acid 0.15%, malic acid 2.25%, propylene glycol 40%, salicylic acid 0.037%; 100 mL, 340 mL

GSL **Logic**™ **Ear Cleaner** (Sanofi)
Solution, xylene 2%, for *dogs, cats*; 60 mL

Oterna™ **Ear and Wound Cleanser** (Coopers Pitman-Moore)
Solution, benzoic acid, malic acid, propylene glycol, salicylic acid; 118 mL

GSL **Malatex**™ (Norton)
Solution, benzoic acid 0.15%, malic acid 2.25%, propylene glycol 40%, salicylic acid 0.0375%; 500 mL

GSL **Sebumol** (Willows Francis)
Ear drops, pure squalane; 7 mL

14 Drugs acting on the

SKIN

14.1 Dermatological vehicles
14.2 Topical antibacterial skin preparations
14.3 Topical antifungal skin preparations
14.4 Topical anti-inflammatory skin preparations
14.5 Antipruritic and keratolytic preparations
14.6 Skin disinfecting and cleansing preparations
14.7 Preparations for warts
14.8 Essential fatty acid preparations

The use of topical preparations acting on the skin is also described in Ectoparasiticides (section 2.2), under Preparations for the care of teats and udders (section 11.2), Drugs acting on the ear (Chapter 13), and Drugs acting on feet (Chapter 15).

14.1 Dermatological vehicles

The skin is amenable to treatment by local application as there is immediate contact between drug and target tissue. Both vehicle and active ingredients are important in treatment. The vehicle affects the degree of hydration of the skin, has a mild anti-inflammatory effect, and may aid the penetration of the active ingredients into the skin.

Before application of a topical preparation, it is important to prepare the area for treatment by clipping away hair or wool and removing contaminating debris with disinfectants or cleansing agents (see section 14.6). The importance of skin preparation and regular application of treatment to the affected area should be stressed to owners.

The tendency for animals to lick the affected area immediately after application can be a major problem, especially in cats, and may result in worsening of the skin condition. Licking

may be reduced by applying the preparation before feeding or exercise, or using methods of restraint such as an Elizabethan collar.

For localised lesions or wounds, formulations are available as powders, sprays, lotions, gels, creams, and ointments. Choice of vehicle depends on the type of lesion and practicability of application.

Creams are either water-miscible and readily removed, or oily and not so easily removed. They should be avoided in exudative lesions.

Aqueous Cream, emulsifying ointment 30%, phenoxyethanol 1%, in freshly boiled and cooled purified water

Ointments are greasy, normally anhydrous, insoluble in water, and more occlusive than creams. They are used for chronic dry lesions and should be avoided in exudative lesions. The more commonly used ointment bases consist of soft paraffin or soft paraffin and liquid paraffin with hard paraffin. Such greasy preparations may not be suitable for pets in household conditions.

Emulsifying Ointment, emulsifying wax 30%, white soft paraffin 50%, liquid paraffin 20%

Hydrous Ointment (oily cream), dried magnesium sulphate 0.5%, phenoxyethanol 1%, water for preparations 48.5%, in wool alcohols ointment

Hydrous Wool Fat (lanolin), wool fat 70% in freshly boiled and cooled purified water

White Soft Paraffin, (white petroleum jelly)

Yellow Soft Paraffin, (yellow petroleum jelly)

Simple Ointment, cetostearyl alcohol 5%, hard paraffin 5%, wool fat 5%, in yellow or white soft paraffin

Lotions are mainly aqueous solutions or suspensions, for application without friction to inflamed unbroken skin. They cool by evaporation, require frequent application, and leave a thin film of drug on the skin. Lotions are used on hairy areas and for lesions with minor exudation and ulceration. Care should be taken with nervous or excitable animals since lotions containing volatile substances can sting on application. 'Shake lotions' such as calamine lotion are used to cool dry scabbed lesions. They leave a film of dry powder.

Pastes are stiff preparations containing a high proportion of finely powdered solids. They are less occlusive than ointments and are used mainly for circumscribed, ulcerated lesions.

Magnesium Sulphate Paste (Morison's Paste), dried magnesium sulphate, after drying, 45 g, phenol 500 mg, anhydrous glycerol 55 g

Compound Zinc Paste, zinc oxide 25%, starch 25%, white soft paraffin 50%

Collodions are painted onto the skin and allowed to dry to leave a flexible film over the site of the application. In veterinary medicine their main use is to 'seal' the teats of non-lactating cows.

Flexible Collodion, castor oil 2.5%, colophony 2.5% in a collodion basis, prepared by dissolving pyroxylin (10%) in a mixture of 3 volumes of ether and 1 volume of alcohol (90%)
Warnings. Highly flammable

Liniments are liquid preparations for external application that contain analgesics and rubefacients (see section 10.4 for preparations).

14.2 Topical antibacterial skin preparations

14.2.1 Antibacterial skin preparations
14.2.2 Preparations for minor skin infections

An infection may be the primary cause of a skin condition or may be secondary to skin trauma or an underlying disorder such as a hormonal imbalance, immunosuppression, or nutritional deficiencies.

Bacteria commonly causing primary skin infections in animals include *Staphylococcus*, *Streptococcus*, and *Proteus* species, *Escherichia coli*, and *Dermatophilus congolensis* ('mycotic' dermatitis).

14.2.1 Antibacterial skin preparations

Antibacterials incorporated into topical preparations include **chlortetracycline** and **oxytetracycline**, which are effective against infections caused by *Bacillus*, *Actinomyces*, *Clostridium*, *Fusiformis*, streptococci, and staphylococci.

Fusidic acid is particularly effective against pyodermas caused by *Staphylococcus aureus*, streptococci, *Actinomyces*, *Neisseria*, and some *Clostridium* species.

Sulphanilamide is effective against common Gram-positive and Gram-negative skin pathogens. **Polynoxylin** has antibacterial and antifungal actions and may act by the release of formaldehyde. It also has antipruritic activity.

Topical antibacterial treatment may be used alone or in combination with systemic therapy. Extended courses of systemic antibacterial treatment may be necessary for skin infections.

In horses, cattle, sheep, and pigs, therapy is based mainly on the penicillins, lincomycin, erythromycin, and potentiated sulphonamides (see section 1.1).

Erythromycin, lincomycin, co-amoxiclav, chloramphenicol, potentiated sulphonamides, and cephalexin (see section 1.1) are indicated for use in dogs and cats.

CHLORTETRACYCLINE HYDROCHLORIDE

Indications. Skin infections, see notes above; hoof lesions (see section 15.1)

PoM **Aureomycin™ Topical Powder** (Cyanamid)
Dusting powder, chlortetracycline hydrochloride 2%, benzocaine 1%; 25 g

PoM **PEP™** (Intervet)
Dusting powder, chlortetracycline hydrochloride 2%, benzocaine 1%; 25 g

FUSIDIC ACID

Indications. Skin infections caused by Gram-positive bacteria, see notes above; otitis externa (see section 13.1)

PoM **Fucidin™** (Leo)
Gel, fusidic acid 2%; 15 g, 30 g
Ointment, sodium fusidate 2%; 15 g, 30 g

OXYTETRACYCLINE HYDROCHLORIDE

Indications. Skin infections, see notes above; hoof lesions, including footrot in sheep (see section 15.1)

PoM **Alamycin™ Aerosol** (Norbrook)
Spray, oxytetracycline hydrochloride 2.5%, suitable dye, for *sheep*; 200 g
Withdrawal Periods. *Sheep*: slaughter withdrawal period nil

PoM **BK-Mycen™ Aerosol** (BK)
Spray, oxytetracycline hydrochloride 2.5%; 200 g

PoM **Duphacycline™ Aerosol** (Duphar)
Spray, oxytetracycline hydrochloride 2.5%, suitable dye, for *sheep*; 200 g
Withdrawal Periods. *Sheep*: slaughter withdrawal period nil

PoM **Embacycline™ Aerosol** (RMB)
Spray, oxytetracycline hydrochloride 2.5%, gentian violet, for *sheep*; 200 g
Withdrawal Periods. *Sheep*: slaughter withdrawal period nil

PoM **Occrycetin™ Aerosol** (Willows Francis)
Spray, oxytetracycline hydrochloride 2.5%, suitable dye, for *sheep*; 200 g
Withdrawal Periods. *Sheep*: slaughter withdrawal period nil

PoM **Oxytetrin™ Aerosol** (Coopers Pitman-Moore)
Spray, oxytetracycline hydrochloride 3.2%, suitable dye, for *sheep*; 160 g
Withdrawal Periods. *Sheep*: slaughter withdrawal period nil, milk withdrawal period nil

PoM **Terramycin™ Aerosol** (Pfizer)
Spray, oxytetracycline hydrochloride 2%, suitable dye, for *sheep*; 200 g
Withdrawal Periods. *Sheep*: slaughter withdrawal period nil, milk withdrawal period nil

POLYNOXYLIN

Indications. Skin infections; otitis externa (see section 13.1)

P **Polynoxylin Gel** (BK)
Polynoxylin 10%; 25 g

SULPHANILAMIDE

Indications. Skin infections, see notes above

PML **Negasunt™** (Bayer)
Dusting powder, coumaphos 3%, propoxur 2%, sulphanilamide 5%; 20 g, 125 g
Withdrawal Periods. Should not be used on *horses* intended for human consumption. *Cattle*: slaughter 28 days, milk 7 days. *Sheep*: slaughter 28 days, milk from treated animals should not be used for human consumption. *Pigs*: slaughter 28 days
Warnings. Lactating cattle should be treated after milking is completed. Powder applied to udders and teats should be washed off before next milking. Harmful to fish

14.2.2 Preparations for minor skin infections

These preparations are used to treat minor skin infections and abrasions, and to prevent infection following surgery, or when dehorning. They are applied as necessary in the form of dusting powders, ointments, or sprays. Preparations containing **benzoic acid**, **cresol**, or **phenols** should not be used on cats (see Prescribing for dogs and cats).

GSL **Aeroclens™** (Battle Hayward & Bower)
Aerosol spray, benzalkonium chloride 1%, chloroxylenol 0.1%; 150 g

PML **Antiseptic Balsam** (Crown)
Liquid, colophony resin 25.79%, phenol 2.15%, raw linseed oil 33.3%, technical white oil 7.83%, turpentine oil 30.93%; 500 mL, 2.5 litres, 5 litres

Cetrimide Cream (Non-proprietary)
Cetrimide 0.5% in a suitable water-miscible basis such as cetostearyl alcohol 5%, liquid paraffin 50% in freshly boiled and cooled purified water

GSL **Cetream™** (Pettifer)
Cream, cetrimide 0.5%, for *horses*; 400 g

GSL **Iodine Spray** (Salsbury)
Available iodine 0.3%; 360 mL

GSL **Iodine Wound Spray** (Lever)
Available iodine 0.3%; 360 mL

PML **Terebene Sheep Balsam** (Battle Hayward & Bower)
Liquid, phenol 4%, turpentine 25%, for *sheep*; 500 mL, 1 litre, other sizes available

GSL **Veterinary Wound Powder** (Alfa Laval)
Dusting powder, chloramine 2%; 125 g

GSL **Veterinary Wound Powder** (Battle Hayward & Bower)
Dusting powder, chloramine 2%; 20 g, 125 g

GSL **Wound Powder** (Crown)
Dusting powder, activated charcoal 64%, camphor 2.5%, iodoform 2.5%; 45 g

GSL **Woundcare Powder** (Animalcare)
Dusting powder, chloramine 2%; 20 g

14.3 Topical antifungal skin preparations

Most fungal infections of the skin and keratin structures of domestic animals are caused by *Trichophyton* and *Microsporum* species. They are commonly referred to as ringworm and are zoonotic infections. *Candida albicans* infection causes mucocutaneous ulcerations in dogs and is rare.

Ringworm is essentially a self-limiting disease. Drug therapy can often shorten the duration of the disease although in some species, notably long-haired cats and dogs, response to treatment may be poor. Paronychial infections may also be refractory to treatment.

The success of drug therapy depends on additional management aimed at reducing and limiting infection such as close clipping the coat of dogs and cats, limiting grooming, isolating the animal, and using antifungal washes on the affected animal and local environment. **Griseofulvin** and **ketoconazole** are used for systemic treatment of ringworm (see section 1.2).

Topical antifungals may be used for the treatment of ringworm, although drug toxicity due to ingestion through grooming, the necessity for clipping of the fur and repeated re-application of the preparation should be taken into account.

Topical preparations containing the imidazoles **enilconazole** and **miconazole** are effective for small areas of infection and may be used in conjunction with griseofulvin for the treatment of ringworm.

Copper naphthenate and **dichlorophen** (see section 15.1) are used for the treatment of ringworm in cattle, and footrot in sheep. **Povidone-iodine** (see section 14.6) is also used as a fungicide. **Natamycin** is an antibiotic having some antifungal activity, which may be used for topical treatment and also for disinfection of the ringworm-contaminated environment and horse tackle. **Tribromometacresol** should not be used in cats as it is a cresol derivative.

BENSULDAZIC ACID

Indications. Ringworm

PML **Defungit™** (Hoechst)
This preparation is now discontinued

Proprietary and non-proprietary medicines that are licensed for human use are printed in small type in The Veterinary Formulary

ENILCONAZOLE

Indications. Ringworm
Dose. *Horses*: *by wash*, 0.2% solution every 3 days for 4 applications
Cattle: *by wash or spray*, 0.2% solution every 3 days for 3-4 applications
Dogs: *by wash*, 0.2% solution every 3 days for 4 applications

P**Imaverol**™ (Janssen)
Liquid concentrate, enilconazole 10%, for *horses, cattle, dogs*; 100 mL, 1 litre.
To be diluted before use
Withdrawal Periods. Should not be used on *horses* intended for human consumption. *Cattle*: slaughter withdrawal period nil, milk withdrawal period nil
Dilute 1 volume in 50 volumes water (= enilconazole 0.2%)

MICONAZOLE

Indications. Ringworm
Dose. *Dogs, cats*: apply daily for up to 6 weeks

PoM**Conoderm**™ (C-Vet)
Cream, miconazole (as nitrate) 2%, for *dogs, cats*; 15 g
Lotion, miconazole (as nitrate) 1%, for *dogs, cats*; 30 mL

NATAMYCIN

Indications. Ringworm
Warnings. Treated animals should not be exposed to sunlight for several hours; use galvanised or plastic containers as natamycin is sensitive to heavy metals such as copper
Dose. *Horses, cattle*: *by spray*, using 1 litre per adult animal, or local application, 0.01% solution, repeat after 4-5 days and again after 14 days if required

PoM**Mycophyt**™ (Mycofarm)
Suspension, powder for reconstitution, natamycin 10%, for *horses, cattle*; 2 g, 10 g
Reconstitute and dilute with 2 litres (for 2-g bottle) water or 10 litres (for 10-g bottle) water (=natamycin 0.01%)

TRIBROMOMETACRESOL

Indications. Ringworm
Contra-indications. Cats
Side-effects. Occasional allergic reactions in horses

P**Tenasol**™ (Willows Francis)
Spray, tribromometacresol 2.5%, salicylic acid 5%, for *horses, cattle, sheep, dogs*; 225 mL, 450 mL

14.4 Topical anti-inflammatory skin preparations

Systemic corticosteroids (see section 7.2.1) are in common use for the control of acute and chronic inflammatory skin disease in all species, but particularly in dogs and cats.

Topical corticosteroid preparations are used mainly to treat limited areas of diseased skin. Repeated use for a prolonged period may cause excessive absorption of these drugs particularly if lesions are abraded or licked. This may result in localised skin atrophy, alopecia, and in some cases depigmentation.

Topical corticosteroids are available as compound preparations with antimicrobials.

In the cat, in preference to topical applications, megestrol acetate is used for its anti-inflammatory effect in the treatment of miliary dermatitis and eosinophilic granuloma complex (see section 8.2.2).

> Operators should wear impervious gloves when applying preparations containing a corticosteroid

COMPOUND ANTI-INFLAMMATORY AND ANTIMICROBIAL PREPARATIONS

PoM**Betsolan**™ (Coopers Pitman-Moore)
Cream, betamethasone sodium phosphate 0.1%, neomycin sulphate 0.5%; 15 g

PoM **Dermobion™** (Willows Francis)
Ointment, chlorophyll paste 2%, cod-liver oil 10%, neomycin sulphate 0.5%, nitrofurazone 0.2%, prednisolone 0.25%; 15 g, 225 g

PoM **Dermobion SA™** (Willows Francis)
Ointment, cod-liver oil 10%, neomycin sulphate 0.5%, nitrofurazone 0.2%, prednisolone 0.25%, for *dogs, cats*; 15 g

PoM **Fucidin™ H** (Leo)
Ointment, hydrocortisone acetate 1%, sodium fusidate 2%; 15 g, 30 g

PoM **Hydrocortisone and Neomycin Cream** (Arnolds)
Hydrocortisone 0.5%, neomycin sulphate 0.5%; 15 g

PoM **Panolog™ Cream** (Ciba-Geigy)
Neomycin (as sulphate) 0.25%, nystatin 100 000 units/g, thiostrepton 2500 units/g, triamcinolone acetonide 0.1%, for *dogs, cats*; 10 g

PoM **Panolog™ Ointment** (Ciba-Geigy)
See section 13.1 for preparation details

PoM **Surolan™** (Janssen)
See section 13.1 for preparation details

PoM **Vetalog™ Plus** (Ciba-Geigy)
Cream, halquinol 0.75%, triamcinolone acetonide 0.025%; 15 g

PoM **Vetsovate™** (Coopers Pitman-Moore)
Cream, betamethasone (as valerate ester) 0.1%, neomycin sulphate 0.5%; 15 g, 30 g

14.5 Antipruritic and keratolytic preparations

Antipruritics are included in some preparations to reduce itching, which may be caused by systemic disease as well as skin disease. Where possible the underlying causes should be treated. Systemic corticosteroids (see section 7.2) may be of benefit in reducing pruritus. Antihistamines (see section 5.2) are sometimes used to control pruritus in allergic skin problems in dogs and cats when sedation may be of value. Keratolytics promote the loosening or separation of the horny layer of the epidermis.

Benzoyl peroxide has keratolytic properties. It is used for the treatment of canine dermatitis, pyoderma, and seborrhoeic dermatitis.

Coal tar and phenol have antipruritic properties, while calamine and zinc oxide act as mild astringents. Salicylic acid and resorcinol have keratolytic and exfoliative properties.

BENZOYL PEROXIDE

Indications. See notes above

P **OxyDex™** (C-Vet)
Gel, benzoyl peroxide 5%, for *dogs*; 30 g
Dose. Apply once or twice daily
Shampoo, benzoyl peroxide 2.5%, for *dogs*; 180 mL, 360 mL

P **OxyDex HP™** (C-Vet)
Shampoo, benzoyl peroxide 5%, for *dogs*; 180 mL

PoM **Paxcutol™** (Virbac)
Shampoo, benzoyl peroxide 2.5%, for *dogs*; 150 mL

COMPOUND ANTIPRURITIC AND KERATOLYTIC PREPARATIONS

GSL **Antiseptic Green Gel** (Battle Hayward & Bower)
Resorcinol 0.5%, for *horses, cattle*; 400 g, 3.5 kg

Coal Tar Solution, BP
Coal tar 20%, polysorbate '80' 5%, in alcohol

GSL **Derasect Tar and Sulphur** (SmithKline Beecham)
Shampoo, coal tar solution 2.5%, colloidal sulphur 5%, salicylic acid 1%, chloroxylenol 1%; 175 mL
Contra-indications. Cats

P **Dermisol™ Cream** (SmithKline Beecham)
See section 13.2 for preparation details

P **Dermisol™ Multicleanse Solution** (SmithKline Beecham)
See section 13.2 for preparation details

GSL **Golden-Coat** (Shep-Fair)
Gel, salicylic acid 1.5%, sulphur 10%, for *dogs, cats*; 50 g

GSL **Golden-Mane** (Shep-Fair)
Gel, salicylic acid 1.5%, sulphur 10%, for *horses*; 350 g

P **Oterna™ Ear and Wound Cleanser** (Coopers Pitman-Moore)
See section 13.2 for preparation details

GSL **Sebolytic** (Virbac)
Shampoo, coal tar 3%, salicylic acid 2%, sulphur 2%, for *dogs*; 200 mL
Contra-indications. Cats

GSL **Sweet Itch Lotion** (Battle Hayward & Bower)
Calamine 12.5%, coal tar solution 12.5%, precipitated sulphur 12.5%, for *horses*; 500 mL

PML **Veterinary Ointment** (Crown)
Liquefied phenol 2.5%, salicylic acid 2%, zinc oxide 15%; 500 g, 2.5 kg

14.6 Skin disinfecting and cleansing preparations

Wound management depends on the nature and site of the damage, the tissues involved, the age of the lesion as well as the species of the patient. Traumatic skin lesions in horses often fail to heal by first intention and may develop granulation tissue, which impedes healing. Treatment is determined by the severity of the wound and the necessity for surgical debridement and repair.

Fresh wounds may be irrigated as a first aid measure with copious amounts of clean water or sodium chloride 0.9% solution to flush out contaminating debris. Infected wounds should be treated with hypertonic solutions such as magnesium sulphate 10% solution or paste (Morison's paste), or sodium chloride 5% to 10% solution.

Penetrating wounds may be flushed with **hydrogen peroxide** 3% or 6% solution to aid the removal of foreign material and aid in the prevention of clostridial infection. Hydrogen peroxide owes its disinfectant action to the ready release of oxygen when applied to tissues. The effect only lasts as long as the oxygen is being released and the antimicrobial effect of liberated oxygen is reduced in the presence of organic matter. Hydrogen peroxide is used to cleanse wounds, especially in inaccessible areas although injection into closed body cavities is dangerous, as the liberated oxygen cannot be released.

Alcohol 70% is commonly used for its solvent properties for the removal of superficial contamination.

Benzalkonium chloride, **cetrimide**, and **povidone-iodine** are used for skin disinfection. These and **cresol** and **selenium sulphide** may also be incorporated into a shampoo basis. Shampoos help to clean the skin and remove crusts and debris when applied daily or weekly depending on the severity of the condition. They are used in the treatment of deep and superficial pyodermas, seborrhoea, and acute moist dermatitis (see also section 14.5).

ALCOHOL

Indications. Skin preparation before injection or surgery
Warnings. Flammable; avoid broken skin

Industrial Methylated Spirit
A mixture of 19 volumes of alcohol of an appropriate strength with 1 volume of approved wood naphtha

Surgical Spirit
Methyl salicylate 0.5 mL, diethyl phthalate 2 mL, castor oil 2.5 mL, Industrial Methylated Spirit to 100 mL

BENZALKONIUM CHLORIDE

Indications. Skin disinfection
Contra-indications. Concurrent use of soaps and anionic detergents

GSL **Marinol™-Blue** (BK)
Liquid concentrate, benzalkonium chloride 50%; 5 litres. To be diluted before use
Dilute 1 volume with 500 volumes water for skin disinfection

GSL **Marinol™-10% Blue** (BK)
Liquid concentrate, benzalkonium chloride 10%, 5 litres. To be diluted before use

Dilute 1 volume with 100 volumes water for skin disinfection

CETRIMIDE

Indications. Skin disinfection; footrot (15.1)
Contra-indications. See under Benzalkonium chloride

Cetrimide Solution
Cetrimide 1% in freshly boiled and cooled purified water
Use undiluted

Cetrimide Solution Strong
Cetrimide 20 to 40%, alcohol (95%) 7.5%, tartrazine 0.0075%
Used to prepare cetrimide solution

See also section 14.2.2

CHLORHEXIDINE GLUCONATE

Indications. Skin disinfection and cleansing
Contra-indications. See under Benzalkonium chloride

GSL **Hibiscrub™ Veterinary** (Coopers Pitman-Moore)
Liquid concentrate, Chlorhexidine Gluconate Solution BP 20% (equivalent to chlorhexidine gluconate 4%), in a surfactant solution; 5 litres. To be diluted before use
Dilute 1 volume with 29 volumes alcohol 70% for skin disinfection
Dilute 1 volume in 1000 volumes water for skin cleansing

GSL **Savlon™ Veterinary Concentrate** (Coopers Pitman-Moore)
Liquid concentrate, Chlorhexidine Gluconate Solution BP 7.5% (equivalent to chlorhexidine gluconate 1.5%), cetrimide 15%; 5 litres. To be diluted before use
Dilute 1 volume with 29 volumes alcohol 70% for skin disinfection
Dilute 1 volume in 100 volumes water for wound cleansing

CRESOL

Indications. Skin cleansing
Contra-indications. Cats

GSL **Animal Shampoo** (Battle Hayward & Bower)
Cresol (as lysol) 1.9%; 500 mL, 1 litre, other sizes available
Dilute 1 volume with 36 volumes water

HEXETIDINE

Indications. Skin cleansing

GSL **Hexocil™** (Parke-Davis)
This preparation is now discontinued

HYDROGEN PEROXIDE

Indications. Skin cleansing and disinfection of wounds

Hydrogen Peroxide Solution 6%
Hydrogen peroxide (20 volumes)
Use undiluted

Hydrogen Peroxide Solution 3%
Hydrogen peroxide (10 volumes)
Use undiluted

IODINE COMPOUNDS

Indications. Skin disinfection
Contra-indications. Concurrent use of other antiseptics or detergents

PoM **Iodine Solution Strong** (Animalcare)
This preparation is now discontinued

GSL **Pevidine™ Antiseptic Solution** (BK)
Solution, available iodine (as povidone-iodine) 1%; 500 mL, 5 litres. May be diluted before use
Use undiluted for wound cleansing
Note. May also be used diluted for intrauterine instillation (see section 8.6)

GSL **Pevidine™ Medicated Wash** (BK)
Solution, available iodine (as povidone-iodine) 0.75%; 100 mL
Use undiluted as a shampoo

GSL **Pevidine™ Surgical Scrub** (BK)
Solution, available iodine (as povidone-iodine) 0.75%; 500 mL, 5 litres
Use undiluted for skin disinfection

See also section 14.2.2

SELENIUM SULPHIDE

Indications. Skin cleansing

PSeleen™ (Sanofi)
Shampoo, selenium sulphide 1%; 150 mL, 1 litre

14.7 Preparations for warts

Papillomatous warts affecting horses, young cattle, and dogs are viral in origin and in most cases are self limiting with spontaneous remission.

Antimony lithium thiomalate is used to hasten resolution of warts and to aid removal of pedunculated lesions as the papillomas are more easily enucleated as they necrose.

Topical applications have limited use as it is often difficult to avoid the spread of the preparation to surrounding delicate tissues thereby causing damage. Preparations containing salicylic acid 20% to 25% should be applied sparingly.

ANTIMONY LITHIUM THIOMALATE

Indications. Removal of pedunculated warts

Contra-indications. Intravenous administration

Side-effects. Transient dullness and hyperthermia

Dose. *Cattle*: *by intramuscular injection*, 900 mg every second day for 8-12 days

Dogs: *by intramuscular injection*, 60 mg and gradually increasing to 150 mg every second day for 8-12 days

PoM **Anthiomaline**™ (RMB)
Injection, antimony lithium thiomalate 60 mg/mL, for *cattle, dogs*; 50 mL
Withdrawal Periods. *Cattle*: slaughter 28 days, milk 7 days

14.8 Essential fatty acid preparations

Essential fatty acids (EFAs) are polyunsaturated fatty acids derived from *cis*-linoleic acid and alpha-linolenic acid. Of particular importance are gamma-linolenic acid (GLA), eicosapentaenoic acid (EPA), and docosahexaenoic acid. GLA, derived from linoleic acid, is a precursor of dihomo-gamma-linolenic acid (DGLA, eicosatrienoic acid).

EFAs are of importance in the maintenance of epidermal barrier function, as phospholipid components of cell membranes, and as precursors of prostaglandins and related compounds. When tissue is damaged, free arachidonic acid is released, which is acted upon by lipoxygenase and cyclo-oxygenase enzymes to produce potent mediators of inflammation. Release of free arachidonic acid is inhibited by glucocorticoids and by the action of prostaglandin E_1. DGLA is a precursor of prostaglandin E_1. Lipoxygenase is inhibited by 15-hydroxydihomo-gamma-linolenic acid, a metabolite of DGLA. EPA can competitively inhibit the formation of arachidonic acid and its conversion to pro-inflammatory substances. Thus the EFAs have potential anti-inflammatory activity.

Production of GLA is limited by the availability of delta-6-desaturase. Deficiency of this enzyme in cats makes them particularly susceptible to some forms of EFA deficiency.

EFA deficiency leads to the development of a dry scurfy coat, hair loss, epidermal peeling and exudation, skin lichenification, and increased susceptibility to infection. Frank EFA deficiency is uncommon in animals fed normal diets but a number of factors can impair absorption and metabolism of EFAs. There is increasing evidence that EFA supplementation can ameliorate allergic skin diseases, particularly atopy in the dog and can lead to improvements in coat condition. Anecdotal reports indicate that it is also effective in miliary dermatitis in cats.

Dietary supplementation with sources of GLA, such as evening primrose oil, and of mixtures of evening primrose oil and marine fish oil, a source of EPA, have been shown to be effective in canine atopy. Although the effect appears to be dose related, optimum dosages and the most effective combinations of these oils have not yet been determined. Daily doses of 132 mg/kg of evening primrose oil and 33 mg/kg of marine fish oil have been used in dogs over periods of one year without ill effects. Side-effects are rare and may include mild and transient diarrhoea and vomiting. These effects can be minimised and absorption of the oils increased if they are given with food. If there is evidence of intolerance to fish then fish oil should be avoided.

The inclusion of biotin and methionine in dermatological preparations may be of benefit where deficiency of these substances may contribute to the skin disorder. See section 15.2 for other preparations containing biotin and methionine.

There are many preparations available. This is not a comprehensive list.

Dermplus™ (C-Vet)
Capsules, docosahexaenoic acid 16.8 mg, eicosapentaenoic acid 25 mg, gamma-linolenic acid 10.2 mg, vitamin E 29.8 mg, for *dogs, cats*; 60
Dose. *Dogs, cats*: 1 capsule/10 kg daily

Dermplus ES™ (C-Vet)
Capsules, docosahexaenoic acid 50 mg, eicosapentaenoic acid 75 mg, gamma-linolenic acid 30 mg, vitamin E 29.8 mg, for *dogs*; 60
Dose. *Dogs*: 1 capsule/25 kg daily

EfaVet™ 1 (Efamol)
Capsules, docosahexaenoic acid 6.8 mg, eicosapentaenoic acid 10.3 mg, gamma-linolenic acid 30.8 mg, linoleic acid 277.2 mg, vitamins, minerals, for *dogs*; 30, 100
Dose. *Dogs*: 1 capsule/10 kg with food

EfaVet™ 2 (Efamol)
Capsules, docosahexaenoic acid 3.4 mg, eicosapentaenoic acid 5.15 mg, gamma-linolenic acid 15.4 mg, linoleic acid 138.6 mg, vitamins, minerals, for *dogs, cats*; 30, 100
Dose. *Dogs, cats*: 1 capsule/5 kg with food

EfaVet™ Regular (Efamol)
Capsules, docosahexaenoic acid 11.6 mg, eicosapentaenoic acid 17.3 mg, gamma-linolenic acid 34.4 mg, linoleic acid 309.6 mg, vitamin E 10 mg, for *dogs*; 50
Dose. *Dogs*: 1 capsule/10 kg with food. This is for maintenance following EfaVet™ 1 or EfaVet™ 2 supplementation

Glavaderm™ (Cambridge VS, Mycofarm)
Capsules, gamma-linolenic acid 43 mg, linoleic acid 298 mg, for *dogs*; 56
Dose. *Dogs*: (up to 15 kg body-weight) 1 capsule daily, (more than 15 kg body-weight) 2 capsules daily

Mirra-Coat™ Daily Care for dogs (Intervet)
Oral powder or liquid, linoleic acid 480 mg, linolenic acid 40 mg/mL, vitamins, for *dogs*; 227 mL, 454 mL, 454 g, 1.1 kg
Dose. *Dogs*: 5 mL/12 kg

Mirra-Coat™ Special Care (Intervet)
Oral powder or liquid, linoleic acid 480 mg, linolenic acid 40 mg/mL, vitamins, biotin, zinc, for *dogs*; 454 g, 1.1 kg; 227 mL, 454 mL
Dose. *Dogs*: 5 mL/12 kg

Mirra-Coat™ for cats (Intervet)
Liquid, arachidonic acid 20 mg, linoleic acid 300 mg, linolenic acid 30 mg/mL, vitamins, biotin, zinc, for *cats*; 114 mL
Dose. *Cats*: 2.5 mL/3 kg

Mirra-Coat™ Equine (Intervet)
Oral powder, polyunsaturated fatty acids 138 mg/g, vitamins, for *horses*; 2.3kg
Dose. *Horses*: 48 g/500 kg

GSL **Norderm™** (SmithKline Beecham)
Liquid, arachidonic acid 29 mg, linoleic acid 365 mg, linolenic acid 55 mg, oleic, palmitoleic, and clupadonic acids 280 mg, lecithins 10.8 mg/mL, vitamins, for *dogs, cats*; 150 mL, 2 litres
Dose. *Dogs, cats*: 1-10 mL

15 Drugs acting on

FEET

15.1 Anti-infective foot preparations
15.2 Hoof care preparations

Treatment of foot conditions necessitates cleaning and trimming of the hoof, removal of deep pus, and curetting of all necrotic material. This is essential before parenteral or topical drugs are used, otherwise therapy may fail. Weather and underfoot conditions may affect the efficacy of local preparations. Bandaging may hasten recovery and will be necessary for the application of treatment in powder form. Parenteral administration of antibiotics, sometimes in addition to topical treatment of the foot lesion, may be necessary for optimal results.

Pododermatitis, a dermatitis of the interdigital skin with under-running of the heel, is commonly called 'footrot' or 'foul in the foot'. Proliferative dermatitis is a proliferative lesion at the back of the pastern. These lesions are commonly named verrucose dermatitis in cattle, and 'strawberry footrot' in sheep.

Footrot in cattle and sheep is caused by the synergistic effect of *Bacteroides nodosus* and *Fusobacterium necrophorum*. *Actinomyces pyogenes* and motile fusiforms are also commonly found in the lesions and contribute to the severity of the condition. Lesions in pigs are primarily caused by abrasions due to poor flooring, and secondary mixed infections.

Proliferative dermatitis in sheep is caused by *Dermatophilus congolensis* and, in cattle, by *F. necrophorum* and is exacerbated by wet and muddy conditions.

Pathogens involved in suppurative hoof lesions include *F. necrophorum*, *A. pyogenes*, *Bacteroides*, and *Escherichia coli*.

The beta-lactam antibacterials (see section 1.1.1) are commonly used for the treatment of foot infections. Procaine penicillin is used, but may be more effective in combination with streptomycin (see section 1.1.3), particularly in cases of footrot in sheep.

Parenteral administration and topical application of tetracyclines (see section 1.1.2) such as chlortetracycline or oxytetracycline are used to treat foot lesions, in particular footrot in cattle, sheep, and pigs.

Sulphadimidine sodium is highly effective in foot infections as are the potentiated sulphonamides (see section 1.1.6).

Metronidazole may be used for irrigation of wounds or as a wet bandage in cases of under-run sole or footrot.

15.1 Anti-infective foot preparations

Foot baths and sprays are common methods of treating foot conditions. Solutions of **cetrimide** or **copper sulphate** can be used for wound cleansing or packing.

Solutions used in foot baths usually contain active ingredients such as **formaldehyde**, copper sulphate, or **zinc sulphate**. Zinc sulphate is less toxic and less irritant than formaldehyde and copper sulphate. Foot baths are used for cattle and sheep. The usual recommendation is to allow the animal to walk through the foot bath slowly.

The active ingredients of sprays include cetrimide, **copper naphthenate**, **dichlorophen**, **chlortetracycline**, and **oxytetracycline**. Cod-liver oil is included in some sprays and this may improve retention of the active ingredient in wet conditions.

CETRIMIDE

Indications. Footrot in sheep; wound cleansing and dressing

Cetrimide Solution
See section 14.6 for preparation details
Cetrimide Solution Strong
See section 14.6 for preparation details
GSL **Footrot Aerosol** (Battle Hayward & Bower)
Spray, cetrimide 6%, diethyl phthalate 2%, for *sheep*; 168 g, 440 g

CHLORTETRACYCLINE HYDROCHLORIDE

See section 14.2.1

COPPER NAPHTHENATE

Indications. Footrot in sheep, hoof lesions in cattle♦ and horses♦, ringworm (14.3)
Warnings. Severe skin lesions occasionally develop in horses

PML **Kopertox**™ (BK, Crown)
Aerosol spray, copper (as naphthenate) 1.25%, for *cattle* (14.3), *sheep*; 294 g
PML **Sprayrem**™ (Cox-Surgical)
Aerosol spray, copper naphthenate 13.5%, cod-liver oil 5%, for *cattle* (14.3), *sheep*; 294 g

COPPER SULPHATE

Indications. Proliferative dermatitis in cattle and sheep, footrot in sheep
Side-effects. Stains wool
Warnings. Toxic, particularly to sheep. Ineffective when solution is dirty. Corrodes metal foot baths
Dose. *Foot bath. Cattle:* copper sulphate 5-10% solution *or* copper sulphate 5%-formaldehyde 10% solution twice daily
Sheep: copper sulphate 5-10% solution
Local application, ointment, powder, or 5% solution

Copper Sulphate
Powder, copper sulphate. To be prepared as a solution for use

Copper Sulphate
Solution, copper sulphate 10%. May be further diluted for use

P **Footrot Ointment** (Crown)
Copper sulphate 46.92%, iron oxide 1.96%, glacial acetic acid 0.9%, for *sheep*; 200 g, 750 g

DICHLOROPHEN

Indications. Footrot in sheep

GSL **Antiseptic Spray** (Ritchey Tagg)
Aerosol spray, dichlorophen 6.5%, suitable dye; 200 g, 400 g
GSL **Footrot Spray** (Crown)
Aerosol spray, dichlorophen 6%, gentian violet 0.3%, for *sheep*; 294 g
GSL **Footrot and Ringworm Spray** (Ritchey Tagg)
Aerosol spray, dichlorophen 6.5%, for *cattle* (14.3), *sheep*; 200 g, 400 g
GSL **Ringworm Aerosol** (Battle Hayward & Bower)
Spray, dichlorophen 3%, undecenoic acid 3%, for *cattle* (14.3); 168 g

FORMALDEHYDE

Indications. Hardening of hooves, footrot in cattle, sheep, and pigs♦
Side-effects. Skin irritation may occur with excessive strength of solution or frequency of use
Warnings. Toxic and irritant. Use in well-ventilated areas. Wear protective clothing in preparation and use of foot bath. Do not use greater than a 10% solution
Dose. *Cattle, sheep, pigs*♦: *foot bath*, 1-3% solution daily for treatment *or* 3-5% solution weekly for prevention
Local application, 5-10% solution

Note. The term formaldehyde is used to describe Formaldehyde Solution BP, also loosely known as formalin.

GSL **Formaldehyde Foot Rot Liquid** (Alfa Laval)
Foot bath, formaldehyde 38%, for *sheep*; 25 litres. To be diluted before use
Dilute 1 volume with 19 volumes water (= formaldehyde 2%)
GSL **Formaldehyde** (Battle Hayward & Bower)
Foot bath, formaldehyde 35%, for *sheep*; 5 litres, 25 litres. To be diluted before use

Dilute 1 volume with 19 volumes water (= formaldehyde 1.75%)

GSL **Formalin** (Micro-Biologicals)
Foot bath, formaldehyde 38%, for *sheep*; 25 litres. To be diluted before use
Dilute 1 volume with 19 volumes water (= formaldehyde 2%)

GSL **Topclip**™ **Formalin** (Ciba-Geigy)
Foot bath, formaldehyde 36.5%, for *cattle*, *sheep*; 25 litres. To be diluted before use
Dilute 1 volume with 19 volumes water (= formaldehyde 1.9%)

OXYTETRACYCLINE HYDROCHLORIDE
See section 14.2.1

ZINC SULPHATE

Indications. Control of footrot in cattle and sheep
Dose. *Foot bath*. *Cattle*: zinc sulphate 10% solution daily *or* zinc sulphate 10%-formaldehyde solution daily. Maximum concentration of formaldehyde should be no greater than 5%. Replenish solution every 30 days
Sheep: zinc sulphate 10% solution after each trimming *or* zinc sulphate 10%-formaldehyde solution after each trimming. Maximum concentration of formaldehyde should be no greater than 5%. Replenish solution every 30 days

PML **Footrite**™ (Crown)
Foot bath, powder for reconstitution, zinc (as sulphate) 28.4%, for *sheep*, 7 kg, 25 kg

PML **Footsure**™ (Young's)
Foot bath, powder for reconstitution, zinc 28.4%, for *sheep*; 25 kg

GSL **Foursure**™ (Synthite)
Foot bath, zinc sulphate (as heptahydrate) 28%, for *sheep*; 20 litres. To be diluted before use

GSL **Golden Hoof**™ (Shep-Fair)
Foot bath, powder for reconstitution, zinc sulphate 99%, for *sheep*; 10 kg, 20 kg

GSL **Golden Hoof Plus**™ (Shep-Fair)
Foot bath, powder for reconstitution, zinc sulphate 99%, wetting agents, for *sheep*; 10 kg, 20 kg

GSL **Hoof-care**™ (Deosan)
Foot bath, powder for reconstitution, zinc sulphate (as heptahydrate) 98%, wetting agents, for *cattle*, *sheep*; 20 kg
Withdrawal Periods. *Cattle*, *sheep*: slaughter withdrawal period nil, milk withdrawal period nil

GSL **Zinc-O-Ped**™ (Battle Hayward & Bower)
Foot bath, powder for reconstitution, zinc sulphate, for *sheep*; 12.5 kg, 20 kg

15.2 Hoof care preparations

Many preparations are said to assist in maintaining the integrity of hoof horn, the efficacy of some being difficult to assess. Beneficial effects have been demonstrated when supplementary **biotin** is added to the diet of biotin-deficient animals. **Methionine** also appears to assist in improving horse hoof horn integrity but its efficacy is better when given in combination with biotin. Application of vegetable oil-based products to the horse hoof will improve appearance of the hoof and probably reduce water loss from the hoof wall and repel salt and corrosive substances. **Tar** or Stockholm tar, which has antiseptic properties, may be used following treatment of an infected frog in the horse or footrot in cattle and sheep. It is used alone or with a packing material to fill defects in the wall, sole, or frog and helps to prevent entry of gravel and reinfection.

BIOTIN

Indications. Biotin-deficiency disorders
Dose. See preparation details

Biocare™ (BK)
Cubes, biotin 7.5 mg/cube, for *horses*; 150
Dose. *Horses*: 7.5-22.5 mg daily

Bio-Ped™ (Battle Hayward & Bower)
Premix, biotin 1.5 mg/g, for *horses*; 300 g

GSL **Biotin** (Arnolds)
Tablets, biotin 50 micrograms, for *dogs*, *cats*; 500

Dose. *Dogs, cats*: 100 micrograms twice daily then 50 micrograms twice weekly

Biotin (Battle Hayward & Bower)
Biotin 750 micrograms/g, for *horses*; 600 g, 1.8 kg

GSL **Biotin** (Micro-Biologicals)
Oral powder, for addition to drinking water, biotin 6.3 mg/g, for *cattle, pigs, poultry*; 20 g

GSL **Equi-Bio**™ (Micro-Biologicals)
Oral powder, for addition to feed, biotin 1.5 mg/g, for *horses*; 300 g
Dose. *Horses*: 5-30 mg daily

Keracare™ (Crown)
Cubes, biotin 7.5 mg, for *horses*; 75
Dose. *Horses*: 7.5-22.5 mg daily

Pedaform™ (C-Vet)
Oral powder, for addition to feed, biotin 1.5 mg/g, for *horses*; 300 g
Dose. *Horses*: 5-30 mg daily

Compound biotin preparations

Biotrition™ (Equine Products)
Oral powder, for addition to feed, biotin 640 micrograms, lysine 1.6 mg, methionine 1.6 mg/g, for *horses*; 500 g, 1.5 kg, 4 kg
Dose. *Horses*: 15-25 g of powder daily

Biotin + Zinc & Methionine (Day Son & Hewitt)
Oral powder, for addition to feed, biotin 1.67 mg, methionine 778 micrograms, zinc (as zinc methionine) 22.2 mg/g, for *horses*; 270 g, 810 g
Dose. *Horses*: 6-15 g of powder daily

Biometh-Z™ (Univet)
Oral powder, for addition to feed, biotin 1 mg, methionine 600 mg, zinc gluconate 67 mg/g, for *horses*; 750 g, 1.5 kg
Dose. *Horses*: 15 g of powder daily

Kera-fac™ (Hand/PH)
Oral powder, for addition to feed, biotin 600 micrograms, calcium 100 micrograms, iron (as sulphate) 2 mg, methionine 200 micrograms, zinc (as sulphate) 4 mg/g, for *horses*; 2.5 kg
Dose. *Horses*: 12.5-37.5 g of powder daily

METHIONINE

Indications. Methionine-deficiency disorders

Methionine (Univet)
Tablets, methionine 250 mg, for *dogs, cats*; 250
Dose. *Dogs, cats*: 250 mg/10 kg 2-3 times daily

Compound methionine preparations

See above, under Compound biotin preparations

TAR
(Stockholm Tar)

Indications. Hoof and horn disorders

Stockholm Tar (Battle Hayward & Bower)
Tar, for *horses, cattle, sheep*; 450 g, 1 kg, other sizes available

TOPICAL HOOF CARE PREPARATIONS

Aintree Antiseptic Hoof Oil (Day Son & Hewitt)
Chloroxylenol 0.1%, pine oil 3%, for *horses*; 500 mL, 5 litres, 25 litres

P **Omniseptine**™ (Lakenlabs)
Ointment, chamomile extract 10%, guaiazulene 0.02%, hexylresorcinol 0.4%, wool fat 28%, for *horses*; 90 g

16 Drugs affecting
NUTRITION AND BODY FLUIDS

16.1 Electrolyte and water replacement solutions
16.2 Plasma substitutes
16.3 Drugs for ketosis
16.4 Minerals
16.5 Vitamins
16.6 Compound multivitamin and mineral preparations
16.7 Special dietary foods for dogs and cats

16.1 Electrolyte and water replacement solutions

16.1.1 Oral solutions
16.1.2 Parenteral solutions

The objectives of fluid therapy, whether oral or parenteral, may include the correction of extracellular fluid (ECF) volume, plasma pH, blood-glucose concentration, plasma concentrations of K^+ and Na^+; restoration of cellular K^+; and the provision of calories.

Any severely dehydrated, shocked, or collapsed animal almost certainly requires parenteral, preferably intravenous, fluid therapy before oral rehydration therapy.

16.1.1 Oral solutions

The effectiveness of oral rehydration therapy depends mainly on the ability to promote intestinal uptake of sodium and water. When reconstituted, oral rehydration preparations consist of isotonic solutions that contain sodium, potassium, and other ions, and glucose. Glycine and anions of fatty acids such as acetate, citrate, and propionate may also be included to facilitate sodium and water uptake. These anions are bicarbonate precursors, which act to repair metabolic acidosis without undermining gastric acidity. Solutions without bicarbonate precursors repair acidosis solely by improving renal perfusion. Oral rehydration solutions are formulated for absorption rather than for the provision of energy. Significant increases in glucose concentration and solution osmolality may lead to hypertonic dehydration and malabsorption diarrhoea. This risk is probably greater in puppies and kittens that are nursed in warm dry surroundings and therefore have greater water losses than in other species such as calves.

The main indication for oral fluid therapy is diarrhoea, which may be accompanied by acidosis. Other uses include post-operative rehydration, an adjunct to intravenous fluid therapy, minimisation of the expected risk of diarrhoea due to stress of transport or weaning, and exertional fluid loss. Concentrated solutions are used in the treatment of pregnancy toxaemia in sheep.

Table 16.1 shows the approximate composition (after reconstitution) of oral rehydration solutions. The volume of fluid and the frequency of administration generally depend on the severity of the condition.

16.1.2 Parenteral solutions

Parenteral solutions essentially restore, by exogenous means, the normal concentrations of natural constituents of ECF. However, idiosyncratic reactions to parenteral fluid constituents may occur in some species, for example, reactions in cats to preservatives in the formulation.

In evaluating an animal for possible fluid therapy, the state of hydration, electrolyte balance, acid-base balance, renal function, and calorific balance should be considered. Evaluation should be based on history, physical examination, and laboratory testing.

The choice of parenteral fluid will depend on the losses that have been incurred. Table 16.2 lists some typical clinical conditions and parenteral solutions that may be appropriate.

The potential effects of parenteral

Table 16.1 Oral rehydration solutions

Product	Na⁺	K⁺	Cl⁻	HCO₃⁻	Precursor†	Glucose %	Ca/Mg	Other components	Species	Reconstitution/dilution details	Pack size
Aminolyte™ (Micro-Biologicals)	85	27	85	0		2.4	+/+	glycine, phosphate	calves, lambs, pigs	Reconstitute paired sachets in 2 litres water	85-g sachets
Anti-Scour™ (Volac)	30	5	23	12		0.8	−/+	organic pulp, phosphate	calves, lambs, piglets	Reconstitute 1 g in 36 mL per kg body-weight for calves, lambs; by addition to feed, 30 g/kg feed for piglets	250 g, 1 kg, other sizes available
BSF Extra™ (SmithKline Beecham)	50	20	39	29	citrate	3.1	−/−	glycine, phosphate	calves	Reconstitute paired sachets in 2 litres water	
Electrosol™ (Arnolds)	115	8	84	46	acetate	2.5	+/+		cattle, pigs, dogs, cats	Dilute 240 mL to 4.5 litres with water	1 litre
Electydral™ (Ciba-Geigy)	80	25	54	50	acetate, propionate	1.4	−/+		calves	Reconstitute 1 sachet in 1.5 litres water	35-g sachets
Ion-Aid™ (RMB)	75	24	75	0		2.3	+/+	glycine, phosphate	calves, pigs, lambs	Reconstitute 2-compartment sachet in 2.3 litres water	85-g sachets
Ionalyte™ (Intervet)	145	11	108	57	acetate	0	+/+		foals, cattle, pigs, dogs, cats	Dilute 1 volume with 15 volumes water	1 litre
IRT Conc™ (Bimeda)	140	10	103	55	acetate	0	+/+		horses, cattle, sheep, pigs	Dilute 1 volume with 19 volumes water	240 mL
Lactolyte™ (Virbac)	77	32	55	40	acetate, propionate	0	+/+	dehydrated whey, phosphate	calves	Reconstitute 1 sachet in 1.5–2.0 litres water	90-g sachets
Lectade™ (SmithKline Beecham)	73	16	73	4	citrate	2.2	−/−	phosphate	horses, calves, pigs, lambs, dogs, cats	Reconstitute small animal paired sachet in 500 mL water; reconstitute large animal sachet in 2–4 litres	Paired sachets
Lectade™ Plus (SmithKline Beecham)	50	20	39	29	citrate	3.1	−/−	glycine, phosphate	calves	Reconstitute paired sachets in 2 litres water	Paired sachets

Table 16.1 Oral rehydration solutions (*continued*)

Product	Na⁺	K⁺	Cl⁻	HCO₃⁻	Pre-cursor†	Glu-cose %	Ca/Mg	Other compo-nents	Species	Reconstitution/dilution details	Pack size
	Millimoles per litre										

Product	Na⁺	K⁺	Cl⁻	HCO₃⁻	Precursor†	Glucose %	Ca/Mg	Other components	Species	Reconstitution/dilution details	Pack size
Liquid Lectade™ (SmithKline Beecham)	74	16	73	13	citrate	2.2	−/−	phosphate	calves, sheep	Dilute 1 volume with 11.5 volumes water; use undiluted for pregnancy toxaemia in sheep (see section 16.3)	960 mL
Life Aid P™ (Norbrook)	76	15	74	2	propion-ate	2.5	−/−	glycine, phosphate	calves, pigs	Reconstitute paired sachets in 2 litres water	Paired sachets
Liquid Life-Aid™ (Norbrook)	79	15	74	2	propion-ate	2.4	−/−	glycine, phosphate	calves, pigs, sheep	Dilute 1 volume with 11.5 volumes water; use undiluted for pregnancy toxaemia in sheep (see section 16.3)	960 mL
Scourproof-V™ (Micro-biologicals)	84	15	48	52	acetate	1.6	−/+	mucopoly-saccharide, wheat bran	calves	Reconstitute 1 sachet in 1.5 litres water	67.2-g sachets

All entries are GSL
† 1 mmol acetate = 1 mmol bicarbonate
 1 mmol citrate = 3 mmol bicarbonate
 1 mmol propionate = 1 mmol bicarbonate

solutions are best judged by comparing the composition to that of normal plasma. Parenteral solutions may be classified according to their clinical use: restoration of ECF volume, specific restoration of plasma volume (see section 16.2), acidifiers, alkalinisers, ECF diluents, maintenance solutions, nutrient solutions, and concentrated additives. Particular solutions may be incompatible with other solutions, for example, calcium – and bicarbonate – containing solutions, or with drugs (see Drug Incompatibilities – Appendix 2). The *restoration of ECF volume* can only be achieved by solutions of plasma-like sodium concentration (130-160 mmol/litre), preferably administered intra-venously. Intravenous infusions used include **sodium chloride 0.9%**, **Hartmann's Solution**, and **Darrow's Solution**. Darrow's solution contains a high potassium concentration and is not suitable for initial restoration of ECF volume in cases of neonatal diarrhoea when, despite potassium depletion, hyperkalaemia is likely as a result of acidosis and poor perfusion of tissues generally and the kidneys in particular. Total fluid deficits in clinically dehydrated animals are likely to be 50-150 mL/kg of which 50% of the deficit should be corrected within 6 hours. Fluids may be administered at a rate of 10 mL/kg per hour for 6 hours; this would provide 50% of the fluid required

Table 16.2 Parenteral fluid therapy for various disorders

Condition	Disturbances	Fluid	Suggested additives
Drought, unable to drink/swallow, diabetes insipidus, polyuric renal failure, pyrexia	primary water depletion	sodium chloride 0.18% + glucose 4%	potassium chloride (10–20 mmol/L) if therapy longer than 3 days
Vomiting	loss of water, H^+, Na^+, Cl^-, K^+; metabolic alkalosis	Ringer's solution or sodium chloride 0.9%	potassium chloride (10–20 mmol/L) if therapy longer than 3 days
Vomiting (bile-stained)	loss of water, H^+, HCO_3^-, Cl^-, Na^+; metabolic acidosis	sodium chloride 0.9%	
Diarrhoea	loss of water, Na^+, HCO_3^-, Cl^-, (K^+ if long term); metabolic acidosis	compound sodium lactate infusion	potassium chloride (10–20 mmol/L) if therapy is prolonged; bicarbonate (1–3 mmol/kg) if condition is severe and therapy is prolonged
Bowel obstruction	loss of water, Na^+, Cl^-, HCO_3^-; metabolic acidosis	plasma expander + compound sodium lactate infusion	bicarbonate (1–3 mmol/kg)
Urethral obstruction, ruptured urinary bladder	accumulation of K^+, H^+; metabolic acidosis	sodium chloride 0.9% + glucose 5% or sodium chloride 0.18% + glucose 4% or sodium chloride 0.9%	bicarbonate (1–3 mmol/kg) if in hypovolaemic shock
Haemorrhage	blood loss; hypovolaemic shock	plasma expander or compound sodium lactate infusion; whole blood if PCV is low	
Burns, peritonitis, pancreatitis	loss of plasma and ECF; hypovolaemic shock	plasma expander + compound sodium lactate infusion	bicarbonate (1–3 mmol/kg)

for a patient with a fluid deficit of 120 mL/kg. Initial treatment of shock may need higher infusion rates of up to 100 mL/kg per hour (less in cats). High infusion rates should only be used for short periods and in the absence of pulmonary or cardiac dysfunction. Cardio-pulmonary function should be monitored during infusion at high rates and restoration of urine output must be confirmed.

Disturbances of plasma-sodium concentration reflect water rather than sodium imbalance. Therefore, hyponatraemia is generally corrected by repair of ECF volume and hypernatraemia by controlled access to water given orally or gradual use of glucose 5% intravenous infusion or sodium chloride 0.45% intravenous infusion, to avoid sudden changes in plasma-sodium concentration.

Acidifiers contain no bicarbonate precursors and are used to repair metabolic alkalosis. They may improve a mild acidosis despite their composition, by increasing ECF volume and thereby improving renal perfusion and function. Intravenous infusions used as acidifiers include **Ringer's Solution** and **sodium chloride 0.9%**.

Alkalinisers are required for the repair of metabolic acidosis. These solutions contain bicarbonate or one of its precursors such as lactate or acetate. Lactate is converted solely in the liver and is not suitable for use in patients with hepatic impairment. **Hartmann's Solution** contains lactate at a concentration similar to normal plasma; higher concentrations of bicarbonate or its precursor may be needed for severe acidosis.

In the absence of measured plasma-bicarbonate deficit, but with a history suggesting metabolic acidosis, an initial dose of bicarbonate of 1-2 mmol/kg may be given and repeated as necessary after some hours.

Correction of hyperkalaemia is facilitated by the correction of metabolic acidosis. Cell-potassium deficits can exist in the presence of hyperkalaemia.

ECF diluents provide a parenteral source of water that is made temporarily isotonic, such as contained in **glucose 5%** intravenous infusion. Calorie content is trivial compared with daily requirements although there is temporary relief of hypoglycaemia.

Maintenance solutions substitute for normal oral intake of water and dietary electrolytes. They contain approximately 20% of the plasma-sodium concentration plus other electrolytes, notably potassium, and sufficient glucose (usually about 4%) for isotonicity. They are intended for intravenous infusion rather than subcutaneous use, which may be important in dehydrated animals because of the low sodium concentration

of such solutions. Examples of maintenance solutions include **Duphalyte™**, and **sodium chloride 0.18% and glucose 4%** intravenous infusion.

Nutrient solutions are intended to provide a nutritionally adequate substitute for the diet where oral intake is not possible, grossly insufficient, or contra-indicated over an extended period. Nutrient solutions are based on high concentrations of glucose or lipid emulsions to provide calories, soya or casein protein hydrolysates or amino acids to provide protein precursors and essential amino acids. Nutrient solutions increase the risk of phlebitis and systemic infections and should only be given intravenously through large veins. At present, there are no nutrient solutions licensed for veterinary use.

Concentrated additives are added to existing solutions to increase the content of one particular ion, for example, bicarbonate or potassium, with minimal change in volume. They must be adequately mixed before being received by the animal. High concentrations of potassium may cause cardiac arrhythmias.

Table 16.3 shows the approximate composition of parenteral fluids licensed for use in veterinary medicine.

GLUCOSE
(Dextrose monohydrate)

Indications. See notes above
Dose. See preparation details and notes above

PoM **Aqupharm™ No 6** (Animalcare)
Intravenous infusion, glucose 5%, for *dogs, cats*; 500 mL, 1 litre

PML **Dextrose 20%** (Bimeda)
Injection, glucose 20%, for *lambs*, 400 mL
Withdrawal Periods. *Lambs*: slaughter withdrawal period nil
Dose. *Lambs*: *by intraperitoneal injection*, 10 mL/kg

PoM **Duphalyte™** (Duphar)
Infusion, amino acids, calcium chloride dihydrate, dexpanthenol, glucose, hydroxocobalamin, magnesium sulphate,

Table 16.3 Composition of parenteral fluids

		Na$^+$	K$^+$	Ca^{2+}	Mg^{2+}	Cl$^-$	HCO$_3^-$	Precursor	Glucose %	Other components
Normal plasma values (in the dog)		145	5	2.5	0.82	100	24			
Intravenous infusions										
Aqupharm™ No 1 (Animalcare)	sodium chloride 0.9% intravenous infusion	150				150				
Aqupharm™ No 3 (Animalcare)	sodium chloride 0.9% + glucose 5% intravenous infusion	150				150			5.0	
Aqupharm™ No 6 (Animalcare)	glucose 5% intravenous infusion								5.0	
Aqupharm™ No 9 (Animalcare)	Ringer's Solution	147	4	2.0		155				
Aqupharm™ No 10 (Animalcare)	Darrow's Solution	121	35			103	53	lactate		
Aqupharm™ No 11 (Animalcare)	compound sodium lactate infusion	131	5	2.0		111	29	lactate		
Aqupharm™ No 18 (Animalcare)	sodium chloride 0.18% + glucose 4%	30				30			4.0	
Calvet™ No 10 (Animalcare)	sodium chloride 0.9% + glucose 5.5% intravenous infusion	150				150			5.5	
Duphalyte™ (Duphar)		18	3	1.0	0.8	5	18	acetate	5	vitamins, amino acids
GS-5.5 (BK, Crown)	sodium chloride 0.9% + glucose 5.5% intravenous infusion	150				150			5.5	
Haemaccel™ (Hoechst)		145	5	6.0		156				polygeline 3.5%
Intraven™ (Ivex)	glucose 5% intravenous infusion								5.0	
	glucose 10% intravenous infusion								10	
	glucose 20% intravenous infusion								20	
	glucose 50% intravenous infusion								50	

Table 16.3 Composition of parenteral fluids (*continued*)

	Millimoles per litre						Pre-cursor	Glucose %	Other components
	Na^+	K^+	Ca^{2+}	Mg^{2+}	Cl^-	HCO_3^-			
sodium chloride 0.45% intravenous infusion	75				75				
sodium chloride 0.9% intravenous infusion	150				150				
sodium chloride 0.18% + glucose 4% intravenous infusion	30				30			4.0	
sodium chloride 0.9% + glucose 5% intravenous infusion	150				150			5.0	
Isolec™ (Ivex)	131	5	2.0		111	29	lactate		
Additives Sodium bicarbonate 1.26%	150					150			
Sodium bicarbonate 8.4%	1000					1000			
Potassium chloride solution, strong		2000			2000				

nicotinamide, potassium chloride, pyridoxine hydrochloride, riboflavine (as sodium phosphate), sodium acetate trihydrate, thiamine hydrochloride, for *horses, cattle, pigs, dogs, cats*; 100 mL, 500 mL

Dose. *Horses: by slow intravenous injection*, up to 2 mL/kg; *foals: by slow intravenous injection*, up to 6 mL/kg

Cattle, pigs: by subcutaneous, slow intravenous, or intraperitoneal injection, up to 2 mL/kg; *calves, piglets: by subcutaneous, slow intravenous, or intraperitoneal injection*, up to 6 mL/kg

Dogs, cats: by subcutaneous or intravenous infusion, up to 10 mL/kg

PoM **Intraven™ Glucose Intravenous Infusion** (Ivex)
Intravenous infusion, glucose 5%; 50 mL, 100 mL, other sizes available

Intravenous infusion, glucose 10%; 500 mL, 1 litre
Intravenous infusion, glucose 20%; 500 mL, 1 litre
Intravenous infusion, glucose 50%; 500 mL

For preparations containing sodium chloride and glucose see under Sodium chloride, below

POTASSIUM CHLORIDE

Indications. See notes above
Warnings. Rapid injection may be cardiotoxic
Dose. Maximum rate 0.5 mmol/kg per hour

PoM **Potassium Chloride Solution, Strong**
Sterile solution, for addition to intravenous

infusion, potassium chloride 150 mg/mL; 10 mL

Note. Must be diluted with not less than 50 times its volume of sodium chloride 0.9% or other suitable diluent and mixed well

SODIUM BICARBONATE

Indications. See notes above
Warnings. Incompatible with calcium-containing solutions (see Drug Incompatibilities – Appendix 2)
Dose. See notes above

PoM **Sodium Bicarbonate Intravenous Infusion**
Injection, for addition to intravenous infusion, sodium bicarbonate 1.26%, 1.4%, 2.74%, 4.2%, 8.4%; various sizes available

SODIUM CHLORIDE

Indications. Dose. See notes above

PoM **Aqupharm™ No 1** (Animalcare)
Intravenous infusion, sodium chloride 0.9%, for *dogs, cats*; 500 mL, 1 litre

PoM **Aqupharm™ No 3** (Animalcare)
Intravenous infusion, sodium chloride 0.9%, glucose 4%, for *dogs, cats*; 500 mL, 1 litre

PoM **Aqupharm™ No 9** (Animalcare)
Intravenous infusion, (Ringer's solution), sodium chloride 0.86%, calcium chloride hexahydrate, potassium chloride, for *dogs, cats*; 500 mL, 1 litre

PoM **Aqupharm™ No 18** (Animalcare)
Intravenous infusion, glucose 4%, sodium chloride 0.18%, for *dogs, cats*; 500 mL, 1 litre

PML **Calvet™ No 10** (Animalcare)
Intravenous infusion, sodium chloride 0.9%, glucose 5.5%, for *cattle, sheep, pigs, dogs, cats*; 400 mL

PML **GS-5.5** (BK, Crown)
Intravenous infusion, sodium chloride 0.9%, glucose 5.5%, for *cattle, sheep, pigs*; 400 mL

PoM **Intraven™ Sodium Chloride Intravenous Infusion** (Ivex)
Intravenous infusion, sodium chloride 0.45%; 500 mL
Intravenous infusion, sodium chloride 0.9%; 50 mL, 100 mL, other sizes available

PoM **Intraven™ Sodium Chloride and Glucose Intravenous Infusion** (Ivex)
Intravenous infusion, sodium chloride 0.18%, glucose 4%; 500 mL, 1 litre
Intravenous infusion, sodium chloride 0.9%, glucose 5%; 500 mL, 1 litre

SODIUM LACTATE

Indications. See notes above
Contra-indications. Hepatic impairment; patients with cardiac arrhythmias
Dose. See notes above

PoM **Aqupharm™ No 10** (Animalcare)
Intravenous infusion, (Darrow's solution), potassium chloride, sodium chloride, sodium lactate, for *dogs, cats*; 1 litre

PoM **Aqupharm™ No 11** (Animalcare)
Intravenous infusion, (compound sodium lactate intravenous infusion), calcium chloride dihydrate, potassium chloride, sodium chloride, sodium lactate, for *dogs, cats*; 500 mL, 1 litre

PoM **Isolec™** (Ivex)
Intravenous infusion, (compound sodium lactate intravenous infusion), bicarbonate (as lactate), calcium, chloride, potassium, sodium, for *horses, cattle*; 3 litres, 5 litres

16.2 Plasma substitutes

Haemorrhage occurs most commonly as a result of trauma but may also occur internally following surgery; rupture of tumours, abdominal ulceration in cattle, or guttural pouch mycosis in horses; or post partum. Haemorrhage may be associated with coagulopathies or platelet abnormalities due to poisoning with warfarin or bracken, or congenital bleeding disorders.

Shock is the failure of adequate perfusion of cells, tissues, and organs. Causes of shock are numerous and include hypovolaemia resulting from haemorrhage, fluid and electrolyte loss due to vomiting and diarrhoea, heat stroke, and burns; toxic shock due to sepsis or endotoxaemia; and vasogenic shock due to traumatic injury, anaphylaxis, or electrocution.

Plasma substitutes such as **gelatin** are artificial colloids that restore circulating volume by mimicking the action of plasma proteins such as albumin.

Plasma substitutes are retained in the circulation longer than electrolyte solutions due to their higher molecular weight. The use of colloids and electrolyte solutions in preference to whole blood in the early stages of shock ensures that the 'sludging phenomena', which occur in the peripheral microcirculation, are minimised.

Severe haemorrhage may lead to hypovolaemia and is life-threatening. Restoration of circulating blood volume with plasma-replacement solutions is a priority before replacing ECF loss. If packed-cell volume (PCV) falls below 150 mL/litre in cattle or 210 mL/litre in dogs and cats, whole blood transfusion should be considered.

Cross-matching of donor and recipient blood is not always possible but, fortunately, reactions are rarely seen in first transfusion animals. A healthy adult animal of the same species as the patient should be used as a donor. One percent of the donor's body-weight is the amount of blood that may be safely taken at one time. Before transfusion, corticosteroids (see section 7.2.1), such as dexamethasone 100 micrograms/kg, may be administered to prevent transfusion reactions such as dyspnoea and pyrexia. Intravenous administration of blood into the patient should be performed slowly. Intraperitoneal transfusion may be of value especially in neonates.

GELATIN

Indications. Shock
Contra-indications. Mixing with citrated blood
Dose. Volume equal to estimated blood loss

PoM **Haemaccel**™ (Hoechst)
Intravenous infusion, polygeline (degraded gelatin, average molecular-weight 35 000) 35 g/litre, with sodium chloride, potassium chloride, and calcium chloride; 500 mL

16.3 Drugs for ketosis
(bovine acetonaemia, ovine pregnancy toxaemia)

Ketosis is caused by accumulation of ketone bodies in the blood and tissues. Depending on the causative agent, the condition is generally self-limiting and responsive to treatment in cattle but often fatal in sheep.

Any factor that causes a reduction in the intake or absorption of dietary carbohydrate precursors can cause ketosis. Secondary ketosis is commonly caused by depressed appetite resulting from a primary disease such as metritis, mastitis, or abomasal displacement.

Normally, carbohydrates in the diet are converted to acetic, butyric, and propionic acids in the rumen. Propionic acid is converted to oxaloacetate, which forms glucose. Acetic and butyric acids are converted via the tricarboxylic acid cycle to produce energy, provided oxaloacetate is available.

An increased utilisation of glucose as in early lactation in cows or in ewes carrying twins or triplets, a reduced ingestion of carbohydrate due to an inadequate diet, or a disease state will result in a decreased amount of available oxaloacetate. Acetic and butyric acids are therefore converted to the ketone bodies acetoacetate and beta-hydroxybutyrate. High concentrations of ketone bodies cause inappetance and further exacerbate the situation. In both species the liver is depleted of glycogen and, especially in sheep, undergoes fatty change.

Treatment is aimed at providing replacement glucose. Immediate relief is achieved by intravenous injection of **glucose**, although response may be transient if treatment is not continued until the negative energy balance is relieved. In addition, glucose precursors such as **propionate** and **propylene glycol** may be given by mouth. Many preparations contain cobalt and iodine as concurrent deficiencies of these minerals may add to the severity of the condition.

Glucocorticoids (see section 7.2.1) aid therapy by causing gluconeogenesis, stimulating appetite, and reducing milk yield in cattle. High doses may induce parturition in early cases of pregnancy toxaemia in ewes. Many ewes also develop metabolic acidosis and treatment with intravenous solutions such as compound sodium lactate infusion or sodium bicarbonate infusion (section 16.1.2) is necessary.

Control of ketosis includes the provision of an adequate and balanced diet before and during the risk period.

GLUCOSE
(Dextrose monohydrate)

Indications. Ketosis
Dose. *Cattle*: *by subcutaneous or slow intravenous injection*, 200-400 g
Sheep: *by subcutaneous or slow intravenous injection*, 50-100 g

PML **Calvet™ No 8** (Animalcare)
Injection, glucose 50%, for *cattle, sheep*; 400 mL

PML **D-50™ No 8** (BK, Crown)
Injection, glucose 50%, for *cattle, sheep*; 400 mL

GLYCEROL

Indications. Ketosis; glaucoma (12.5)
Dose. Ketosis.
Cattle: 500 mL twice daily for 2-3 days
Sheep: 3 mL/kg (maximum dose 120 mL)

GSL **Glycerol** (Non-proprietary)
PML **Twin-Lamb Remedy** (Battle Hayward & Bower)
Oral liquid, calcium glycerophosphate 20 mg, glucose 530 mg, glycerol 0.38 mL/mL, for *sheep*; 150 mL
Dose. *Sheep*: 150 mL and repeated after 12 hours if required

PROPYLENE GLYCOL

Indications. Ketosis
Dose. See preparation details

GSL **Acetade** (C-Vet)
Oral liquid, propylene glycol containing cobalt sulphate 990 micrograms, potassium iodide 1.76 mg/mL, for *cattle, sheep*; 1 litre, 5 litres
Dose. *Cattle*: 200 mL twice daily for 1 day then 100 mL twice daily for 3 days
Sheep: 100 mL daily

GSL **Forketos™** (Arnolds)
Oral solution, propylene glycol 800 mg, choline chloride 20.3 mg, cobalt sulphate 1 mg, potassium iodide 1.76 mg/mL, for *cattle, sheep*; 1 litre, 25 litres
Dose. *Cattle*: 114-227 mL daily *Sheep*: 114 mL daily

GSL **Ketofree™** (Intervet)
Oral liquid, for addition to drinking water or feed or to prepare an oral solution, propylene glycol 80 mg, choline chloride 20 mg, potassium iodide 1.78 mg/mL, for *cattle, sheep*; 1 litre
Dose. *Cattle*: 227 mL twice daily for 1 day then 114 mL twice daily for 3 days *Sheep*: 114 mL daily

GSL **Ketol™** (Intervet)
Oral liquid, propylene glycol 0.8 mL, choline chloride 20 mg, potassium iodide 1.78 mg/mL, for *cattle, sheep*; 1 litre, 23 litres
Dose. *Cattle*: 225 mL twice daily for 1 day then 115 mL twice daily for 3 days *Sheep*: 115 mL daily

GSL **Ketosaid™** (Norbrook)
Oral liquid, propylene glycol 0.99 mL/mL, for *cattle, sheep*; 1 litre, 2 litres, other sizes available
Withdrawal Periods. *Cattle, sheep*: slaughter withdrawal period nil, milk withdrawal period nil
Dose. *Cattle*: 200 mL twice daily for 1 day then 100 mL twice daily for 3 days *Sheep*: 100 mL daily for 4 days

GSL **Ketosis™** (Crown)
Oral liquid, propylene glycol containing cobalt sulphate 990 micrograms, potassium iodide 1.76 mg/mL, for *cattle, sheep*; 1 litre, 5 litres
Dose. *Cattle*: 200 mL twice daily for 1 day then 100 mL twice daily for 3 days *Sheep*: 100 mL daily

GSL **Liquid Lectade™** (SmithKline Beecham)
See Table 16.1 for preparation details
Dose. *Sheep*: pregnancy toxaemia, 160 mL, repeat every 4-8 hours as necessary

GSL **Liquid Life-Aid™** (Norbrook)
See Table 16.1 for preparation details
Dose. *Sheep*: pregnancy toxaemia, 160 mL, repeat 3-6 times daily as necessary

GSL **Twin Lamb**™ (Trilanco)
Oral liquid, propylene glycol containing cobalt sulphate 990 micrograms, potassium iodide 1.76 mg/mL, for *sheep*; 1 litre
Dose. *Sheep*: 100 mL daily

16.4 Minerals

16.4.1   Calcium
16.4.2   Cobalt
16.4.3   Copper
16.4.4   Iodine
16.4.5   Iron
16.4.6   Magnesium
16.4.7   Manganese
16.4.8   Phosphorus
16.4.9   Selenium
16.4.10 Sodium
16.4.11 Zinc
16.4.12 Compound mineral
            preparations

The need for treatment with the major minerals is restricted almost entirely to calcium, magnesium, and phosphorus. Magnesium and phosphorus deficiencies are often associated with hypocalcaemia. Severe sodium deficiency in cattle occurs occasionally but deficiencies of the other major mineral elements such as potassium and sulphur are rare.

The diets of ruminants often contain insufficient concentrations of trace elements and primary deficiencies of cobalt, copper, and selenium may occur. Interference with the absorption of these trace elements by sulphate, molybdenum, or iron can result in secondary deficiencies. A primary iron deficiency is almost entirely restricted to the rapidly growing piglet.

A wide variety of therapeutic preparations are available for the treatment and prevention of mineral deficiency diseases.

16.4.1 Calcium

In dairy cows, short-term calcium imbalance almost always occurs at, or soon after, parturition when lactation more than doubles the animal's requirement for calcium. This increased demand is not always balanced by an increase in the intestinal absorption of calcium or by the mobilisation of calcium from bone and the concentration of calcium in the plasma may fall. In ewes, a similar imbalance can occur in late pregnancy and in bitches eclampsia may occur in late pregnancy or early lactation. In beef cattle and sheep, hypocalcaemia may occur when animals are fed a diet high in oxalate-containing plants. Hypocalcaemia is rarely seen in mares but may be precipitated by stress, such as during foal heat or transport.

Signs of hypocalcaemia in cattle are characterised by a short period of excitement and tetany, and muscle tremor of the head and limbs. The animal becomes stiff in gait. The stiffness is followed by muscular weakness and ataxia leading to sternal recumbency and a characteristic kinking of the neck. In sheep the signs are similar to those in cattle but most cases occur in the last month of pregnancy and may be confused with signs of pregnancy toxaemia (see section 16.3). In mares lactation tetany results in tetanic convulsions after a period of stiffness and incoordination. In dogs hypocalcaemia is characterised by behavioural aberrations, muscle twitches, ataxia, paresis, and ultimately tetany and grand mal seizures.

In hypocalcaemia, the amount of calcium provided therapeutically is usually insufficient to provide for the increased output, but the objective of therapy is to correct the imbalance in the short term and to stimulate homoeostatic mechanisms to adapt to the increased requirements for calcium. In most cases an almost immediate and dramatic response follows intravenous infusion of calcium in all species. Calcium borogluconate is routinely used in ruminants at concentrations of either 20 or 40 percent. The amount of calcium provided therapeutically is small in comparison with the animal's daily requirement and it is essential to ensure that appetite is maintained. If eclampsia occurs in bitches, ideally pups should not be allowed to suckle the dam but should be hand reared.

In cattle, a volume of calcium injection equal to that administered intravenously may also be administered by subcutaneous injection. Subcutaneous injection of calcium in dogs and cats may cause necrosis at the site of injection and in cattle subcutaneous swelling may persist for several days.

The absorption of calcium from the gastro-intestinal tract and mobilisation of calcium from bone may be accelerated by calcitriol (see section 16.5.4). This vitamin may be used for the prevention of hypocalcaemia in dairy cattle. In dogs and cats, oral calcium supplementation during the latter stages of pregnancy may prevent hypocalcaemia.

CALCIUM SALTS

Indications. Prevention and treatment of hypocalcaemia
Side-effects. Persistent swelling or necrosis at injection site, see notes above
Dose. Expressed as calcium
Treatment. *Horses, cattle: by subcutaneous or slow intravenous injection*, 3-12 g according to the patient's response, dependent on clinical signs and blood analysis
Sheep, goats, pigs: by subcutaneous or slow intravenous injection, 0.5-1.5 g according to the patient's response, dependent on clinical signs and blood analysis
Dogs: by slow intravenous injection, 75-500 mg according to the patient's response, dependent on clinical signs and blood analysis
Prophylaxis. *Dogs, cats*: see oral preparation details

Note. 1 mg calcium ≡ 11.2 mg calcium gluconate ≡ 13.2 mg calcium borogluconate

Oral preparations

Canovel Calcium Tablets (SmithKline Beecham)
Tablets, calcium, for *dogs, cats*; 30, 150
Dose. *Dogs*: (less than 9 kg body-weight) ½ tablet daily; (more than 9 kg) 1 tablet/9 kg daily
Cats: ½ tablet daily

See also section 16.5.4

Parenteral preparations

PoM **Calcium Gluconate** (Non-proprietary)
Injection, calcium (as gluconate) 8.9 mg/mL (≡ calcium gluconate 10%); 5 mL, 10 mL

PML **Calc™ No 1** (BK)
Injection, calcium 15.2 mg/mL, for *cattle, sheep*; 400 mL

PML **Calc™ No 2** (BK)
Injection, calcium 30.4 mg/mL, for *cattle, sheep*; 400 mL

PML **Calcibor™ CBG 20%** (Arnolds)
Injection, calcium (as borogluconate) 15.2 mg/mL (≡ calcium borogluconate 20%), for *cattle, sheep, pigs*; 400 mL

PML **Calcibor™ CBG 40%** (Arnolds)
Injection, calcium (as borogluconate) 30.4 mg/mL (≡ calcium borogluconate 40%), for *cattle, sheep, pigs*; 400 mL

PML **Calciject™ 40** (Norbrook)
Injection, calcium (as borogluconate) 30.4 mg/mL (≡ calcium borogluconate 40%), for *horses, cattle, sheep, goats, pigs, dogs*; 400 mL

PML **Calvet™ No 1** (Animalcare)
Injection, calcium (as borogluconate) 15.2 mg/mL (≡ calcium borogluconate 20%), for *cattle, sheep*; 400 mL

PML **Calvet™ No 2** (Animalcare)
Injection, calcium (as borogluconate) 30.4 mg/mL (≡ calcium borogluconate 40%), for *cattle, sheep*; 400 mL

PML **CBG-20™** (Crown)
Injection, calcium 15.2 mg/mL, for *cattle, sheep*; 400 mL

PML **CBG-40™** (Crown)
Injection, calcium 30.4 mg/mL, for *cattle, sheep*; 400 mL

PML **Flexopax™ No 1** (BK)
Injection, calcium (as gluconate) 15.2 mg/mL (≡ calcium borogluconate 20%), for *cattle, sheep, pigs, dogs*; 400 mL

PML **Flexopax™ No 2** (BK)
Injection, calcium (as gluconate) 30.4 mg/mL (≡ calcium borogluconate 40%), for *cattle, sheep, pigs*; 400 mL

PML **Supercal™ 20%** (Bimeda)
Injection, calcium (as borogluconate) 14.84 mg/mL (≡ calcium borogluconate 19.6%), for *cattle, sheep*; 400 mL

PML **Supercal™ 40%** (Bimeda)
Injection, calcium (as borogluconate) 29.68 mg/mL (≡ calcium borogluconate 39.2%), for *cattle, sheep*; 400 mL

Compound calcium preparations

PML **Calcitad™ 50** (BK)
Injection, calcium borogluconate 429 mg, calcium gluconate 31 mg, calcium hydroxide 13.2 mg, magnesium chloride 65 mg, phosphorylethanolamine 6 mg/mL, for *cattle, dogs*; 100 mL
Dose. *Cattle*: by *subcutaneous or slow intravenous injection*, 100 mL
Dogs: by *subcutaneous, intramuscular, or slow intravenous injection*, 3-10 mL

PML **Maxacal™** (Crown)
Injection, calcium borogluconate 429 mg, calcium gluconate 31 mg, calcium hydroxide 13.2 mg, magnesium chloride 65 mg, phosphorylethanolamine 6 mg/mL, for *cattle*; 100 mL
Dose. *Cattle*: by *subcutaneous or slow intravenous injection*, 100 mL

See also section 16.4.12.1

16.4.2 Cobalt

Cobalt is an essential trace element. It is a component of cyanocobalamin and hydroxocobalamin, which are forms of vitamin B_{12} (see section 16.5.2). Vitamin B_{12} is synthesised by the microflora in the gastro-intestinal tract of ruminants and therefore cobalt supplements need to be given by mouth.
Cobalt deficiency predominantly affects young growing ruminants. The signs of cobalt deficiency in ruminants are not specific. There is a decrease of appetite, loss of body-weight, and emaciation with anaemia. Pica often develops and growth and wool production decline. Prevention of deficiency can be provided by a slow-release ruminal bolus containing cobalt oxide. Alternatively, cobalt may be included as a component of anthelmintic preparations.

COBALT OXIDE

Indications. Prevention and treatment of cobalt deficiency

Contra-indications. Administration of ruminal boluses to animals under 8 weeks of age
Dose. See preparation details

GSL **Cobalt Pellets** (Cox-Surgical)
Ruminal bolus, s/r, cobalt oxide 3 g, for *sheep*; 100
Dose. *Sheep*: one 3-g ruminal bolus
Ruminal bolus, s/r, cobalt oxide 9 g, for *cattle*; 30
Dose. *Cattle*: one 9-g ruminal bolus

Permaco™ C (Coopers Pitman-Moore)
Ruminal bolus, s/r, cobalt (as oxide) 6.3 g, for *cattle*; 30
Dose. *Cattle*: one 6.3-g ruminal bolus with concurrent administration of a grinder

Permaco™ S (Coopers Pitman-Moore)
Ruminal bolus, s/r, cobalt (as oxide) 2.1 g, for *sheep*; 100
Dose. *Sheep*: one 2.1-g ruminal bolus with concurrent administration of a grinder

16.4.3 Copper

Copper deficiency is common in ruminants and affects predominantly young growing animals. Primary deficiency may occur owing to inadequate dietary copper and secondary deficiency because of high levels of molybdenum, iron, or sulphate in the diet.
Signs of copper deficiency include inhibition of growth in the immature animal, discoloration of the hair, and dysfunction of the central nervous system with demyelination in neonatal lambs, which is commonly termed 'swayback'.
In cattle, primary and secondary copper deficiency can cause unthriftiness, loss of coat colour, and diarrhoea. 'Pine' is sometimes used to describe unthriftiness due to copper or cobalt deficiency in calves. If the deficiency is prolonged, the structure of the collagen is altered resulting in deformity of long bones. In sheep, copper deficiency is usually associated with enzootic ataxia due to demyelination. There are structural changes in the wool and it becomes discoloured.

Treatment of hypocuprosis is by parenteral injection of copper salts. Care should be taken to avoid overdosing sheep, which are susceptible to copper toxicity. Copper salts such as calcium copperedetate and cuproxoline are rapidly mobilised from the site of intramuscular or subcutaneous administration and may be toxic in sheep. The recommended doses for sheep provide only a small amount of copper. Preparations based on methionine or heptonate complexes are not so readily mobilised from the site of injection and are more commonly used in sheep.

The oral administration of copper can also correct copper deficiencies but more slowly than parenteral treatment because of the time taken for intestinal absorption and its possible inhibition by sulphates, iron, and molybdenum. Slow-release preparations based on copper oxide are available.

Any excess copper provided by either oral or parenteral preparations is stored in body tissues predominantly in the liver. In sheep, the concentration of copper in the liver can become so high that there may be a sudden release of copper into the blood causing intravascular haemolysis leading to a haemolytic crisis and death.

COPPER SALTS

Indications. Prevention and treatment of hypocuprosis

Contra-indications. Concurrent administration of other medicines including copper-containing preparations but excluding vaccines. Hepatic or renal impairment

Warnings. Administer only to animals at risk or suffering from hypocuprosis; sheep are particularly susceptible to copper toxicity

Dose. See preparation details

Oral preparations

PML **Copacaps**™ **Cattle** (RMB)
Ruminal bolus, s/r, copper (as oxide) 8.8 g, for *cattle*; 50
Dose. *Cattle*: (100-200 kg body-weight) one 8.8-g ruminal bolus; (more than

200 kg body-weight) two 8.8-g ruminal boluses

PML **Copacaps**™ **Ewe/Calf** (RMB)
Ruminal bolus, s/r, copper (as oxide) 2.1 g, for *calves, sheep*; 30
Dose. *Calves*: one 2.1-g ruminal bolus per 25 kg body-weight (maximum dose 8 ruminal boluses)
Sheep: two 2.1-g ruminal boluses; *lambs*: (20-40 kg body-weight) one 2.1-g ruminal bolus

PML **Copacaps**™ **Lamb** (RMB)
Ruminal bolus, s/r, copper (as oxide) 1.1 g, for *lambs*; 30
Dose. *Lambs*: (10-20 kg body-weight) one 1.1-g ruminal bolus

Copasure A™ (Deosan)
Ruminal bolus, copper (as oxide) 21.25 g, for *cattle*; 24
Dose. *Cattle*: (150-350 kg body-weight) one 21.25-g ruminal bolus; (more than 350 kg body-weight) one or two 21.25-g ruminal boluses

Copasure C™ (Deosan)
Ruminal bolus, copper (as oxide) 10.625 g, for *calves*; 254
Dose. *Calves*: one 10.625-g ruminal bolus

PML **Coppinox**™ (Animax)
Ruminal bolus, s/r, copper (as oxide) 23 g, for *cattle*; 24
Dose. *Cattle*: (less than 350 kg body-weight) one 23-g ruminal bolus; (more than 350 kg body-weight) two 23-g ruminal boluses

PML **Copporal** (SmithKline Beecham)
Ruminal bolus, s/r, copper (as oxide) 1.7 g, 3.4 g, 20.4 g, for *cattle, sheep*; 1.7-g ruminal bolus 100, 3.4-g ruminal bolus 50, 20.4-g ruminal bolus 24
Dose. *Cattle*: (less than 100 kg body-weight) two 3.4-g ruminal boluses; (100-300 kg body-weight) one 20.4-g ruminal bolus; (more than 300 kg body-weight) one or two 20.4-g ruminal boluses
Sheep: one 3.4-g ruminal bolus; *lambs*: one 1.7-g ruminal bolus

PML **Copprite**™ (SmithKline Beecham)
Ruminal bolus, s/r, copper (as oxide) 1.7 g, 3.4 g, 20.4 g, for *cattle, sheep*; 1.7-g ruminal bolus 100, 3.4-g ruminal bolus 50, 20.4-g ruminal bolus 24
Dose. *Cattle*: (less than 100 kg body-weight) two 3.4-g ruminal boluses; (100-

300 kg body-weight) one 20.4-g ruminal bolus; (more than 300 kg body-weight) one or two 20.4-g ruminal boluses
Sheep: one 3.4-g ruminal bolus; *lambs*: one 1.7-g ruminal bolus

Parenteral preparations

PML **Bo-Jec Copper**™ (Young's)
Injection, copper (as calcium copperedetate) 50 mg/mL, for *cattle*; 2 mL
Dose. *Cattle: by subcutaneous injection*, (less than 18 months of age) 50 mg; (more than 18 months of age) 100 mg

PML **Bovicoppa**™ (BK)
Injection, copper (as calcium copperedetate) 50 mg/mL, for *cattle*; 2 mL
Dose. *Cattle: by subcutaneous injection*, (less than 18 months of age) 50-100 mg; (more than 18 months of age) 100-200 mg

PML **Copamex**™ (Crown)
Injection, copper (as methionine complex) 20 mg/mL, for *cattle, sheep*; 100 mL, 250 mL
Dose. *Cattle: by intramuscular injection*, 40-120 mg
Sheep: by subcutaneous or intramuscular injection, 40 mg; *lambs: by subcutaneous or intramuscular injection*, 10 mg

PML **Copavet**™ (C-Vet)
Injection, copper (as methionine complex) 20 mg/mL, for *cattle, sheep*; 50 mL, 100 mL, 250 mL
Dose. *Cattle: by intramuscular injection*, 40-120 mg
Sheep: by subcutaneous or intramuscular injection, 40 mg; *lambs: by subcutaneous or intramuscular injection*, 10 mg

PML **Coppaclear**™ (Crown)
Injection, copper (as heptonate) 12.5 mg/mL, for *sheep*; 100 mL
Dose. *Sheep: by intramuscular injection*, 25 mg

PoM **Coprin**™ (Coopers Pitman-Moore)
Injection, copper (as calcium copperedetate) 100 mg/dose, for *cattle*; single-dose applicator
Withdrawal Periods. *Cattle*: slaughter withdrawal period nil, milk withdrawal period nil
Dose. *Cattle: by subcutaneous injection*, (less than 100 kg body-weight) ½ dose, (more than 100 kg body-weight) 1-2 doses every 4 months as necessary

PML **Cujec**™ (Coopers Pitman-Moore)
Injection, copper (as cuproxoline) 6 mg/mL, for *cattle, sheep*; 100 mL
Withdrawal Periods. *Cattle, sheep*: slaughter withdrawal period nil, milk withdrawal period nil
Dose. *Cattle: by subcutaneous injection*, 12-60 mg
Sheep: by subcutaneous injection, 6-12 mg

PML **Cuvine**™ (BK)
Injection, copper (as heptonate) 12.5 mg/mL, for *sheep*; 100 mL
Dose. *Sheep: by intramuscular injection*, 25 mg

PML **New Swaycop**™ (Young's)
Injection, copper (as heptonate) 12.5 mg/mL, for *sheep*; 100 mL
Dose. *Sheep: by intramuscular injection*, 25 mg

16.4.4 Iodine

Dietary iodine is required for the synthesis of tri-iodothyronine and thyroxine by the thyroid gland. A deficiency results in compensatory hyperplasia of the thyroid gland, alopecia, prolonged gestation, and a raised incidence of stillbirths and weak offspring. All species may be affected, especially herbivores consuming only forage grown in regions where the soil is deficient in iodine.

Many concentrated foods and mineral supplements (see section 16.6) contain sufficient iodine to ensure that the overall dietary concentration exceeds 1 mg/kg feed. This concentration is the minimum required, although greater concentrations may be needed if the diet also contains kale, rapeseed, linseed, groundnut, or soybean.

16.4.5 Iron

Acute iron deficiency affects piglets that are maintained under conditions of intensive husbandry and rely on an all milk diet. The piglet's requirement for approximately 7 mg of iron daily is not provided by the milk diet alone. Acute hypochromic anaemia develops within the first 3 weeks of life and clinical signs appear at 3 to 6 weeks of age. The piglets appear pale and are often hairy in appearance. Their food intake and growth rate decline and diarrhoea is common.

Iron deficiency may occur in any species as a result of chronic blood loss associated either with gastro-intestinal parasites or ectoparasites.

Iron supplementation is commonly required for the prevention of iron deficiency anaemia in suckling piglets. In piglets, iron is always administered in the form of a complex such as iron dextran or gleptoferron, in order to avoid the toxic effects caused by ions of free iron.

Iron supplements are usually administered in the first week of life. The iron is stored in body tissues until required for haematopoiesis. Occasionally, there may be residual staining of the tissues at, or near, the site of injection.

IRON SALTS

Indications. Prevention and treatment of iron-deficiency anaemia
Side-effects. See notes above
Dose. *Horses, cattle, sheep*: see preparation details
Piglets: *by intramuscular injection*, 200 mg
Dogs, cats, mink, poultry: see preparation details

PML **10% Iron Dextran** (Battle Hayward & Bower, Crown)
Injection, iron dextran 100 mg/mL, for *piglets*; 100 mL

PML **Ferrofax™ 10 Plus** (C-Vet)
Injection, iron (as iron dextran) 100 mg, cyanocobalamin 100 micrograms/mL, for *piglets*; 100 mL

PML **Ferromax™** (Crown)
Injection, iron (as iron dextran) 100 mg/mL, for *piglets*; 100 mL

PML **Ferromax™ Plus** (Crown)
Injection, iron (as iron dextran) 100 mg, cyanocobalamin 100 micrograms/mL, for *piglets*; 100 mL

PML **Gleptosil™** (Fisons)
Injection, iron (as gleptoferron) 200 mg/mL, for *piglets*; 100 mL

PML **Heptomer™** (Animalcare)
Injection, iron (as gleptoferron) 200 mg/mL, for *piglets*; 100 mL

PML **Imposil™ 200** (Fisons)
Injection, iron (as iron dextran) 100 mg/mL, for *horses, cattle, sheep, piglets, puppies, kittens, mink*; 100 mL
Dose. *By intramuscular injection*. Treatment.
Horses: up to 1 g as a divided dose, repeat after 1 week or every month as necessary
Cattle: 10 mg/kg; *calves*: 1 g, repeat every week as necessary
Sheep: 500 mg, repeat every week as necessary; *lambs*: 300 mg, repeat every week as necessary
Pigs: 10 mg/kg
Dogs, cats, mink, fur bearing animals: 25 mg/kg, repeat every week as necessary
Prevention. *Calves*: 1 g, repeat at 4-6 weeks of age
Lambs: 300 mg
Piglets: 200 mg before 3 days of age
Puppies, kittens, mink, fur bearing animals: 25 mg every week as necessary

PML **Iron Dextran** (Hand/PH)
Injection, iron (as iron dextran) 200 mg/mL, for *piglets*; 100 mL

PML **Leodex™ 10%** (Leo)
Injection, iron (as iron dextran) 100 mg/mL, for *piglets*; 100 mL

PML **Leodex™ 20%** (Leo)
Injection, iron (as iron dextran) 200 mg/mL, for *piglets*; 100 mL

PML **Leodex™ 10% Plus** (Leo)
Injection, iron (as iron dextran) 100 mg, cyanocobalamin 100 micrograms/mL, for *piglets*; 100 mL

PML **Microdex™** (Micro-Biologicals)
Injection, iron (as iron dextran) 100 mg/mL, for *piglets*; 100 mL

GSL **Poultry Tonic** (Battle Hayward & Bower)
Oral liquid, ferrous phosphate 300 mg/mL, for *chickens, turkeys, ducks, geese*; 200 mL, 500 mL
Dose. *Poultry*: 220 mL/100 litres drinking water; *by addition to feed*, 5 mL per 6 birds

PML **Ruby Iron Dextran 10%** (Spencer)
Injection, iron (as iron dextran) 100 mg/mL, for *piglets*; 100 mL

PML **Scordex**™ (Crown)
Injection, iron (as iron dextran) 200 mg/mL, for *piglets*; 100 mL

PML **Tri-Dex**™ (Trilanco)
Injection, iron (as iron dextran) 100 mg/mL, for *piglets*; 100 mL

PML **Tri-Dex**™ EC (Trilanco)
Injection, iron (as iron dextran) 100 mg/mL, for *piglets*; 100 mL

PML **Tri-Dex**™ **Plus** (Trilanco)
Injection, cyanocobalamin 100 micrograms, iron (as iron dextran) 100 mg/mL, for *piglets*; 100 mL

PML **Veterinary Iron Injection** (Animalcare)
Injection, iron (as iron dextran) 100 mg/mL, for *piglets*; 100 mL

16.4.6 Magnesium

Acute magnesium deficiency associated with hypomagnesaemia is most common in lactating ruminants. The animals become ataxic and collapse, with tetanic convulsions of the limbs and neck. Opisthotonos and nystagmus may occur. Chronic magnesium deficiency is also common, and may be associated with a decreased appetite and a reduction in milk yield, which may be confused with ketosis.

Treatment of acute magnesium deficiency is difficult and the husbandry and management of ruminants should be designed to avoid the onset of the acute disease. Intravenous administration of magnesium salts may precipitate terminal convulsions in sheep and cattle. The acute disease is almost always due to a long-term dietary deficiency of magnesium. It is essential to provide continuous magnesium supplements to the animal.

Temporary supplementation may be provided by subcutaneous administration of magnesium but other methods are required for long-term maintenance. Oral supplementation methods, which may be used both prophylactically or therapeutically, include slow-release magnesium alloy ruminal boluses or the addition of magnesium compounds either to the drinking water or to the feed.

MAGNESIUM SALTS

Indications. Prevention and treatment of hypomagnesaemia
Warnings. Intravenous administration of magnesium salts may precipitate seizures
Dose. *Cattle*: *by mouth*, see preparation details; *by subcutaneous injection*, 50-100 g of magnesium sulphate according to the patient's response
Sheep: *by mouth*, see preparation details; *by subcutaneous injection*, 12.5-25.0 g of magnesium sulphate according to the patient's response

Oral preparations

Rumag Aqua™ (Rumenco)
Oral solution, for addition to drinking water, magnesium 50 mg/mL, for *cattle*; 25 litres
Dose. *Cattle*: *by addition to drinking water*, 0.33 litre/animal daily

Rumag Sugalic™ (Rumenco)
Oral liquid, for addition to feed, magnesium 35 mg/mL in molasses base, for *cattle*; 25 litres, 120 litres
Dose. *Cattle*: by addition to feed, 0.5 litre/animal daily

PML **Rumbul**™ (Agrimin)
Ruminal bolus, s/r, magnesium (as magnesium/aluminium/copper alloy) 15 g, for *calves, sheep*; 20
Dose. *Calves*: two 15-g boluses
Sheep: one 15-g bolus
Ruminal bolus, s/r, magnesium (as magnesium/aluminium/copper alloy) 40 g, for *cattle*; 10
Dose. *Cattle*: two 40-g boluses, repeat after 4 weeks if required

Parenteral preparations

PML **Calvet**™ **No 9** (Animalcare)
Injection, magnesium sulphate 250 mg/mL, for *cattle*; 400 mL

PML **Magnesium Sulphate** (Arnolds)
Injection, magnesium sulphate 250 mg/mL, for *cattle*; 400 mL

PML **Magnesium Sulphate** (Bimeda)
Injection, magnesium sulphate 250 mg/mL, for *cattle, sheep, pigs*; 400 mL

PML **Magnesium Sulphate** (Norbrook)
Injection, magnesium sulphate 250 mg/mL, for *cattle, sheep*; 400 mL

PML **MS-25** (Crown)
Injection, magnesium sulphate 250 mg/ mL, for *cattle*; 400 mL

PML **MS-25 No 9** (BK)
Injection, magnesium sulphate 250 mg/ mL, for *cattle*; 400 mL

16.4.7 Manganese

A deficiency of manganese is uncommon, but may occur if the diet contains less than 20 mg manganese per kg feed or high concentrations of calcium and phosphorus. The clinical signs of deficiency include poor growth, weakness, infertility, birth of stillborn or weak offspring, and an increase in the proportion of male offspring. Most concentrated foods and dietary supplements contain manganese. Deficiency is most likely to occur in herbivores consuming only herbage grown in regions where the soil is deficient in manganese and high in calcium.

16.4.8 Phosphorus

Acute phosphorus deficiency is uncommon in farm animals but hypophosphataemia may occur in association with acute hypocalcaemia. Phosphorus deficiency in the lactating cow has been associated with the development of postparturient haemoglobinuria after the onset of acute haemolysis. Cows may be affected during the first 4 weeks of lactation. More commonly, phosphorus deficiency causes chronic hypophosphataemia, which may result in skeletal defects, lameness, and low milk production.

Treatment with compound preparations (see section 16.4.12.1) is usually effective. Phosphorus-containing preparations may be used if animals fail to respond to calcium therapy.

Chronic hypophosphataemia may occur in ruminants being fed a diet containing inadequate phosphorus and increasing the phosphorus content of the feed should alleviate any clinical signs.

PHOSPHORUS SALTS

Indications. Treatment and prevention of hypophosphataemia

Warnings. Avoid perivascular injection
Dose. See preparation details

PML **Coforta™ 10** (Bayer)
Injection, butafosfan 100 mg, cyanocobalamin 50 micrograms/mL, for *horses, cattle, sheep, goats, pigs, dogs, cats, poultry*; 100 mL
Dose. *By subcutaneous or intramuscular injection*. *Horses, cattle*: 10-25 mL; *foals, calves*: 5-12 mL
Sheep, goats: 2.5-5.0 mL; *lambs*: 1.5-2.5 mL
Pigs: 2.5-10.0 mL; *piglets*: 1.0-2.5 mL
Dogs: 0.5-5.0 mL
Cats: 0.5-2.5 mL
Poultry: 1.0 mL

PoM **Double Phosphorus™** (Arnolds)
Injection, calcium hypophosphite 48.4 mg, glucose 200 mg/mL, for *cattle*; 400 mL
Dose. *Cattle: by slow intravenous injection*, up to 400 mL

PoM **Foston™** (Hoechst)
Injection, phosphorus (as toldimfos) 140 mg/mL, for *horses, cattle, sheep, pigs, dogs, cats*; 50 mL
Dose. Acute hypophosphataemia. *By subcutaneous, intramuscular, or intravenous injection*.
Horses, cattle: 10-25 mL; *foals, calves*: 5 mL
Sheep, pigs: 5 mL
Dogs, cats: 1-3 mL
Chronic hypophosphataemia. *By subcutaneous or intramuscular injection*.
Horses, cattle, sheep, pigs: 2.5-5.0 mL every 2 days for 5-10 doses
Dogs, cats: 1-2 mL every 2 days for 5-10 doses

> Proprietary and non-proprietary medicines that are licensed for human use are printed in small type in The Veterinary Formulary

16.4.9 Selenium

The essential role of selenium is as part of the enzyme glutathione peroxidase whose function is to prevent free radical damage to tissues. Disease is limited almost entirely to young growing animals and the adequacy of their selenium supply can be assessed by measuring the activity of glutathione peroxidase in the blood. There is a complex interaction between the requirements for selenium and vitamin E. Either nutrient may substitute, in part, for the other.

Primary selenium deficiency is associated with infertility in sheep and with muscular degeneration in young growing animals, which may lead to cardiac, respiratory, or skeletal myodegeneration. Moderate selenium deficiency results in illthrift, reduced growth rate, and the animal's immunocompetence may be compromised.

Confirmed deficiencies can be treated by the parenteral administration of selenium salts, but amounts greater than 450 micrograms of readily available selenium per kg body-weight may cause acute toxicity in sheep.

For prevention of selenium deficiency, depot preparations are available.

SELENIUM SALTS

Indications. Selenium deficiency
Dose. See preparation details

PoM **Deposel**™ (BK)
Depot injection (oily), selenium (as barium selenate) 50 mg/mL, for *cattle, sheep*; 5 mL
Dose. *Cattle, sheep*: *by subcutaneous injection*, 1 mg/kg

PoM **Selendale**™ (Arnolds)
Injection, selenium (as sodium selenite) 2.5 mg/mL, for *calves, lambs*; 50 mL
Withdrawal Periods. *Calves, lambs*: slaughter one month, milk from treated animals should not be used for human consumption
Dose. *Calves*: *by subcutaneous injection*, 50 micrograms/kg
Lambs: *by subcutaneous injection*, 250 micrograms within one week of birth, then 1.25-2.5 mg after 4 weeks

Accidental self-injection with oil-based preparations can cause severe vascular spasm and prompt medical attention is essential

16.4.10 Sodium

Sodium is an essential electrolyte. The concentration of sodium in extracellular fluid is controlled by hormonal mechanisms. Concentrated food contains added salt for palatability and stock receiving this diet are unlikely to become sodium deficient.

Therefore, sodium deficiency is unusual in species other than grazing herbivores not receiving concentrated feed supplements. Many pastures in the UK provide less than the required 1.5 g per kg feed to avoid deficiency. The requirement is higher for lactating animals and animals with mastitis owing to the loss of sodium in the milk.

Sodium deficiency occurs in high yielding cattle subsisting solely on a grass-based diet. The body's initial response to sodium deficiency, beyond that which can be countered by sodium conservation, is to reduce the extracellular fluid volume. This results in polycythaemia and an increase in packed-cell volume and haemoglobin concentration, which is commonly observed in grazing cattle in the UK during summer. Greater deprivation results in pica for salt, and ultimately polyuria and polydipsia due to renal failure. Prevention and treatment are achieved by providing salt blocks or compound mineral feed blocks (see section 16.6).

16.4.11 Zinc

Zinc has been shown experimentally to be important in the hepatic synthesis of protein, and severe zinc deficiency may lead to growth cessation. Pigs and certain breeds of cattle may exhibit clinical signs of zinc deficiency when their diet contains less than 50 mg per kg and over 5 g per kg of calcium. Parakeratosis develops with the skin becoming crusty and cracked, and growth is also depressed. Supplementation of the diet with at least 100 mg of zinc per kg feed is usually effective in treating and preventing deficiency.

Dermatoses as a result of zinc deficiency may occur in dogs and cats. Deficiencies in puppies and certain breeds such as Siberian huskies have been reported. High levels of cereals in the diet may result in zinc deficiency in the dog.

16.4.12 Compound mineral preparations

16.4.12.1 Calcium, magnesium, and phosphorus preparations

16.4.12.2 Compound trace element preparations

16.4.12.1 CALCIUM, MAGNESIUM AND PHOSPHORUS PREPARATIONS

Compound mineral preparations containing calcium with magnesium, or calcium with magnesium and phosphorus may be beneficial for the treatment of hypocalcaemia in certain areas of known mineral deficiency. Some cases of milk fever in cows may be associated with subclinical hypomagnesaemia before calving, and cows that relapse repeatedly after treatment with calcium solutions may be hypophosphataemic. The precise biochemistry of the disorder should be determined by blood analysis before treatment. Sheep may exhibit similarly complicated biochemical abnormalities for which compound mineral preparations may be beneficial.

Compound mineral preparations are often given by subcutaneous administration shortly before calving for the prevention of milk fever.

CALCIUM and MAGNESIUM

PML **Calc™ No 7** (BK)
Injection, calcium 22.8 mg, magnesium 4.65 mg/mL, for *cattle, sheep*; 400 mL
Dose. *Cattle*: *by subcutaneous or slow intravenous injection*, 400 mL
Sheep: *by subcutaneous or slow intravenous injection*, 35-75 mL

PML **Calvet™ No 7** (Animalcare)
Injection, calcium (as borogluconate) 22.8 mg, magnesium (as chloride) 4.65 mg/mL, for *cattle, sheep*; 400 mL
Dose. *Cattle*: *by subcutaneous or slow intravenous injection*, 400 mL
Sheep: *by subcutaneous or slow intravenous injection*, 35-75 mL

PML **CM-30** (Crown)
Injection, calcium 22.8 mg, magnesium 4.65 mg/mL, for *cattle, sheep*; 400 mL
Dose. *Cattle*: *by subcutaneous or slow intravenous injection*, 400 mL
Sheep: *by subcutaneous or slow intravenous injection*, 35-75 mL

CALCIUM, MAGNESIUM, and PHOSPHORUS

PML **Calc™ No 3** (BK)
Injection, calcium (as borogluconate) 15.2 mg, magnesium 3.25 mg and phosphorus 8.46 mg (as magnesium hypophosphite)/mL, for *cattle, sheep*; 400 mL
Dose. *Cattle*: *by subcutaneous or slow intravenous injection*, 400-800 mL
Sheep: *by subcutaneous or intravenous injection*, 50-100 mL

PML **Calc™ No 4** (BK)
Injection, calcium 22.8 mg, magnesium 2.04 mg, phosphorus 5.32 mg/mL, for *cattle*; 400 mL
Dose. *Cattle*: *by subcutaneous or slow intravenous injection*, 200-400 mL

PML **Calc™ No 5** (BK)
Injection, calcium 30.4 mg, magnesium 2.04 mg, phosphorus 5.32 mg, for *cattle*; 400 mL
Dose. *Cattle*: *by subcutaneous or slow intravenous injection*, 150-400 mL

PML **Calc™ No 6** (BK)
Injection, calcium (as borogluconate) 15.2 mg, glucose 200 mg, magnesium 4.65 mg and phosphorus 12.1 mg (as magnesium hypophosphite)/mL, for *cattle, sheep*; 400 mL
Dose. *Cattle*: *by subcutaneous or slow intravenous injection*, 200-400 mL
Sheep: *by subcutaneous or slow intravenous injection*, 25-80 mL

PML **Calcibor™ CMP 20** (Arnolds)
Injection, calcium borogluconate 200 mg, magnesium hypophosphite 30 mg/mL, for *cattle, sheep, pigs*; 400 mL
Dose. *Cattle*: *by subcutaneous or slow intravenous injection*, 200-400 mL
Sheep, pigs: *by subcutaneous or slow intravenous injection*, 50-100 mL

PML **Calcibor™ CMP 30** (Arnolds)
Injection, calcium borogluconate 300 mg, magnesium hypophosphite 30 mg, for *cattle*; 400 mL

Dose. *Cattle*: *by slow intravenous injection*, 200-400 mL

PML Calcibor™ CMP 40 (Arnolds)
Injection, calcium borogluconate 400 mg, magnesium hypophosphite 30 mg/mL, for *cattle*; 400 mL
Dose. *Cattle*: *by slow intravenous injection*, 200-400 mL

PML Calcibor™ CMP & D (Arnolds)
Injection, calcium borogluconate 200 mg, glucose 50 mg, magnesium hypophosphite 30 mg/mL, for *cattle, sheep, pigs*; 400 mL
Dose. *Cattle*: *by subcutaneous or slow intravenous injection*, 200-400 mL
Sheep, pigs: *by subcutaneous or slow intravenous injection*, 50-100 mL

PML Calciject™ 30 + 3 (Norbrook)
Injection, calcium borogluconate 300 mg, magnesium hypophosphite 30 mg/mL, for *horses, cattle, sheep, pigs, goats, dogs*; 400 mL
Dose. *By subcutaneous or slow intravenous injection*. *Horses*: 150-300 mL
Cattle: 150-400 mL
Sheep, goats, pigs: 15-50 mL
Dogs: 3-15 mL

PML Calciject™ 40 MP (Norbrook)
Injection, calcium borogluconate 400 mg, magnesium hypophosphite 50 mg/mL, for *cattle, sheep, pigs*; 400 mL
Dose. *Cattle*: *by subcutaneous or slow intravenous injection*, 200-400 mL
Sheep, pigs: *by subcutaneous or slow intravenous injection*, 20-50 mL

PML Calciject™ PMD (Norbrook)
Injection, calcium borogluconate 200 mg, glucose 200 mg, magnesium hypophosphite 50 mg/mL, for *horses, cattle, sheep, goats, pigs*; 400 mL
Dose. *By subcutaneous or slow intravenous injection*. *Horses*: 150-300 mL
Cattle: 200-400 mL
Sheep, goats, pigs: 15-50 mL

PML Calvet™ No 3 (Animalcare)
Injection, calcium (as borogluconate) 15.2 mg, magnesium 3.25 mg and phosphorus 8.46 mg (as magnesium hypophosphite)/mL, for *cattle, sheep*; 400 mL
Dose. *Cattle*: *by subcutaneous or slow intravenous injection*, 400-800 mL

Sheep: *by subcutaneous or slow intravenous injection*, 50-100 mL

PML Calvet™ No 5 (Animalcare)
Injection, calcium (as borogluconate) 30.4 mg, magnesium 2.04 mg and phosphorus 5.32 mg (as magnesium hypophosphite)/mL, for *cattle*; 400 mL
Dose. *Cattle*: *by subcutaneous or slow intravenous injection*, 150-400 mL

PML Calvet™ No 6 (Animalcare)
Injection, calcium (as borogluconate) 15.2 mg, glucose 200 mg, magnesium 4.65 mg and phosphorus 12.1 mg (as magnesium hypophosphite)/mL, for *cattle, sheep*; 400 mL
Dose. *Cattle*: *by subcutaneous or slow intravenous injection*, 200-400 mL
Sheep: *by subcutaneous or slow intravenous injection*, 25-80 mL

PML CMP-20 (Crown)
Injection, calcium (as borogluconate) 15.2 mg, magnesium 3.25 mg and phosphorus 8.46 mg (as magnesium hypophosphite)/mL, for *cattle*; 400 mL
Dose. *Cattle*: *by subcutaneous or slow intravenous injection*, 400-800 mL

PML CMP-30 (Crown)
Injection, calcium 22.8 mg, magnesium 2.04 mg, phosphorus 5.32 mg/mL, for *cattle*; 400 mL
Dose. *Cattle*: *by subcutaneous or slow intravenous injection*, 200-400 mL

PML CMP-40 (Crown)
Injection, calcium 30.4 mg, magnesium 2.04 mg, phosphorus 5.32 mg/mL, for *cattle*; 400 mL
Dose. *Cattle*: *by subcutaneous or slow intravenous injection*, 150-400 mL

PML CMPD-20 (Crown)
Injection, calcium (as borogluconate) 15.2 mg, glucose 200 mg, magnesium 4.65 mg and phosphorus 12.1 mg (as magnesium hypophosphite)/mL, for *cattle, sheep*; 400 mL
Dose. *Cattle*: *by subcutaneous or slow intravenous injection*, 200-400 mL
Sheep: *by subcutaneous or slow intravenous injection*, 25-80 mL

PML Flexopax™ No 3 (BK)
Injection, calcium (as gluconate) 15.5 mg, magnesium hypophosphite 22.2 mg/mL, for *cattle, sheep*; 400 mL

Dose. *Cattle*: *by subcutaneous or slow intravenous injection*, 400-800 mL
Sheep: *by subcutaneous or slow intravenous injection*, 50-100 mL

PML **Flexopax™ No 6** (BK)
Injection, anhydrous glucose 181.8 mg, calcium (as gluconate) 15.5 mg, magnesium hypophosphite 22.2 mg/mL, for *cattle*; 400 mL
Dose. *Cattle*: *by subcutaneous or slow intravenous injection*, 200-400 mL

PML **Supercal™ 20% PM** (Bimeda)
Injection, calcium (as borogluconate) 14.84 mg, magnesium 2.78 mg and phosphorus 7.08 mg (as magnesium hypophosphite)/mL, for *cattle, sheep*; 400 mL
Dose. *Cattle, sheep*: *by subcutaneous, slow intravenous, or intraperitoneal injection*, 0.5-1.5 mL/kg

PML **Supercal™ 25% PMD** (Bimeda)
Injection, calcium (as borogluconate) 18.54 mg, glucose 200 mg, magnesium 4.63 mg and phosphorus 11.8 mg (as magnesium hypophosphite)/mL, for *cattle, sheep*; 400 mL
Dose. *Cattle, sheep*: *by subcutaneous, slow intravenous, or intraperitoneal injection*, 0.4-1.2 mL/kg

PML **Supercal™ 30% PM** (Bimeda)
Injection, calcium (as borogluconate) 22.26 mg, magnesium 2.78 mg and phosphorus 7.08 mg (as magnesium hypophosphite)/mL, for *cattle, sheep*; 400 mL
Dose. *Cattle, sheep*: *by subcutaneous, slow intravenous, or intraperitoneal injection*, 0.34-1.0 mL/kg

PML **Supercal™ 40% PM** (Bimeda)
Injection, calcium (as borogluconate) 29.68 mg, magnesium 2.78 mg and phosphorus 7.08 mg (as magnesium hypophosphite)/mL, for *cattle, sheep*; 400 mL
Dose. *Cattle, sheep*: *by subcutaneous, slow intravenous, or intraperitoneal injection*, 0.25-0.76 mL/kg

16.4.12.2 COMPOUND TRACE ELEMENT PREPARATIONS

It is not unusual for young growing animals to be deficient in copper, cobalt, and selenium. Treatment or prophylaxis with preparations containing combinations of the 3 elements is advisable provided that the possibility of copper toxicity in sheep is considered.

PoM **Copacobal™** (C-Vet)
Oral solution, for dilution, cobalt chloride 80 mg, copper sulphate 213 mg, glycerol 632 mg/mL, for *cattle, sheep*; 100 mL, 1 litre. To be diluted before use
Cattle and sheep oral solution. Dilute 1 volume with 4 volumes water
Lamb oral solution. Dilute 1 volume with 9 volumes water
Dose. *Cattle*: 15 mL of diluted solution in spring and autumn
Sheep: 5-10 mL of diluted solution in spring and autumn; *lambs*: 5 mL of diluted solution at 8 weeks of age and again in autumn

Trace Element Tablets (Battle Hayward & Bower)
Tablets, cobalt 32 mg, copper 56 mg, iron 265 mg, magnesium 8.5 mg, manganese 56 mg, for *cattle, sheep*; 100, 250, other sizes available
Dose. *Cattle*: 4 tablets
Sheep: 1 tablet

16.5 Vitamins

16.5.1 Vitamin A
16.5.2 Vitamin B
16.5.3 Vitamin C
16.5.4 Vitamin D
16.5.5 Vitamin E
16.5.6 Vitamin K
16.5.7 Multivitamin preparations

Vitamins are used for the prevention and treatment of specific deficiency diseases and when the diet is known to be vitamin deficient. They are also often used for general supportive therapy without sufficient evidence of a beneficial effect. The administration of excessive amounts, particularly of vitamins A or D, can be harmful and may cause pathological changes.

16.5.1 Vitamin A

Vitamin A and its precursor beta carotene are present in growing plants which form the primary source of the vitamin. Much of the vitamin content of the forage can be lost if its conservation and storage are poor. Deficiency is commonest in cattle fed only poor quality hay in winter. The liver can store large quantities of vitamin A and provides a reserve of the vitamin, particularly for carnivores. Diets deficient in vitamin A produce no ill effect until the liver stores are depleted and the plasma concentration falls below 220 units per litre. The daily requirement of vitamin A is about 35 units per kg bodyweight.

A deficiency of vitamin A interferes with bone growth, with the maintenance of tissues, particularly secretory epithelial tissue, and with the growth of the embryo. In young animals, deficiency arrests growth of the skull causing neurological effects such as blindness due to pressure on the growing brain and cranial nerve roots. Older animals may develop a rough coat with scaly, cracked skin, and dry mucous membranes. They may fail to grow and reproduce and may exhibit neurological dysfunction. Animals of all ages may develop night blindness due to a deficiency of retinal rhodopsin.

Dietary supplementation or parenteral administration are convenient ways to prevent, and to some extent reverse, the effects of the deficiency, although the neurological deficits due to cranial growth inhibition may not be completely reversible. Overdosage from excessive dietary intake of liver most commonly occurs in cats and dogs and may result in vertebral fusion.

VITAMIN A
(Retinol)

Indications. Hypovitaminosis A
Side-effects. Excessive dosage may result in vertebral fusion in dogs and cats
Dose. *By intramuscular injection. Cattle*: 300000 units every 1-3 days; *calves*: 50000-150000 units every 3-4 days from 4-6 weeks of age
Sheep: 150000 units daily
Pigs: 50000-150000 units 3 weeks before farrowing; *piglets*: 100000 units

Dogs, cats: 10000-100000 units every 3 days

PML**Multivet™ A** (C-Vet)
Injection, vitamin A 100000 units/mL, for *cattle, sheep, pigs, dogs, cats*; 50 mL

16.5.2 Vitamin B

The complex of B vitamins includes thiamine (B_1), nicotinic acid (niacin), riboflavine, choline, pantothenic acid, pyridoxine (B_6), biotin (see section 15.2), folic acid, and vitamin B_{12}. All of these can be synthesised by the microflora in the gastro-intestinal tract of ruminants and deficiencies are therefore uncommon among herbivores. Deficiencies affect the nervous, alimentary, and epidermal systems.

Vitamin B_{12} is a collective term for the cobalamins of which **cyanocobalamin** and **hydroxocobalamin** are the principal compounds. They are cobalt-containing vitamins. Ruminants are able to convert cobalt to vitamin B_{12} in the rumen. Therefore, deficiency of vitamin B_{12} occurs in these species when cobalt is deficient in the diet. In carnivores, vitamin B_{12} deficiency may occur as a result of inadequate absorption of the vitamin from the gastro-intestinal tract or increased body requirements.

In all species, cobalamins are required for maintenance of tissues, protein synthesis, and haematopoiesis. Clinical signs of deficiency include anorexia, unthriftiness, anaemia, and incoordination.

Thiamine deficiency may occur due to dietary deficiency or destruction of the vitamin by thiaminase. A nutritional deficiency is unlikely in herbivores but may occur in carnivores when vitamins are destroyed by excessive heating during processing. Secondary thiamine deficiency may occur in carnivores, because of the thiaminase present in fish, and in horses because of the thiaminase present in bracken.

Secondary thiamine deficiency can be treated successfully with thiamine supplements if the therapy is started shortly after the onset of clinical signs. Thiamine may be used in the treatment of cerebrocortical necrosis in cattle and sheep.

CYANOCOBALAMIN

Indications. Treatment of vitamin B$_{12}$ deficiency

Dose. *By intramuscular injection. Horses, cattle*: 1-3 mg 1-2 times weekly; *foals, calves*: 0.5-1.5 mg 1-2 times weekly
Sheep, pigs, goats: 250-750 micrograms 1-2 times weekly
Dogs, cats: 250-500 micrograms 1-2 times weekly
Small pet birds: see preparation details

PoM **Cyano™ 12-1000** (Bimeda)
Injection, cyanocobalamin 1 mg/mL, for *cattle, sheep, pigs*; 50 mL

PML **Intravit™ 12** (Norbrook)
Injection, cyanocobalamin 500 micrograms/mL, for *horses, cattle, sheep, goats, pigs, dogs, cats*; 100 mL

Multivet™ B$_{12}$ (C-Vet)
PoM *Injection*, cyanocobalamin 250 micrograms/mL, for *horses, cattle, sheep, pigs, dogs, cats*; 50 mL
PML *Injection*, cyanocobalamin 1 mg/mL, for *horses, cattle, sheep, pigs*; 50 mL

PoM **Ornimed™ B$_{12}$** (LAB)
Medicated feed, cyanocobalamin 4 micrograms/g, for *small pet birds*; 10 g
Dose. *Small pet birds*: 6 micrograms daily

PoM **Vitamin B$_{12}$** (Animalcare)
Injection, cyanocobalamin 250 micrograms/mL, 1 mg/mL, for *horses, cattle, sheep, pigs, dogs, cats*; 50 mL

PML **Vitamin B$_{12}$** (Battle Hayward & Bower)
Injection, cyanocobalamin 250 micrograms/mL, for *horses, cattle, sheep, pigs*; 100 mL
Withdrawal Periods. *Cattle*: slaughter withdrawal period nil, milk withdrawal period nil. *Sheep, pigs*: slaughter withdrawal period nil
Note. May also be administered by subcutaneous injection

PML **Vitamin B$_{12}$** (Crown)
Injection, cyanocobalamin 250 micrograms/mL, 1 mg/mL, for *horses, cattle, sheep, pigs*; 250-micrograms/mL vial 100 mL; 1-mg/mL vial 50 mL

Note. May also be administered by subcutaneous injection

PoM **Vitamin B$_{12}$** (Univet)
Injection, cyanocobalamin 1 mg/mL, for *horses, cattle, sheep, pigs*; 50 mL

PoM **Vitbee™** (Arnolds)
Injection, cyanocobalamin 250 micrograms/mL, 1 mg/mL, for *horses, cattle, sheep, pigs*; 50 mL

THIAMINE
(Vitamin B$_1$)

Indications. Treatment of thiamine deficiency
Dose. *Horses: by subcutaneous, intramuscular, or slow intravenous injection*, 0.25-1.25 mg/kg twice daily for up to 7 days
Cattle, sheep: by subcutaneous, intramuscular, or slow intravenous injection, 5-10 mg/kg, repeat every 3 hours as necessary
Cats[♦]: *by intramuscular injection*, 50 mg 1-2 times daily

PoM **Vitamin B1** (Bimeda)
Injection, thiamine hydrochloride 100 mg/mL, for *horses, cattle, sheep*; 50 mL

16.5.3 Vitamin C
(Ascorbic acid)

Ascorbic acid is synthesised by all animals except the primates and guinea pigs. Deficiency may occur in these species when the diet contains inadequate supplies of fresh fruit and vegetables or food is stored incorrectly.

16.5.4 Vitamin D

The term vitamin D is used for a range of compounds including ergocalciferol (calciferol, vitamin D$_2$), cholecalciferol (vitamin D$_3$), alfacalcidol (1α-hydroxycholecalciferol), and calcitriol (1,25-dihydroxycholecalciferol).
Cholecalciferol is synthesised from the sterols present in skin on exposure to sunlight. It may be converted to calcitriol in the liver and kidney. Calcitriol is 10 times as potent as cholecalciferol.
Vitamin D enhances the absorption of calcium from the intestine and acts,

together with parathyroid hormone and calcitonin, to regulate the processes of bone resorption and formation during remodelling of the skeleton.

The increased absorption of calcium after administration of vitamin D is used in ewes to provide for the proper skeletal calcification of lambs before birth, and in cows to prevent clinical hypocalcaemia, which may occur at calving due to the onset of lactation. The timing of the injection of vitamin D is most important and for optimum effectiveness should fall between 8 and 2 days before calving. A deficiency of cholecalciferol results in the failure of bone to calcify correctly and leads to rickets in young animals and osteomalacia in adults. These conditions may be treated and prevented by administration of cholecalciferol either parenterally or in the diet.

Excessive administration of cholecalciferol or other forms of vitamin D may result in metastatic calcification of the major blood vessels, the kidney, and other organs.

ALFACALCIDOL
(1α-Hydroxycholecalciferol)

Indications. See notes above
Side-effects. Excessive dosage may result in calcification of blood vessels and organs, see notes above
Dose. See preparation details

PoM **Vetalpha™** (BK)
Injection, alfacalcidol 35 micrograms/mL, for *cattle*; 10 mL
Withdrawal Periods. *Cattle*: slaughter 3 days, milk 72 hours
Dose. *Cattle*: *by subcutaneous injection*, 350 micrograms 24-48 hours before calving. Repeat once only after 72-96 hours if calving has not occurred

CHOLECALCIFEROL
(Vitamin D₃)

Indications. See notes above
Side-effects. See under Alfacalcidol
Dose. See preparation details

PML **Duphafral™ D₃ 1000** (Duphar)
Injection, cholecalciferol 25 mg/mL, for *cattle*; 10 mL

Dose. *Cattle*: *by intramuscular injection*, 250 mg 2-8 days before calving

PML **Suntax™ D₃** (Crown)
Injection, cholecalciferol 6.25 mg/mL, for *cattle, sheep*; 100 mL
Dose: *By subcutaneous or intramuscular injection*. *Cattle*: 9.40-31.25 mg; *calves*: 6.25 mg
Sheep: 6.25-12.5 mg 8-10 weeks before lambing; *lambs*: 3.125-6.25 mg

PML **Super-Suntax™** (C-Vet)
Injection, cholecalciferol 6.25 mg/mL, for *cattle, sheep*; 100 mL
Dose. *By subcutaneous or intramuscular injection*. *Cattle*: 12.5-31.25 mg
Sheep: 6.25-12.5 mg 8-10 weeks before lambing; *lambs*: 3.125 mg

Compound calcium and vitamin D preparations

P **Collo-Cal™ D** (C-Vet)
Oral solution, colloidal calcium oleate 7.5 mg, vitamin D 1.75 micrograms/mL, for *dogs*; 100 mL, 500 mL, 2 litres
Dose. *Dogs*: 0.5-1.0 mL/kg

Efficalcium™ (Virbac)
Tablets, calcium 545 mg, cholecalciferol 3.75 micrograms, fluoride 875 micrograms, phosphorus 345 mg, for *dogs, cats*; 100
Dose. *Dogs*: ½-2 tablets daily

Pet-Cal™ (SmithKline Beecham)
Tablets, calcium hydrogen phosphate 2.04 g, cholecalciferol 5 micrograms, for *dogs, cats*; 30, 150
Dose. *Dogs*: (less than 9 kg body-weight) ½ tablet daily; (more than 9 kg body-weight) 1 tablet per 9 kg body-weight daily
Cats: ½ tablet daily

16.5.5 Vitamin E
(Tocopherols)

Vitamin E is present in growing plants and in cereals. It is an antoxidant and is necessary for the stability of muscular tissue. It has a similar role to selenium (see section 16.4.9) and each can to some extent replace the other.

A deficiency occurs most commonly in young ruminants receiving a diet of poor quality hay, straw, and roots. Muscles that are deficient in vitamin E become stiff, swollen, and painful, and degenerative changes become visible microscopically. The disease is called 'white muscle disease'. Both skeletal and heart muscle are susceptible. Parenteral therapy with vitamin E, selenium, or both produces a complete restoration of health. Prophylaxis requires a daily intake of approximately 1 g of vitamin E for cows, 150 mg for calves, 75 mg for ewes, and 25 mg for lambs.

ALPHA TOCOPHEROLS

Indications. See notes above
Dose. See preparation details

Note. Vitamin E 1 mg = *dl*-alpha tocopheryl acetate 1 unit = *d*-alpha tocopheryl acid succinate 1.21 units

GSL **Tocovite™** (Arnolds)
Tablets, vitamin E (as *d*-alpha tocopheryl acid succinate) 41 mg, 83 mg, 165 mg, for *horses, calves, lambs, dogs*; 100
Dose. *Horses*: 0.83-2.48 g daily
Calves: 165-248 mg daily
Lambs, dogs: 41-83 mg daily

GSL **Vita-E Succinate™** (Bioglan)
Tablets, scored, vitamin E (as *d*-alpha tocopheryl acid succinate) 41 mg, 165 mg, for *dogs*; 100, 500
Dose. *Dogs*: 41-330 mg daily
Oral powder, for addition to feed, vitamin E (as *d*-alpha tocopheryl acid succinate) 330 mg/g, for *horses*; 82.6 g
Dose. *Horses*: 0.83-1.65 g daily

GSL **Vitamin E** (Duphar)
Tablets, vitamin E (as *d*-alpha tocopheryl acid succinate) 41 mg; 250
Dose. 1.6-8.3 mg/kg daily

Compound Selenium and Vitamin E preparations

PoM **Dystosel™** (Intervet)
Injection, selenium (as potassium selenate) 1.5 mg, vitamin E (as *dl*-alpha tocopheryl acetate) 68 mg/mL, for *calves, sheep, pigs*; 50 mL
Withdrawal Periods. *Calves*: slaughter 8 weeks. *Sheep*: slaughter 8 weeks, milk from treated animals should not be used for human consumption. *Pigs*: slaughter 8 weeks

Dose. *By subcutaneous or intramuscular injection*.
Calves: 0.02-0.04 mL/kg, repeat after 2-4 weeks if required
Ewes: 0.04 mL/kg; *lambs*: 0.5-1.0 mL, repeat after 2-4 weeks if required
Pigs: 0.04 mL/kg, repeat after 2-4 weeks if required

PoM **Vitenium™** (C-Vet)
Injection, selenium (as sodium selenite) 500 micrograms, vitamin E (as *dl*-alpha tocopheryl acetate) 150 mg/mL, for *horses, cattle, sheep, pigs*; 100 mL
Dose. *Horses: by intramuscular injection*, up to 20 mL; *foals*: 2-5 mL
Cattle: by subcutaneous or intramuscular injection, up to 15 mL; *calves*: 2-5 mL
Sheep: by subcutaneous or intramuscular injection, up to 5 mL; *lambs*: 0.5-3.0 mL
Pigs: by subcutaneous or intramuscular injection, up to 5 mL; *piglets*: 0.5-2.0 mL

PoM **Vitesel™** (Norbrook)
Injection, *dl*-alpha tocopheryl acetate 68 mg, selenium (as potassium selenate) 1.5 mg/mL, for *calves, sheep, pigs*; 50 mL
Withdrawal Periods. *Calves, sheep, pigs*: slaughter 8 weeks
Dose. *By subcutaneous or intramuscular injection*. *Calves*: 0.02-0.04 mL/kg, repeat after 2-4 weeks if required
Ewes: 0.04 mL/kg; *lambs*: 0.5-1.0 mL, repeat after 2-4 weeks if required
Pigs: 0.04 mL/kg, repeat after 2-4 weeks if required

See also section 16.4.9 for preparations containing selenium

16.5.6 Vitamin K

Vitamin K is necessary for the production of blood clotting factors and proteins necessary for the normal calcification of bone.

Oral coumarin anticoagulants, found in many rodenticides, act by interfering with vitamin K metabolism in the hepatic cells and their effects can be antagonised by giving vitamin K. **Phytomenadione** (vitamin K_1) is initially given by intravenous injection, followed by oral treatment for up to 5 days. In severe cases, blood transfusion may be required. **Menadione** (vitamin K_3) is included in some compound preparations.

PHYTOMENADIONE
(Vitamin K₁)

Indications. See notes above
Dose. *Dogs*: *by intravenous or intramuscular injection*, 10-30 mg, repeat daily for 2 days
Cats: initially, *by intravenous injection*, 1-2 mg/kg, repeat after 6 hours. Then, *by intramuscular injection*, 1-2 mg/kg once daily for 2 days, then *by mouth*, 1-2 mg/kg daily for 3-5 days

Konakion™ (Roche)
P *Tablets*, phytomenadione 10 mg; 25
PoM *Injection*, phytomenadione 2 mg/mL, 10 mg/mL; 2-mg/mL vial 0.5 mL; 10-mg/mL vial 1 mL

Proprietary and non-proprietary medicines that are licensed for human use are printed in small type in The Veterinary Formulary

16.5.7 Multivitamin preparations

Multivitamin preparations may be used for the prevention and treatment of vitamin deficiencies, particularly during periods of illness, convalescence, stress, and unthriftiness.

There are many preparations available. This is not a comprehensive list.

Oral preparations

P **Abidec™** (Parke-Davis)
This preparation is now discontinued

PML **Vital™** (Crown)
Oral solution, cholecalciferol 37.5 micrograms, cyanocobalamin 50 micrograms, dexpanthenol 10 mg, nicotinamide 35 mg, pyridoxine hydrochloride 3 mg, riboflavine 3 mg, thiamine hydrochloride 10 mg, vitamin A 15 000 units, vitamin E 6 mg/mL, for *cattle, sheep, pigs*; 200 mL

PML **Vitasol™** (Micro-Biologicals)
Oral liquid, cholecalciferol 18.75 micrograms, cyanocobalamin 2.5 micrograms,

vitamin A 12 500 units, vitamin E 50 mg/mL, for *calves, pigs, poultry*; 1 litre

Parenteral preparations

PML **A-Pek™ Plus** (Crown)
Injection, cholecalciferol 1.88 mg, vitamin A 500 000 units, vitamin E (as *dl*-alpha tocopherol acetate) 50 mg/mL, for *cattle, sheep, pigs*; 100 mL

PoM **Bimavite™ Plus** (Bimeda)
Injection, ascorbic acid 70 mg, nicotinamide 22.5 mg, pyridoxine hydrochloride 7 mg, riboflavine (as phosphate) 800 micrograms, thiamine hydrochloride 35 mg/mL, for *horses, cattle, sheep, goats, pigs, dogs, cats*; 50 mL

PoM **Combivit™** (Norbrook)
Injection, ascorbic acid 70 mg, nicotinamide 23 mg, pyridoxine hydrochloride 7 mg, riboflavine sodium phosphate 500 micrograms, thiamine hydrochloride 35 mg/mL, for *horses, cattle, sheep, goats, pigs, dogs, cats*; 50 mL, 100 mL

PML **Duphafral™ Ade Forte** (Duphar)
Injection, cholecalciferol 1.25 mg, vitamin A 500 000 units, vitamin E 50 units/mL, for *cattle, sheep, pigs*; 50 mL

PoM **Duphafral™ Extravite** (Duphar)
Injection, ascorbic acid 70 mg, nicotinamide 23 mg, pyridoxine hydrochloride 7 mg, riboflavine sodium phosphate 500 micrograms, thiamine hydrochloride 35 mg/mL, for *horses, cattle, sheep, goats, pigs, dogs, cats*; 50 mL, 100 mL

PoM **Duphafral™ Multivitamin** (Duphar)
Injection, cholecalciferol 187.5 micrograms, cyanocobalamin 20 micrograms, dexpanthenol 25 mg, nicotinamide 35 mg, pyridoxine hydrochloride 3 mg, riboflavine 5 mg, thiamine hydrochloride 10 mg, vitamin A 15 000 units, vitamin E 20 mg/mL, for *calves, lambs, piglets*; 100 mL

PML **Multivet™** (C-Vet)
Injection, cholecalciferol 25 micrograms, dexpanthenol 25 mg, nicotinamide 35 mg, pyridoxine hydrochloride 3 mg, riboflavine 5 mg, thiamine hydrochloride 10 mg, vitamin A 15 000 units, vitamin B₁₂ 50 micrograms, vitamin E 20 mg/mL, for *calves, lambs, piglets*; 100 mL

PoM **Multivet™ 4BC** (C-Vet)
Injection, ascorbic acid 70 mg, nicotinamide 23 mg, pyridoxine hydrochloride 7 mg, riboflavine sodium phosphate 500 micrograms, thiamine hydrochloride 35 mg/mL, for *horses, cattle, sheep, goats, pigs, dogs, cats*; 50 mL, 100 mL

PML **Multivitamin** (Arnolds)
Injection, cholecalciferol 25 micrograms, cyanocobalamin 50 micrograms, dexpanthenol 25 mg, nicotinamide 35 mg, pyridoxine hydrochloride 3 mg, riboflavine sodium phosphate 5 mg, thiamine hydrochloride 10 mg, vitamin A 15 000 units, vitamin B_{12} 50 micrograms, vitamin E 20 mg/mL, for *horses, cattle, sheep, goats, pigs, dogs, cats*; 100 mL

PML **Multivitamin** (Bimeda)
Injection, cholecalciferol 25 micrograms, cyanocobalamin 50 micrograms, dexpanthenol 25 mg, nicotinamide 35 mg, pyridoxine hydrochloride 3 mg, riboflavine 5 mg, thiamine hydrochloride 10 mg, vitamin A 15 000 units, vitamin E 20 mg/mL, for *cattle, sheep, pigs*; 100 mL

PML **Multivitamin** (Norbrook)
Injection, cholecalciferol 25 micrograms, cyanocobalamin 50 micrograms, dexpanthenol 25 mg, nicotinamide 35 mg, pyridoxine hydrochloride 3 mg, riboflavine sodium phosphate 5 mg, thiamine hydrochloride 10 mg, vitamin A 15 000 units, vitamin E 20 mg/mL, for *horses, cattle, sheep, goats, pigs, dogs, cats*; 100 mL

PoM **Pabrinex™-Vet** (Paines & Byrne)
Injection, ascorbic acid 70 mg, nicotinamide 23 mg, pyridoxine hydrochloride 7 mg, riboflavine sodium phosphate 700 micrograms, thiamine hydrochloride 35 mg/mL, for *horses, cattle, sheep, dogs, cats*; 50 mL

PoM **Parentrovite™** (SmithKline Beecham)
This preparation is now discontinued

PoM **Polyvit™** (Univet)
Injection, ascorbic acid 70 mg, nicotinamide 23 mg, pyridoxine hydrochloride 7 mg, riboflavine sodium phosphate 700 micrograms, thiamine hydrochloride 35 mg/mL, for *horses, cattle, sheep, dogs, cats*; 50 mL

PoM **Poten™ 4B-C** (Intervet)
Injection, ascorbic acid 70 mg, nicotinamide 22.5 mg, pyridoxine hydrochloride 7 mg, riboflavine 800 micrograms, thiamine hydrochloride 35 mg/mL, for *horses, cattle, sheep, goats, pigs, dogs, cats*; 50 mL

PML **Tri-Ade™** (Trilanco)
Injection, cholecalciferol 1.88 mg, vitamin A 500 000 units, vitamin E 50 mg/mL, for *cattle, sheep, pigs*; 100 mL

PML **Vetrivite™ Plus** (C-Vet)
Injection, cholecalciferol 1.88 mg, vitamin A 500 000 units, vitamin E 50 units/mL, for *cattle, sheep, pigs*; 50 mL

PML **Vital™ Multivitamin** (Crown)
Injection, cholecalciferol 25 micrograms, cyanocobalamin 50 micrograms, dexpanthenol 25 mg, nicotinamide 35 mg, pyridoxine hydrochloride 3 mg, riboflavine 5 mg, thiamine hydrochloride 10 mg, vitamin A 15 000 units, vitamin E 20 mg/mL, for *calves, lambs, piglets*; 100 mL

PML **Vitamin AD_3E** (Animalcare)
This preparation is now discontinued

PML **Vitamin A D & E** (Fisons)
Injection, cholecalciferol 1.25 mg, vitamin A 500 000 units, vitamin E 50 units/mL, for *cattle, sheep, pigs*; 50 mL

16.6 Compound multivitamin and mineral preparations

Compound multivitamin and mineral preparations are used as general tonics or supplements, although their therapeutic efficacy has not been established. Some oral liquid preparations may contain caffeine and care should be taken if administering them to horses or dogs used in competitions (see Prescribing for animals used in competitions).

There are many preparations available. This is not a comprehensive list.

Oral preparations

All-Trace™ (Agrimin)
Ruminal bolus, cholecalciferol, cobalt, copper, iodine, manganese, selenium, sulphur, vitamin A, vitamin E, zinc, for *cattle*; 20

Canovel™ **Vitamin Mineral** (SmithKline Beecham)
Tablets, calcium pantothenate, cobalt, copper, ergocalciferol, iodine, iron, manganese, nicotinic acid, phosphorus, pyridoxine hydrochloride, riboflavine, selenium, sodium chloride, sugars, thiamine hydrochloride, vitamin A, vitamin E, yeast, zinc, for *dogs*; 50

Collotone™ (Harkers)
Oral solution, for addition to drinking water, caffeine citrate, green ferric ammonium citrate, iron and magnesium citrate, sodium glycerophosphate, thiamine hydrochloride, for *pigeons*; 200 mL

PML **Collovet**™ (C-Vet)
Oral liquid, caffeine citrate, copper chloride, green ferric ammonium citrate, iron and manganese citrate, potassium glycerophosphate solution, sodium glycerophosphate solution, thiamine hydrochloride, for *horses, cattle, pigs, dogs, cats, mink, birds*; 500 mL, 2 litres

Convital R™ (Bimeda)
Oral liquid, calcium, cholecalciferol, cobalt, copper, iodine, iron, magnesium, manganese, nicotinic acid, phosphorus, potassium, pyridoxine, riboflavine, sodium, thiamine, vitamin A, vitamin E, zinc, for *horses*; 4.5 litres

Duphasol™ **13/6** (Duphar)
Oral powder, ascorbic acid, biotin, cholecalciferol, cobalt, copper, cyanocobalamin, folic acid, iodine, iron, manganese, menadione, nicotinic acid, pantothenic acid, pyridoxine hydrochloride, riboflavine, thiamine hydrochloride, vitamin A, vitamin E, zinc, for *cattle, sheep, pigs, poultry*; 100 g

Equisup™ **23** (Univet)
Oral powder, ascorbic acid, biotin, cholecalciferol, choline, cobalt, copper, cyanocobalamin, dexpanthenol, folic acid, iodine, iron, lysine, manganese, menadione, methionine, nicotinic acid, pyridoxine, riboflavine, selenium, thiamine, vitamin A, vitamin E, zinc, for *horses*; 1.5 kg

Equisup Selco-V™ (Univet)
Oral liquid, cholecalciferol, cobalt, cyanocobalamin, selenium, thiamine hydrochloride, vitamin A, vitamin E, for *horses, cattle, sheep*; 1 litre

Equi-ton™ (Intervet)
Oral liquid, cholecalciferol, choline bitartrate, cyanocobalamin, dexpanthenol, ferric ammonium citrate, inositol, nicotinamide, pyridoxine hydrochloride, riboflavine, thiamine hydrochloride, vitamin A, vitamin E, for *horses*; 1 litre

Leo Cud™ (Leo)
Oral powder, casein, cholecalciferol, cobalt sulphate, copper sulphate, maize starch, manganese dioxide, methionine, nicotinamide, riboflavine, sodium bicarbonate, sodium phosphate, sodium propionate, thiamine hydrochloride, vitamin A, dried yeast, skimmed milk powder, for *cattle, sheep, goats*; 80 g, 160 g

Methisal™ (Univet)
Oral powder, for addition to feed, calcium carbonate, methionine, potassium chloride, sodium chloride, zinc gluconate, for *horses*; 2 kg

Minivit™ (Univet)
Oral solution, ascorbic acid, cholecalciferol, dexpanthenol, menadione, nicotinamide, pyridoxine hydrochloride, riboflavine, thiamine hydrochloride, vitamin A, vitamin E, for *puppies, kittens, rodents, birds, tortoises*; 7 mL

Mostivit™ **Plus** (Crown)
Oral liquid, cholecalciferol, cobalt, cyanocobalamin, selenium, vitamin A, vitamin E, for *horses, cattle, sheep*; 500 mL, 1 litre, 2 litres

Nutri-Plus™ (Virbac)
Oral gel, calcium pantothenate, cholecalciferol, cyanocobalamin, folic acid, iodine, iron, magnesium, manganese, nicotinamide, pyridoxine hydrochloride, riboflavine, thiamine hydrochloride, vitamin A, vitamin E, for *dogs, cats*; 120.5 g

Pardivit™ (Bayer)
Oral liquid, cholecalciferol, cobalt, selenium, vitamin A, vitamin E, for *cattle, sheep*; 500 mL, 1 litre

Pet-Tabs™ (SmithKline Beecham)
Tablets, calcium, cobalt, copper, cyanocobalamin, ergocalciferol, iodine, iron, linoleic acid, magnesium, manganese, nicotinic acid, phosphorus, pyridoxine hydrochloride, riboflavine, thiamine mononitrate, vitamin A, vitamin E, zinc, for *dogs*; 50, 150

Pet-Tabs™ Feline (SmithKline Beecham)
Tablets, calcium pantothenate, choline, cobalt, copper, ergocalciferol, inositol, iodine, iron, linoleic acid, magnesium, manganese, nicotinic acid, phosphorus, pyridoxine hydrochloride, riboflavine, thiamine mononitrate, vitamin A, vitamin E, zinc, for *cats*; 100

Pigeon Minerals (Harkers)
Oral powder, cholecalciferol, calcium, cobalt, copper, iodine, iron, magnesium, manganese, phosphorus, riboflavine, sodium chloride, vitamin A, zinc, for *pigeons*; 1 kg

PML **Proviton™** (Crown)
Oral powder, casein, cobalt sulphate, dried yeast, glucose, methionine, sodium bicarbonate, sodium phosphate, starch, vitamin A, for *cattle, sheep*; 100 g

SA-37™ (Intervet)
Tablets, arachidonic acid, ascorbic acid, biotin, calcium, cholecalciferol, choline, cobalt, copper, cyanocobalamin, dexpanthenol, folic acid, iodine, iron, lecithin, linoleic acid, linolenic acid, manganese, nicotinic acid, phosphorus, potassium, pyridoxine hydrochloride, riboflavine, thiamine hydrochloride, vitamin A, vitamin E, vitamin K, zinc, for *dogs, cats*; 100, 500
Oral powder, arachidonic acid, ascorbic acid, biotin, calcium, cholecalciferol, choline, cobalt, copper, cyanocobalamin, dexpanthenol, folic acid, iodine, iron, lecithin, linoleic acid, linolenic acid, manganese, nicotinic acid, phosphorus, potassium, pyridoxine hydrochloride, riboflavine, thiamine hydrochloride, vitamin A, vitamin E, vitamin K, zinc, for *dogs, cats, pet birds*; 100 g, 200 g, 2 kg

Trelenium™ (C-Vet)
Oral liquid, cholecalciferol, cobalt, selenium, vitamin A, vitamin E, for *horses, cattle, sheep*; 500 mL

PML **Veterinary Tonic** (Crown)
Oral liquid, caffeine citrate, green ferric ammonium citrate, iron and manganese citrate, potassium glycerophosphate, sodium glycerophosphate, thiamine hydrochloride, for *horses, cattle, pigs, dogs, cats, mink, birds*; 1 litre

Vins Plus™ (Univet)
Oral liquid, cyanocobalamin, folic acid, pyridoxine hydrochloride, iron, for *horses, dogs*; 100 mL, 1 litre

Vionate™ (Ciba-Geigy)
Oral powder, calcium, calcium pantothenate, cholecalciferol, choline chloride, cobalt, copper, cyanocobalamin, folic acid, iodine, iron, magnesium, manganese, menadione, nicotinic acid, phosphorus, pyridoxine hydrochloride, riboflavine, sodium chloride, thiamine hydrochloride, vitamin A, vitamin E, for *horses, dogs, cats, birds, mink, chinchillas, rabbits, reptiles*; 120 g, 1 kg, 4 kg

GSL **Vi-Sorbin™** (SmithKline Beecham)
Oral liquid, cyanocobalamin, ferric pyrophosphate, folic acid, pyridoxine hydrochloride, sorbitol, for *horses, calves, dogs, cats*; 1 litre

Parenteral preparations

PoM **Haemo 15™** (Arnolds)
Injection, biotin, choline chloride, cobalt gluconate, copper gluconate, cyanocobalamin, dexpanthenol, ferric ammonium citrate, glycine, inositol, lysine hydrochloride, nicotinamide, pyridoxine hydrochloride, racemethionine, riboflavine sodium phosphate, for *horses*; 100 mL

PoM **Vitatrace™** (Univet)
Injection, cobalt gluconate, copper gluconate, cyanocobalamin, dexpanthenol, ferric ammonium citrate, nicotinamide, pyridoxine hydrochloride, riboflavine, thiamine hydrochloride, for *horses, cattle, sheep, pigs, dogs, cats*; 100 mL

16.7 Special dietary foods for dogs and cats

Modification of nutrient intake is a useful adjunct in the management of many diseases, and in some cases is essential for successful treatment.

Despite the need to control specific nutrient levels, the diet must provide the animal with its daily requirement for energy and other essential nutrients. Diets intended for long-term maintenance should not result in a nutritional deficiency. Only complete diets have been included in this section.

Special diets for small animals (also known as prescription diets) do not require licensing under the Medicines Act 1968 unless overt therapeutic or preventive claims are made for the preparation.

A diet should be selected only if it has the specific nutritional characteristics to manage the individual case. Invariably, more than one nutritional component should be considered, and accurate diagnosis is crucial to the correct choice of diet.

Tables 16.4 and 16.5 state the content of main constituents such as protein, fat, and fibre, and minerals including calcium, magnesium, phosphorus, and calcium. Metabolisable energy in kilocalories per 100 g of dried feed is also listed. Other information on protein derivatives is noted where necessary. When selecting the correct diet, these factors should be taken into consideration. The manufacturers' claims for the use of therapeutic diets vary considerably. The main clinical conditions that may benefit from dietary management are discussed below.

The quantity of protein in a diet and its source may vary. Low protein diets usually contain highly digestible protein sources. Limited protein intake permits reduced protein metabolism and excretion, which may be helpful in the maintenance of animals with conditions such as renal or hepatic impairment, or for older animals.

The objectives of dietary management of renal impairment are to adjust the intake of protein, electrolytes, and water to the optimum level that the kidney is able to tolerate. Calorific requirements should be met with non-protein nutrients such as fat and carbohydrate. A reduction in sodium and phosphorus

intake may be advised and there may be an increased requirement for water-soluble vitamins if there is significant urinary loss.

Highly digestible diets are indicated in liver disease, providing 2 to 3 g of protein per kg body-weight daily. Low protein diets are necessary in the presence of hepatic encephalopathy. Foods containing a high purine content should be avoided.

In pancreatic insufficiency, treatment involves the substitution of the deficient digestive enzymes. Dietary management should include a moderate fat content, easily digestible carbohydrates, and protein of a high biological value.

Congestive heart failure may necessitate the adjustment of calorie intake, depending on whether the animal is obese or cachectic. Protein intake should be reduced in the presence of compromised cardiac or renal function unless plasma-protein concentration continues to fall. If increased protein intake is given to try to stabilise plasma-protein concentrations, the latter should be monitored carefully. If there is no improvement in blood-protein concentrations following increased protein intake, the animal should be put onto a lower protein diet. Dietary sodium should also be restricted according to the severity of the cardiac condition. Cats with dilated cardiomyopathy have similar nutritional requirements, but with extra taurine.

Special diets have an important role in the treatment of canine urolithiasis. Management of struvite uroliths includes the use of diets containing low protein and minerals, particularly magnesium and phosphorus, which produce urine acidification. Low protein diets are also advocated for cystine calculi. Urate deposits are controlled with diets that contain a low purine and protein content, and produce alkalinisation of the urine. Calcium oxalate calculi are also managed by alkalinisation of the urine and reduction of dietary calcium and oxalate. Feline urologic syndrome and struvite urolithiasis require a reduction in the magnesium content of the diet and acidification of the urine.

Table 16.4 Special diet preparations for dogs

Preparation	Pro-tein %	Fat %	Fibre %	Energy kcal/100 g	Cal-cium %	Mag-nesium %	Phos-phorus %	Sodium %	Comments
Liquid and canned feeds									
Canine Concentration diet (Pedigree)	36.7	25.9	3.4	133	1.5	0.1	1.2	0.9	
Canine Low Calorie diet (Pedigree)	52.9	21.7	2.2	56	2.6	0.2	2.1	0.9	
Canine Low Fat diet (Pedigree)	34.4	5.4	2.2	97	1.8	0.2	1.5	0.9	
Canine Low Protein diet (Pedigree)	16.7	31.1	1.5	133	0.8	0.1	0.5	0.3	
Canine Selected Protein diet (Pedigree)	30.0	28.9	1.3	104	2.2	0.1	1.8	0.9	Protein derived from chicken and rice
Canistar High Digestibility diet (RMB)	27.0	15.0	0.6	450					
Canistar High Protein diet (RMB)	33.2	32.8	0.4	520					
Canistar Low Calorie diet (RMB)	25.0	8.0	6.2	388					
Canistar Low Protein diet (RMB)	16.5	30.3	0.4	542					
Liquivite Special Care (Creg)	5.6	3.5	0.1	55					Liquid preparation
Prescription dict Canine C/D (Hill's)	22.8	24.0	0.3	490	0.6	0.07	0.44	0.25	
Prescription diet Canine D/D (Hill's)	26.7	21.6	3.4	460	0.54		0.41	0.51	Protein derived from mutton, rice, gluten free
Prescription diet Canine G/D (Hill's)	17.7	19.2	6.1	450	0.6		0.42	0.23	
Prescription diet Canine H/D (Hill's)	17.3	28.8	0.7	520	0.54		0.43	0.09	
Prescription diet Canine I/D (Hill's)	25.4	14.7	0.7	430	1.2		0.9	0.5	

Table 16.4 Special diet preparations for dogs (*continued*)

Preparation	Pro-tein %	Fat %	Fibre %	Energy kcal/ 100 g	Cal-cium %	Mag-nesium %	Phos-phorus %	Sodium %	Comments
Prescription diet Canine K/D (Hill's)	16.1	27.3	0.7	510	0.82		0.26	0.22	
Prescription diet Canine P/D (Hill's)	31.4	26.1	1.0	490	1.24		1.14	0.57	
Prescription diet Canine R/D (Hill's)	25.6	7.0	25.2	240	0.50		0.36	0.3	
Prescription diet Canine S/D (Hill's)	7.6	26.2	2.4	510	0.27	0.017	0.12	1.2	Protein derived from egg and liver, gluten free
Prescription diet Canine U/D (Hill's)	10.4	27.2	1.4	530	0.39	0.03	0.14	0.24	Protein derived from rice and casein, gluten free
Prescription diet Canine W/D (Hill's)	16.2	12.1	13.2	360	0.45		0.38	0.22	
Dry Feeds Canistar High Digestibility diet (RMB)	33.4	17.8	2.0	454					
Canistar Low Calorie diet (RMB)	30.0	6.7	7.8	367					
Canistar Low Protein diet (RMB)	16.7	18.9	3.4	463					
Doggy Lo-Calorie diet (Leo)	22.0	5.0	7.0	330	1.2		1.0		
Doggy Lo-Protein diet (Leo)	17.0	7.0	3.0		0.6	0.13	0.5	0.28	
Prescription diet Canine C/D (Hill's)	22.2	21.4	2.4	470	0.81	0.1	0.52	0.29	
Prescription diet Canine D/D (Hill's)	16.3	12.0	1.5	430	0.51		0.36	0.3	Protein derived from rice and egg
Prescription diet Canine G/D (Hill's)	19.0	13.6	7.1	410	0.68		0.47	0.28	

Table 16.4 Special diet preparations for dogs (*continued*)

Preparation	Protein %	Fat %	Fibre %	Energy kcal/ 100 g	Calcium %	Magnesium %	Phosphorus %	Sodium %	Comments
Prescription diet Canine H/D (Hill's)	17.5	21.2	1.1	460	0.77		0.55	0.06	
Prescription diet Canine I/D (Hill's)	27.3	14.5	0.9	430	1.4		1.1	0.5	
Prescription diet Canine K/D (Hill's)	14.8	19.8	0.9	470	0.78		0.28	0.23	Protein derived from egg, maize, rice, and whey
Prescription diet Canine P/D (Hill's)	32.3	23.1	3.3	460	1.75		1.32	0.34	
Prescription diet Canine R/D (Hill's)	25.0	7.0	21.8	250	1.1		0.7	0.3	
Prescription diet Canine U/D (Hill's)	9.5	21.0	2.2	500	0.4	0.04	0.13	0.26	Protein derived from egg, maize, rice, and whey; gluten free
Prescription diet Canine W/D (Hill's)	16.9	7.4	16.4	310	0.55		0.48	0.23	
Rite-Weight diet (Wafcol)	20.0	3.0	6.0	310	1.3	0.03	0.9	0.43	
Special '21' (Wafcol)	21.0	6.0	5.0	337	1.5	0.04	1.4	0.23	Protein derived from meat, maize, and soya; gluten free
Vegetarian diet (Wafcol)	20.0	8.0	8.0	347	1.3	0.03	0.9	0.43	Protein derived from maize and soya
Veteran diet (Wafcol)	16.0	8.0	5.0	354	1.5	0.04	1.4	0.39	

Table 16.5 Special diet preparations for cats

Preparation	Pro-tein %	Fat %	Fibre %	Energy kcal/ 100 g	Cal-cium %	Mag-nesium %	Phos-phorus %	Sodium %	Comments
Liquid and canned feeds									
Feline Concentration diet (Pedigree)	45.8	37.5	1.3	112	2.0	0.1	1.7	0.8	
Feline Low Calorie diet (Pedigree)	53.5	22.2	2.1	55	2.0	0.1	2.2	1.0	
Feline pH Control diet (Pedigree)	42.0	41.1	1.6	93	0.7	0.08	0.6	0.3	
Felistar High Protein diet (RMB)	45.0	32.5	8.4	444					
Felistar Low Calorie diet (RMB)	42.5	10.0	8.0	309					
Felistar Low Mineral diet (RMB)	39.5	31.0	0.4	438					
Liquivite Special Care (Creg)	5.6	3.5	0.1	55					Liquid preparation
Prescription diet Feline C/D (Hill's)	43.9	29.8	1.4	500	0.8	0.07	0.7	0.38	
Prescription diet Feline H/D (Hill's)	43.0	26.6	1.7	470	0.82	0.07	0.78	0.24	
Prescription diet Feline K/D (Hill's)	30.4	42.9	0.7	570	0.61	0.07	0.46	0.4	
Prescription diet Feline P/D (Hill's)	50.0	31.8	1.3	510	1.1	0.12	0.9	0.48	
Prescription diet Feline R/D (Hill's)	34.2	8.4	28.3	290	0.59	0.051	0.51	0.42	
Prescription diet Feline S/D (Hill's)	41.4	34.1	1.4	520	0.69	0.058	0.55	0.79	
Prescription diet Feline W/D (Hill's)	42.8	16.7	12.4	360	0.76	0.07	0.68	0.48	

Table 16.5 Special diet preparation for cats (*continued*)

Preparation	Pro-tein %	Fat %	Fibre %	Energy kcal/ 100 g	Cal-cium %	Mag-nesium %	Phos-phorus %	Sodium %	Comments
Dry feeds									
Felistar Low Calorie diet (RMB)	35.6	10.0	8.4	323					
Felistar Low Mineral diet (RMB)	33.4	22.3	2.4	418					
Prescription diet Feline C/D (Hill's)	35.2	26.0	1.8	490	0.8	0.08	0.7	0.46	
Prescription diet Feline K/D (Hill's)	28.6	27.8	1.6	490	0.79	0.07	0.47	0.25	potassium 0.78%
Prescription diet Feline P/D (Hill's)	40.0	27.8	1.3	490	1.3	0.1	1.0	0.49	
Prescription diet Feline R/D (Hill's)	38.0	8.2	18.5	320	0.85	0.066	0.65	0.4	
Prescription diet Feline S/D (Hill's)	35.0	26.4	1.1	480	0.68	0.055	0.58	0.76	
Prescription diet Feline W/D (Hill's)	39.0	9.4	10.1	340	0.73	0.066	0.66	0.34	

In the management of obesity during initial weight reduction, calorific intake should be reduced to 60 percent of the calculated maintenance needs for the dog, and 66 percent of the maintenance needs for the cat. An increase in dietary fibre intake may be advocated. In anorexia, the requirements for energy, protein, and fat are increased. If anorexia is secondary to other dietary requirements, force feeding may be necessary. Liquid diets may be useful for the anorexic animal and also during a convalescent period such as following surgery.

The control of diet in patients with particular gastro-intestinal disorders may help to manage the condition. Animals that are prone to constipation should be fed twice daily with a diet containing up to 10 percent fibre on a dry matter basis, which may aid water retention in the colon and also stimulate peristalsis following feeding. The diet should also have a low fat content and ingestion of bones, feathers, and skin should be restricted. For dogs, regular exercise taken about half to one hour after feeding will assist in encouraging defecation and improve gastro-intestinal muscle tone.

Dietary management may also be used as an adjunct to therapy in patients with diarrhoea. All food, except water, should be withheld for 24 hours, then small feeds provided 4 to 6 times daily. An easily digestible diet should be provided and one that contains high biological value protein at 4 g/kg body-weight daily; less than 15 percent fat on a dry weight basis for dogs; less than 1.5 percent fibre on a dry weight basis; and less than 10 percent sucrose and lactose as the carbohydrate source. In cases of severe diarrhoea or when vomiting accompanies diarrhoea, parenteral electrolyte and water replacement (see section 16.1) should be considered.

The commonest manifestations of food-induced allergy in the dog are as skin lesions. Dietary management involves the identification of a balanced diet that does not contain the protein source causing the allergic response. This is achieved by feeding hypoallergenic diets. Provocative exposure to different protein sources may be required to confirm the diagnosis.

17 GROWTH PROMOTERS

17.1 Antibacterial growth promoters
17.2 Other growth promoters

Growth promoters are added to feed or milk replacer in small quantities of up to 100 g per tonne to stimulate growth-rate, to improve feed conversion efficiency, or both. Growth promoters are most widely used in pig and poultry diets and increasingly in rations for intensively-reared cattle and the diets of fur-bearing animals. Individual animals may receive widely varying doses when growth promoters are incorporated into feed blocks.

17.1 Antibacterial growth promoters

The major growth promoters available are antibacterial compounds, mainly those that are not used for therapeutic or prophylactic purposes. Most are active against Gram-positive bacteria.

Antibacterial growth promoters may increase live-weight gain by 3 to 5 percent in poultry, pigs, and calves and up to 10 percent in ruminating cattle. The resultant increased feed conversion efficiency reduces the time and quantity of feed required to raise the animal.

Antibacterial growth promoters are not absorbed from the gastro-intestinal tract to any great extent and therefore plasma-drug concentrations are low. Not all antibacterial drugs possess growth-promoting activity. Their growth promoting potential does not appear to be related to their chemical structure.

In ruminants, the primary site of action is on the microflora of the rumen, enhancing the microbial production of the gluconeogenic fatty acid propionate at the expense of acetate and butyrate. In monogastric species the mode of action is not clear but a number of theories have been advanced. Growth promoters may act by suppressing harmful bacterial metabolites, potentially pathogenic organisms, or competition between organisms. Alternatively, growth promoters may act by altering metabolic activity or enhancing the intestinal absorption of nutrients.

Growth promoters may be administered to calves, lambs, and pigs up to 6 months of age. In poultry, these drugs are usually given up to 9 to 12 weeks of age, excluding those licensed for use in layer hens.

Avoparcin is a glycopeptide antibiotic. It may be administered to broiler chickens, turkeys, pigs, calves, lambs, growing-finishing cattle, and lactating dairy cattle. **Avilamycin** is used as a growth promoter in pigs.

Bacitracin zinc is a polypeptide antibiotic. In animals, it is now only used for growth-promoting purposes.

Bambermycin is a phosphorus-containing glycolipid antibiotic. It is used as a growth promoter in cattle, pigs, and poultry.

Monensin is an ionophore polyether antibiotic. It is used as an anticoccidial in poultry (see section 1.4.1). Monensin is used as a growth promoter in beef cattle and dairy heifers up to the time of first service. Cattle beginning monensin treatment within 60 days of slaughter should receive only half the normal dose. **Salinomycin** is also used for prevention of coccidiosis in poultry, and for growth promotion in pigs.

Spiramycin is a macrolide antibiotic and is active against Gram-positive bacteria and mycoplasmas. **Tylosin** is also a macrolide antibiotic. It is used in pigs.

Virginiamycin is a peptolide antibiotic, which acts against Gram-positive organisms by inhibiting protein synthesis.

AVILAMYCIN

Indications. To improve growth-rate and feed conversion efficiency

Contra-indications. Do not use simultaneously with other antibacterial growth promoters
Dose. *Pigs*: (up to 16 weeks of age) 20-40 g/tonne feed; (16-24 weeks of age) 10-20 g/tonne feed

PML**Maxus™ 100** (Elanco)
Premix, avilamycin 100 g/kg, for *pigs*; 25 kg
Withdrawal Periods. *Pigs*: slaughter withdrawal period nil

AVOPARCIN

Indications. To improve growth-rate and feed conversion efficiency
Contra-indications. See under Avilamycin
Dose. *Cattle*: (up to 24 weeks of age) 15-40 g/tonne feed; *growing-finishing cattle*: 15-30 g/tonne complete feed; *by addition to supplementary feed or feed block*, maximum dose, (less than 100 kg body-weight) 103 mg/100 kg body-weight, (more than 100 kg body-weight) 103 mg/100 kg and increase dose by 4.3 mg/10 kg body-weight; *lactating dairy cattle*: 4-10 g/tonne complete feed; *by addition to supplementary feed or feed block*, 50-100 mg/animal
Lambs: (up to 16 weeks of age) 10-20 g/tonne feed
Pigs: (up to 16 weeks of age) 10-40 g/tonne feed; (16-24 weeks of age) 5-20 g/tonne feed
Broiler chickens: 7.5-15.0 g/tonne feed
Turkeys: 10-20 g/tonne feed

PML**Avoparcin** (Hand/PH)
Premix, avoparcin 20 g/kg, for *cattle*, *pigs*, *broiler chickens*, *turkeys*; 1 kg, 20 kg
Withdrawal Periods. *Cattle, pigs, poultry*: slaughter withdrawal period nil
Premix, avoparcin 50 g/kg, for *cattle*, *pigs*, *broiler chickens*, *turkeys*; 20 kg
Withdrawal Periods. *Cattle, pigs, poultry*: slaughter withdrawal period nil

PML**Avotan™ 50** (Cyanamid)
Oral Powder, for addition to feed, avoparcin 50 g/kg, for *cattle*, *lambs*, *pigs*, *broiler chickens*, *turkeys*; 20 kg
Withdrawal Periods. *Cattle*: slaughter withdrawal period nil, milk withdrawal

period nil. *Lambs, pigs, poultry*: slaughter withdrawal period nil

PML**Avotan™ Super** (Cyanamid)
Oral powder, for addition to feed, avoparcin 100 g/kg, for *cattle*, *lambs*, *pigs*, *broiler chickens*, *turkeys*; 20 kg
Withdrawal Periods. *Cattle*: slaughter withdrawal period nil, milk withdrawal period nil. *Lambs, pigs, poultry*: slaughter withdrawal period nil

PML**Avotan™ Super G** (Cyanamid)
Oral granules, for addition to feed, avoparcin 100 g/kg, for *cattle*, *lambs*, *pigs*, *broiler chickens*, *turkeys*; 20 kg
Withdrawal Periods. *Cattle*: slaughter withdrawal period nil, milk withdrawal period nil. *Lambs, pigs, poultry*: slaughter withdrawal period nil

BACITRACIN ZINC

Indications. To improve growth-rate, feed conversion efficiency, and egg production
Contra-indications. See under Avilamycin. Adult breeding stock
Dose. *Calves, lambs, pigs*: (up to 16 weeks of age) 5-50 g/tonne feed; (16-24 weeks of age) 5-20 g/tonne feed; *by addition to milk replacer*, 5-80 g/tonne feed
Layer hens: 15-100 g/tonne feed
Broiler chickens, turkeys: (up to 4 weeks of age) 5-50 g/tonne feed; (5-26 weeks of age) 5-20 g/tonne feed
Rabbits, mink: 5-20 g/tonne feed

PML**Albac™ Feed Supplement** (Rosen)
Oral powder, for addition to feed, bacitracin zinc 100 g/kg, for *calves*, *lambs, pigs, broiler chickens, layer hens, turkeys, rabbits, mink*; 25 kg
Oral powder, for addition to feed, bacitracin zinc 150 g/kg, for *calves*, *lambs, pigs, broiler chickens, layer hens, turkeys, rabbits, mink*; 25 kg

PML**Albac™ Lactodispersible** (Rosen)
Oral powder, for addition to milk replacer, bacitracin zinc 100 g/kg, for *calves, lambs, pigs*; 25 kg

PML**ZB-100™** (Hand/PH)
Oral powder, for addition to feed, bacitracin zinc 100 g/kg, for *calves*,

lambs, pigs, chickens, turkeys, rabbits bred for fur, mink; 25 kg
Withdrawal Periods. *Calves, lambs, pigs, poultry*: slaughter withdrawal period nil

PML **Zinc Bacitracin** (Roussel)
Premix, bacitracin (as bacitracin zinc) 100 g/kg, for *calves, pigs, poultry*; 25 kg

BAMBERMYCIN

Indications. To improve growth-rate and feed conversion efficiency
Contra-indications. See under Avilamycin. Ducks, geese, or pigeons; adult breeding stock
Dose. *Cattle*: (up to 24 weeks of age) 6-16 g/tonne feed or milk replacer; (fattening cattle) 2-10 g/tonne complete feed; *by addition to supplementary feed*, maximum dose, 40 mg/100 kg body-weight, more than 100 kg body-weight, increase dose by 1.5 mg/10 kg body-weight; 80 mg/kg feed block
Pigs: 1-20 g/tonne feed; 10-25 g/tonne milk replacer
Layer hens: 2-5 g/tonne feed
Broiler chickens: (up to 16 weeks of age) 1-20 g/tonne feed
Turkeys: (up to 26 weeks of age) 1-20 g/tonne feed
Fur-bearing animals: 2-4 g/tonne feed

PML **Bambermycin** (Hand/PH)
Oral powder, for addition to feed or milk replacer, bambermycin 5 g/kg, for *cattle, pigs, broiler chickens, layer hens, turkeys, fur-bearing animals*; 25 kg
Withdrawal Periods. *Cattle, pigs, poultry*: slaughter withdrawal period nil
Oral powder, for addition to feed or milk replacer, bambermycin 20 g/kg, for *cattle, pigs, broiler chickens, layer hens, turkeys, fur-bearing animals*; 3 kg, 25 kg
Withdrawal Periods. *Cattle, pigs, poultry*: slaughter withdrawal period nil
Oral powder, for addition to feed or milk replacer, bambermycin 40 g/kg, for *cattle, pigs, broiler chickens, layer hens, turkeys, fur-bearing animals*; 25 kg
Withdrawal Periods. *Cattle, pigs, poultry*: slaughter withdrawal period nil

PML **Flavomycin**™ (Hoechst)
Premix, bambermycin 5 g/kg, for *cattle, pigs, poultry*; 25 kg

Withdrawal Periods. *Cattle, pigs, poultry*: slaughter withdrawal period nil
Premix, bambermycin 80 g/kg, for *cattle, pigs, poultry*; 25 kg
Withdrawal Periods. *Cattle, pigs, poultry*: slaughter withdrawal period nil

MONENSIN

Indications. To improve growth-rate and feed conversion efficiency in cattle; prophylaxis of coccidiosis in poultry (see section 1.4.1)
Contra-indications. See under Avilamycin
Warnings. Should not be given within 7 days before or after the administration of tiamulin (see Drug Interactions – Appendix 1). Toxic to horses
Dose. *Cattle*: 20-40 g/tonne complete feed; *by addition to supplementary feed*, maximum dose, (less than 100 kg body-weight) 140 mg/100 kg body-weight, (more than 100 kg body-weight) 140 mg/100 kg body-weight and increase dose by 6 mg/10 kg; *by intra-ruminal administration*, (more than 200 kg body-weight) one 16.5-g bolus, repeat after 5 months

Oral preparations

PML **Monensin-20 Ruminant** (Hand/PH)
Premix, monensin (as monensin sodium) 20 g/kg for *cattle*; 2 kg, 20 kg
Withdrawal Periods. *Cattle*: slaughter withdrawal period nil

PML **Monensin-100 Ruminant** (Hand/PH)
This preparation is now discontinued

PML **Romensin**™ (Elanco)
Premix, monensin (as monensin sodium) 100 g/kg, for *cattle*; 25 kg
Withdrawal Periods. *Cattle*: slaughter withdrawal period nil

Slow-release oral preparations

PML **Romensin**™ **RDD** (Elanco)
Ruminal bolus, s/r, monensin (as monensin sodium) 16.5 g, for *cattle*; 10
Withdrawal Periods. *Cattle*: slaughter withdrawal period nil

SALINOMYCIN SODIUM

Indications. To improve growth-rate and feed conversion efficiency in pigs;

prophylaxis of coccidiosis in poultry (see section 1.4.1)
Contra-indications. Side-effects. Warnings. Not to be given within 7 days before or after the administration of tiamulin (see Drug Interactions – Appendix 1). Toxic to horses. Should not be used in turkeys
Dose. *Pigs*: (up to 16 weeks of age) 30-60 g/tonne feed; (up to 24 weeks of age) 15-30 g/tonne feed

PML **Salocin™ 120** (Hoechst)
Oral granules, for addition to feed, salinomycin sodium 120 g/kg, for *pigs*; 25 kg
Withdrawal periods. *Pigs*: slaughter withdrawal period nil

SPIRAMYCIN

Indications. To improve growth-rate and feed conversion efficiency
Contra-indications. See under Avilamycin. Layer hens; adult breeding stock
Dose. *Calves, lambs, kids*: (up to 16 weeks of age) 5-50 g/tonne feed; (16-24 weeks of age) 5-20 g/tonne feed; *by addition to milk replacer*, (up to 24 weeks of age) 5-80 g/tonne
Pigs: (up to 16 weeks of age) 5-50 g/tonne feed; (16-24 weeks of age) 5-20 g/tonne feed; *by addition to milk replacer*, (up to 12 weeks of age) 5-80 g/tonne
Poultry, fur-bearing animals: 5-20 g/tonne feed

PML **Spira 200** (Rhône-Poulenc AN)
Oral powder, for addition to feed, spiramycin (as embonate) 200 g/kg, for *calves, lambs, kids, pigs, broiler chickens, turkeys, fur-bearing animals*; 25 kg
Withdrawal Periods. *Calves, lambs, kids, pigs poultry*: slaughter withdrawal period nil

PML **Spira 200 L** (Rhône-Poulenc AN)
Oral powder, for addition to milk replacer, spiramycin (as embonate) 200 g/kg, for *calves, lambs, kids, piglets*; 25 kg

TYLOSIN

Indications. To improve growth-rate and feed conversion efficiency

Contra-indications. See under Avilamycin
Dose. *Pigs*: (up to 16 weeks of age) 10-40 g/tonne feed; (16-24 weeks of age) 10-20 g/tonne feed

PML **Tylamix™** (Elanco)
Premix, tylosin (as phosphate) 100 g/kg, for *pigs*; 25 kg
Withdrawal Periods. *Pigs*: slaughter withdrawal period nil
Premix, tylosin 250 g/kg, for *pigs*; 50 kg
Withdrawal Periods. *Pigs*: slaughter withdrawal period nil

PML **Tylosin-20** (Hand/PH)
Premix, tylosin (as phosphate) 20 g/kg, for *pigs*; 2 kg, 25 kg
Withdrawal Periods. *Pigs*: slaughter withdrawal period nil

PML **Tylosin-100** (Hand/PH)
Premix, tylosin (as phosphate) 100 g/kg, for *pigs*; 25 kg
Withdrawal Periods. *Pigs*: slaughter withdrawal period nil

PML **Tylosin 250 Abchem™** (A B Pharmaceuticals)
Premix, tylosin (as phosphate) 250 g/kg, for *pigs*; 25 kg
Withdrawal Periods. *Pigs*: slaughter withdrawal period nil

VIRGINIAMYCIN

Indications. To improve growth-rate, feed conversion efficiency, and egg production
Contra-indications. See under Avilamycin. Ducks, geese, or pigeons; adult breeding stock; pigs over 6 months of age
Dose. *Calves*: (up to 16 weeks of age) 5-50 g/tonne feed; (16-24 weeks of age) 5-20 g/tonne feed; 5-80 g/tonne milk replacer
Pigs: (up to 16 weeks of age) 5-50 g/tonne feed; (16-24 weeks of age) 5–20 g/tonne feed; 5-80 g/tonne milk replacer
Layer hens: 20 g/tonne feed
Broiler chickens: (up to 9 weeks of age) 20 g/tonne feed
Turkeys: (up to 8 weeks of age) 20 g/tonne feed; (8-16 weeks of age) 5 g/tonne feed

PML **Stafac™ 20** (SmithKline Beecham)
Oral powder, for addition to feed, virginiamycin 20 g/kg, for *calves, pigs, broiler chickens, layer hens, turkeys*; 2 kg, 25 kg
Withdrawal Periods. *Calves, pigs, poultry*: slaughter withdrawal period nil

PML **Stafac™ 100** (SmithKline Beecham)
Oral powder, for addition to feed, virginiamycin 100 g/kg, for *calves, pigs, broiler chickens, layer hens, turkeys*; 25 kg
Withdrawal Periods. *Calves, pigs, poultry*: slaughter withdrawal period nil

PML **Stafac™ 500** (SmithKline Beecham)
Oral powder, for addition to feed, virginiamycin 500 g/kg, for *calves, pigs, broiler chickens, layer hens, turkeys*; 25 kg
Withdrawal Periods. *Calves, pigs, poultry*: slaughter withdrawal period nil

PoM **Stafac™ 500** (SmithKline Beecham)
Oral powder, for addition to feed virginiamycin 500 g/kg, for *layer and breeding chickens*; 25 kg
Withdrawal Periods. *Poultry*: slaughter withdrawal period nil, egg withdrawal period nil

PML **Stafac™ S-400** (SmithKline Beecham)
Oral powder, for addition to milk replacer, virginiamycin 400 g/kg, for *calves*; 25 kg
Withdrawal Periods. *Calves*: slaughter withdrawal period nil

PML **Virginiamycin-20** (Hand/PH)
Oral powder, for addition to feed, virginiamycin 20 g/kg, for *calves, pigs, poultry*; 2 kg, 25 kg
Withdrawal Periods. *Calves, pigs*: slaughter withdrawal period nil. *Poultry*: slaughter withdrawal period nil, egg withdrawal period nil

17.2 Other growth promoters

Certain **copper** salts may be incorporated into the diet of pigs in excess of nutritional requirements and have a growth-promoting effect. The efficacy of copper as a growth promoter is probably related to its antimicrobial activity. Some reports have shown that copper and antibiotics have an additive effect and they may be combined in pig feeds.

Arsenical compounds have been used for many years as growth promoters in pig and poultry diets but, in general, have now been superseded by the use of antibiotics.

COPPER

Indications. To improve growth-rate and feed conversion efficiency
Warnings. Care should be taken that sheep do not have access to effluent from treated pigs
Dose. *Pigs*: (up to 16 weeks of age) 175 g/tonne feed; (17-24 weeks of age) 100 g/tonne feed

PML **Copper Carbonate** (UKASTA)
Oral powder, for addition to feed, copper (as copper carbonate) 551 g/kg, for *pigs*
Withdrawal Periods. *Pigs*: slaughter withdrawal period nil

PML **Copper Sulphate** (UKASTA)
Oral powder, for addition to feed, copper (as copper sulphate) 254 g/kg, for *pigs*
Withdrawal Periods. *Pigs*: slaughter withdrawal period nil

PML **Cupric Oxide** (UKASTA)
Oral powder, for addition to feed, copper (as cupric oxide) 785 g/kg, for *pigs*
Withdrawal Periods. *Pigs*: slaughter withdrawal period nil

18 VACCINES and IMMUNOLOGICAL PREPARATIONS

Immunity in animals may be acquired by either passive or active means. **Passive immunity** occurs by the transfer of maternal antibodies to offspring or by the injection of antiserum to an animal of any age. Domestic mammals acquire passive immunity by intestinal absorption of antibodies from colostrum ingested within the first few hours of life. In birds, maternal antibody is transferred to the yolk, from where the developing chick absorbs it. The degree of protection conferred depends upon the amount and specificity of the immunoglobulins transferred. Passive immunity lasts only as long as antibodies remain reactive in the blood after which the animal loses any resistance to infection. Generally, passive immunity persists from 3 to 12 weeks. Maternally-acquired antibodies may interfere with the production of active immunity.

Commercially available preparations of antisera are usually produced by immunising horses or cattle to obtain sera containing the appropriate immunoglobulins or antitoxic globulins. Such preparations are frequently used to provide temporary protection, for example, with tetanus antitoxin. The injection of antiserum, especially if repeated a number of times, may produce hypersensitivity reactions. The potency of an antitoxic serum is expressed in terms of the International Unit (IU) defined by the World Health Organization and abbreviated to 'unit' in The Veterinary Formulary.

Active immunity develops as a result of infection with a micro-organism, or by administration of a vaccine prepared from live or inactivated organisms, or from detoxified exotoxins produced by organisms.

Live vaccines may be nonpathogenic forms of the infecting organism, such as in Marek's disease, or modified forms of the organism, for example orf virus. They stimulate production of antibodies either locally or systemically. Local antibodies may be stimulated by vaccines that promote immunity at mucosal surfaces, such as the nasal or intestinal mucosae. Living bacteria or viruses in vaccines colonise and replicate on the surface of the appropriate mucosa. Immunity derived from such vaccines develops rapidly and they may be used to protect noninfected animals during a herd outbreak of a disease such as infectious bovine rhinotracheitis.

The degree of protection afforded by live vaccines varies depending upon the antigen and the animal and is usually high and of long duration, although it is generally less than that following natural infection. Immunity usually develops slowly as it depends on the ability of the living micro-organism to multiply in the tissues of the host and stimulate immunoglobulin production.

Antibodies, especially maternally-derived, may inhibit the replication of the live micro-organism in the vaccine and thus interfere with the process of immunisation. Therefore, further doses of vaccine may be recommended, at suitable intervals to allow interfering antibodies to decline.

Inactivated vaccines contain sufficient antigen to stimulate immunoglobulins but generally require 2 doses, with an appropriate interval between, in order to produce a satisfactory immune response and protection. These vaccines contain adjuvants that enhance the immune reaction. Adjuvants commonly used are aluminium hydroxide or aluminium phosphate or an appropriate mineral oil such as liquid paraffin. Therefore, inactivated vaccines may cause local irritation and swelling at the site of injection. The organisms within inactivated vaccines do not replicate. These vaccines must always be administered by injection into a body tissue or cavity, as recommended. Booster doses of inactivated vaccines, often administered annually, are usually employed to maintain an enduring immunity.

Toxoids are toxins treated by heat or chemical means to destroy their deleterious properties without destroying their ability to stimulate the formation of antibodies, for example tetanus toxoid. Toxoids usually contain adjuvants.

Autogenous vaccines are prepared from cultures of material derived from a lesion of the animal to be vaccinated, for example wart vaccines.

Contra-indications and side-effects of vaccines. The possibility of undesirable side-effects should be considered when vaccines are used. Unhealthy or febrile animals should not be vaccinated. Animals should not be vaccinated within 3 to 4 weeks of receiving immunosuppressive drugs. When administering vaccines derived from bacteria, care should be taken in the use of antibacterials. When herds or flocks are being vaccinated with live vaccines, the transmission of infection due to the organism in the vaccine should be borne in mind, for example the introduction of orf virus into a susceptible flock. With vaccines containing live herpesviruses the probability of latent infections and their effects on future export of animals from the herd may require consideration. Some live vaccines, such as feline panleucopenia virus, may be able to cross the placenta and cause fetal abnormalities. In general, inactivated vaccines should be used in pregnant animals. Some inactivated vaccines may cause a transient swelling at the injection site.

Temporary clinical signs, such as coughing may be seen after administration of some vaccines, such as canine tracheobronchitis vaccine. Occasionally, animals exhibit a hypersensitivity reaction post-vaccination. Adrenaline (see section 4.5) or corticosteroids (see section 7.2.1) should be administered promptly.

Accidental self-injection with oil-based vaccines can cause intense vascular spasm and prompt medical attention is essential. A copy of the warning given in the product leaflet or data sheet should be shown to the doctor (or nurse) on duty.

Storage and handling of vaccines. Care must be taken to store all vaccines and other immunological preparations under the conditions recommended by the manufacturer, otherwise the preparation may become denatured and totally ineffective. Refrigerated storage at 2°C to 8°C is usually necessary. Unless otherwise specified, vaccines should not be frozen and should be protected from light. Some vaccines, such as Marek's disease vaccine are stored in solid carbon dioxide or in liquid nitrogen. Live antigens may be inactivated by disinfectants or alcohol and these substances must not be used to sterilise syringes.

Only sterile needles and syringes should be used for vaccination and injections given with aseptic precautions to avoid the possibility of abscess formation or the transmission of incidental infections. The repeated use of single needles and syringes within herds and flocks is undesirable. Containers that have held live vaccines can be potentially hazardous and should be made safe in accordance with Health and Safety Executive recommendations.

Injectable vaccines should be reconstituted as recommended by the manufacturer and liquid preparations should always be adequately shaken before use to ensure uniformity of the material to be injected.

18.1 Immunological preparations for horses

Vaccines available for the immunisation of horses include tetanus, equine influenza virus, and equine herpesvirus 1.

It is advisable that horses are always vaccinated against tetanus. In addition, the Jockey Club and Fédération Equestre Internationale (FEI) require horses to be vaccinated regularly against equine influenza. Vaccination against the equine herpesvirus that causes rhinopneumonitis and abortion is sometimes recommended. In special circumstances vaccination against rabies, salmonellosis, and *Escherichia coli* infection is practised.

Generally, vaccines are either injected subcutaneously or intramuscularly, into the neck or breast region dependent on the antigen present in the vaccine.

With some vaccines there is a recommendation to avoid strenuous exercise particularly following primary vaccination. Local and systemic adverse reactions have been reported especially with influenza vaccines.

18.1.1 Anthrax

No proprietary vaccine is available against anthrax (see section 18.2.1)

18.1.2 Equine herpesvirus 1

Infection with equine herpesvirus 1 may cause respiratory disease, abortion, neonatal death, and paresis. The respiratory form, known as equine viral rhinopneumonitis, is characterised by mild fever, coughing, nasal discharge, and conjunctivitis.

Inactivated and live vaccines are available. Either vaccine may be used in foals and pregnant mares. The live vaccine is intended only for protection against the respiratory form of the infection. All horses over 3 months of age should be vaccinated. An initial dose should be given and repeated after 4 to 8 weeks. Thereafter, all animals at risk should be vaccinated with a single dose every 3 months. Pregnant mares should be vaccinated after the second month of pregnancy. Immunity following natural infection lasts only a few months. Similarly, protection after vaccination is limited and frequent revaccination is necessary.

The inactivated vaccine is used in healthy pregnant mares as an aid in prevention of abortion. Pregnant mares are vaccinated during the fifth, seventh, and ninth months of pregnancy. Previously unvaccinated mares more than 5 months pregnant should be vaccinated immediately and then every 2 months until foaling. Maiden or barren mares in stable or pasture contact with pregnant mares should be vaccinated similarly. Other horses in contact with vaccinated pregnant mares, should be vaccinated at the time of contact, followed by a further dose 3 to 4 weeks later. A third dose should be given 6 months later followed by a booster dose every 12 months.

Indications. Vaccination against equine herpesvirus 1

Contra-indications. Side-effects. Warnings. See notes at beginning of chapter

Dose. See preparation details, see notes above for vaccination programmes

Live vaccines

PoM **Rhinomune**™ (SmithKline Beecham) *Injection*, powder for reconstitution, equine rhinopneumonitis vaccine, living, prepared from virus strain RAC-H, for *horses*; 1-dose vial

Dose. *Horses: by intramuscular injection*, 1 dose

Inactivated vaccines

PoM **Pneumabort-K**™ (ScanVet)
Injection, equine rhinopneumonitis vaccine, inactivated, prepared from virus, containing a suitable oil as adjuvant, for *horses*; 2 mL
Dose. *Horses*: by intramuscular injection, 2 mL

> Accidental self-injection with oil-based vaccines can cause severe vascular spasm and prompt medical attention is essential

18.1.3 Equine influenza

Equine influenza is a respiratory disease caused by Orthomyxoviridae type A influenza viruses. The disease is characterised by a mild fever and a persistent cough. Vaccination against equine influenza is required for horses entering property or competing under the rules of the Jockey Club or the FEI. Certification by a veterinary surgeon that the horse is correctly vaccinated and pictorially identified is necessary.
The initial vaccination course consists of 2 injections given 4 to 6 weeks apart. Further doses are given 6 and 12 months after the primary course. Foals born to vaccinated mares should not be vaccinated before 3 months of age. It is usually recommended that booster doses be given every 12 months thereafter, although shorter intervals, such as every 6 months, have been advocated. To comply with the rules of the Jockey Club and FEI, revaccination must be completed annually (see under Prescribing for animals used in competitions).
Alternatively, combined equine influenza virus and tetanus vaccines (see section 18.1.6) may be used for the initial vaccination course and every alternate annual booster vaccination.
Indications. Vaccination against equine influenza
Contra-indications. Side-effects. Warnings. See notes at beginning of chapter
Dose. See preparation details, see notes above for vaccination programmes

PoM **Duvaxyn**™ **IE** (Duphar)
Injection, equine influenza vaccine, inactivated, prepared from influenza A virus strains Equi/1 Prague, Equi/2 Miami, Equi/2 Kentucky 81, for *horses*; 1 mL
Dose. *Horses*: by intramuscular injection, 1 mL

PoM **Equinplus**™ (Coopers Pitman-Moore)
Injection, equine influenza vaccine, inactivated, prepared from influenza A virus strains Equi/1 Prague, Equi/2 Miami, Equi/2 Kentucky, for *horses*; 1-dose vial
Dose. *Horses*: by intramuscular injection, 1 dose

PoM **Prevac**™ (Hoechst)
Injection, equine influenza vaccine, inactivated, prepared from influenza A virus strains Equi/1 Prague 56, Equi/2 Miami 63, Equi/2 Fontainebleau 79, containing aluminium hydroxide as adjuvant, for *horses, donkeys, other Equidae*; 2 mL
Dose. *Horses, donkeys, other Equidae*: by intramuscular injection, 2 mL

See also section 18.1.6

18.1.4 Rabies

See section 18.4.6

18.1.5 Tetanus

Tetanus is caused by the toxin of *Clostridium tetani* and may affect all species. Animals are affected when wounds become infected with clostridial spores. Clinical signs include hyperaesthesia, tetany, and tonic convulsions. Horses are most susceptible to the neurotoxin.
Immunity to tetanus is generated by a primary course consisting of 2 doses of toxoid given approximately 4 to 6 weeks apart. A further dose should be given 12 months after the primary course, followed by booster doses every 2 to 3 years for horses and annually for other species. Previously immunised pregnant mares should be given a booster dose about one month before foaling. Foals from immunised mares will generally

not require to be vaccinated until 4 months of age. However, foals whose immune status is doubtful should be given tetanus antitoxin shortly after birth and again at 6 weeks of age, when a primary vaccination course may be commenced.

Animals that have not been vaccinated or whose immune status is doubtful should be given antitoxin prophylactically when exposed to risk of infection, for example, following injury. If desired, toxoid may be given simultaneously at a separate injection site using a different syringe. The antitoxin may be given at the site of injury or point of entry of the infection, if known. When used for treatment, antitoxin should initially be given intravenously. Repeat treatment daily as necessary.

Indications. Prevention and treatment of tetanus

Contra-indications. Side-effects. Warnings. See notes at beginning of chapter

Dose. See preparation details, see notes above for vaccination programmes

Antitoxins

PoM **Tetanus Antitoxin Concentrated** (Coopers Pitman-Moore)

Injection, prepared from *Clostridium tetani* antitoxin, containing 500 units/mL; for *horses, cattle, sheep, pigs*; 10 mL, 50 mL

Dose. Treatment. Initial dose *by intravenous injection* then *by subcutaneous injection*.

Horses, cattle: 100000 units, then 50000 units daily; *calves*: 15000 units, then 7500 units daily

Sheep, pigs: 15000 units, then 7500 units daily

Prophylaxis. *By subcutaneous injection*.

Horses, cattle: 3000 units; *calves*: 500 units

Sheep, pigs: 500 units

PoM **Tetanus Antitoxin** (C-Vet)

Injection, prepared from *Clostridium tetani* antitoxin, containing 1500 units/mL, for *horses, cattle, sheep, pigs, dogs*; 2 mL, 10 mL, 50 mL

Dose. Treatment. *By slow intravenous injection*. *Horses, cattle*: 150000 units daily; *calves*: 25000 units daily

Sheep, pigs: 25000 units daily; *lambs, piglets*: 12500 units daily

Dogs: 12500 units daily

Prophylaxis. *By subcutaneous or intramuscular injection*.

Horses, cattle: 3000 units; *calves*: 500 units

Sheep, pigs: 500 units; *lambs, piglets*: 250 units

Dogs: 250 units

PoM **Tetanus Antitoxin Behringwerke** (Hoechst)

Injection, prepared from *Clostridium tetani* antitoxin, containing 1000 units/mL, for *horses, cattle, sheep, pigs, dogs*; 50 mL

Dose. Treatment. *Horses, cattle*: *by epidural or intravenous injection*, 30000 units, with concurrent administration of 15000 units given *by subcutaneous or intramuscular injection*

Prophylaxis. *By subcutaneous or intramuscular injection*.

Horses, cattle: 7500 units; *foals, calves*: 3000 units

Sheep, pigs: up to 3000 units

Dogs: 500-1000 units

Vaccines

PoM **Duvaxyn™ T** (Duphar)

Injection, tetanus vaccine, inactivated, prepared from *Clostridium tetani* toxoid, containing aluminium phosphate as adjuvant, for *horses, ponies*; 1 mL

Dose. *Horses, ponies*: *by intramuscular injection*, 1 mL

PoM **Tetanus Toxoid** (Coopers Pitman-Moore)

Injection, tetanus vaccine, inactivated, prepared from *Clostridium tetani* toxoid, containing aluminium phosphate as adjuvant, for *horses, cattle, sheep*; 2 mL

Dose. *Horses*: *by intramuscular injection*, 2 mL

Cattle, sheep: *by subcutaneous injection*, 2 mL

PoM **Tetanus Toxoid** (C-Vet)

Injection, tetanus vaccine, inactivated, prepared from *Clostridium tetani* toxoid, containing a suitable aluminium salt as adjuvant, for *horses, other mammalian species*; 1 mL

Dose. *Horses*: *by intramuscular injection*, 1 mL

Other mammalian species: *by sub-cutaneous or intramuscular injection*, 1 mL

PoM **Tetanus Toxoid Concentrated** (Hoechst)
Injection, tetanus vaccine, inactivated, prepared from *Clostridium tetani* toxoid, containing aluminium hydroxide as adjuvant, for *horses, other mammalian species*; 1 mL
Dose. *Horses, other mammalian species*: *by subcutaneous or intramuscular injection*, 1 mL

PoM **Thorovax**™ (Coopers Pitman-Moore)
Injection, tetanus vaccine, inactivated, prepared from *Clostridium tetani* toxoid, containing aluminium phosphate as adjuvant, for *horses, other mammalian species*; 2 mL
Dose. *Horses*: *by intramuscular injection*, 2 mL
Cattle, sheep, pigs: *by subcutaneous injection*, 2 mL
Dogs, cats: *by subcutaneous injection*, 1 mL

See also section 18.1.6

18.1.6 Combination vaccines for horses

PoM **Duvaxyn**™ **IE-T** (Duphar)
Injection, combined equine influenza and tetanus vaccine, inactivated, prepared from influenza A virus strains Equi/1 Prague, Equi/2 Miami, Equi/2 Kentucky 81, *Clostridium tetani* toxoid, containing aluminium phosphate as adjuvant, for *horses*; 1-dose vial
Dose. *Horses*: *by intramuscular injection*, 1 dose, see section 18.1.3 for vaccination programmes

PoM **Equinplus**™-**T** (Coopers Pitman-Moore)
Injection, combined equine influenza and tetanus vaccine, inactivated, prepared from influenza A virus strains Equi/1 Prague, Equi/2 Miami, Equi/2 Kentucky, *Clostridium tetani* toxoid, containing aluminium phosphate as adjuvant, for *horses*; 1-dose vial
Dose. *Horses*: *by intramuscular injection*, 1 dose, see section 18.1.3 for vaccination programmes

PoM **Prevac**™ **T** (Hoechst)
Injection, combined equine influenza and tetanus vaccine, inactivated, prepared from influenza A virus strains Equi/1 Prague 56, Equi/2 Miami 63, Equi/2 Fontainebleau 79, *Clostridium tetani* toxoid, containing aluminium hydroxide as adjuvant, for *horses, donkeys, other Equidae*; 2 mL
Dose. *Horses, donkeys, other Equidae*: *by intramuscular injection*, 2 mL, see section 18.1.3 for vaccination programmes

18.2 Immunological preparations for cattle, sheep, and goats

18.2.1   Anthrax
18.2.2   Bovine viral pneumonia
18.2.3   Clostridial infections
18.2.4   Contagious pustular dermatitis
18.2.5   Enteritis
18.2.6   Enzootic ovine abortion
18.2.7   Erysipelas
18.2.8   Footrot
18.2.9   Leptospirosis
18.2.10 Louping ill
18.2.11 Lungworm
18.2.12 Pasteurellosis
18.2.13 Rabies

The immunisation programme used for ruminants depends on the management system, location, and the history of the herd or flock.
Cattle are often vaccinated against blackleg and tetanus but, in some herds, immunisation against other conditions, such as anthrax, 'husk' (lungworm disease), rotavirus, and infectious bovine rhinotracheitis (IBR) is also necessary.
Sheep flocks are generally vaccinated to prevent clostridial diseases but vaccination against other diseases, such as chlamydial abortion and louping ill, is sometimes necessary depending on the flock and its history. Goat vaccination is similar to that adopted for sheep.
In cattle, the site for vaccination by subcutaneous injection is usually the neck, while for intramuscular injection, the gluteal muscle region is used. For sheep, the anterior third of the neck is usually recommended. With prep-

arations in multidose containers, frequent changes of needle are necessary.

18.2.1 Anthrax

Anthrax is caused by spores of *Bacillus anthracis* and characterised by sudden death. Anthrax is a zoonotic infection. No commercial vaccine is available for routine vaccination of horses, ruminants, and pigs. MAFF should be contacted for information regarding emergency supplies.

18.2.2 Bovine viral pneumonia

Enzootic pneumonia in calves may be primarily caused by viruses, with secondary bacterial invasion, and exacerbation by inadequate housing and ventilation. Causative viruses include adenovirus, herpesvirus, parainfluenza virus 3 (PI3), respiratory syncytial virus (RSV), reovirus, and rhinovirus.

18.2.2.1 Bovine parainfluenzavirus
18.2.2.2 Bovine herpesvirus
18.2.2.3 Respiratory syncytial virus
18.2.2.4 Combination vaccines for bovine viral pneumonia

18.2.2.1 BOVINE PARAINFLUENZAVIRUS

Depending on the age of the calf and therefore the amount of maternally-derived antibody, the vaccine is administered intranasally either as a single dose at 12 weeks of age or more, or as a vaccination course with one dose being given at 3 weeks of age followed by a second dose at 10 weeks of age.

Indications. Vaccination against bovine parainfluenzavirus
Contra-indications. Side-effects. Warnings. See notes at beginning of chapter
Dose. See preparation details, see notes above for vaccination programmes

PoM **Imuresp**™ (SmithKline Beecham) Intranasal solution, powder for reconstitution, PI3 vaccine, living, prepared from virus strain RLB 103ts, for *calves, growing cattle*; 2 mL
Dose. *Calves, growing cattle: by intranasal application*, 2 mL into one nostril
See also section 18.2.2.4

18.2.2.2 BOVINE HERPESVIRUS

Bovine herpesvirus 1 is the causative agent of infectious bovine rhinotracheitis (IBR) characterised by an upper respiratory-tract infection, which may lead to pneumonia. The virus may also cause infectious pustular vulvovaginitis. Vaccination provides immunity against both the respiratory and genital forms of the disease. Calves of any age may be vaccinated but if under 3 months old, revaccination at this age is recommended. Annual revaccination is advised.

The vaccine will not prevent the disease in cattle that are already infected but it may reduce disease in a developing outbreak. Protection develops within 40 to 72 hours coinciding with the presence of interferon in nasal secretions. Antibodies are detectable in serum and nasal secretions by day 10 post-vaccination. Maternally-derived antibody does not prevent development of active immunity following vaccination in calves.

Cattle that have been vaccinated become sero-positive and thus may be unacceptable for export. Following vaccination, some cattle develop pyrexia and clinical signs of respiratory disease, which may last 3 to 5 days.

Indications. Vaccination against infectious bovine rhinotracheitis
Contra-indications. Side-effects. Warnings. See notes at beginning of chapter
Dose. See preparation details, see notes above for vaccination programmes

PoM **Tracherine**™ (SmithKline Beecham) *Intranasal solution*, powder for reconstitution, IBR vaccine, living, prepared from virus strain RLB 106 ts, for *cattle*; 2 mL
Dose. *Cattle: by intranasal application*, 2 mL into one nostril

See also section 18.2.2.4

18.2.2.3 RESPIRATORY SYNCYTIAL VIRUS

A live virus vaccine is available for the immunisation of calves against respiratory syncytial virus disease

(RSV). The vaccine may be used simultaneously with bovine para-influenzavirus vaccine and infectious bovine rhinotracheitis vaccine. Calves are vaccinated twice with an interval of 3 weeks between doses. Calves under 4 months of age should be vaccinated similarly with an additional vaccination at 4 months.

Indications. Vaccination against respiratory syncytial virus
Contra-indications. **Side-effects**. **Warnings**. See notes at beginning of chapter
Dose. See preparation details, see notes above for vaccination programmes

PoM **Rispoval RS™** (SmithKline Beecham)
Injection, powder for reconstitution, RSV vaccine, living, prepared from bovine virus, for *calves*; 5-dose vial
Dose. *Calves*: by intramuscular injection, 2 mL

18.2.2.4 COMBINATION VACCINES FOR BOVINE VIRAL PNEUMONIA

PML **Bo-Vax Pneumonia™** (Young's)
Injection, bovine viral pneumonia vaccine, inactivated, prepared from bovine adenovirus 3, bovine reovirus 1, bovine viral diarrhoea, IBR, PI3, for *calves*; 25 mL
Dose. *Calves*: by intramuscular injection, 2 mL at 4, 6, and 12 weeks of age, repeat as a single dose after 12 months if required

PoM **Imuresp™ RP** (SmithKline Beecham)
Intranasal solution, powder for reconstitution, combined IBR and PI3 vaccine, living, prepared from IBR virus strain RLB 106 ts, PI3 virus strain RLB 103 ts, for *calves, growing cattle*; 1-dose vial, 5-dose vial
Dose. *Calves, growing cattle*: by intranasal application, 2 mL into one nostril, see under section 18.2.2.1 for vaccination programmes

PoM **Pneumovac™ Plus** (C-Vet)
Injection, bovine viral pneumonia vaccine, inactivated, prepared from bovine adenovirus 3, bovine reovirus 1, bovine viral diarrhoea, IBR, PI3, for *calves*; 25 mL

Dose. *Calves*: by intramuscular injection, 2 mL at 4, 6, and 12 weeks of age, repeat as a single dose after 12 months if required

---

18.2.3 Clostridial infections

Sheep are routinely vaccinated against clostridial infections and vaccination is recommended for cattle and goats.
The exotoxins produced by clostridial species exhibit a variety of pathogenic effects. *Cl. chauvoei* (*Cl. feseri*) causes blackleg disease and post-parturient gangrene in sheep. *Cl. haemolyticum* (*Cl. novyi* type D) is the causative agent of bacillary haemoglobinuria and *Cl. novyi* (*Cl. oedematiens*) causes black disease. The various serotypes of *Cl. perfringens* (*Cl. welchii*) cause different diseases; type B causes lamb dysentery, type C causes struck, and type D causes pulpy kidney disease. Exotoxins of *Cl. septicum* lead to braxy and *Cl. tetani* exotoxins cause tetanus (see section 18.1.5).
Single and multicomponent vaccines are available. See Table 18.1 for an alphabetical list of vaccines and the clostridial infections they confer immunity against. Several clostridial infections may frequently occur in an area. Therefore, it is common practice to vaccinate routinely with combination vaccines capable of producing immunity to 4 to 8 clostridial infections. The vaccination programmes may vary with manufacturers' recommendations.
Antitoxins are available for passive immunisation of sheep and lambs and to prevent infection in cattle and goats where these species are at risk. The preparations may be expected to confer passive immunity for 3 to 4 weeks.
The available *Cl. perfringens* antitoxins contain either individual antitoxic globulins or a combination of antitoxic globulins. They are able to neutralise either the beta toxin or the beta and epsilon toxins produced by *Cl. perfringens* type B, the beta toxin produced by type C, or the the epsilon toxin produced by type D.
Vaccination programmes for multicomponent **vaccines** may vary with the

degree of risk in an area. Generally, sheep and lambs are given 2 doses with an interval of 4 to 6 weeks between doses and this primary course is completed 3 to 4 weeks before a period of risk such as lambing. For subsequent pregnancies, ewes are given a single injection 3 to 4 weeks before lambing. Lambs born to vaccinated ewes are protected by maternally-derived antibodies for up to 16 weeks of age, after which they should receive 2 doses of vaccine with an interval of 4 to 6 weeks between doses. Lambs, if born to unvaccinated ewes, should generally be vaccinated in the first 2 weeks of life, and again 4 to 6 weeks later. A booster dose each autumn is recommended but in areas of higher risk, a booster dose every 6 months may be appropriate.

For cattle, 2 doses are given separated by an interval of 3 to 4 weeks and administered 3 to 4 weeks before a period of risk. Annual booster doses are recommended. For pigs, 2 doses are given separated by an interval of at least 2 weeks.

Indications. Prevention and treatment of clostridial infections
Contra-indications. Side-effects. Warnings. See notes at beginning of chapter
Dose. See preparation details, see notes above for vaccination programmes

Antitoxins

PML **Lamb Dysentery and Pulpy Kidney Antiserum** (Coopers Pitman-Moore)
Injection, prepared from *Cl. perfringens* type B, C, and D antitoxins, containing beta antitoxin 2000 units, epsilon antitoxin 200 units/mL, for *sheep*; 50 mL
Dose. *Sheep*: *by subcutaneous injection*, (16-45 kg body-weight) 3-8 mL, (45 kg body-weight or more) 8 mL; *lambs*: *by subcutaneous injection*, (up to 16 kg body-weight) 3 mL

PML **Lambisan™** (Hoechst)
Injection, combined lamb dysentery, pulpy kidney, and struck antiserum, prepared from *Cl. perfringens* type B and D antitoxins, containing beta antitoxin 1200 units, epsilon antitoxin

120 units/mL, for *calves, sheep, piglets*; 100 mL
Dose. *Calves*: *by subcutaneous or intramuscular injection*, 25 mL
Sheep: *by subcutaneous or intramuscular injection*, 12.5 mL; *lambs*: *by subcutaneous or intramuscular injection*, 5 mL
Piglets: *by subcutaneous or intramuscular injection*, 5 mL

PML **Pulpy Kidney Antiserum** (Hoechst)
Injection, prepared from *Cl. perfringens* type D antitoxin, containing 300 units/mL, for *cattle, sheep, goats*; 100 mL
Dose. *Cattle*: *by subcutaneous or intramuscular injection*, 3000 units
Sheep, goats: *by subcutaneous or intramuscular injection*, 1500 units; *lambs*: *by subcutaneous or intramuscular injection*, 600 units

PML **Ryvac™ LD** (Young's)
Injection, combined lamb dysentery, pulpy kidney, and struck antiserum, prepared from *Cl. perfringens* type B and D antitoxins, containing beta antitoxin 1200 units, epsilon antitoxin 120 units/mL, for *lambs*; 100 mL
Dose. *Lambs*: *by subcutaneous or intramuscular injection*, 5 mL

Vaccines

PML **Blackleg Vaccine** (Coopers Pitman-Moore)
Injection, inactivated, prepared from *Cl. chauvoei* toxoid, containing alum as adjuvant, for *cattle, sheep*; 50 mL
Dose. *Cattle*: *by subcutaneous injection*, 2 mL
Sheep: *by subcutaneous injection*, 1 mL

PML **Blackleg Vaccine** (Hoechst)
Injection, inactivated, prepared from *Cl. chauvoei* toxoid, containing aluminium hydroxide as adjuvant, for *cattle, sheep*; 50 mL
Dose. *Cattle, sheep*: *by subcutaneous or intramuscular injection*, 2 mL

PML **Braxy/Blackleg Vaccine** (Hoechst)
Injection, inactivated, prepared from *Cl. chauvoei* toxoid, *Cl. septicum* toxoid, containing aluminium hydroxide as adjuvant, for *cattle, sheep*; 50 mL, 100 mL
Dose. *Cattle, sheep*: *by subcutaneous injection*, 2 mL

Table 18.1 Immunological preparations for clostridial infections

	Bacillary haemoglobinuria	Black disease	Black-leg	Braxy	Lamb dysentery	Pulpy kidney	Struck	Teta-nus	Other infections
Antitoxins									
Lamb Dysentery and Pulpy Kidney Antiserum (Coopers Pitman-Moore)					+	+	+		
Lambisan™ (Hoechst)					+	+	+		
Pulpy Kidney Antiserum (Hoechst)						+			
Ryvac™ LD (Young's)					+	+	+		
Tetanus Antitoxin (Coopers Pitman-Moore)								+	
Tetanus Antitoxin (C-Vet)								+	
Tetanus Antitoxin Behringwerke (Hoechst)								+	
Vaccines									
Blackleg Vaccine (Coopers Pitman-Moore)			+						
Blackleg Vaccine (Hoechst)			+						
Braxy/Blackleg Vaccine (Hoechst)			+	+					
Covexin™ 8 (Coopers Pitman-Moore)	+	+	+	+	+	+	+	+	
Duvaxyn™ (Duphar)								+	
Heptavac™ (Hoechst)		+	+	+	+	+	+	+	
Heptavac-P™ (Hoechst)		+	+	+	+	+	+	+	Pasteurellosis
Lambivac™ (Hoechst)					+	+	+	+	
Nilvax™ (Coopers Pitman-Moore)	+	+	+	+	+	+	+	+	Gastro-intestinal roundworms and lungworms in sheep

Table 18.1 Immunological preparations for clostridial infections (*continued*)

	Bacillary haemoglobinuria	Black disease	Black-leg	Braxy	Lamb dysentery	Pulpy kidney	Struck	Tetanus	Other infections
Ovivac™ (Hoechst)			+	+		+		+	
Ovivac-P™ (Hoechst)			+	+		+		+	Pasteurellosis
Pulpy Kidney and Tetanus Vaccine (Coopers Pitman-Moore)						+		+	
Pulpy Kidney and Tetanus Vaccine (Hoechst)						+		+	
Quadrivexin™ (Coopers Pitman-Moore)					+	+	+	+	
Ryvac™ 4 (Young's)			+	+		+		+	
Ryvac™ 5P (Young's)			+	+		+		+	Pasteurellosis
Ryvac™ 7 (Young's)	+	+	+	+	+	+	+	+	
Ryvac™ 7P (Young's)	+	+	+	+	+	+	+	+	Pasteurellosis
Ryvac™ LD+ (Young's)					+	+	+	+	
Tasvax™ 8 (Coopers Pitman-Moore)	+	+	+	+	+	+	+	+	
Tasvax™ Gold (Coopers Pitman-Moore)		+	+	+		+		+	
Tetanus Toxoid (Coopers Pitman-Moore)								+	
Tetanus Toxoid (C-Vet)								+	
Tetanus Toxoid (Hoechst)								+	
Thorovax™ (Coopers Pitman-Moore)								+	
Tribovax™-T (Coopers Pitman-Moore)	+	+	+	+				+	
Trivexin™ T (Coopers Pitman-Moore)			+	+		+		+	

PML **Covexin™ 8** (Coopers Pitman-Moore)
Injection, combined bacillary haemoglobinuria, black disease, blackleg, braxy, lamb dysentery, pulpy kidney, struck, and tetanus vaccine, inactivated, prepared from *Cl. chauvoei* toxoid, *Cl. haemolyticum* toxoid, *Cl. novyi* toxoid, *Cl. perfringens* type B, C, and D toxoids, *Cl. septicum* toxoid, *Cl. tetani* toxoid, containing alum as adjuvant, for *cattle, sheep*; 100 mL, 250 mL, 500 mL
Dose. *Cattle: by subcutaneous injection*, 5 mL
Sheep: by subcutaneous injection, initial dose 5 mL then 2 mL; *lambs: by subcutaneous injection*, 2 mL

PML **Heptavac™** (Hoechst)
Injection, combined black disease, blackleg, braxy, lamb dysentery, pulpy kidney, struck, and tetanus vaccine, inactivated, prepared from *Cl. chauvoei* toxoid, *Cl. novyi* toxoid, *Cl. perfringens* type B, C, and D toxoids, *Cl. septicum* toxoid, *Cl. tetani* toxoid, containing aluminium hydroxide as adjuvant, for *sheep*; 50 mL, 100 mL, other sizes available
Dose. *Sheep: by subcutaneous injection*, 2 mL

PML **Heptavac-P™** (Hoechst)
Injection, combined black disease, blackleg, braxy, lamb dysentery, pasteurellosis, pulpy kidney, struck, and tetanus vaccine, inactivated, prepared from *Cl. chauvoei* toxoid, *Cl. novyi* toxoid, *Cl. perfringens* type B, C, and D toxoids, *Cl. septicum* toxoid, *Cl. tetani* toxoid, antigens of *P. haemolytica* serotypes A, T, containing aluminium hydroxide as adjuvant, for *sheep*; 50 mL, 100 mL, other sizes available
Dose. *Sheep: by subcutaneous injection*, 2 mL

PML **Lambivac™** (Hoechst)
Injection, combined lamb dysentery, pulpy kidney, struck, and tetanus vaccine, inactivated, prepared from *Cl. perfringens* type B, C, and D toxoids, *Cl. tetani* toxoid, containing aluminium hydroxide as adjuvant, for *cattle, sheep, goats, pigs*; 50 mL, 100 mL
Dose. *Cattle, sheep, goats, pigs: by subcutaneous injection*, 2 mL

PML **Nilvax™** (Coopers Pitman-Moore)
Injection, combined bacillary haemoglobinuria, black disease, blackleg, braxy, lamb dysentery, pulpy kidney, struck, and tetanus vaccine, inactivated, prepared from *Cl. chauvoei* toxoid, *Cl. haemolyticum* toxoid, *Cl. novyi* toxoid, *Cl. perfringens* type C and D toxoids, *Cl. septicum* toxoid, *Cl. tetani* toxoid, containing a suitable aluminium salt as adjuvant, levamisole (as phosphate) 68 mg/mL, for *sheep*; 100 mL, 500 mL
Withdrawal Periods. *Sheep*: slaughter 3 days, milk 7 days
Dose. *By subcutaneous injection. Sheep*: (30-44 kg body-weight) 3.5 mL; (45-54 kg body-weight) 4.0 mL; (55-69 kg body-weight) 5.0 mL; (70-79 kg body-weight) 6.0 mL; (80-95 kg body-weight) 7.0 mL

PML **Ovivac™** (Hoechst)
Injection, combined blackleg, braxy, pulpy kidney, and tetanus vaccine, inactivated, prepared from *Cl. chauvoei* toxoid, *Cl. perfringens* type D toxoid, *Cl. septicum* toxoid, *Cl. tetani* toxoid, containing aluminium hydroxide as adjuvant, for *sheep*; 50 mL, 100 mL
Dose. *Sheep: by subcutaneous injection*, 2 mL

PML **Ovivac-P™** (Hoechst)
Injection, combined blackleg, braxy, pasteurellosis, pulpy kidney, and tetanus vaccine, inactivated, prepared from *Cl. chauvoei* toxoid, *Cl. perfringens* type D toxoid, *Cl. septicum* toxoid, *Cl. tetani* toxoid, antigens of *P. haemolytica* serotypes A, and T, containing aluminium hydroxide as adjuvant, for *sheep*; 100 mL, 500 mL
Dose. *Sheep: by subcutaneous injection*, 2 mL

PML **Pulpy Kidney and Tetanus Vaccine** (Coopers Pitman-Moore)
Injection, inactivated, prepared from *Cl. perfringens* type D toxoid, *Cl. tetani* toxoid, containing alum as adjuvant, for *sheep*; 100 mL, 250 mL
Dose. *Sheep: by subcutaneous injection*, 2 mL

PML **Pulpy Kidney and Tetanus Vaccine** (Hoechst)
Injection, inactivated, prepared from *Cl. perfringens* type D toxoid, *Cl. tetani* toxoid, containing aluminium hydroxide

as adjuvant, for *cattle, sheep, goats*; 50 mL, 100 mL, 250 mL

Dose. *Cattle, sheep, goats*: *by sub-cutaneous injection*, 2 mL

PML **Quadrivexin**™ (Coopers Pitman-Moore)

Injection, combined lamb dysentery, pulpy kidney, struck, and tetanus vaccine, inactivated, prepared from *Cl. perfringens* type B, C, and D toxoids, *Cl. tetani* toxoid, containing alum as adjuvant, for *sheep*; 100 mL

Dose. *Sheep*: *by subcutaneous injection*, 2 mL

PML **Ryvac**™ 4 (Young's)

Injection, combined blackleg, braxy, pulpy kidney, and tetanus vaccine, inactivated, prepared from *Cl. chauvoei* toxoid, *Cl. perfringens* type D toxoid, *Cl. septicum* toxoid, *Cl. tetani* toxoid, containing aluminium hydroxide as adjuvant, for *sheep*; 100 mL

Dose. *Sheep*: *by subcutaneous injection*, 2 mL

PML **Ryvac**™ 5P (Young's)

Injection, combined blackleg, braxy, pasteurellosis, pulpy kidney, and tetanus vaccine, inactivated, prepared from *Cl. chauvoei* toxoid, *Cl. perfringens* type D toxoid, *Cl. septicum* toxoid, *Cl. tetani* toxoid, antigens of *P. haemolytica* serotypes A, and T, containing aluminium hydroxide as adjuvant, for *sheep*; 100 mL, 500 mL

Dose. *Sheep*: *by subcutaneous injection*, 2 mL

PML **Ryvac**™ 7 (Young's)

Injection, combined black disease, blackleg, braxy, lamb dysentery, pulpy kidney, struck, and tetanus vaccine, inactivated, prepared from *Cl. chauvoei* toxoid, *Cl. novyi* toxoid, *Cl. perfringens* type B, C, and D toxoids, *Cl. septicum* toxoid, *Cl. tetani* toxoid, containing aluminium hydroxide as adjuvant, for *sheep*; 100 mL, 250 mL, 500 mL

Dose. *Sheep*: *by subcutaneous injection*, 2 mL

PML **Ryvac**™ 7P (Young's)

Injection, combined black disease, blackleg, braxy, lamb dysentery, pasteurellosis, pulpy kidney, struck, and tetanus vaccine, inactivated, prepared from *Cl.*

chauvoei toxoid, *Cl. novyi* toxoid, *Cl. perfringens* type B, C, and D toxoids, *Cl. septicum* toxoid, *Cl. tetani* toxoid, antigens of *P. haemolytica* serotypes A, T, containing aluminium hydroxide as adjuvant, for *sheep*; 50 mL, 100 mL, other sizes available

Dose. *Sheep*: *by subcutaneous injection*, 2 mL

PML **Ryvac**™ LD+ (Young's)

Injection, combined lamb dysentery, pulpy kidney, struck, and tetanus vaccine, inactivated, prepared from *Cl. perfringens* type B, C, and D toxoids, *Cl. tetani* toxoid, containing aluminium hydroxide as adjuvant, for *sheep*; 100 mL

Dose. *Sheep*: *by subcutaneous injection*, 2 mL

PML **Tasvax**™ 8 (Coopers Pitman-Moore)

Injection, combined bacillary haemo-globinuria, black disease, blackleg, braxy, lamb dysentery, pulpy kidney, struck, and tetanus vaccine, inactivated, prepared from *Cl. chauvoei* toxoid, *Cl. haemolyticum* toxoid, *Cl. novyi* toxoid, *Cl. perfringens* type C and D toxoids, *Cl. septicum* toxoid, *Cl. tetani* toxoid, containing aluminium hydroxide as adjuvant, for *cattle, sheep, goats*; 50 mL, 100 mL, other sizes available

Dose. *Cattle*: *by subcutaneous injection*, 4 mL

Sheep, goats: *by subcutaneous injection*, 2 mL

PML **Tasvax**™ Gold (Coopers Pitman-Moore)

Injection, combined black disease, blackleg, braxy, pulpy kidney, and tetanus vaccine, inactivated, prepared from *Cl. chauvoei* toxoid, *Cl. novyi* toxoid, *Cl. perfringens* type D toxoid, *Cl. septicum* toxoid, *Cl. tetani* toxoid, containing a suitable aluminium salt as adjuvant, for *cattle, sheep*; 100 mL, 200 mL

Dose. *Cattle*: *by subcutaneous injection*, 4 mL

Sheep: *by subcutaneous injection*, 2 mL

PML **Tribovax**™-T (Coopers Pitman-Moore)

Injection, combined bacillary haemo-globinuria, black disease, blackleg, braxy, and tetanus vaccine, inactivated, prepared from *Cl. chauvoei* toxoid, *Cl.*

haemolyticum toxoid, *Cl. novyi* toxoid, *Cl. septicum* toxoid, *Cl. tetani* toxoid, containing alum as adjuvant, for *cattle*; 50 mL
Dose. *Cattle*: *by subcutaneous injection*, 2 mL

PML **Trivexin™   T** (Coopers Pitman-Moore)
Injection, combined blackleg, braxy, pulpy kidney, and tetanus vaccine, inactivated, prepared from *Cl. chauvoei* toxoid, *Cl. perfringens* type D toxoid, *Cl. septicum* toxoid, *Cl. tetani* toxoid, containing alum as adjuvant, for *sheep*; 100 mL
Dose. *Sheep*: *by subcutaneous injection*, 2 mL

18.2.4 Contagious pustular dermatitis
(Contagious ecthyma)

Contagious pustular dermatitis, commonly known as orf, is caused by a poxvirus and characterised by scabby, pustular lesions mainly on the muzzle and lips. The disease affects sheep and goats and is a zoonotic infection.
The vaccine is used in sheep and lambs 2 to 3 weeks before the expected period of disease risk. Revaccination should be given every 5 to 12 months depending on the degree of challenge in the area. The vaccine should not be used on farms or in flocks where orf is not a problem, nor used to vaccinate ewes less than 6 weeks before lambing. Vaccinated sheep develop mild lesions of orf at the site of vaccination. This is usually the inside of the thigh or axilla and the vaccine is administered by scarification.

Indications. Vaccination against contagious pustular dermatitis
Contra-indications. Use on farms where the disease is not endemic. Vaccination of ewes less than 6 weeks before lambing or during lactation; see also notes at beginning of chapter
Side-effects. **Warnings**. See notes above and at beginning of chapter
Dose. See preparation details, see notes above for vaccination programmes

PoM **Scabivax™** (Coopers Pitman-Moore)
Liquid for scarification, contagious pustular dermatitis vaccine, living, prepared from scab material from sheep infected with modified virus, for *sheep*; 50-dose vial
Dose. *Sheep*: *by scarification*, 1 application

18.2.5 Enteritis

Enteritis in ruminants may be caused by many organisms including bacteria, viruses, and parasites. Antisera and vaccines are available for the prevention and treatment of enteritis caused by *Escherichia coli*, *Salmonella*, *Pasteurella*, and rotavirus, and by clostridial organisms (see section 18.2.3). Vaccines may contain either serotypes of a single bacterium or a combination of bacterial serotypes.
18.2.5.1 *Escherichia coli* infections
18.2.5.2 Salmonellosis
18.2.5.3 Combination immunological preparations for enteritis in cattle and sheep

18.2.5.1 ESCHERICHIA COLI INFECTIONS

Indications. Vaccination against *E. coli*
Contra-indications. **Side-effects**. **Warnings**. See notes at beginning of chapter
Dose. See preparation details
PML **Coliovac™** (Hoechst)
Injection, *E. coli* vaccine, inactivated, prepared from *E. coli* O antigens 8, 9, 11, 15, 20, 26, 35, 78, 86, 101, 115, 137; K antigens 30, 32, 35, B41, 60, 61, V79, 80, 85, 99, V165; F41 antigen, K99 antigen, containing aluminium hydroxide as adjuvant, for *sheep*; 100 mL, 250 mL
Dose. *Sheep*: *by subcutaneous injection*, 2 mL, repeat dose after at least 2 weeks. The second dose should be given 3-4 weeks before lambing. Annual revaccination 3-4 weeks before lambing

18.2.5.2 SALMONELLOSIS

Salmonellosis is a zoonotic disease. Several forms of the disease occur including abortion, acute or chronic enteritis, and septicaemia. A vaccine is available for immunisation of young calves against disease caused by *Salmonella dublin*. Some degree of protection is also afforded against *S. typhimurium*, but this is less durable. Calves should be vaccinated about a week before exposure to infection or as soon as they arrive on premises known to be infected.

Indications. Vaccination against salmonellosis
Contra-indications. Side-effects. Warnings. See notes at beginning of chapter
Dose. See preparation details, see notes above for vaccination programmes

PoM **Mellavax™** (Coopers Pitman-Moore)
Injection, powder for reconstitution, salmonellosis vaccine, living, prepared from *S. dublin* strain HWS 51, for *calves*; 5-dose vial
Dose. *Calves: by subcutaneous injection*, 1 dose

18.2.5.3 COMBINATION IMMUNOLOGICAL PREPARATIONS FOR ENTERITIS IN CATTLE AND SHEEP

Antisera are used prophylactically and therapeutically especially in young ruminants for enteric infections caused by certain serotypes of *E. coli*. Repeated daily administration of antigen may be necessary for treatment. Antisera are given soon after birth or before periods of challenge and may be administered at intervals of 10 to 14 days during periods of risk.
Vaccines contain important antigens of *E. coli*, such as K99 or selected, inactivated serotypes. Vaccines also contain *Salmonella* species, *P. multocida* serotypes, or rotavirus. Initial vaccination of cattle and sheep may involve a course of 2 vaccine doses given at an interval of 14 to 21 days. Previously unvaccinated cows and ewes should be vaccinated, with the second dose administered not less than 3 weeks before calving or the lambing season. Thereafter, pregnant animals may be given an annual booster approximately 3 weeks before the expected date of parturition.

Indications. Vaccination against enteritis
Contra-indications. Side-effects. Warnings. See notes at beginning of chapter
Dose. See preparation details, see notes above for vaccination programmes

Antisera

PML **Bovisan™ DPS** (Hoechst)
Injection, combined *E. coli, Pasteurella*, and *Salmonella* antiserum, prepared from *E. coli, P. multocida* Roberts types 1, 2, 3, 4, *S. dublin, S. typhimurium*, for *calves, sheep*; 100 mL
Dose. Treatment. *By subcutaneous or intramuscular injection.*
Calves: 40 mL
Sheep: 10 mL
Prophylaxis. *By subcutaneous or intramuscular injection.*
Calves: 20 mL
Sheep: 5 mL

PML **Ecosan™** (Hoechst)
Injection, combined *E. coli* and *Salmonella* antiserum, prepared from *E. coli, S. dublin, S. enteritidis, S. typhimurium*, for *calves, sheep*; 100 mL
Dose. Treatment. *By subcutaneous, intramuscular, or intravenous injection.*
Calves: 20 mL
Sheep: 10 mL
Prophylaxis. *By subcutaneous, intramuscular, or intravenous injection.*
Calves: 10 mL
Sheep: 5 mL

Antisera-vaccine combinations

PML **Grovax™** (Hoechst)
Injection, combined *E. coli, Diplococcus, Pasteurella*, and *Salmonella* antiserum/vaccine, inactivated, prepared from *D. pneumoniae* strains types 8, 18, 19, 22, 33, selected *E. coli* serotypes, *P. multocida* Roberts types 1, 2, 3, 4, *S. dublin, S. typhimurium*, in combination with antisera to the same organisms, and containing cobalt, copper, iodine, iron, zinc as trace elements, for *cattle*; 100 mL
Dose. Treatment. *Calves: by subcutaneous injection*, 40 mL
Prophylaxis. *Cattle: by subcutaneous injection*, 40 mL, repeat dose at least 2 weeks before calving in pregnant animals; *calves: by subcutaneous injection*, 20-30 mL

Vaccines

PML Bovivac™ (Hoechst)
Injection, combined *E. coli* and *Salmonella* vaccine, inactivated, prepared from *E. coli* serotypes, *S. dublin* strains, *S. typhimurium* strains, containing aluminium hydroxide as adjuvant, for *cattle, sheep*; 50 mL
Dose. *Cattle*: by subcutaneous injection, 5 mL; *calves*: by subcutaneous injection, 2 mL
Sheep: by subcutaneous injection, 2 mL; *lambs*: by subcutaneous injection, 1 mL

PML Bovivac™ Plus (Hoechst)
Injection, combined *E. coli*, *Pasteurella*, and *Salmonella* vaccine, inactivated, prepared from *E. coli* serotypes, *P. multocida* Roberts types 1, 2, 3, 4, *S. dublin* strains, *S. typhimurium* strains, containing aluminium hydroxide as adjuvant, for *cattle*; 50 mL
Dose. *Cattle*: by subcutaneous injection, 5 mL; *calves*: by subcutaneous injection, 2 mL

PoM Rotavec™ K99 (Coopers Pitman-Moore)
Injection, combined bovine rotavirus and *E. coli* vaccine, inactivated, prepared from virus antigens, *E. coli* K99 antigens, containing aluminium hydroxide and a light mineral oil as adjuvants, for *cattle*; 5 mL, 20 mL
Dose. *Cattle*: by intramuscular injection, 1 mL as a single dose between 12 and 4 weeks before calving

18.2.6 Enzootic ovine abortion

Chlamydia psittaci infection causes late abortion in sheep. The vaccine is administered subcutaneously into the chest wall behind the shoulder. All breeding stock should be vaccinated in late summer or early autumn before service and a booster dose given after 3 years.

Indications. Vaccination against enzootic ovine abortion
Contra-indications. Side-effects. Warnings. See notes at beginning of chapter
Dose. See preparation details, see notes above for vaccination programmes

PML Ovine Enzootic Abortion (Coopers Pitman-Moore)
Injection, inactivated, prepared from ovine *Chlamydia* strains A22, S26/3 grown on yolk-sac membranes, containing light liquid paraffin as adjuvant, for *sheep*; 20 mL
Dose. *Sheep*: by subcutaneous injection, 1 mL

18.2.7 Erysipelas

Infection with *Erysipelothrix rhusiopathiae* (*Ery. insidiosa*) occurs in lambs and in older sheep as a joint infection and bacteraemia and arises, for example, after dipping in contaminated baths. Sheep may be vaccinated to increase their immunity. Two doses are given at an interval of 2 to 6 weeks, with the second dose administered 2 weeks before the expected period of risk. In pregnant ewes, the second dose is given 3 weeks before lambing. See section 18.3.5 for erysipelas in pigs and section 18.6.7 for erysipelas in turkeys.

Indications. Vaccination against erysipelas
Contra-indications. Side-effects. Warnings. See notes at beginning of chapter
Dose. See preparation details, see notes above for vaccination programmes

PML Erysorb™ ST (Hoechst)
Injection, erysipelas vaccine, inactivated, prepared from *Ery. rhusiopathiae*, containing aluminium hydroxide as adjuvant, for *sheep, turkeys* (18.6.7); 50 mL, 100 mL
Dose. *Sheep*: by subcutaneous injection, 2 mL

18.2.8 Footrot

Vaccination against footrot in sheep should be part of an overall foot care programme (see Chapter 15). Timing of vaccination is important and should be carried out before the expected period of disease risk, which is generally in autumn, spring, and before housing. Available vaccines are prepared from *Bacteroides (Fusiformis) nodosus*. Two doses are given at an interval of 4 to 8 weeks. Lambs over 2 weeks of age may be vaccinated, but not ewes between 6 weeks before and 2 weeks after lambing, nor lactating ewes. Booster doses should be given every 6 months. A persistent reaction, lasting for several weeks, may occur at the site of injection. Therefore vaccination should be avoided within 2 months of shearing or before sale or showing.

Indications. Vaccination against footrot
Contra-indications. Vaccination of lambs under 2 weeks of age, see notes above
Side-effects. Warnings. See notes at beginning of chapter
Dose. See preparation details, see notes above for vaccination programmes

PML **Clovax**™ (Coopers Pitman-Moore)
Injection, footrot vaccine, inactivated, prepared from *B. nodosus*, containing alum as adjuvant, for *sheep*; 50 mL, 250 mL
Dose. *Sheep*: *by subcutaneous injection*, 2 mL

PML **Footvax**™ (Coopers Pitman-Moore)
Injection, footrot vaccine, inactivated, prepared from *B. nodosus* strains, containing a suitable oil as adjuvant, for *sheep*; 50 mL
Dose. *Sheep*: *by subcutaneous injection*, 1 mL

PML **Vaxall Norot**™ (Janssen, Webster)
Injection, footrot vaccine, inactivated, prepared from *B. nodosus*, containing a suitable adjuvant, for *sheep*; 50 mL
Dose. *Sheep*: *by subcutaneous injection*, 1 mL

> **Accidental self-injection with oil-based vaccines can cause severe vascular spasm and prompt medical attention is essential**

18.2.9 Leptospirosis

Leptospirosis is caused by serotypes of *Leptospira interrogans*. The organism is zoonotic and pathogenicity varies between the species. In cattle, leptospirosis is characterised by subacute febrile illness or abortion. Infection in calves may cause acute haemolytic anaemia with jaundice and haemoglobinuria, and an interstitial nephritis.

A primary vaccination course of 2 vaccinations 4 to 6 weeks apart is given after 5 months of age. If calves are vaccinated before 5 months of age, a further course should be given starting at that age. The course should be completed before the main season of transmission of leptospirosis caused by *Leptospira interrogans* serovar *hardjo*. A single annual booster injection is recommended.

Vaccinated cattle may be positive for diagnostic tests and therefore may be unacceptable for export to some countries.

Indications. Vaccination against leptospirosis
Contra-indications. Side-effects. Warnings. See notes at beginning of chapter and notes above
Dose. See preparation details, see notes above for vaccination programmes

PoM **Leptavoid**™-**H** (Coopers Pitman-Moore)
Injection, leptospirosis vaccine, inactivated, prepared from *L. interrogans* serovar *hardjo*, containing alum as adjuvant, for *cattle*; 20 mL, 50 mL
Dose. *Cattle*: *by subcutaneous injection*, 2 mL

18.2.10 Louping ill

Louping ill is caused by a *Flavivirus* transmitted by ticks of the species *Ixodes ricinus*. The disease is characterised by fever, gait abnormalities, and convulsions.

Initial vaccinations for cattle should be completed 2 weeks, and for sheep and goats 4 weeks, before exposure to infection is expected. In cattle, 2 vaccinations are given with an interval of 3 weeks to 6 months. In sheep and goats, a single dose suffices. The vaccination course should be completed before the last month of pregnancy for cows, ewes, and does being immunised for the first time. Colostral immunity transferred to lambs will give protection for 2 to 3 months. A booster dose should be given to cattle every 12 months and to sheep and goats every 2 years.

Indications. Vaccination against louping ill
Contra-indications. Side-effects. Warnings. See notes at beginning of chapter
Dose. See preparation details, see notes above for vaccination programmes

PML **Louping-Ill Vaccine** (Coopers Pitman-Moore)
Injection, inactivated, prepared from virus grown on tissue culture, containing a suitable mineral oil as adjuvant, for *cattle, sheep, goats*; 20 mL
Dose. *Cattle*: *by subcutaneous injection*, 2 mL
Sheep, goats: *by subcutaneous injection*, 1 mL

> Accidental self-injection with oil-based vaccines can cause severe vascular spasm and prompt medical attention is essential

18.2.11 Lungworm

Lungworm (husk, bovine verminous pneumonia) infection may lead to pneumonia with secondary bacterial invasion. The vaccine is a suspension of live, partially inactivated, larvae of *Dictyocaulus viviparus*. The larvae induce immunity while migrating from the gut to the lung where they are destroyed. The vaccination course, given to cattle over 8 weeks of age, consists of 2 doses given at an interval of 4 weeks. Following the second dose, cattle should be kept away from contaminated pasture for 2 weeks.
Transient bouts of coughing may occur 7 to 10 days after vaccination. Occasionally, respiratory disease may be precipitated in animals with subclinical infectious pneumonia. Use of other live vaccines and anthelmintics is restricted before and after lungworm vaccination. Vaccinated stock should not be placed with unvaccinated animals on the same pasture.
The shelf-life of the vaccine is short, such that when stored at 2°C to 6°C, the larvae may be expected to survive for 45 days.

Indications. Vaccination against lungworm

Contra-indications. Vaccination with other live vaccines 14 days before or after vaccination against lungworm; use of sustained-release anthelmintics until 14 days after second dose of lungworm vaccine or use of other endoparasiticides 7 days before until 10 days after vaccination against lungworm; use of ivermectin-containing preparations 4 weeks before and up to 10 days after second dose of lungworm vaccine; see also notes at beginning of chapter
Side-effects. Transient coughing
Dose. See preparation details, see notes above for vaccination programmes

PoM **Dictol**™ (Coopers Pitman-Moore)
Oral suspension, lungworm vaccine, living, prepared from third-stage *D. viviparus* larvae, for *calves*; 25 mL
Dose. *Calves*: 25 mL

PoM **Huskvac**™ (Intervet)
Oral suspension, lungworm vaccine, living, prepared from third-stage *D. viviparus* larvae, for *calves*; 25 mL
Dose. *Calves*: 25 mL

18.2.12 Pasteurellosis

Pasteurella haemolytica and *P. multocida* may cause either a septicaemic or pneumonic form of pasteurellosis. Antisera and vaccines are available for the prevention and treatment of pasteurellosis in cattle, sheep, goats, and pigs. Vaccines for *P. haemolytica* contain biotypes A and T. *P. multocida* vaccines contain serotypes 1 (or B), 2 (or A), 3 (or C), or 4 (or D). Vaccines are also available that contain *Actinomyces pyogenes* and staphylococcal organisms, which may be used to prevent bacterial pneumonia of multiple cause.
Antisera are given soon after birth or before periods of challenge and may be administered at intervals of 10 to 14 days during periods of risk. For treatment, administer one dose and repeat after 24 hours as necessary.
Vaccines are usually given as a course with the second dose administered approximately 4 weeks after the initial dose and at least 2 weeks before the disease is expected to appear. Revaccination is recommended before

an expected seasonal outbreak. A single booster dose every 12 months is recommended except in locations where the disease is severe when a second vaccination should be given approximately 4 weeks after the first. For sheep, vaccination programmes are completed 3 to 4 weeks before lambing.

Indications. Vaccination against pasteurellosis
Contra-indications. **Side-effects**. **Warnings**. See notes at beginning of chapter
Dose. See preparation details, see notes above for vaccination programmes

Antisera

PML **Haemosan**™ (Hoechst)
Injection, Pasteurella antiserum, prepared from P. haemolytica serotypes A1, A2, T3, T4, A6, A7, A9, T10, T15, and P. multocida Roberts types 1, 2, 3, 4, for cattle, sheep; 100 mL
Dose. Treatment. By subcutaneous or intramuscular injection.
Cattle: at least 80 mL; calves: at least 40 mL
Sheep: at least 20 mL; lambs: at least 10 mL
Prophylaxis. By subcutaneous or intramuscular injection.
Cattle: 40 mL; calves: 20 mL
Sheep: 10 mL; lambs: 5 mL

PML **Bovisan**™ DPS (Hoechst)
See section 18.2.5.3 for preparation details

Vaccines

PML **Carovax**™ (Coopers Pitman-Moore)
Injection, pasteurellosis vaccine, inactivated, prepared from P. haemolytica, P. multocida Roberts types 2, 3, 4, containing alum as adjuvant, for sheep, pigs; 100 mL, 500 mL
Contra-indications. Cattle
Dose. Sheep, pigs: by subcutaneous injection, 2 mL

PML **Ovipast**™ (Hoechst)
Injection, pasteurellosis vaccine, inactivated, prepared from P. haemolytica serotypes A, T, containing aluminium hydroxide as adjuvant, for sheep; 100 mL, 500 mL
Dose. Sheep: by subcutaneous injection, 2 mL

PML **Ryvac**™ P (Young's)
Injection, pasteurellosis vaccine, inactivated, prepared from P. haemolytica serotypes A, T, containing aluminium hydroxide as adjuvant, for sheep; 100 mL
Dose. Sheep: by subcutaneous injection, 2 mL

18.2.12.1 COMBINATION VACCINES FOR PASTEURELLOSIS AND OTHER BACTERIAL INFECTIONS

PML **Pastacidin**™ (Hoechst)
Injection, combined Actinomyces pyogenes, Pasteurella, and Staphylococcus vaccine, inactivated, prepared from A. pyogenes, P. haemolytica, P. multocida Roberts types 1, 2, 3, 4, Staph. albus, Staph. aureus, containing aluminium hydroxide as adjuvant, for cattle, sheep, pigs; 50 mL
Dose. Cattle: by subcutaneous injection, 2 mL
Sheep, pigs: by subcutaneous injection, 1 mL

See also sections 18.2.3 and 18.2.5.3

18.2.13 Rabies

See section 18.4.6

18.3 Immunological preparations for pigs

18.3.1 Anthrax
18.3.2 Atrophic rhinitis
18.3.3 Aujeszky's disease
18.3.4 Enteritis
18.3.5 Erysipelas
18.3.6 Pasteurellosis
18.3.7 Porcine parvovirus
18.3.8 Tetanus

Immunisation programmes used for pigs depend upon which diseases are liable to be encountered in the herd. Pigs are generally vaccinated against erysipelas. Vaccination against parvovirus infection is also usual in breeding herds. Immunisation against E. coli and Cl. perfringens infections is frequently practised. Subcutaneous and intramuscular injections are usually given behind the ear in adult pigs, and in the flank or axillary region in piglets.

18.3.1 Anthrax

No proprietary vaccine is available against anthrax (see section 18.2.1)

18.3.2 Atrophic rhinitis

The aetiology of atrophic rhinitis is unclear. Immunisation against the bacterial components of atrophic rhinitis syndrome is possible with inactivated vaccines prepared from cultures of *Bordetella bronchiseptica* and *Pasteurella multocida*.

Sows or gilts are given a primary course of 2 doses during the first pregnancy, starting up to 6 weeks before farrowing, and a single booster injection during each subsequent pregnancy, to provide passive protection for the piglets.

Vaccination of piglets may also be carried out at or before weaning, depending on the degree of passive protection. If the sow is unvaccinated, piglets should be vaccinated at one week and 3 to 4 weeks of age. If the sow has been previously vaccinated, piglets should be vaccinated at weaning and 6 weeks later.

Indications. Vaccination against atrophic rhinitis
Contra-indications. Side-effects. Warnings. See notes at beginning of chapter
Dose. See preparation details, see notes above for vaccination programmes

PML **Delsuvac™ Ar-Tox** (Mycofarm)
Injection, atrophic rhinitis vaccine, inactivated, prepared from *B. bronchiseptica*, *P. multocida* toxoid, containing a suitable oil as adjuvant, for *pigs*; 20 mL, 50 mL
Dose. *Pigs*: *by intramuscular injection*, 2 mL

PML **Nobi-Vac™ AR-T** (Intervet)
Injection, atrophic rhinitis vaccine, inactivated, prepared from *B. bronchiseptica*, *P. multocida* toxoid, containing a suitable oil as adjuvant, for *pigs*; 20 mL, 50 mL

Dose. *Pigs*: *by intramuscular injection*, 2 mL

> **Accidental self-injection with oil-based vaccines can cause severe vascular spasm and prompt medical attention is essential**

PoM **Suvaxyn™ Rhinitis** (Duphar)
Injection, atrophic rhinitis vaccine, inactivated, prepared from *B. bronchiseptica*, for *pigs*; 100 mL
Dose. *Pigs*: *by subcutaneous or intramuscular (preferred) injection*, 1 mL

18.3.3 Aujeszky's disease

Aujeszky's disease is caused by a herpesvirus and is characterised by respiratory, reproductive, and nervous signs. In Britain, a slaughter and eradication policy is in operation for the control of Aujeszky's disease. A live vaccine is available in Northern Ireland for administration to healthy piglets and consists of a course of 2 doses. The first dose is given at 5 to 6 weeks of age and the second vaccination 3 weeks later.

Indications. Vaccination against Aujeszky's disease
Contra-indications. Side-effects. Warnings. Not for use in Britain (see above). See also notes at beginning of chapter
Dose. See preparation details, see notes above for vaccination programmes

PoM **Suvaxyn™ Aujeszky** (Duphar)
Injection, powder for reconstitution, Aujeszky's disease vaccine, living, prepared from virus strain Bartha K61, for *pigs*; 50-dose vial
Dose. *Pigs*: *by intramuscular injection*, 1 dose

18.3.4 Enteritis

18.3.4.1 *Escherichia coli* infections
18.3.4.2 Combination immunological preparations for enteritis in pigs

Enteritis in neonatal and young pigs may be caused by bacteria including *E. coli*, *Pasteurella*, and *Salmonella* species, *Cl. perfringens* enterotoxin, viruses, parasites, and influenced by inadequate housing or management procedures.

18.3.4.1 *ESCHERICHIA COLI* INFECTIONS

Vaccines are available for the protection of piglets against *E. coli* infections, which contain selected serotypes of strains of the organism or important antigens. Combination preparations are also available.

Sows and gilts are vaccinated to provide passive immunity for piglets. Females should not be vaccinated less than 2 to 3 weeks prior to farrowing. Oral vaccines should not be used in the last 8 weeks of gestation.

Indications. Vaccination against *E. coli* infection

Contra-indications. Side-effects. Warnings. See notes at beginning of chapter and notes above

Dose. See preparation details

Parenteral vaccines

PML **Delsuvac™ Coli-5** (Mycofarm)
Injection, *E. coli* vaccine, inactivated, prepared from *E. coli* LT toxoid and antigens K88ab, K88ac, K99, 987P, containing a suitable oil as adjuvant, for *pigs*; 50 mL
Dose. *Pigs: by intramuscular injection*, 2 mL 5-6 weeks before farrowing, repeat not less than 2 weeks before farrowing. Revaccinate every 6 months

PML **Nobi-Vac™ Porcol-5** (Intervet)
Injection, *E. coli* vaccine, inactivated, prepared from *E. coli* LT toxoid and antigens K88ab, K88ac, K99, 987P, containing a suitable oil as adjuvant, for *pigs*; 20 mL, 50 mL
Dose. *Pigs: by intramuscular injection*, 2 mL

PML **Porcovac™ AT** (Hoechst)
Injection, *E. coli* vaccine, inactivated, prepared from *E. coli* serotypes of porcine origin, containing aluminium hydroxide as adjuvant, for *pigs*; 50 mL, 100 mL
Dose. *Pigs: by subcutaneous or intramuscular injection*, 5 mL at service *or* up to 6 weeks before farrowing, repeat not less than 3 weeks before farrowing; *piglets: by subcutaneous or intramuscular injection*, 2 mL, repeat after 10-14 days

PML **Sow Intagen™ O/I** (Unifeeds)
Injection, *E. coli* vaccine, inactivated, prepared from *E. coli* and associated polysaccharide antigens, for *pigs*; 2 mL
Dose. *Pigs: by intramuscular injection*, 2 mL as a single dose 15-24 days before farrowing

PML **Suvaxyn™ E.Coli P4** (Duphar)
Injection, *E. coli* vaccine, inactivated, prepared from *E. coli* antigens containing high concentrations of antigens F41, K88, K99, 987P, containing a suitable adjuvant, for *pigs*; 20 mL
Dose. *Pigs: by intramuscular injection*, 2 mL at 4 weeks and 2 weeks before farrowing, thereafter revaccinate 2 weeks before each farrowing

> **Accidental self-injection with oil-based vaccines can cause severe vascular spasm and prompt medical attention is essential**

Oral vaccines

PML **Pig Intagen™** (Unifeeds)
Premix, *E. coli* vaccine, inactivated, prepared from residues and extracts of *E. coli* serotypes, for *pigs*; 15 kg
Dose. *Pigs*: (up to 4 weeks of age) 10 kg/tonne feed; (4-6 weeks of age) 5 kg/tonne feed; (6-12 weeks of age) 2.5 kg/tonne feed; (adults) 1.5 kg/tonne feed

18.3.4.2 COMBINATION IMMUNOLOGICAL PREPARATIONS FOR ENTERITIS IN PIGS

Antisera-vaccine combinations

PML **Serovax™** (Hoechst)
Injection, combined *Diplococcus*, *E. coli*, *Pasteurella*, *Salmonella*, and *Streptococcus* antiserum/vaccine, inactivated, prepared from *D. pneumoniae* types 8, 18, 19, 22, 33, *E. coli* serotypes of porcine origin, *S. cholerae-suis* strains, *P. multocida* Roberts types 2, 4, *Streptococcus* Lancefield's group C, in combination with *E. coli* antiserum and containing cobalt, copper, iodine, iron, zinc, for *pigs*; 100 mL

Dose. Treatment. *Piglets*: *by subcutaneous or intramuscular injection*, 5 mL, repeat dose after 1-2 days if required Prophylaxis. *Pigs*: *by subcutaneous injection*, 5-15 mL, repeat dose after 10-14 days or at least 2 weeks before farrowing; *piglets*: *by subcutaneous or intramuscular injection*, 3 mL, repeat · dose after 10-14 days

Vaccines

PML **Gletvax™ 5** (Coopers Pitman-Moore)
Injection, combined *E. coli*, enterotoxaemia vaccine, inactivated, prepared from *E. coli* antigens K88ab, K88ac, K99, 987P, *Cl. perfringens* type C toxoid, containing aluminium hydroxide as adjuvant, for *pigs*; 50 mL
Withdrawal Periods. *Pigs*: slaughter withdrawal period nil
Dose. *Pigs*: *by subcutaneous or intramuscular injection*, 5 mL at service *or* up to 6 weeks before farrowing, repeat dose 2 weeks before farrowing. Thereafter revaccinate 2 weeks before farrowing

PML **Lambisan™** (Hoechst)
See section 18.2.3 for preparation details

PML **Lambivac™** (Hoechst)
See section 18.2.3 for preparation details

18.3.5 Erysipelas

In pigs, erysipelas is characterised by either an acute septicaemia or a chronic arthritis. The disease is caused by *Erysipelothrix rhusiopathiae* (*Ery. insidiosa*). Vaccination consists of a course of 2 doses with an interval of 3 to 4 weeks. Revaccination is usually necessary every 6 to 12 months. Piglets may be vaccinated at 4 to 7 days of age and the dose repeated 2 to 3 weeks later. Sows should not be vaccinated in the last 4 weeks of gestation.

Indications. Vaccination against erysipelas
Contra-indications. Side-effects. Warnings. See notes at beginning of chapter and notes above
Dose. See preparation details, see notes above for vaccination programmes

PML **Erysorb™ Plus** (Hoechst)
Injection, erysipelas vaccine, inactivated, prepared from *Ery. rhusiopathiae* serotypes 1, 2, containing aluminium hydroxide as adjuvant, for *pigs*; 50 mL, 100 mL
Dose. *Pigs*: *by subcutaneous injection*, 2 mL

PML **Ferrovac™ Ery** (Crown)
Injection, erysipelas vaccine, inactivated, prepared from *Ery. rhusiopathiae* strains and antigens, containing aluminium hydroxide as adjuvant, for *pigs*; 50 mL
Contra-indications. Piglets under 12 weeks of age
Dose. *Pigs*: *by subcutaneous injection*, 2 mL

PML **Suvaxyn™ Erysipelas** (Duphar)
Injection, erysipelas vaccine, inactivated, prepared from *Ery. rhusiopathiae* strains, containing a suitable adjuvant, for *pigs, turkeys* (see section 18.6.7); 100 mL
Dose. *Pigs*: *by subcutaneous injection*, 2 mL

PML **Swine Erysipelas** (Coopers Pitman-Moore)
Injection, inactivated, prepared from *Ery. rhusiopathiae* cultures, containing aluminium hydroxide as adjuvant, for *pigs*; 50 mL, 100 mL
Contra-indications. Pregnant animals
Dose. *Pigs*: *by subcutaneous injection*, 2 mL

18.3.6 Pasteurellosis

PML **Carovax™** (Coopers Pitman-Moore)
See section 18.2.12 for preparation details

PML **Pastacidin™** (Hoechst)
See section 18.2.12.1 for preparation details

18.3.7 Porcine parvovirus

Porcine parvovirus infection causes abortion and infertility. Vaccines are used in breeding pigs. For boars, 2 doses are given, the first at 6 to 7 months of age and the second 6 months later with booster doses every 1 to 2 years depending on the vaccine. Sows are given a single dose 2 weeks before service, while gilts of at least 6 months of age are given a single dose 2 to 8 weeks before the first service. Subsequent booster doses are given at least 2 weeks before service every 1 to 2 years. These measures are usually necessary to maintain immunity in the breeding herd.

Indications. Vaccination against porcine parvovirus infection
Contra-indications. **Side-effects**. **Warnings**. See notes at beginning of chapter
Dose. See preparation details, see notes above for vaccination programmes

PoM **Delsuvac™ Parvo** (Mycofarm)
Injection, porcine parvovirus vaccine, inactivated, prepared from virus, containing a suitable oil as adjuvant, for *pigs*; 20 mL, 50 mL
Dose. *Pigs*: *by intramuscular injection*, 2 mL

PoM **Pig Parvovirus Vaccine** (Coopers Pitman-Moore)
Injection, inactivated, prepared from virus grown on porcine tissue culture, containing a suitable adjuvant, for *pigs*; 20 mL
Dose. *Pigs*: *by intramuscular injection*, 2 mL

PoM **Porculin™ Parvo** (Coopers Pitman-Moore)
Injection, porcine parvovirus vaccine, inactivated, prepared from virus grown on porcine tissue culture, containing a suitable oil as adjuvant, for *pigs*; 20 mL
Dose. *Pigs*: *by intramuscular injection*, 2 mL

PoM **Suvaxyn™ Parvo** (Duphar)
Injection, porcine parvovirus vaccine, inactivated, prepared from virus grown on porcine tissue culture, containing a suitable adjuvant, for *pigs*; 20 mL
Dose. *Pigs*: *by intramuscular injection*, 2 mL

PoM **Suvaxyn™ Parvo 2** (Duphar)
Injection, porcine parvovirus vaccine, inactivated, prepared from virus grown on porcine tissue culture, containing a suitable oil as adjuvant, for *pigs*; 20 mL

Dose. *Pigs*: *by intramuscular injection*, 2 mL

> Accidental self-injection with oil-based vaccines can cause severe vascular spasm and prompt medical attention is essential

18.3.8 Tetanus

See section 18.1.5

18.4 Immunological preparations for dogs

18.4.1 Canine distemper
18.4.2 Canine parvovirus
18.4.3 Infectious canine hepatitis
18.4.4 Infectious tracheobronchitis
18.4.5 Leptospirosis
18.4.6 Rabies
18.4.7 Tetanus
18.4.8 Combination vaccines for dogs
18.4.9 Combination immunoglobulins for dogs

Many factors such as the animal's age, health, and maturity, the presence of maternally-derived antibodies, the antigenic mass of the vaccine used, and the presence of infection in the environment may affect fixed canine vaccination programmes. It is now considered better to devise schedules appropriate to individual circumstances. This should be taken into account when interpreting the guidelines in the text below or the manufacturer's recommendations.

The National Greyhound Racing Club require that racing greyhounds are vaccinated against distemper, leptospirosis, and parvovirus (see Prescribing for animals used in competitions).

18.4.1 Canine distemper

Canine distemper virus (CDV) causes a highly infectious disease of dogs and other carnivores, which is characterised by respiratory, alimentary, and occasionally, nervous signs. Respiratory signs alone may occur and distemper virus can be involved in the kennel cough syndrome.

The presence of maternally-derived antibody in puppies will interfere with successful immunisation. Generally, maternally-derived antibody will have declined to non-interfering levels by 12 weeks of age, although some individuals will have lost this immunity by 8 to 9 weeks of age. Thus, where there is low risk of exposure, with puppies in isolation, one vaccination at 12 weeks of age should provide sufficient protection. An additional later vaccination may be necessary when puppies are born to bitches that experienced an active infection or had been vaccinated just before pregnancy. Where young puppies are at risk, earlier vaccination schedules should be used. Accordingly, an initial dose may be given at 6 to 8 weeks of age, and repeated at 12 weeks. Some authorities advise routine vaccination at 9 and 12 weeks in all cases in order to reduce the immunity gap.

Where high and unavoidable levels of challenge virus are likely, such as in a pet shop or stray dogs' home, active immunity should be induced in puppies as early as possible. Measles vaccine and some canine distemper vaccines can overcome low to moderate levels of maternally-derived antibody. Measles vaccine may be used from 5 to 6 weeks of age, or canine distemper vaccine from 6 weeks, but puppies should still be vaccinated at 12 weeks of age with canine distemper vaccine.

An initial booster vaccination should be given at one year of age and theoretically distemper titres should last for several years. Recommendations for revaccination for complete protection vary from 1 to 2 years.

Non-domestic carnivore species that are susceptible to canine distemper include foxes, mink, ferrets, and exotic zoo species. In general, clinical signs resemble those of distemper in domestic dogs. Information from manufacturers should be sought before using vaccines in these species. Quarantine measures, good hygiene, and good management are also important in a control programme.

Indications. Vaccination against canine distemper virus (CDV) infection
Contra-indications. Vaccination of puppies under 6 weeks of age

Side-effects. Warnings. See notes at beginning of chapter
Dose. See preparation details, see notes above for vaccination programmes

PoM **Kavak**™ **D** (Duphar)
Injection, powder for reconstitution, CDV vaccine, living, prepared from virus grown on tissue culture, for *dogs*; 1-dose vial
Note. May be reconstituted with Kavak™ i-HLP, i-HL, L, i-LP, or Parvo
Dose. *Dogs*: *by subcutaneous or intramuscular injection*, 1 dose

PoM **Nobi-Vac**™ **D** (Intervet)
Injection, powder for reconstitution, CDV vaccine, living, prepared from virus grown on cell-line tissue culture, for *dogs*; 1-dose vial
Note. May be reconstituted with Nobi-Vac™ L
Dose. *Dogs*: *by subcutaneous injection*, 1 dose

PoM **Vaxitas**™ **D** (Coopers Pitman-Moore)
Injection, powder for reconstitution, CDV vaccine, living, prepared from virus grown on cell-line tissue culture, for *dogs*; 1-dose vial
Note. May be reconstituted with Vaxitas™ L, KHL, K Parvo L, or K Parvo
Dose. *Dogs*: *by subcutaneous injection*, 1 dose

See also section 18.4.8

18.4.1.1 MEASLES

Measles virus is related to canine distemper virus. Measles vaccine may be used to protect puppies from 5 to 6 weeks of age against early exposure to canine distemper (see above).

Indications. Primary vaccination against canine distemper
Contra-indications. Vaccination of puppies under 5 weeks of age
Side-effects. Warnings. See notes at beginning of chapter
Dose. *Dogs*: (5-12 weeks of age) *by intramuscular injection*, 1 dose

PoM **Kavak**™ **M** (Duphar)
Injection, powder for reconstitution, CDV vaccine, living, prepared from measles virus grown on tissue culture, for *dogs*; 1-dose vial

Note. May be reconstituted with Kavak™ L, Parvo, i-LP, or i-HLP

See also section 18.4.8

18.4.2 Canine parvovirus

Canine parvovirus (CPV) infection is an enteric disease that first appeared in the canine population in 1978. The main target sites for multiplication of virus are the lymphatic tissues and intestinal epithelium, and, in neonatal puppies, the myocardium. Myocarditis is rare because most bitches are now immune, puppies being protected by maternally-derived antibody. In older dogs, disease signs may vary from subclinical infection to severe haemorrhagic enteritis.

CPV is closely related to feline pan-leucopenia virus (FPV) and, initially, FPV vaccines were used to protect dogs. However, these have now been superseded by homologous CPV vaccines, which generally induce a longer-lasting and more consistent response.

Most problems with CPV vaccination have arisen because of the high level of challenge virus in the environment, and because low levels of maternally-derived antibody may interfere with vaccination but not protect against infection. Puppies may become susceptible before they can respond to vaccination. In addition, the duration of maternally-derived anti-bodies to CPV may be quite variable and sometimes long-lasting, anything from 4 to 20 weeks, depending on the level of immunity in the dam.

The duration of maternally-derived antibody in puppies may be predicted using a normograph based on the bitch's titre and a known antibody half-life of approximately 9 days. However, where practicable, each puppy's antibody level should be assessed individually to determine the optimum age for vac-cination since there may be great variability in colostral intake between puppies within a litter.

Alternatively, puppies may be vac-cinated repeatedly at 2 to 4 week intervals between 6 and 12 or 18 weeks of age, the precise timing depending on when the puppy is presented, the exposure risk, and the vaccine used. Although immunity following modified live vaccine administration is probably of longer duration, annual booster vaccination is recommended.

Some live vaccines may induce a viraemia and, therefore, inactivated vaccines may be used for pregnant bitches to boost the puppies' antibody levels if required.

CPV is extremely resistant in the environment. Adequate disinfection procedures, in addition to vaccination, are essential if a clinical case occurs.

Indications. Vaccination against canine parvovirus (CPV) infection
Contra-indications. Pregnant bitches should not be vaccinated with some live vaccines
Side-effects. Warnings. See notes at beginning of chapter
Dose. See preparation details, see notes above for vaccination programmes

Live vaccines

PoM **Boostervac™ CPv** (C-Vet)
Injection, CPV vaccine, living, prepared from virus of canine origin, for *dogs*; 1 mL
Dose. *Dogs: by subcutaneous or intra-muscular injection*, 1 mL

PoM **Caniffa™ P** (RMB)
Injection, powder for reconstitution, CPV vaccine, living, prepared from virus Cornell strain CPV C780916, for *dogs*; 1-dose vial
Note. May be reconstituted with Can-iffa™ L
Dose. *Dogs: by subcutaneous or intra-muscular injection*, 1 dose

PoM **Delcavac™ P** (Mycofarm)
Injection, powder for reconstitution, CPV vaccine, living, prepared from virus grown on cell-line tissue culture, for *dogs*; 1-dose vial
Note. May be reconstituted with Del-cavac™ L
Dose. *Dogs: by subcutaneous injection*, 1 dose

PoM **Nobi-Vac™ Parvo-C** (Intervet)
Injection, powder for reconstitution, CPV vaccine, living, prepared from virus grown on cell-line tissue culture, for *dogs*; 1-dose vial

Note. May be reconstituted with Nobi-Vac™ L

Dose. *Dogs*: *by subcutaneous injection*, 1 dose

PoM **Vanguard™ CPV** (SmithKline Beecham)
Injection, CPV vaccine, living, prepared from virus grown on NL-DK-1 established canine cell line, for *dogs*; 1 mL
Dose. *Dogs*: *by subcutaneous injection*, 1 mL

PoM **Vaxitas™ Parvo** (Coopers Pitman-Moore)
Injection, powder for reconstitution, CPV vaccine, living, prepared from virus grown on cell-line tissue culture, for *dogs*; 1-dose vial
Note. May be reconstituted with Vaxitas™ L
Dose. *Dogs*: *by subcutaneous injection*, 1 dose

PoM **Vaxitas™ Parvo** (Liquid) (Coopers Pitman-Moore)
Injection, CPV vaccine, living, prepared from virus grown on cell-line tissue culture, for *dogs*; 1-dose syringe
Dose. *Dogs*: *by subcutaneous injection*, 1 dose

Inactivated vaccines

PoM **Canilep™-Parvo** (Coopers Pitman-Moore)
Injection, CPV vaccine, inactivated, prepared from virus grown on a cell line, containing a suitable adjuvant, for *dogs*; 1-dose vial
Dose. *Dogs*: *by subcutaneous injection*, 1 dose

PoM **Kavak™ Parvo** (Duphar)
Injection, CPV vaccine, inactivated, prepared from virus grown on a cell line, containing a suitable adjuvant, for *dogs*; 1-dose vial
Dose. *Dogs*: *by subcutaneous or intramuscular injection*, 1 dose

PoM **Vaxitas™ K Parvo** (Coopers Pitman-Moore)
Injection, CPV vaccine, inactivated, prepared from virus grown on cell-line tissue culture, containing aluminium hydroxide as adjuvant, for *dogs*; 1-dose syringe

Dose. *Dogs*: *by subcutaneous injection*, 1 dose

See also section 18.4.8

18.4.3 Infectious canine hepatitis

Infectious canine hepatitis (ICH) is caused by canine adenovirus type 1 (CAV 1). The virus has a predilection for hepatic cells, vascular endothelium, and lymphoid tissue. Disease signs may vary from inapparent to a severe form characterised by depression, anorexia, thirst, abdominal pain, and vomiting. In some cases, sudden death may occur, especially in young puppies, and the virus may be involved in the 'fading puppy' syndrome.

Transient corneal opacity or 'blue eye' may occur in some dogs 1 to 3 weeks after acute ICH infection. This is due to virus-antibody complexes and generally heals spontaneously, although complications and, occasionally, blindness may result in some cases. In many recovered animals, the virus persists in the kidney and may be shed in the urine for at least 6 months.

In the UK, CAV 1 is also regarded as a possible cause of kennel cough. The closely related CAV 2, which does not cause ICH, is also involved in the aetiology of kennel cough.

Originally, modified live CAV 1 vaccines were used to control ICH, but in a small percentage of dogs the vaccines induced ocular lesions similar to those seen in the natural disease. Since dogs vaccinated with CAV 2 become immune to both CAV 1 and CAV 2 infection, and CAV 2 vaccines have the advantages that they do not induce 'blue eye', possible viral persistence with lesions in the kidney, and viral excretion in the urine, CAV 2 has replaced CAV 1 in most live canine adenovirus vaccines.

Vaccination may be carried out from 6 to 8 weeks of age, but a second dose should always be given at 12 weeks of age. In general, maternally-derived antibody appears less of a problem in ICH compared to the other major canine viral infections. Since the disease has been well controlled by vaccination, there is little challenge virus in the environment, and the virus-host immunity balance is generally stable. Immunity following live virus vaccination probably lasts several years, but booster vaccinations every 1 to 2 years are recommended. Inactivated vaccines are also available, which may be given to pregnant animals. The immunity induced is not so long-lasting and annual boosters are required.

Indications. Vaccination against infectious canine hepatitis

Contra-indications. **Side-effects**. **Warnings**. See notes at beginning of chapter and above

Dose. See preparation details, see notes above for vaccination programmes

See section 18.4.8 for preparation details

18.4.4 Infectious tracheobronchitis

Canine infectious tracheobronchitis, commonly called the 'kennel cough' syndrome, is mainly caused by *Bordetella bronchiseptica*, although a number of viruses are also implicated. The disease tends to occur where dogs are congregated together. The bacteria appear to attach specifically to cilia of the trachea and bronchi, and persist in the dog several months after infection. However, coughing occurs predominantly only in the first week or two after infection, when bacterial growth is greatest.

Viruses such as CDV, canine adenovirus types 1 and 2, canine parainfluenza (PI) virus, and canine herpesvirus may also be involved in the aetiology of the disease. Combination vaccines are available against several of these viruses (see section 18.4.8).

Originally, systemic vaccination against *B. bronchiseptica* was found not to be consistently satisfactory, and adverse reactions at the injection site were common. Intranasal vaccines are reasonably effective, with few side-effects, although individuals may experience transient coughing a few days after vaccination. The vaccine appears to induce good local immunity and is not interfered with by maternally-derived antibody. Therefore puppies over 2 weeks of age may be vaccinated.

Immunity takes 5 days or more to develop and thus dogs should be isolated during this period. Revaccination every 6 to 10 months is recommended, depending on potential exposure. Dogs under treatment with antibiotics should not be vaccinated.

Indications. Vaccination against infectious tracheobronchitis

Contra-indications. **Side-effects**. **Warnings**. See notes at beginning of chapter, transient coughing after vaccination

Dose. *Dogs*: (2 weeks of age or more) *by intranasal instillation*, one dose into 1 nostril or half dose into each nostril, see notes above for vaccination programmes

PoM **Intrac**™ (Schering-Plough)
Injection, powder for reconstitution, infectious tracheobronchitis vaccine, living, prepared from *B. bronchiseptica* strain S 55, for *dogs*; 1-dose vial

18.4.5 Leptospirosis

Leptospirosis in the dog is predominantly caused by the 2 serotypes of *Leptospira interrogans*, *L. interrogans* serovar *canicola* (primary host, the dog) or *L. interrogans* serovar *icterohaemorrhagiae* (primary host, the rat). The disease is characterised by acute haemorrhage, hepatitis and jaundice, or acute interstitial nephritis. Often infection is subclinical. Leptospirosis is a zoonotic infection.

Maternally-derived immunity to *Leptospira interrogans* is not a problem in puppies with respect to vaccination, as it is absent by 8 weeks of age. The vaccine is an inactivated vaccine and 2 doses are required 2 to 6 weeks apart for primary vaccination, starting at about 8 weeks of age. Annual boosters are required.

Although the organism may be spread by direct contact with an infected animal, the main infection source is from urine or urine-contaminated water or soil. Recovered animals may shed leptospirae into the urine for some time. Thus, while vaccination is generally effective in controlling the disease, if a clinical case occurs, antibiotic therapy should be given to eliminate the organism, supported by disinfection of contaminated premises.

Indications. Vaccination against leptospirosis

Contra-indications. Side-effects. Warnings. See notes at beginning of chapter

Dose. See preparation details, see notes above for vaccination programmes

PoM **Boostervac™ L** (C-Vet)
Injection, leptospirosis vaccine, inactivated, prepared from antigens of *L. interrogans* serotypes, for *dogs*; 1 mL
Dose. *Dogs*: *by subcutaneous or intramuscular injection*, 1 mL

PoM **Caniffa™ L** (RMB)
Injection, leptospirosis vaccine, inactivated, prepared from *L. interrogans* serotypes, for *dogs*; 1-dose vial
Dose. *Dogs*: *by subcutaneous or intramuscular injection*, 1 dose

PoM **Delcavac™ L** (Mycofarm)
Injection, leptospirosis vaccine, inactivated, prepared from *L. interrogans* serotypes, for *dogs*; 1 mL

Dose. *Dogs*: *by subcutaneous injection*, 1 mL

PoM **Kavak™ L** (Duphar)
Injection, leptospirosis vaccine, inactivated, prepared from *L. interrogans* serotypes, for *dogs*; 1-dose vial
Dose. *Dogs*: *by subcutaneous or intramuscular injection*, 1 dose

PoM **Nobi-Vac™ L** (Intervet)
Injection, leptospirosis vaccine, inactivated, prepared from *L. interrogans* serotypes, for *dogs*; 1 mL
Dose. *Dogs*: *by subcutaneous injection*, 1 mL

PoM **Vanguard™ Lepto ci** (SmithKline Beecham)
Injection, leptospirosis vaccine, inactivated, prepared from *L. interrogans* serotypes, for *dogs*; 1 mL
Dose. *Dogs*: *by subcutaneous or intramuscular injection*, 1 mL

PoM **Vaxitas™ L (sf)** (Coopers Pitman-Moore)
Injection, leptospirosis vaccine, inacti-

Table 18.2 Combination vaccines for dogs (see section 18.4.8)

	Canine distemper virus	Canine parvovirus	Infectious canine hepatitis	Leptospirosis	Parainfluenza	Measles
Boostervac™ CPvL (C-Vet)		+		+		
Boostervac™ DHPi (C-Vet)	+		+		+	
Caniffa™ DH (RMB)	+		+			
Caniffa™ DHP (RMB)	+	+	+			
Canilep™-DHL (Coopers Pitman-Moore)	+		+	+		
Canilep™-DHLP (Coopers Pitman-Moore)	+	+	+	+		
Canilep™-HL (Coopers Pitman-Moore)			+	+		
Canilep™-HLP (Coopers Pitman-Moore)		+	+	+		

Table 18.2 Combination vaccines for dogs (*continued*)

	Canine distemper virus	Canine parvovirus	Infectious canine hepatitis	Leptospirosis	Parainfluenza	Measles
Delcavac™ DA2 (Mycofarm)	+		+			
Delcavac™ DP (Mycofarm)	+	+				
Delcavac™ DA2P (Mycofarm)	+	+	+			
Delcavac™ DA2PPi (Mycofarm)	+	+	+		+	
Kavak™ DA$_2$ (Duphar)	+		+			
Kavak™ i-HL (Duphar)			+	+		
Kavak™ i-HLP (Duphar)		+	+	+		
Kavak™ i-LP (Duphar)		+		+		
Nobi-Vac™ DH 2 (Intervet)	+		+			
Nobi-Vac™ DHP (Intervet)	+	+	+			
Nobi-Vac™ DHPPi (Intervet)	+	+	+		+	
Nobi-Vac™ Puppy DP (Intervet)	+	+				
Vanguard™ 7 (SmithKline Beecham)	+	+	+	+	+	
Vanguard CPV-L (SmithKline Beecham)		+		+		
Vaxitas™ DA$_2$ (Coopers Pitman-Moore)	+		+			
Vaxitas™ DA2 Parvo (Coopers Pitman-Moore)	+	+	+			
Vaxitas™ K Parvo L (Coopers Pitman-Moore)		+		+		

vated, prepared from *L. interrogans*
serotypes, for *dogs*; 1-dose syringe
Dose. *Dogs*: *by subcutaneous injection*,
1 dose

See also section 18.4.8

18.4.6 Rabies

Rabies is a neurotropic disease capable
of affecting virtually all mammals. It
exists world-wide, except in places such
as the UK and Australasia where it has
been excluded by rigorous quarantine.
In countries where the disease is
enzootic, a number of species including
dogs, jackals, racoons, and bats are
possible reservoir hosts. In Europe, the
red fox is the most important species
involved, and may serve as a source of
infection for other animals, including
dogs and cats, and thence to man.

Animals entering quarantine are
required to be vaccinated with an
approved vaccine. Animals may also be
vaccinated if they are going abroad.

**Supplies of rabies vaccine in the UK
are only available through veterinary
surgeons against authorisations by
DVO's of MAFF or DA (N. Ireland).
The use of the vaccine in dogs and cats
is restricted to quarantine kennels and
animals about to be exported.**

18.4.7 Tetanus

See section 18.1.5

18.4.8 Combination vaccines for dogs

An alphabetical list of combination
vaccines for dogs and the infections to
which their confer immunity is given in
Table 18.2.

PoM **Boostervac™ CPvL** (C-Vet)
Injection, combined living CPV and
inactivated leptospirosis vaccine, prepared from CPV grown on an established
cell line, *L. interrogans* serotypes, for
dogs; 1 mL
Dose. *Dogs*: *by subcutaneous or intramuscular injection*, 1 mL, see manufacturer   details   for   vaccination
programmes

PoM **Boostervac™ DHPi** (C-Vet)
Injection, powder for reconstitution,
combined CDV, ICH, and PI vaccine,
living, prepared from CDV, ICH virus,
PI virus grown on an established cell
line, for *dogs*; 1-dose vial
Note. May be reconstituted with
Boostervac™ CPvL, CPv, or L
Dose. *Dogs*: *by subcutaneous or intramuscular injection*, 1 dose, see manufacturer   details   for   vaccination
programmes

PoM **Caniffa™ DH** (RMB)
Injection, powder for reconstitution,
combined CDV and ICH vaccine, living,
prepared from egg-adapted CDV strain
passaged through a vero cell culture
system, non-oncogenic clone of CAV_2
Manhattan strain Toronto A26 adapted
to a canine renal cell-tissue culture
system, for *dogs*; 1-dose vial
Note. May be reconstituted with Can-
iffa™ L
Dose. *Dogs*: *by subcutaneous injection*,
1 dose, see manufacturer details for
vaccination programmes

PoM **Caniffa™ DHP** (RMB)
Injection, powder for reconstitution,
combined CDV, CPV, and ICH vaccine,
living, prepared from egg-adapted CDV
strain passaged through a vero cell
culture system, CPV Cornell strain CPV
C780916, non-oncogenic clone of CAV_2
Manhattan strain Toronto A26 adapted
to a canine renal tissue culture system,
for *dogs*; 1-dose vial
Note. May be reconstituted with Can-
iffa™ L
Dose. *Dogs*: *by subcutaneous injection*,
1 dose, see manufacturer details for
vaccination programmes

PoM **Canilep™-DHL** (Coopers Pitman-
Moore)
Injection, 2 fractions for reconstitution,
combined living CDV, and inactivated
ICH and leptospirosis vaccine, prepared
from CDV grown on cell culture,
antigens of ICH virus grown on cell
culture, antigens of *L. interrogans*
serotypes for *dogs*; two 1-dose vials
Dose. *Dogs*: *by subcutaneous injection*,
1 combined dose, see manufacturer
details for vaccination programmes

PoM **Canilep™-DHLP** (Coopers Pitman-Moore)
Injection, 2 fractions for reconstitution, combined living CDV, and inactivated CPV, ICH, and leptospirosis vaccine, prepared from CDV grown on cell culture, antigens of CPV grown on a cell line, antigens of ICH virus grown on cell culture, antigens of *L. interrogans* serotypes, for *dogs*; two 1-dose vials
Dose. *Dogs*: *by subcutaneous injection*, 1 combined dose, see manufacturer details for vaccination programmes

PoM **Canilep™-HL** (Coopers Pitman-Moore)
Injection, combined ICH and leptospirosis vaccine, inactivated, prepared from antigens of ICH virus grown on cell culture, antigens of *L. interrogans* serotypes, for *dogs*; 1-dose vial
Dose. *Dogs*: *by subcutaneous injection*, 1 dose, see manufacturer details for vaccination programmes

PoM **Canilep™-HLP** (Coopers Pitman-Moore)
Injection, combined CPV, ICH, and leptospirosis vaccine, inactivated, prepared from antigens of CPV grown on a cell line, antigens of ICH virus grown on cell culture, antigens of *L. interrogans* serotypes, for *dogs*; 1-dose vial
Dose. *Dogs*: *by subcutaneous injection*, 1 dose, see manufacturer details for vaccination programmes

PoM **Delcavac™ DA2** (Mycofarm)
Injection, powder for reconstitution, combined CDV and ICH vaccine, living, prepared from CDV strain Onderstepoort grown on cell-line tissue culture, CAV_2 strain grown on cell-line tissue culture, for *dogs*; 1-dose vial
Note. May be reconstituted with Delcavac™ L
Dose. *Dogs*: *by subcutaneous injection*, 1 dose, see manufacturer details for vaccination programmes

PoM **Delcavac™ DA2P** (Mycofarm)
Injection, powder for reconstitution, combined CDV, CPV, and ICH vaccine, living, prepared from CDV strain Onderstepoort, CPV, CAV_2, all grown on cell-line tissue culture, for *dogs*; 1-dose vial

Note. May be reconstituted with Delcavac™ L
Dose. *Dogs*: *by subcutaneous injection*, 1 dose, see manufacturer details for vaccination programmes

PoM **Delcavac™ DA2PPi** (Mycofarm)
Injection, powder for reconstitution, combined CDV, CPV, ICH, and PI vaccine, living, prepared from CDV strain Onderstepoort, CPV, CAV_2, and PI virus, all grown on cell-line tissue culture, for *dogs*; 1-dose vial
Note. May be reconstituted with Delcavac™ L
Dose. *Dogs*: *by subcutaneous injection*, 1 dose, see manufacturer details for vaccination programmes

PoM **Delcavac™ DP** (Mycofarm)
Injection, powder for reconstitution, combined CDV and CPV vaccine, living, prepared from CDV strain Onderstepoort grown on cell-line tissue culture, CPV grown on cell-line tissue culture, for *dogs*; 1-dose vial
Dose. *Dogs*: *by subcutaneous injection*, 1 dose, see manufacturer details for vaccination programmes

PoM **Kavak™ DA₂** (Duphar)
Injection, powder for reconstitution, combined CDV and ICH vaccine, living, prepared from CDV, CAV_2, for *dogs*; 1-dose vial
Note. May be reconstituted with Kavak™ i-LP, L, or Parvo
Dose. *Dogs*: *by subcutaneous or intramuscular injection*, 1 dose, see manufacturer details for vaccination programmes

PoM **Kavak™ i-HL** (Duphar)
Injection, combined ICH and leptospirosis vaccine, inactivated, prepared from ICH virus, *L. interrogans* serotypes, for *dogs*; 1-dose vial
Dose. *Dogs*: *by subcutaneous or intramuscular injection*, 1 dose, see manufacturer details for vaccination programmes

PoM **Kavak™ i-HLP** (Duphar)
Injection, combined CPV, ICH, and leptospirosis vaccine, inactivated, prepared from CPV grown on a continuous cell line, ICH virus grown on a continuous cell line, *L. interrogans*

serotypes grown in an artificial medium, containing a suitable adjuvant, for *dogs*; 1-dose vial
Dose. *Dogs*: *by subcutaneous or intramuscular injection*, 1 dose, see manufacturer details for vaccination programmes

PoM **Kavak™ i-LP** (Duphar)
Injection, combined CPV and leptospirosis vaccine, inactivated, prepared from CPV grown on a continuous cell line, *L. interrogans* serotypes grown on an artificial medium, containing a suitable adjuvant, for *dogs*; 1-dose vial
Dose. *Dogs*: *by subcutaneous or intramuscular injection*, 1 dose, see manufacturer details for vaccination programmes

PoM **Nobi-Vac™ DH2** (Intervet)
Injection, powder for reconstitution, combined CDV and ICH vaccine, living, prepared from CDV strain grown on cell-line tissue culture, CAV_2 strain grown on cell-line tissue culture, for *dogs*; 1-dose vial
Note. May be reconstituted with Nobi-Vac™ L
Dose. *Dogs*: *by subcutaneous injection*, 1 dose, see manufacturer details for vaccination programmes

PoM **Nobi-Vac™ DHP** (Intervet)
Injection, powder for reconstitution, combined CDV, CPV, and ICH vaccine, living, prepared from CDV, CPV, CAV_2, all grown on cell-line tissue culture, for *dogs*; 1-dose vial
Note. May be reconstituted with Nobi-vac™ L
Dose. *Dogs*: *by subcutaneous injection*, 1 dose, see manufacturer details for vaccination programmes

PoM **Nobi-Vac™ DHPPi** (Intervet)
Injection, powder for reconstitution, combined CDV, CPV, ICH, and PI vaccine, living, prepared from CDV, CPV, CAV_2, and PI virus, all grown on cell-line tissue culture, for *dogs*; 1-dose vial
Note. May be reconstituted with Nobi-Vac™ L
Dose. *Dogs*: *by subcutaneous injection*, 1 dose, see manufacturer details for vaccination programmes

PoM **Nobi-Vac™ Puppy DP** (Intervet)
Injection, powder for reconstitution, combined CDV and CPV vaccine, living, prepared from CDV grown on cell-line tissue culture, CPV grown on cell-line tissue culture, for *puppies*; 1-dose vial
Dose. *Puppies*: *by subcutaneous injection*, 1 dose, see manufacturer details for vaccination programmes

PoM **Vanguard™ 7** (SmithKline Beecham)
Injection, 2 fractions for reconstitution, living CDV, CPV, ICH, and PI, and inactivated leptospirosis vaccine, prepared from CDV strain Snyder-Hill, CPV strain NL-35-D, CAV_2 strain CAV-2 Manhattan, PI virus NL-CPI-5 strain, grown on an established canine cell line, *L. interrogans* serotypes, for *dogs*; two 1-dose vials
Dose. *Dogs*: *by subcutaneous injection*, 1 combined dose, see manufacturer details for vaccination programmes

PoM **Vanguard™ CPV-L** (SmithKline Beecham)
Injection, combined living CPV and inactivated leptospirosis vaccine, prepared from CPV strain NL-35-D, *L. interrogans* serotypes, for *dogs*; 1 mL
Dose. *Dogs*: *by subcutaneous injection*, 1 mL, see manufacturer details for vaccination programmes

PoM **Vaxitas™ DA₂** (Coopers Pitman-Moore)
Injection, powder for reconstitution, combined CDV and ICH vaccine, living, prepared from CDV grown on cell-line tissue culture, CAV_2 strain grown on cell-line tissue culture, for *dogs*; 1-dose vial
Note. May be reconstituted with Vaxitas™ L, K Parvo L, K Parvo
Dose. *Dogs*: *by subcutaneous injection*, 1 dose, see manufacturer details for vaccination programmes

PoM **Vaxitas™ DA2 Parvo** (Coopers Pitman-Moore)
Injection, powder for reconstitution, combined CDV, CPV, and ICH vaccine, living, prepared from CDV, CPV, CAV_2, all grown on cell-line tissue culture, for *dogs*; 1-dose vial
Note. May be reconstituted with Vaxitas™ L

Dose. *Dogs*: *by subcutaneous injection*, 1 dose, see manufacturer details for vaccination programmes

PoM **Vaxitas™ K Parvo L** (Coopers Pitman-Moore)
Injection, combined CPV and leptospirosis vaccine, inactivated, prepared from CPV grown on cell-line tissue culture, *L. interrogans* serotypes, containing aluminium hydroxide as adjuvant, for *dogs*; 1-dose syringe
Dose. *Dogs*: *by subcutaneous injection*, 1 dose, see manufacturer details for vaccination programmes

> Accidental self-injection with oil-based vaccines can cause severe vascular spasm and prompt medical attention is essential

18.4.9 Combination immunoglobulins for dogs

PoM **Maxagloban™ P** (Hoechst)
Injection, combined CDV, CPV, ICH, and leptospirosis immunoglobulin, prepared from canine serum containing neutralising antibodies to CDV, CPV, ICH virus, and *L. interrogans* serotypes, for *dogs, foxes, ferrets, mink, other exotic Canidae, and Mustelidae*; 5 mL
Dose. Treatment of CDV, ICH, or leptospirosis infections
Dogs, ferrets, foxes, mink, other Canidae, Mustelidae: *by subcutaneous or intramuscular injection*, 0.4 mL/kg
Treatment of parvovirus infections.
Dogs: *by subcutaneous or intramuscular injection*, 1 mL/kg, repeat every 3 days
Prophylaxis of CDV, ICH, or leptospirosis infections
Dogs, ferrets, foxes, mink, other Canidae, Mustelidae: *by subcutaneous or intramuscular injection*, 0.2 mL/kg
Prophylaxis of parvovirus infection.
Dogs: *by subcutaneous or intramuscular injection*, 1 mL/kg

18.5 Immunological preparations for cats

18.5.1 Feline panleucopenia
18.5.2 Feline viral respiratory disease complex
18.5.3 Rabies
18.5.4 Combination vaccines for cats

18.5.1 Feline panleucopenia

Feline panleucopenia (FPL), or feline infectious enteritis, is a highly infectious, ubiquitous disease affecting not only the domestic cat but other Felidae, and also some other species such as mink. There is only one serotype of the virus and it is highly immunogenic. Where vaccination has been carried out, it has been extremely successful in controlling the disease.

Both live and inactivated vaccines are available, and although antibody titres may be slightly lower with inactivated vaccines, both types confer adequate immunity. Live vaccines probably induce a more rapid onset of protection, and are more likely to be able to overcome low levels of maternally-derived antibody. Inactivated vaccines have the advantage that they may be safely administered to pregnant queens or to kittens less than 4 weeks of age. Live vaccines are contra-indicated in this situation because feline panleucopenia virus may cross the placenta and induce cerebellar hypoplasia in fetal or newborn kittens.

Vaccination should not be performed in unhealthy or immunosuppressed animals, especially with live vaccines since wild-type panleucopenia virus itself is immunosuppressive.

In most kittens, maternally-derived antibody has declined to non-interfering levels by 12 weeks of age. Thus from this age onwards, for most vaccines, one dose is usually sufficient. Where maternally-derived antibody is likely to be unusually high, an additional dose should be given at 16 weeks. Young kittens from 6 weeks of age onwards may be vaccinated, but require additional doses at 2 to 4 week intervals, ensuring the last dose is at 12 weeks or later.

Antibody titres, following vaccination with live vaccine, have been shown to persist for at least 4 years, and for over one year following administration of inactivated vaccines. An initial booster vaccination at one year of age is, however, advisable, with revaccination every 1 to 2 years thereafter, particularly in high risk situations or where natural boosting is unlikely.

Following an outbreak of disease, vaccination should be accompanied by thorough cleansing of premises with an appropriate disinfectant, since the virus is extremely stable and there are usually high levels of virus in the environment.

Indications. Vaccination against feline panleucopenia (FPL)
Contra-indications. Side-effects. Warnings. See notes above, see notes at beginning of chapter
Dose. See preparation details, see notes above for vaccination programmes

Live vaccines

PoM **Feliniffa**™ **P** (RMB)
Injection, powder for reconstitution, FPL vaccine, living, prepared from virus, for *cats*; 1-dose vial
Note. May be reconstituted with Feliniffa™ RC
Dose. *Cats*: *by subcutaneous injection*, 1 dose

PoM **Feli-Pan**™ **MLV** (C-Vet)
Injection, FPL vaccine, living, prepared from virus grown on an established cell line of feline origin, for *cats*; 1-dose vial
Dose. *Cats*: *by subcutaneous or intramuscular injection*, 1 dose

PoM **Felocell**™ (SmithKline Beecham)
Injection, powder for reconstitution, FPL vaccine, living, prepared from virus strain 'Snow Leopard' grown on NLFK-1 feline kidney cell line, for *cats*; 1-dose vial
Dose. *Cats*: *by subcutaneous or intramuscular injection*, 1 dose

PoM **Katavac**™ **P** (Duphar)
Injection, powder for reconstitution, FPL vaccine, living, prepared from virus grown on tissue culture, for *cats*; 1-dose vial
Dose. *Cats*: *by subcutaneous or intramuscular injection*, 1 dose

PoM **Nobi-Vac**™ **FPL** (Intervet)
Injection, FPL vaccine, living, prepared from virus grown on cell-line tissue culture, for *cats*; 1-dose vial
Dose. *Cats*: *by subcutaneous or intramuscular injection*, 1 dose

PoM **Vaxicat**™ **P** (Coopers Pitman-Moore)
Injection, powder for reconstitution, FPL vaccine, living, prepared from virus grown on cell-line tissue culture, for *cats*; 1-dose vial
Dose. *Cats*: *by subcutaneous injection*, 1 dose

See also section 18.5.4

Inactivated vaccines

PoM **Feli-Pan**™ (C-Vet)
Injection, FPL vaccine, inactivated, prepared from virus-bearing tissue culture fluids infected with FPL virus, for *cats*; 1-dose vial
Dose. *Cats*: *by subcutaneous or intramuscular injection*, 1 dose

PoM **Felocine**™ (SmithKline Beecham)
Injection, FPL vaccine, inactivated, prepared from virus, for *cats*; 1 mL
Dose. *Cats*: *by subcutaneous or intramuscular injection*, 1 mL

PoM **Katavac**™ **iP** (Duphar)
Injection, FPL vaccine, inactivated, prepared from tissue culture of feline origin infected with virus, for *cats*; 1-dose vial
Dose. *Cats*: *by subcutaneous or intramuscular injection*, 1 dose

PoM **Purtect**™ **kP** (Coopers Pitman-Moore)
Injection, FPL vaccine, inactivated, prepared from virus grown on a feline cell line, for *cats*; 1-dose vial
Dose. *Cats*: *by subcutaneous injection*, 1 dose

PoM **Vaxicat**™ **kP** (Coopers Pitman-Moore)
Injection, FPL vaccine, inactivated, prepared from virus grown on cell-line tissue culture, containing aluminium hydroxide as adjuvant, for *cats*; 1-dose syringe
Dose. *Cats*: *by subcutaneous injection*, 1 dose

See also section 18.5.4

18.5.2 Feline viral respiratory disease complex

Feline viral rhinotracheitis (FVR) virus, (feline herpesvirus 1), and feline calicivirus are the 2 main causes of upper respiratory-tract disease in cats and account for approximately 80 percent of cases. Feline calicivirus infection is generally milder than FVR and is often associated with mouth ulceration. There is only one strain of FVR virus, but there are a number of strains of feline calicivirus. Most are closely related antigenically, and strains selected for vaccine use have broad antigenicity. Nevertheless, current vaccines do not protect against some strains and widespread use of particular vaccines may encourage selection for these.

Live and inactivated systemic vaccines, and live intranasal vaccines are available. In previously healthy, unexposed cats, all types of vaccine induce reasonable protection against disease, though not necessarily against infection. However, both respiratory viruses are extremely widespread and clinically healthy carriers are common. Thus management measures, such as early weaning and isolation, are often necessary to ensure kittens are not already incubating the disease, or perhaps are already carriers at the time of vaccination.

Live systemic vaccines are normally quite safe but should be administered carefully. There are occasional reports that if the vaccine is inadvertently given via the respiratory route, for example, if a cat licks the injection site or an aerosol is made with the syringe, then respiratory signs may develop. Thus in completely virus-free colonies of cats an inactivated vaccine might be preferable. Live intranasal vaccine may cause transient mild sneezing, and occasionally other signs. However, it induces rapid protection, in 2 to 4 days, and so is specifically indicated during a disease outbreak or in stray cat homes. It is inadvisable to vaccinate pregnant queens with live vaccines.

In general, kittens should be vaccinated with systemic vaccines initially at 9 weeks of age, when in most cases maternally-derived antibody has declined to non-interfering levels. A second dose is given 3 to 4 weeks later. However, the duration of maternally-derived antibody can be quite variable; for FVR, antibody may last for 2 to 10 weeks and for feline calicivirus, antibody may persist for up to 14 weeks. However, little work has been done in relating maternally-derived antibody levels to either protection or interference with vaccination.

Intranasal vaccination should be initiated at 12 weeks of age. Although not licensed in the UK for earlier use, in some cases intranasal vaccine may be useful for controlling disease in very young kittens because it is not interfered with by maternally-derived antibody. Earlier vaccination schedules may also be initiated with systemic vaccines, vaccinating at 3 to 4 week intervals until 12 weeks of age.

Annual revaccination is usually recommended, but in some high risk situations, vaccination every 6 months may be advisable.

Indications. Vaccination against feline calicivirus infection and feline viral rhinotracheitis (FVR)
Contra-indications. Side-effects. Warnings. See notes above, see notes at beginning of chapter
Dose. See preparation details, see notes above for vaccination programmes

Live vaccines

PoM **Feliflu™ (FVR-C)** (C-Vet)
Injection, powder for reconstitution, combined feline calicivirus and FVR vaccine, living, prepared from viruses grown on an established cell line of feline origin, for *cats*; 1-dose vial
Note. May be reconstituted with Felipan™ MLV
Dose. *Cats*: *by subcutaneous or intramuscular injection*, 1 dose

PoM **Felocell Flu™** (SmithKline Beecham)
Injection, powder for reconstitution, combined feline calicivirus and FVR vaccine, living, prepared from FVR virus strain FVRm, calicivirus strain F9, grown on NLFK-1 feline kidney cell line, for *cats*; 1-dose vial

Dose. *Cats*: *by subcutaneous or intra-muscular injection*, 1 dose

PoM **FR-FC™** (Webster)
Injection, powder for reconstitution, combined feline calicivirus and FVR vaccine, living, prepared from viruses grown on a cell line, for *cats*; 1-dose vial
Dose. *Cats*: *by subcutaneous injection*, 1 dose

PoM **Katavac™ CHI** (Duphar)
Injection, powder for reconstitution, combined feline calicivirus and FVR vaccine, living, prepared from viruses grown on an established feline cell line, for *cats*; 1-dose vial
Note. May be reconstituted with Kata-vac™ iP
Dose. *Cats*: *by subcutaneous or intra-muscular injection*, 1 dose

PoM **Katavac™ CHN** (Duphar)
Intranasal solution, powder for recon-stitution, combined feline calicivirus and FVR vaccine, living, prepared from viruses grown on the Crandell cell line, for *cats*; 1-dose vial
Dose. *Cats*: *by intranasal instillation*, 0.5 mL of reconstituted solution into each nostril

PoM **Purtect™ RC** (Coopers Pitman-Moore)
Injection, powder for reconstitution, combined feline calicivirus and FVR vaccine, living, prepared from viruses grown separately on feline cell lines, for *cats*; 1-dose vial
Note. May be reconstituted with Pur-tect™ kP
Dose. *Cats*: *by subcutaneous injection*, 1 dose

Inactivated vaccines

PoM **Feliniffa™ RC** (RMB)
Injection, combined feline calicivirus and FVR vaccine, inactivated, containing a suitable oil as adjuvant, for *cats*; 1-dose vial
Dose. *Cats*: *by subcutaneous injection*, 1 dose

See also section 18.5.4

> Accidental self-injection with oil-based vaccines can cause severe vascular spasm and prompt medical attention is essential

18.5.3 Rabies

See section 18.4.6

18.5.4 Combination vaccines for cats

PoM **Delcavac™ FPRC** (Mycofarm)
Injection, powder for reconstitution, combined feline calicivirus, FPL, and FVR vaccine, living, prepared from viruses grown on cell-line tissue culture, for *cats*; 1-dose vial
Dose. *Cats*: *by subcutaneous or intra-muscular injection*, 1 dose, see manu-facturer details for vaccination programmes

PoM **Feline 3™** (Webster)
Injection, powder for reconstitution, combined feline calicivirus, FPL, and FVR vaccine, living, prepared from viruses grown on a cell line, for *cats*; 1-dose vial
Dose. *Cats*: *by subcutaneous injection*, 1 dose

PoM **Felocell™ CVR** (SmithKline Beecham)
Injection, powder for reconstitution, combined feline calicivirus, FPL, and FVR vaccine, living, prepared from FPL virus strain 'Snow Leopard', FVR virus strain FVRm, feline calicivirus strain F9, grown on NLFK-1 feline kidney cell line, for *cats*; 1-dose vial
Dose. *Cats*: *by subcutaneous or intra-muscular injection*, 1 dose, see manu-facturer details for vaccination programmes

PoM **Katavac™ Plus** (Duphar)
Injection, 2 fractions for reconstitution, combined live feline calicivirus and FVR, and inactivated FPL vaccine, prepared from feline calicivirus and FVR virus grown on an established feline cell line, tissue culture of feline origin infected with FPL, for *cats*; two 1-dose vials
Dose. *Cats*: *by subcutaneous or intra-muscular injection*, 1 combined dose, see manufacturer details for vaccination programmes

PoM **Nobi-Vac™ Tricat** (Intervet)
Injection, powder for reconstitution, combined feline calicivirus, FPL, and

FVR vaccine, living, prepared from viruses grown on cell-line tissue culture, for *cats*; 1-dose vial

Dose. *Cats*: *by subcutaneous or intramuscular injection*, 1 dose, see manufacturer details for vaccination programmes

PoM **Purtect™ RCkP** (Coopers Pitman-Moore)

Injection, 2 fractions for reconstitution, combined live feline calicivirus and FVR, and inactivated FPL vaccine, prepared from viruses grown on feline cell lines, for *cats*; two 1-dose vials

Dose. *Cats*: *by subcutaneous injection*, 1 combined dose, see manufacturer details for vaccination programmes

18.6 Immunological preparations for birds

18.6.1 Avian infectious bronchitis
18.6.2 Avian encephalomyelitis
18.6.3 Avian infectious bursal disease
18.6.4 Duck virus hepatitis
18.6.5 Duck septicaemia
18.6.6 Egg drop syndrome 1976
18.6.7 Erysipelas
18.6.8 Fowl pox
18.6.9 Infectious laryngotracheitis
18.6.10 Marek's disease
18.6.11 Newcastle disease
18.6.12 Paramyxovirus 3 disease
18.6.13 Pasteurellosis
18.6.14 Pigeon paramyxovirus
18.6.15 Turkey rhinotracheitis
18.6.16 Combination vaccines for birds

Vaccine administration. Vaccines may be given to birds in the drinking water, by spraying, by beak dipping, by intranasal or intra-ocular instillation, by injection, or by wingstab or footstab techniques.

When giving live virus vaccines in the **drinking water** it is advisable to add skimmed milk powder, at the rate of 2 to 4 g/litre, to the water that is to be used to dilute the vaccine. This prolongs the life of the virus. Whole milk should not be used for this purpose because the fat content may cause blockages in automatic drinking systems.

Before vaccination, water is withheld for 2 hours and drink dispensers are checked to ensure that there are sufficient available so that all birds are able to drink the vaccine within one hour. The lighting is dimmed and about half the total volume of diluted vaccine is used to fill the drink dispensers. The lighting is then restored. The drink dispensers are replenished where necessary with the remaining diluted vaccine until the birds have drunk all or most of the vaccine. Normal water supply is then made available.

The amount of water required varies with age, and can be calculated as follows:

Age of birds (days)	Drinking water required per 1000 birds (litres)
1–7	2–4
14–32	9–11
35–49	13–18
56 and over	20–22

Live virus vaccines may be administered by **spraying**. The vaccine is diluted using freshly boiled and cooled purified water, and the diluted vaccine is sprayed over the birds using machinery adjusted to suit the particular environment and requirements. Operators should wear suitable face masks, preferably the Siebe-Gorman type.

Coarse spraying in the hatchery is suitable for day-old chicks. Although it may be used for older housed birds, it is less effective. For use on chicks, the vaccine is diluted in 300 to 400 mL of water at 25°C. This is sufficient for 1000 birds. When spraying, ensure that all the birds are wetted. Allow them to stand in their boxes to dry, avoiding draughts.

Older birds are penned together in groups in dim light. The vaccine is diluted in water at a rate of 1 to 1.5 litres per 1000 doses. The birds are sprayed from a distance of approximately

45 centimetres from above ensuring that droplets fall on them. Allow the birds to dry for 10 to 15 minutes, avoiding direct heat as this may affect the efficacy of the vaccine.

Aerosol spraying is used on birds that are 10 days of age or over. The vaccine is diluted in 30 to 40 mL of water per 1000 doses. After preparing the vaccine and machines, dim the lighting and switch off the ventilation. Then spray over the heads of the birds for about 2 minutes for 5000 birds, keeping the ventilation and lights off for a total time of 10 minutes. Longer periods without ventilation may stress the birds.

Another method of vaccination is by **intranasal** or **intra-ocular instillation**. One thousand vaccine doses are diluted in 40 to 50 mL of sterile water at 25°C such that one drop contains the required dose. The vaccine is then instilled into one eye or one nostril. In the latter case, the other nostril is held closed until the bird has inhaled the vaccine. **Beak dipping** is suitable for day-old chicks only. One thousand vaccine doses are reconstituted in 150 mL of water and placed in a shallow dish. The beak of each bird is dipped into the solution. This vaccination method is not as effective as intranasal or intra-ocular instillation.

Vaccines may also be administered by **injection**. Intramuscular injection of an inactivated oil-based vaccine is usually given into the breast or thigh muscles. Other vaccine solutions may be given by subcutaneous or intramuscular injection into the fold of the skin at the back of the neck in poultry or the base of the neck in pigeons. Pigeons should not be fed for 12 hours before vaccination as a distended crop may distort the anatomy of the injection site. The **wingstab** technique is used for fowl pox vaccine and the method of administration is described under section 18.6.8. Duck virus hepatitis vaccine is given by the **footstab** technique and described in section 18.6.4.

It is important that a veterinarian with experience in dealing with poultry should be consulted as vaccination programmes for these species vary from site to site.

18.6.1 Avian infectious bronchitis

Live virus vaccines are available for vaccination against avian infectious bronchitis, which are either highly attenuated (H120) or less attenuated (H52). The figures indicate the number of eggs through which the strains are passed to produce the desired degree of attenuation. Inactivated oil-based vaccines are also available.

All vaccination programmes should commence with the H120-attenuated live vaccine at day-old or 3 weeks of age, followed by a booster dose at 7 weeks of age. At 16 to 18 weeks of age, an H52 vaccine or an inactivated vaccine is used. There should be an interval of at least 6 weeks between administration of the live vaccine and vaccination with the inactivated preparation. The H52 vaccine should not be used in conjunction with the inactivated vaccine.

Indications. Vaccination against avian infectious bronchitis

Contra-indications. Use of H52 or inactivated vaccine for primary vaccination, or on premises where primary vaccination has not been carried out

Side-effects. Warnings. See notes at beginning of chapter

Dose. See preparation details, see notes at beginning of section 18.6 for methods of administration, see notes above for vaccination programmes

Live vaccines

PML **IBMM Vaccine** (Salsbury)
By addition to drinking water, spraying, by intranasal or intra-ocular instillation, powder for reconstitution, avian infectious bronchitis vaccine, living, prepared from virus modified Mass. strain, for *chickens*; 1000-dose vial

PML **Nobilis H-52** (Intervet)
By addition to drinking water, powder for reconstitution, avian infectious bronchitis vaccine, living, prepared from virus strain Mass. type H52, for *chickens* 1000-dose vial

Withdrawal Periods. *Poultry*: slaughter withdrawal period nil, egg withdrawal period nil

PML**Nobilis H-120** (Intervet)
By addition to drinking water, powder for reconstitution, avian infectious bronchitis vaccine, living, prepared from virus strain Mass. type H120, for *chickens*; 1000-dose vial, 2500-dose vial
Withdrawal Periods. *Poultry*: slaughter withdrawal period nil, egg withdrawal period nil
Note. May be administered by spraying to day-old chicks after prior consultation with manufacturer

PML**Poulvac**™ **H52** (Duphar)
By addition to drinking water, powder for reconstitution, avian infectious bronchitis vaccine, living, prepared from virus Mass. strain H52, for *chickens*; 1000-dose vial, 2500-dose vial
Withdrawal Periods. *Poultry*: slaughter withdrawal period nil, egg withdrawal period nil

PML**Poulvac**™ **H120** (Duphar)
By addition to drinking water, coarse or aerosol spraying, powder for reconstitution, avian infectious bronchitis vaccine, living, prepared from virus Mass. strain H120, for *chickens*; 1000-dose vial, 2500-dose vial, 5000-dose vial
Withdrawal Periods. *Poultry*: slaughter withdrawal period nil, egg withdrawal period nil

Inactivated vaccines

> Accidental self-injection with oil-based vaccines can cause severe vascular spasm and prompt medical attention is essential

PML**Iblin**™ (Coopers Pitman-Moore)
Injection, avian infectious bronchitis vaccine, inactivated, prepared from virus Mass. strain M41 grown in eggs, containing a suitable oil as adjuvant, for *chickens*; 500 mL
Withdrawal Periods. *Poultry*: slaughter withdrawal period nil, egg withdrawal period nil
Dose. *Poultry*: *by intramuscular injection*, 0.5 mL

PML**Iblin Bivalent**™ (Coopers Pitman-Moore)
Injection, avian infectious bronchitis vaccine, inactivated, prepared from virus strains GV101 and M41 grown in eggs, containing a suitable oil as adjuvant, for *chickens*; 500 mL
Withdrawal Periods. *Poultry*: slaughter withdrawal period nil, egg withdrawal period nil
Dose. *Poultry*: *by intramuscular injection*, 0.5 mL

See also section 18.6.16

18.6.2 Avian encephalomyelitis

Live virus vaccines are available for vaccination against avian encephalomyelitis. These vaccines are normally administered by dilution in drinking water, but may also be given by coarse spraying. All breeders and laying hens should be vaccinated between 10 and 16 weeks of age.

Indications. Vaccination against avian encephalomyelitis
Contra-indications. Eggs for hatching should not be taken for the first 4-5 weeks after vaccination; see also notes at beginning of chapter
Side-effects. Warnings. May cause a clinical reaction in chicks; decreased egg production in older birds; see also notes at beginning of chapter
Dose. See notes at beginning of section 18.6 for methods of administration, see notes above for vaccination programmes

PML**AE (Lyophilised)** (Salsbury)
By addition to drinking water, powder for reconstitution, avian encephalomyelitis vaccine, living, prepared from virus, for *chickens between 10 weeks of age and 4 weeks before laying*; 1000-dose vial

PML**AE Nobilis** (Intervet)
By addition to drinking water, powder for reconstitution, avian encephalomyelitis vaccine, living, prepared from virus strain Calnek 1143, for *chickens 8 weeks of age and over*; 500-dose vial, 1000-dose vial

18.6.3 Avian infectious bursal disease

Live virus vaccines and inactivated oil-based vaccines are available as monovalent and polyvalent preparations.

The live vaccines may be given by incorporating them in the drinking water, by spraying, by intra-ocular instillation, by subcutaneous or intra-muscular injection. Vaccines formulated to be administered by intramuscular injection may only be given by that route. Similarly, the preparations formulated to be given by the other techniques are unsuitable for intramuscular injection.

Broilers with no maternally-derived antibodies may be vaccinated at one day old with live virus vaccine. Birds with maternally-derived antibodies are vaccinated at 4 to 5 weeks of age. Breeding stock receive live virus vaccine at 4 to 5 weeks and, in some cases at 8 weeks, followed by inactivated vaccine at 16 to 18 weeks of age. Replacement stock receive inactivated vaccine at 4 to 5 weeks of age.

Problems have been experienced in the UK with an acute, highly virulent infectious bursal disease virus infection. This infection is afforded no protection by live vaccines generally available. **Gumboro™ Nobilis Strain D78** (Intervet) and **Poulvac™ Bursine 2** (Duphar) may be used under an Animal Test Certificate to aid in control of this infection. Consult manufacturers for further information.

Indications. Vaccination against avian infectious bursal disease
Contra-indications. Side-effects. Warnings. See notes at beginning of chapter
Dose. See preparation details, see notes at beginning of section 18.6 for methods of administration, see notes above for vaccination programme

Live vaccines

PML **Gumboro™ Disease Nobilis** (Intervet)
By addition to drinking water or spraying, powder for reconstitution, infectious bursal disease vaccine, living, prepared from virus, for *day-old chicks, chickens 4 weeks of age*; 500-dose vial, 1000-dose vial
Withdrawal Periods. *Poultry*: slaughter withdrawal period nil, egg withdrawal period nil
Injection, powder for reconstitution, infectious bursal disease vaccine, living,

prepared from virus, for *day-old chicks*; 1000-dose vial
Withdrawal Periods. *Poultry*: slaughter withdrawal period nil, egg withdrawal period nil
Dose. *Poultry*: by intramuscular injection, 1 dose

Inactivated vaccines

PML **Maternalin™** (Coopers Pitman-Moore)
Injection, infectious bursal disease vaccine, inactivated, prepared from virus strain 52/70, grown in chicken bursal tissue, containing a suitable oil as adjuvant, for *chickens 18-20 weeks of age*; 250 mL, 500 mL
Withdrawal Periods. *Poultry*: slaughter withdrawal period nil
Dose. *Poultry*: by intramuscular injection, 0.5 mL

See also section 18.6.16

18.6.4 Duck virus hepatitis

A live virus vaccine is available for administration to susceptible day-old ducklings by footstab technique. The vaccine is administered by using a needle, which is gently stabbed through the footweb and slowly withdrawn.

PML **Duck hepatitis virus** (Animal Health Trust)
Injection, duck virus hepatitis vaccine, living, prepared from virus strain Rispen H53 grown in chicken eggs, for *day-old ducklings*; 2 mL, 4 mL
Dose. *Ducks*: by footstab, 0.004 mL
Note. This vaccine is only available to members of the Duck Producers Association

18.6.5 Duck septicaemia

Duck septicaemia is caused by *Pasteurella anatipestifer* (*Moraxella anatipestifer*). Autogenous inactivated vaccines may be made by licensed laboratories for use on individual farms where this condition is a problem.

18.6.6 Egg drop syndrome 1976

Egg drop syndrome 1976 is characterised by a fall in egg production with loss of shell strength and pigmentation. Inactivated oil-based vaccines are available for vaccination of replacement breeding and layer flocks, before commencement of lay. Birds are vaccinated at 14 to 18 weeks of age. One vaccination is usually sufficient to provide immunity, although in some circumstances a second vaccination may be necessary.

Indications. Vaccination against egg drop syndrome 1976
Contra-indications. Side-effects. Warnings. See notes at beginning of chapter
Dose. See preparation details, see notes above for vaccination programmes

PML **Edsilin**™ (Coopers Pitman-Moore)
Injection, egg drop syndrome 1976 vaccine, inactivated, prepared from avian adenovirus, containing a suitable oil as adjuvant, for *chickens 16-20 weeks of age*; 500 mL
Dose. *Poultry: by intramuscular injection*, 0.5 mL

PML **Nobi-Vac**™ **EDS 76** (Intervet)
Injection, egg drop syndrome 1976 vaccine, inactivated, prepared from adenovirus strain BC14, containing a suitable oil as adjuvant, for *chickens 14-18 weeks of age*; 1000-dose vial
Dose. *Poultry: by subcutaneous injection*, 0.5 mL

> Accidental self-injection with oil-based vaccines can cause severe vascular spasm and prompt medical attention is essential

18.6.7 Erysipelas

Erysipelothrix rhusiopathiae (*Ery. insidiosa*) causes infection in turkeys. Birds are vaccinated before they reach 14 weeks of age.
Indications. Vaccination against erysipelas
Contra-indications. Side-effects. Warnings. See notes at beginning of chapter
Dose. See preparation details

PML **Erysorb**™ **ST** (Hoechst)
Injection, erysipelas vaccine, inactivated, prepared from *Ery. rhusiopathiae* strains, containing aluminium hydroxide as adjuvant, for *sheep* (18.2.7), *turkeys over 6 weeks of age*; 50 mL, 100 mL

Dose. *Turkeys: by subcutaneous or intramuscular injection*, 0.5 mL, repeat dose after 2-6 weeks

PML **Suvaxyn**™ **Erysipelas** (Duphar)
Injection, erysipelas vaccine, inactivated, prepared from *Ery. rhusiopathiae* strains, containing a suitable adjuvant, for *pigs* (18.3.5), *turkeys over 8 weeks of age*; 100 mL
Dose. *Turkeys: by subcutaneous injection*, (up to 4.5 kg body-weight) 0.5 mL, (more than 4.5 kg body-weight) 1 mL. Repeat dose every 3 months

See also section 18.6.16

18.6.8 Fowl pox

A freeze-dried live virus vaccine is available. This is a preparation derived from cell cultures or eggs infected either with a suitable strain of pigeon pox virus or with a suitably attenuated strain of fowl pox virus or of turkey pox virus. The reconstituted vaccine deteriorates rapidly and only one vial should be prepared for use at a time.

Replacement pullets and breeders may be vaccinated at any time after 6 weeks of age, by the wingstab technique. This will provide immunity throughout the laying period. The vaccine should not be used in birds under 6 weeks of age, and in laying birds.

To carry out vaccination, the bird is held with the wing spread up, the needle is dipped in the vaccine and used to puncture the wing web, avoiding blood vessels, bones, muscles, and feathers. A 'take' has occurred where there is an initial swelling at the vaccination site that increases over the following 4 to 5 days, until a scab has formed. Birds showing no evidence of a 'take' should be revaccinated.

Turkeys should be vaccinated on the outer surface of the thigh, after first removing a few feathers. The wingstab technique is not suitable for these birds because they sleep with their heads under the wings and facial lesions may develop.

The duration and depth of immunity is variable and may be overcome by stress or a virulent challenge.

Indications. Vaccination against fowl pox

Contra-indications. Birds younger than 6 weeks, layer hens

Dose. See notes above for method of administration and vaccination programmes

PML **Poxine**™ (Salsbury)
Injection, powder for reconstitution, fowl pox vaccine, living, prepared from virus grown in chick embryo, for *chickens 6-16 weeks of age*; 500-dose vial

18.6.9 Infectious laryngotracheitis

A freeze-dried live vaccine is available for administration to chickens over 4 weeks of age. The vaccine is usually given by intra-ocular instillation. Incorporation into the drinking water is less effective, while use of the spraying method may result in severe losses.

If rearing and laying sites are contaminated, the first vaccination at 4 to 5 weeks of age will need boosting with a further vaccination at 16 to 20 weeks of age. If there are no problems on the rearing site, birds are vaccinated by intra-ocular instillation when they are moved to the laying farms. All birds on the site should be vaccinated.

Vaccinated birds should not be taken to a site where there are any non-vaccinated birds as the virus is shed from vaccinated birds during the laying period.

Indications. Vaccination against infectious laryngotracheitis

Contra-indications. Side-effects. Warnings. See notes at beginning of chapter

Dose. See notes at beginning of section 18.6 for methods of administration, see notes above for vaccination programmes

PML **L T Vaccine** (Salsbury)
By intra-ocular instillation, infectious laryngotracheitis vaccine, living, for *chickens 4 weeks of age*; 1000-dose vial

18.6.10 Marek's disease

'Wet' cell-associated live vaccines prepared from turkey herpesvirus, from attenuated Marek's virus, or from nonpathogenic Marek's viruses, are available. The vaccines are stored in ampoules in liquid nitrogen and under these conditions ($-196.5°C$) may be expected to retain their potency for 2 years. The diluent supplied by the manufacturer is stored at 2°C to 6°C. When required for use, the vaccine is rapidly thawed in water at 37°C and then mixed gently with the diluent using a wide bore needle to avoid damage to the vaccine. Reconstituted vaccine should be used within one hour. Because of the nature of the storage conditions, ampoules may shatter, and operators handling these vaccines should be suitably protected, in particular from the possibility of glass particles penetrating the eyes.

As an alternative to storage in liquid nitrogen, the vaccine may be stored in solid carbon dioxide in which case it may be expected to retain its potency for one month from date of purchase. Freeze-dried lyophilised 'dry' live vaccines are also available, which are easier to handle.

Chicks are usually vaccinated at day-old in the hatchery. Vaccination is occasionally repeated at 3 to 4 weeks of age. In conditions of severe challenge, the 'wet' vaccines are more effective than the 'dry' vaccines. In some circumstances, day-old chicks may need to be given a dose of each.

A vaccine is available from MAFF for chicks to be exported and under authorisation by DVO.

Indications. Vaccination against Marek's disease

Contra-indications. Side-effects. Warnings. See notes above, see notes at beginning of chapter

Dose. See preparation details, see notes above for vaccination programmes

PML **Delvax**™ **Marek THV Cell Associated** (Mycofarm)
Injection, powder for reconstitution, Marek's disease vaccine, living, deep-frozen, prepared from turkey herpesvirus strain FC126 grown on chick embryo fibroblast tissue cultures, *day-old chicks, chickens 3 weeks of age*; 250-

dose vial, 500-dose vial, other sizes available
Dose. *Poultry*: *by intramuscular injection*, 0.2 mL

PML **Delvax™ Marek THV Freeze Dried** (Mycofarm)
Injection, powder for reconstitution, Marek's disease vaccine, living, freeze-dried, prepared from turkey herpesvirus strain FC126 grown on chick embryo fibroblast tissue cultures, for *day-old chicks, chickens 3 weeks of age*; 250-dose vial, 500-dose vial, other sizes available
Dose. *Poultry*: *by intramuscular injection*, 0.2 mL

PML **Marexine™ (MD)** (Intervet)
Injection, powder for reconstitution, Marek's disease vaccine, living, prepared from Marek's disease virus strain HPRS-16, for *day-old chicks, chickens up to 3 weeks of age*; 250-dose vial, 500-dose vial, 1000-dose vial
Dose. *Poultry*: *by intramuscular injection*, 0.1 mL

PML **Marexine™ THV** (Intervet)
Injection, powder for reconstitution, Marek's disease vaccine, living, freeze-dried, prepared from turkey herpesvirus strain PB-THV 1, for *day-old chicks, chickens 3 weeks of age*; 250-dose vial, 500-dose vial, other sizes available
Withdrawal Periods. *Poultry*: slaughter withdrawal period nil
Dose. *Poultry*: *by intramuscular injection*, 0.1 mL

PML **Marexine™ THV/CA** (Intervet)
Injection, powder for reconstitution, Marek's disease vaccine, living, cell associated, prepared from turkey herpesvirus strain PB-THV 1, for *day-old chicks, chickens up to 3 weeks of age*; 250-dose vial, 500-dose vial, other sizes available
Dose. *Poultry*: *by intramuscular injection*, 0.1 mL

PML **MD-VAC (Frozen Wet)** (Salsbury)
Injection, powder for reconstitution, Marek's disease vaccine, living, deep-frozen, prepared from turkey herpesvirus Witter strain, for *day-old chicks*; 1000-dose vial
Withdrawal Periods. *Poultry*: slaughter withdrawal period nil

Dose. *Poultry*: *by intramuscular injection*, 0.2 mL

PML **MD-VAC (Lyophilised)** (Salsbury)
Injection, powder for reconstitution, Marek's disease vaccine, living, freeze-dried, prepared from turkey herpesvirus grown on chicken tissue culture, for *day-old chicks*; 1000-dose vial
Dose. *Poultry*: *by subcutaneous or intramuscular injection*, 0.1 mL

18.6.11 Newcastle disease

Live freeze-dried vaccines and oil-based inactivated vaccines are available for vaccination against Newcastle disease. Vaccination programmes depend upon the degree of challenge in any geographical area. In areas of low challenge or no challenge, chicken and turkey broilers are not vaccinated. Replacement pullets receive a live virus vaccine at 3 weeks and 10 weeks of age, followed by an inactivated vaccine between 16 and 18 weeks of age. In areas of high challenge, broilers are vaccinated with live vaccines at day-old, 3 weeks, and 5 weeks of age. Replacement pullets receive the same regimen followed by a further course of live vaccine at 10 weeks and inactivated vaccine at 16 weeks. Revaccination with live vaccine during lay may be necessary in exceptional circumstances. In severe challenge areas, the day-old chick may be given the live vaccine by intra-ocular instillation simultaneously with an intramuscular injection of the inactivated vaccine. The latter is ineffective without the former. Administration of the live vaccine by the aerosol spraying method is more effective than when given via the drinking water. More birds are covered and a more rapid immune response is produced in the bird.

Indications. Vaccination against Newcastle disease
Contra-indications. Side-effects. Warnings. See notes at beginning of chapter
Dose. See preparation details, see notes at beginning of section 18.6 for methods of administration, see notes above for vaccination programmes

Live vaccines

PML Hitchner B1 (Salsbury)
By addition to drinking water, spraying, intranasal, or intra-ocular instillation, powder for reconstitution, Newcastle disease vaccine, living, prepared from virus strain Hitchner B1, for *chickens, turkeys, game birds*; 1000-dose vial

PML Hitchner B1 Nobilis (Intervet)
By addition to drinking water, spraying or beak dipping, powder for reconstitution, Newcastle disease vaccine, living, prepared from virus strain Hitchner B1, for *chickens*; 1000-dose vial, 2500-dose vial
Withdrawal Periods. *Poultry*: slaughter withdrawal period nil, egg withdrawal period nil

Inactivated vaccines

Accidental self-injection with oil-based vaccines can cause severe vascular spasm and prompt medical attention is essential

PML Newcadin™ (Coopers Pitman-Moore)
Injection, Newcastle disease vaccine, inactivated, prepared from virus Ulster strain grown in eggs, containing a suitable oil as adjuvant, for *broilers, layer hens, turkeys*; 500 mL
Dose. *Layer hens, turkeys*: by intramuscular injection, 0.5 mL
Broilers, birds to be slaughtered within 28 days: by subcutaneous injection, 0.5 mL

PML Newcadin™ 25 (Coopers Pitman-Moore)
Injection, Newcastle disease vaccine, inactivated, prepared from virus Ulster strain grown in eggs, containing a suitable oil as adjuvant, for *chickens, turkeys*; 500 mL
Withdrawal Periods. *Poultry*: slaughter withdrawal period nil
Dose. *Chickens*: by subcutaneous or intramuscular injection, 0.25 mL
Turkeys: by subcutaneous or intramuscular injection, 0.5 mL

PML Newcadin™ Day-Old (Coopers Pitman-Moore)
Injection, Newcastle disease vaccine, inactivated, prepared from virus Ulster strain grown in eggs, containing a suitable oil as adjuvant, for *1-4 day-old chicks*; 250 mL
Withdrawal Periods. *Poultry*: slaughter withdrawal period nil
Dose. *Poultry*: by subcutaneous or intramuscular injection, 0.1 mL simultaneously with Hitchner B1 Newcastle disease vaccine

PML Newcavac™ Nobilis (Intervet)
Injection, Newcastle disease vaccine, inactivated, prepared from virus, containing a suitable oil as adjuvant, for *chickens, turkeys, guinea fowl, pheasants, ducks*; 1000-dose vial
Dose. *Poultry, game birds*: by subcutaneous or intramuscular injection, 0.5 mL

See also section 18.6.16

18.6.12 Paramyxovirus 3 disease

An oil-based, inactivated, vaccine is available for administration to breeding turkeys. The second of the 2 doses required is given not less than 2 weeks before commencement of laying.

Indications. Vaccination against paramyxovirus 3 disease
Side-effects. A small proportion of birds may show a low serological response to Newcastle disease virus antigen if they have not received prior vaccination with Newcastle disease vaccine
Dose. See preparation details, see notes above for vaccination programmes

PML PMV₃™ (Coopers Pitman-Moore)
Injection, paramyxovirus 3 disease vaccine, inactivated, prepared from avian virus grown in eggs, containing a suitable oil as adjuvant, for *breeding turkeys*; 250 mL
Withdrawal Periods. *Poultry*: slaughter withdrawal period nil
Dose. *Poultry*: by intramuscular injection, 0.5 mL, repeat dose after 4-6 weeks

18.6.13 Pasteurellosis

Inactivated vaccines for pasteurellosis alone and combination vaccines against erysipelas and pasteurellosis are available. The latter appears to give better protection against pasteurellosis than the former. They are mainly used in turkeys, although they are occasionally necessary for broiler breeder flocks and pheasants.

Turkey breeding flocks are vaccinated at 12, 16, and 28 weeks of age. Occasionally this has to be brought forward, if challenge occurs at an earlier age. There is very little protection from the first dose of vaccine. It is inadvisable to give the oil-based vaccine to birds in lay.

Autogenous vaccines may be prepared by licensed laboratories where the *Pasteurella* serotype is not covered by those in the commercial vaccines.

Indications. Vaccination against pasteurellosis
Contra-indications. Birds in lay
Side-effects. Warnings. See notes at beginning of chapter
Dose. See preparation details, see notes above for vaccination programmes

PML **Pabac**™ (Salsbury)
Injection, pasteurellosis vaccine, inactivated, prepared from multivalent types of *Pasteurella multocida*, containing a suitable oil as adjuvant, for *chickens, turkeys, geese, pheasants, ducks*; 500 mL
Withdrawal Periods. *Poultry, game birds*: slaughter 6 weeks
Dose. *Poultry, game birds*: *by subcutaneous injection*, 0.5 mL, repeat dose after 4-5 weeks

See also section 18.6.16

18.6.14 Pigeon paramyxovirus

Pigeons may be vaccinated at any time over 3 weeks of age by subcutaneous injection at the base of the neck with an aqueous inactivated vaccine. All pigeons in the loft should be vaccinated. Vaccination should be carried out at least 2 weeks before the beginning of the racing season or show season. A booster vaccination should be given every 12 months.

Live Newcastle disease vaccine (see section 18.6.11) Hitchner B1 strain may be administered by intra-ocular instillation to stimulate a rapid immune response against paramyxovirus. Live vaccine gives protection for a short period only and re-vaccination should be carried out every 3 months. This vaccine should not be given in the drinking water to pigeons as they may receive an inadequate dose by this method.

During an acute outbreak of paramyxovirus disease the live vaccine is given by intra-ocular instillation simultaneously with an injection of the inactivated vaccine.

Indications. Vaccination against pigeon paramyxovirus infection
Contra-indications. Side-effects. Warnings. See notes at beginning of chapter
Dose. See preparation details, see notes above for vaccination programmes

P† **Colombovac**™ **PMV** (Duphar, Salsbury)
Injection, pigeon paramyxovirus vaccine, inactivated, prepared from avian paramyxovirus serotype 1 strain PMV-1, containing a suitable adjuvant, for *pigeons*; 10 mL, 20 mL
Withdrawal Periods. *Pigeons*: slaughter withdrawal period nil
Dose. *Pigeons*: *by subcutaneous injection*, 0.2 mL
†PoM in Northern Ireland

P **Nobi-Vac**™ **Paramyxo** (Intervet)
Injection, pigeon paramyxovirus vaccine, inactivated, prepared from virus serotype 1, containing a suitable oil as adjuvant, for *pigeons*; 20 mL, 50 mL
Dose. *Pigeons*: *by subcutaneous injection*, 0.25 mL

P† **Paramyx**™ **1** (Harkers)
Injection, pigeon paramyxovirus 1 vaccine, inactivated, containing a suitable oil as adjuvant, for *pigeons*; 25 mL
Dose. *Pigeons*: *by subcutaneous injection*, 0.5 mL, repeat dose after 4-6 weeks
†PoM in Northern Ireland

18.6.15 Turkey rhinotracheitis

A live virus vaccine is available for the protection of fattening turkeys against turkey rhinotracheitis (TRT). The birds are vaccinated between day-old and 9 days of age. This will provide immunity to the virus for approximately 14 weeks.

Indications. Vaccination against turkey rhinotracheitis
Contra-indications. Side-effects. Warnings. See notes at beginning of chapter
Dose. See notes at beginning of section 18.6 for methods of administration, see notes above for vaccination programme

PoM **Turkadin**™ (Coopers Pitman-Moore)
By spraying, powder for reconstitution, turkey rhinotracheitis vaccine, living, prepared from virus, for *turkeys*; 1000-dose vial, 2000-dose vial
Withdrawal Periods. *Poultry*: slaughter withdrawal period nil

18.6.16 Combination vaccines for birds

An alphabetical list of combination vaccines for poultry and the infections to which they confer immunity is given in Table 18.3.

PML **Ibinac**™ **ND** (Salsbury)
Injection, combined avian infectious bronchitis and Newcastle disease vaccine, inactivated, prepared from avian infectious bronchitis virus strain Mass. 41, Newcastle disease virus Ulster strain, grown in eggs, containing a suitable oil as adjuvant, for *chickens 16-20 weeks of age*; 500 mL
Dose. *Poultry*: *by intramuscular injection*, 0.5 mL

PML **Maridin**™ (Coopers Pitman-Moore)
Injection, combined avian infectious bursal disease and Newcastle disease vaccine, inactivated, prepared from avian infectious bursal disease virus grown on chicken bursal tissue, Newcastle disease virus grown in eggs, containing a suitable oil as adjuvant, for *chickens 18-20 weeks of age*; 500 mL
Withdrawal Periods. *Poultry*: slaughter withdrawal period nil
Dose. *Poultry*: *by intramuscular injection*, 0.5 mL

PML **Maternalin**™ **Plus** (Coopers Pitman-Moore)
Injection, combined avian infectious bronchitis and avian infectious bursal

disease vaccine, inactivated, prepared from avian infectious bronchitis virus grown in eggs, and avian bursal disease virus grown on chicken bursal tissue, containing a suitable oil as adjuvant, for *chickens 18-20 weeks of age*; 250 mL
Withdrawal Periods. *Poultry*: slaughter withdrawal period nil
Dose. *Poultry*: *by intramuscular injection*, 0.5 mL

PML **Myxilin**™ (Coopers Pitman-Moore)
Injection, combined avian infectious bronchitis and Newcastle disease vaccine, inactivated, prepared from avian infectious bronchitis virus strain Mass. 41 and Newcastle disease virus Ulster strain, grown in eggs, containing a suitable oil as adjuvant, for *chickens 16-20 weeks of age*; 500 mL
Dose. *Poultry*: *by intramuscular injection*, 0.5 mL

PML **Myxilin**™ **EDS** (Coopers Pitman-Moore)
Injection, combined avian infectious bronchitis, egg drop syndrome 1976, and Newcastle disease vaccine, inactivated, prepared from viruses, containing a suitable oil as adjuvant, for *chickens 16-20 weeks of age*; 500 mL
Withdrawal Periods. *Poultry*: slaughter withdrawal period nil
Dose. *Poultry*: *by intramuscular injection*, 0.5 mL

PML **Newcavac**™ **Nobilis + EDS '76** (Intervet)
Injection, combined egg drop syndrome 1976 and Newcastle disease vaccine, inactivated, prepared from adenovirus strain BC14, Newcastle disease strain Clone 30, containing a suitable oil as adjuvant, for *chickens 14-18 weeks of age*; 1000-dose vial
Dose. *Poultry*: *by subcutaneous or intramuscular injection*, 0.5 mL

PML **Nobi-Vac**™ **IB + G + ND** (Intervet)
Injection, combined avian infectious bronchitis, avian infectious bursal disease, and Newcastle disease vaccine, inactivated, prepared from avian infectious bronchitis virus Mass. strain, avian infectious bursal disease virus immunogenic strain, and Newcastle disease virus strain Clone 30, containing

Table 18.3 Combination vaccines for poultry

	Avian infectious bronchitis	Avian infectious bursal disease	Egg drop syndrome 1976	Erysipelas	Newcastle disease	Pasteurellosis
Ibinac™ ND (Salsbury)	+				+	
Maridin™ (Coopers Pitman-Moore)		+			+	
Maternalin™ Plus (Coopers Pitman-Moore)	+	+				
Myxilin™ (Coopers Pitman-Moore)	+				+	
Myxilin™ EDS (Coopers Pitman-Moore)	+		+		+	
Newcavac™ Nobilis + EDS '76 (Intervet)			+		+	
Nobi-Vac™ IB + G + ND (Intervet)	+	+			+	
Nobi-Vac™ IB + ND + EDS (Intervet)	+		+		+	
Pasteurella-Erysipelas Vaccine (Hoechst)				+		+
Ultravac™ (Coopers Pitman-Moore)	+	+			+	

a suitable oil as adjuvant, for *chickens 14-20 weeks of age*; 1000-dose vial
Dose. *Poultry*: *by subcutaneous or intramuscular injection*, 0.5 mL

PML **Nobi-Vac™ IB + ND + EDS** (Intervet)
Injection, combined avian infectious bronchitis, egg drop syndrome 1976, and Newcastle disease vaccine, inactivated, prepared from avian infectious bronchitis virus Mass. strain, adenovirus strain BC14, Newcastle disease virus strain Clone 30, containing a suitable oil

as adjuvant, for *chickens 14-20 weeks of age*; 1000-dose vial
Dose. *Poultry*: *by subcutaneous or intramuscular injection*, 0.5 mL

PML **Pasteurella-Erysipelas Vaccine** (Hoechst)
Injection, inactivated, prepared from *Ery. rhusiopathiae* strains, *P. multocida* Roberts types 2, 4 of avian origin, containing aluminium hydroxide as adjuvant, for *turkeys*; 250 mL, 500 mL
Dose. *Poults more than 6 weeks of*

age: *by subcutaneous or intramuscular injection*, 0.5 mL, repeat dose after 3-4 weeks
Adults: *by subcutaneous or intramuscular injection*, 1 mL, repeat dose after 3-4 weeks

PML **Ultravac™** (Coopers Pitman-Moore)
Injection, combined avian infectious bronchitis, avian infectious bursal disease, and Newcastle disease vaccine, inactivated, prepared from infectious bursal disease virus grown on chicken bursal tissue, avian infectious bronchitis virus and Newcastle disease virus grown separately in eggs, containing a suitable oil as adjuvant, for *chickens 18-20 weeks of age*; 500 mL
Withdrawal Periods. *Poultry*: slaughter withdrawal period nil
Dose. *Poultry*: *by intramuscular injection*, 0.5 mL

18.7 Immunological preparations for rabbits

18.7.1 Myxomatosis

Myxomatosis infection affects rabbits and hares, although the English hare is not susceptible to the disease. The disease is caused by myxoma virus, which resembles fibroma virus contained in the vaccine. The virus is transmitted from wild rabbits by mosquitoes and rabbit fleas to domestic animals. Myxomatosis may be fatal and prevention by vaccination is practised. Control during an outbreak also includes use of ectoparasiticides (see section 2.2.2).

Indications. Vaccination against myxomatosis
Side-effects. Occasional local reactions at injection site
Dose. *Rabbits*: routine vaccination, 0.5-mL dose of vaccine reconstituted in 5.5 mL of diluent. Revaccinate every 9-12 months
Vaccination during an active outbreak, 0.2-mL dose of vaccine reconstituted in 2.5 mL diluent, see notes above

PoM **Weyvak™** (Mansi)
Injection, powder for reconstitution, myxomatosis vaccine, living, prepared

from fibroma virus, for *rabbits over 2 weeks of age*; 5-mL vial
Note. Vaccine should be discarded 3 hours after reconstitution

18.8 Immunological preparations for fish

18.8.1 Enteric redmouth disease
18.8.2 Furunculosis
18.8.3 Vibriosis
18.8.4 Combination vaccines for fish

Vaccines are available for the control of enteric redmouth disease caused by *Yersinia ruckeri*, vibriosis caused by *Vibrio anguillarum*, and furunculosis caused by *Aeromonas salmonicida* in Atlantic salmon and rainbow trout.
Vaccines are administered to fish by intraperitoneal injection (see Prescribing for fish), by dipping in a vaccine solution, or by passing under a spray of vaccine solution. Fish should be anaesthetised before vaccination by injection (see Prescribing for fish).
An annual revaccination is recommended against redmouth and vibriosis. At water temperatures of 10°C immunity will develop within 14 to 21 days but will take longer at lower temperatures.

18.8.1 Enteric redmouth disease

PML **AquaVac™ ERM** (AVL)
By dip or spray, enteric redmouth vaccine, prepared from *Y. ruckeri* strain Hagerman, for *rainbow trout*; 550 mL, 1 litre
Dose. *Fish*: dilute 1 volume with 9 volumes water.
By dip (fish 1 g body-weight or more), for 30 seconds
By spray, allow 5 seconds exposure to spray delivered at a rate of 750 mL/ minute. Repeat after 14-21 days for fish of less than 1 g body-weight

PML **Ermogen™** (Vetrepharm)
By dip, spray, or injection, enteric redmouth vaccine, inactivated, prepared from *Y. ruckeri* strain YR22, for *rainbow trout*; 1 litre

Dose. *Fish*: dilute 1 volume with 9 volumes water.
By dip, for 30 seconds
By spray, allow 2-5 seconds exposure to spray
Dilute 1 volume with 9 volumes sodium chloride intravenous infusion 0.9%.
By intraperitoneal injection, 0.1 mL to anaesthetised fish

The water temperature of the vaccine solution should not vary more than 2°C to 5°C from the water temperature in the original holding facility

18.8.2 Furunculosis

Furogen™ (Vetrepharm)
PML *By dip*, furunculosis vaccine, inactivated, prepared from *A. salmonicida* strains AS27, AS57, for *Atlantic salmon and rainbow trout 5 g body-weight or more*; 1 litre
Dose. *Fish*: dilute 1 volume with 9 volumes water.
By dip, for 60 seconds
PoM *Injection*, furunculosis vaccine, inactivated, prepared from *A. salmonicida* strain AS27, for *Atlantic salmon 35 g body-weight or more*; 1 litre
Dose. *Fish*: by intraperitoneal injection, 0.1 mL to anaesthetised fish

PML **AquaVac**™   **Furovac-Immersion** (AVL)
By dip, furunculosis vaccine, prepared from *A. salmonicida* strains, for *Atlantic salmon 20 g body-weight or more*; 500 mL, 1 litre
Dose. *Fish*: dilute 1 volume with 9 volumes water.
By dip, for 60 seconds

PoM **AquaVac**™ **Furovac IJ** (AVL)
Injection, furunculosis vaccine, prepared from *A. salmonicida*, containing a suitable adjuvant, for *fish*; 250 mL, 1 litre
Dose. *Fish*: (5-454 g body-weight) *by intraperitoneal injection*, 0.1 mL to anaesthetised fish; (more than 454 g body-weight) *by intraperitoneal injection*, 0.2 mL to anaesthetised fish

See also section 18.8.4

18.8.3 Vibriosis

PML **AquaVac**™ **Vibrio** (AVL)
By dip or spray, vibriosis vaccine, prepared from *V. anguillarum* biotypes I, II, for *rainbow trout*; 550 mL, 1 litre
Dose. *Fish*: dilute 1 volume with 9 volumes water.
By dip, (fish 2 g body-weight or more) 30 seconds
By spray, allow 5 seconds exposure to spray delivered at a rate of 750 mL/ minute. Repeat after 14-21 days for fish of less than 2 g body-weight

See also section 18.8.4

18.8.4 Combination vaccines for fish

PoM **AquaVac**™ **Vibrio-Furovac IJ** (AVL)
Injection, combined furunculosis and vibriosis vaccine, prepared from *A. salmonicida, V. anguillarum* biotypes I, II, containing a suitable adjuvant, for *fish*; 250 mL, 1 litre
Dose. *Fish*: (5-454 g body-weight) *by intraperitoneal injection*, 0.1 mL to anaesthetised fish; (more than 454 g body-weight) *by intraperitoneal injection*, 0.2 mL to anaesthetised fish

Appendix 1: Drug Interactions

In veterinary practice, multiple drug therapy is frequently used. It is important to realise that particular combinations of drugs may interact rather than exert their independent effects. The interaction may result either in a loss of therapeutic activity or an increase in the toxic or side-effects of one or both of the drugs.

Drug interactions *in vivo* may be either pharmacodynamic or pharmacokinetic. A **pharmacodynamic** interaction occurs when one drug has an agonistic or antagonistic action on an effect of the other drug. An interaction may occur when 2 drugs act at the same receptor site or when they act at different receptor sites that both produce similar effects on a tissue. This type of interaction is normally predictable on the basis of the mechanism of drug action and may be expected in all cases of concurrent administration of the 2 drugs. Furthermore, it can be expected to occur with all similar drugs within a particular group. An example of this type of interaction is that between amino-glycoside antibiotics and non-depolarising muscle relaxants, at the neuromuscular junction, leading to an enhanced neuromuscular blockade.

A **pharmacokinetic** interaction occurs when one drug interferes with the absorption, distribution, metabolism, or excretion of another drug. This type of interaction may not be seen in every case of co-administration and may depend on variables such as the state of health or age of the patient and the time interval between administration of the 2 drugs. There may also be differences in susceptibility to such interactions between various species.

Drug interaction at the site of sub-cutaneous, intramuscular, or intravenous injection is rare and the majority of interactions affecting absorption are seen following oral administration. Absorption of drugs from the gastro-intestinal tract will depend on their solubility and degree of ionisation. Factors that affect these parameters may modify the extent of drug absorption. The absorption of tetracyclines from the gastro-intestinal tract can be reduced in the presence of various metal ions, with which they form insoluble chelates.

The absorption of a drug may be dependent on its gastro-intestinal transit time. A drug that increases gastro-intestinal motility may adversely affect the absorption of another drug. This usually leads to lower plasma-drug concentrations being achieved resulting in apparent therapeutic failure. Less frequently, an interaction may occur in which a reduction in gastro-intestinal motility may lead to higher plasma-drug concentrations resulting in toxicity.

Interactions affecting drug distribution are often associated with the action of one drug on the plasma-protein binding of another. Plasma-protein binding sites are non-specific and any drug that binds to plasma proteins is capable of displacing another, thereby increasing the proportion of free drug able to diffuse from plasma to its site of action. However, it is only drugs that exhibit a high degree of protein binding that demonstrate an increase in effect when displaced. This becomes particularly significant if the drug displaced has a low therapeutic index. An example of this type of drug is warfarin, which may be displaced by compounds such as sulphonamides or non-steroidal anti-inflammatory drugs, leading to an enhanced anticoagulant effect and a risk of haemorrhage.

Interactions affecting drug metabolism may occur in the liver. The presence of some drugs in the liver can result in an increase in the liver enzyme concentration after only a few days. Induction of the hepatic microsomal enzyme system by one drug can gradually increase the rate of metabolism of another, resulting in lower plasma-drug concentrations and reduced effect. For example, administration of phenobarbitone may lead to the increased metabolism of drugs including griseofulvin, phenytoin, and hydrocortisone and consequently a reduction in their therapeutic activity.

More rarely, inhibition of liver enzymes may occur. For example, chloramphenicol may increase the effects of barbiturates by inhibiting their breakdown by liver enzymes. This may continue for several weeks after treatment with chloramphenicol has ceased.

Interactions affecting drug excretion may be seen when a drug or an active metabolite is excreted in the urine. Drugs that cause alkalinisation of the urine will facilitate the ionisation of weak acids and increase their excretion and conversely reduce the excretion of weak bases. Drugs that acidify urine will have the opposite effects.

Drugs that render the urine more alkaline include sodium bicarbonate and sodium citrate, while ammonium chloride or ascorbic acid will make the urine more acidic. Examples of drugs that are weak bases include quinine, pethidine, and amphetamine, and weak acids include sulphonamides, salicylates, and phenylbutazone.

Considering the frequent use of multiple drug therapy in veterinary medicine, it is surprising how infrequently drug interactions are reported. This may be because non-fatal interactions are not considered noteworthy, that therapeutic failure is accepted, or that interactions are not considered as a cause of adverse effects. However, if practitioners consider the general pharmacology of the drugs involved when they are using multiple drug therapy then it should be possible to reduce the incidence of drug interactions. Undoubtably, many interactions remain to be discovered and any suspected interaction should be reported to the manufacturer and the Veterinary Medicines Directorate (see General guidance on prescribing).

List of drug interactions

The following is an alphabetical list of drugs and their interactions. To avoid excessive cross-referencing, each drug or group is listed in the alphabetical list and also against the drug or group with which it interacts.

Acepromazine see Phenothiazine derivatives

Acetazolamide
Aspirin: reduced excretion of acetazolamide
Corticosteroids, corticotrophin: increased risk of hypokalaemia
Diuretics: increased risk of hypokalaemia with loop and thiazide diuretics
Quinidine: increased plasma-quinidine concentration reported rarely

Adrenaline see Sympathomimetics

Allopurinol
Cyclophosphamide: enhanced bone-marrow toxicity
Mercaptopurine: enhanced effect of mercaptopurine

Altrenogest see Progestogens

Aluminium hydroxide see Antacids

Ambutonium see Antimuscarinic drugs

Amiloride see Diuretics

Aminoglycosides
Amphotericin: increased risk of nephrotoxicity
Cephalothin and possibly other cephalosporins: increased risk of nephrotoxicity
Cisplatin: increased risk of nephrotoxicity and possibly ototoxicity
Diuretics: increased risk of ototoxicity with loop diuretics
Ether: enhanced neuromuscular blockade
Muscle relaxants: enhanced neuromuscular blockade with non-depolarising muscle relaxants
Methoxyflurane: enhanced neuromuscular blockade; increased risk of nephrotoxicity
Neostigmine: antagonism of interacting drug

Amphotericin
Aminoglycosides: increased risk of nephrotoxicity
Anabolic steroids
Warfarin: enhanced anticoagulant effect
Antacids
Aspirin: large doses of antacids increase aspirin excretion
Chlorpromazine, ketoconazole, penicillamine, tetracyclines: antacids cause reduced absorption of interacting drug
Quinidine: increased plasma-quinidine concentration reported rarely
Anti-arrhythmic drugs
Combinations of 2 or more anti-arrhythmic drugs: enhanced myocardial depression
See also under individual drugs
Anticholinesterase compounds *see* Organophosphorus compounds
See also under individual drugs
Antidiabetic drugs
Beta blockers: enhanced hypoglycaemic effect
Corticosteroids, corticotrophin, progestogens: antagonism of hypoglycaemic effect
Diuretics: antagonism of hypoglycaemic effect with loop and thiazide diuretics
Antiepileptic drugs
Phenothiazine derivatives: antagonism of anticonvulsant effect
See also under individual drugs
Antihistamines
Combination with any other CNS depressant drug: enhanced depressant effects
Antimuscarinic drugs
Ketoconazole: reduced ketoconazole absorption
Metoclopramide: antagonism as interacting drugs have opposing effects on gastro-intestinal motility
Phenothiazine derivatives: reduced plasma-phenothiazine concentration
Apramycin *see* Aminoglycosides
Aspirin
Acetazolamide: reduced excretion of acetazolamide
Antacids: large doses of antacids increase aspirin excretion
Diuretics: antagonism of diuretic effect with spironolactone
Heparin: enhanced anticoagulant effect
Methotrexate: reduced methotrexate excretion

Metoclopramide: increased aspirin absorption
Phenytoin: transient potentiation
Warfarin: increased risk of bleeding due to antiplatelet effect
Atenolol *see* Beta blockers
Atropine *see* Antimuscarinic drugs
Barbiturates
Corticosteroids, corticotrophin: increased risk of potassium loss; increased corticosteroid metabolism
Chloramphenicol, progestogens, theophylline: barbiturates cause reduced plasma concentration of interacting drug
Warfarin: reduced anticoagulant effect
See also under individual drugs *and* Antiepileptic drugs
Bendrofluazide *see* Diuretics
Benzhexol *see* Antimuscarinic drugs
Beta blockers
Antidiabetic drugs: enhanced hypoglycaemic effect
Chlorpromazine: increased plasma-chlorpromazine concentration
Cimetidine: increased plasma-beta blocker concentration
Diuretics: increased risk of ventricular arrhythmias in the presence of hypokalaemia
Lignocaine and similar anti-arrhythmic drugs: increased risk of myocardial depression and bradycardia
Neostigmine: antagonism of interacting drug
Sympathomimetics: enhanced hypertensive effect, especially with non-selective beta blockers
Verapamil: atrioventricular block
Betamethasone *see* Corticosteroids
Boldenone *see* Anabolic steroids
Bromocriptine
Metoclopramide: antagonism of hypoprolactinaemic effect
Bromophos *see* Organophosphorus compounds
Buprenorphine *see* Opioid analgesics
Butorphanol *see* Opioid analgesics
Calcium salts
Cardiac glycosides: large doses of intravenous calcium can precipitate arrhythmias
Diuretics: increased risk of hypercalcaemia with thiazide diuretics
Tetracyclines: reduced absorption of interacting drugs

Captopril
Diuretics: increased risk of hyperkalaemia with potassium-sparing diuretics
Carbaryl
Combinations of 2 or more compounds with anticholinesterase activity such as organophosphorus compounds: enhanced toxicity
Cardiac glycosides
Calcium salts: large doses of intravenous calcium can precipitate arrhythmias
Diuretics: increased toxicity if hypokalaemia occurs; enhanced effect of digoxin with spironolactone
Muscle relaxants: arrhythmias with depolarising muscle relaxants
Phenobarbitone, phenytoin: reduced effect of digitoxin
Quinidine: enhanced effect of digoxin
Cephalothin and possibly other cephalosporins
Aminoglycosides: increased risk of nephrotoxicity
Diuretics: enhanced nephrotoxicity with loop diuretics
Chloramphenicol
Barbiturates: reduced plasma-chloramphenicol concentration
Phenytoin: reduced phenytoin metabolism
Sulphonylureas: enhanced hypoglycaemic effect
Warfarin: enhanced anticoagulant effect
Chlorfenvinphos see Organophosphorus compounds
Chlorpromazine
Antacids: reduced absorption of chlorpromazine
Beta blockers: increased plasma-chlorpromazine concentration
Chlorpropamide see Sulphonylureas *and* Antidiabetic drugs
Chlorpyrifos see Organophosphorus compounds
Cimetidine
Beta blockers, diazepam, fluorouracil, metronidazole, pethidine, propranolol, quinidine, theophylline: cimetidine causes increased plasma concentration of interacting drug
Ketoconazole: reduced ketoconazole absorption
Lignocaine: increased risk of lignocaine toxicity
Phenytoin: reduced phenytoin metabolism
Warfarin: enhanced anticoagulant effect
Cisplatin
Aminoglycosides: increased risk of nephrotoxicity and possibly ototoxicity

CNS depressants
Antihistamines, opioid analgesics, phenothiazine derivatives: enhanced depressant effects
Corticosteroids
Acetazolamide: increased risk of hypokalaemia
Antidiabetic drugs: antagonism of hypoglycaemic effect
Barbiturates, phenytoin: increased risk of potassium loss; increased corticosteroid metabolism
Diuretics: antagonism of diuretic effect; increased risk of hypokalaemia with loop and thiazide diuretics
Metoclopramide: aggression
Co-trimazine see Sulphonamides, potentiated
Co-trimoxazole see Sulphonamides, potentiated
Coumaphos see Organophosphorus compounds
Cyclophosphamide
Allopurinol: enhanced bone-marrow toxicity
Cyclopropane
Sympathomimetics: arrhythmias with adrenaline or isoprenaline
Cythioate see Organophosphorus compounds
Detomidine
Potentiated sulphonamides: increased risk of cardiac arrhythmias
Dexamethasone see Corticosteroids
Diazepam
Cimetidine: increased plasma-diazepam concentration
Phenytoin: reduced phenytoin metabolism
Diazinon see Organophosphorus compounds
Dichlorvos see Organophosphorus compounds
Digitoxin see Cardiac glycosides
Digoxin see Cardiac glycosides
Dihydrostreptomycin see Aminoglycosides
Diuretics
Acetazolamide: increased risk of hypokalaemia with loop and thiazide diuretics
Aminoglycosides: enhanced ototoxicity with loop diuretics
Antidiabetic drugs: antagonism of hypoglycaemic effect with loop and thiazide diuretics
Aspirin: antagonism of diuretic effect of spironolactone

Beta blockers: increased risk of ventricular arrhythmias in the presence of hypokalaemia

Calcium salts: increased risk of hypercalcaemia with thiazide diuretics

Captopril, potassium supplements: increased risk of hyperkalaemia with potassium-sparing diuretics

Cardiac glycosides: increased toxicity if hypokalaemia occurs; enhanced effect of digoxin with spironolactone

Cephalothin and possibly other cephalosporins: increased risk of nephrotoxicity with loop diuretics

Corticosteroids, corticotrophin: antagonism of diuretic effect; increased risk of hypokalaemia with loop and thiazide diuretics

Lignocaine: lignocaine effect antagonised by hypokalaemia with loop and thiazide diuretics

NSAIDs: antagonism of diuretic effect; increased risk of hyperkalaemia with potassium-sparing diuretics

Oestrogens: antagonism of diuretic effect

Quinidine: toxicity of quinidine increased by hypokalaemia with loop and thiazide diuretics

Dobutamine *see* Sympathomimetics

Doxapram

Cyclopropane, enflurane, halothane, isoflurane, methoxyflurane: increased risk of cardiac arrhythmias

Ecothiopate

Muscle relaxants: enhanced neuromuscular blockade with depolarising muscle relaxants

Enflurane

Sympathomimetics: arrhythmias with adrenaline or isoprenaline

Erythromycin

Theophylline: increased plasma-theophylline concentration

Warfarin: enhanced anticoagulant effect

Ether

Aminoglycosides: enhanced neuromuscular blockade

Ethinyloestradiol *see* Oestrogens

Ethyloestrenol *see* Anabolic steroids

Etorphine *see* Opioid analgesics

Fentanyl *see* Opioid analgesics

Flumethasone *see* Corticosteroids

Fluorogestone *see* Progestogens

Fluorouracil

Cimetidine: increased plasma-fluorouracil concentration

Framycetin *see* Aminoglycosides

Frusemide *see* Diuretics

General anaesthetics

Beta blockers, chlorpromazine: enhanced hypotensive effect

Gentamicin *see* Aminoglycosides

Glibenclamide *see* Sulphonylureas *and* Antidiabetic drugs

Glipizide *see* Sulphonylureas *and* Antidiabetic drugs

Glycopyrronium *see* Antimuscarinic drugs

Griseofulvin

Phenobarbitone: increased griseofulvin metabolism

Progestogens: reduced plasma-progestogen concentration

Warfarin: reduced anticoagulant effect

Halothane

Sympathomimetics: arrhythmias with adrenaline or isoprenaline

Haloxon *see* Organophosphorus compounds

Heparin

Aspirin: enhanced anticoagulant effect

Hydrochlorothiazide *see* Diuretics

Hydrocortisone *see* Corticosteroids

Hyoscine *see* Antimuscarinic drugs

Iodofenphos *see* Organophosphorus compounds

Iron salts

Penicillamine: reduced penicillamine absorption

Tetracyclines, zinc salts: reduced absorption of interacting drugs

Isoflurane

Sympathomimetics: arrhythmias with adrenaline or isoprenaline

Isoprenaline *see* Sympathomimetics

Kaolin mixtures

Lincomycin: reduced lincomycin absorption

Ketoconazole

Antacids, antimuscarinic drugs, cimetidine, ranitidine: reduced ketoconazole absorption

Phenytoin: increased plasma-phenytoin concentration; reduced plasma-ketoconazole concentration

Warfarin: enhanced anticoagulant effect

Lignocaine

Beta blockers: increased risk of myocardial depression and bradycardia

Cimetidine: increased risk of lignocaine toxicity

Diuretics: lignocaine effect antagonised by hypokalaemia with loop and thiazide diuretics

Lincomycin

Kaolin mixtures: reduced lincomycin absorption

Muscle relaxants: enhanced neuromuscular blockade with non-depolarising muscle relaxants

Neostigmine: antagonism of interacting drug

Maduramicin

Tiamulin: severe growth retardation

Magnesium salts

Muscle relaxants: enhanced neuromuscular blockade with non-depolarising muscle relaxants

Tetracyclines: reduced absorption of interacting drugs

Malathion *see* Organophosphorus compounds

Medroxyprogesterone *see* Progestogens

Megestrol *see* Progestogens

Mercaptopurine

Allopurinol: enhanced effect of mercaptopurine

Methadone *see* Opioid analgesics

Methohexitone *see* Barbiturates

Methotrexate

Aspirin, phenylbutazone: reduced methotrexate excretion

Phenytoin: enhanced anti-folate effect

Methoxyflurane

Aminoglycosides: enhanced neuromuscular blockade; nephrotoxicity

Sympathomimetics: arrhythmias with adrenaline or isoprenaline

Methylprednisolone *see* Corticosteroids

Metoclopramide

Antimuscarinic drugs, opioid analgesics: antagonism as interacting drugs have opposing effects on gastro-intestinal motility

Aspirin: increased aspirin absorption

Bromocriptine: antagonism of hypoprolactinaemic effect

Corticosteroids, corticotrophin: aggression

Paracetamol: increased paracetamol absorption

Phenothiazine derivatives: increased risk of extrapyramidal effects

Metoprolol *see* Beta blockers

Metronidazole

Cimetidine: increased plasma-metronidazole concentration

Phenobarbitone: increased metabolism of metronidazole

Phenytoin: reduced phenytoin metabolism

Warfarin: enhanced anticoagulant effect

Miconazole

Phenytoin: reduced phenytoin metabolism

Sulphonylureas: enhanced hypoglycaemic effect

Warfarin: enhanced anticoagulant effect

Monensin

Tiamulin: reduced monensin metabolism; severe growth retardation

Morphine *see* Opioid analgesics

Muscle relaxants

Aminoglycosides, lincomycin, magnesium salts, polymyxin B sulphate: enhanced neuromuscular blockade with non-depolarising muscle relaxants

Cardiac glycosides: arrhythmias with depolarising muscle relaxants

Ecothiopate, neostigmine, organophosphorus compounds: enhanced neuromuscular blockade with depolarising muscle relaxants

Quinidine: enhanced neuromuscular blockade

Nadolol *see* Beta blockers

Nalidixic acid

Warfarin: enhanced anticoagulant effect

Nandrolone *see* Anabolic steroids

Narasin

Tiamulin: severe growth retardation

Neomycin

Phenoxymethylpenicillin: reduced penicillin absorption

Warfarin: enhanced anticoagulant effect

Neostigmine

Aminoglycosides, beta blockers, lincomycin, quinidine: antagonism of neostigmine

Muscle relaxants: enhanced neuromuscular blockade with depolarising muscle relaxants

Oestradiol *see* Oestrogens

Oestrogens

Diuretics: antagonism of diuretic effect

Opioid analgesics

Metoclopramide: antagonism as interacting drugs have opposing effects on gastro-intestinal motility

Combination with any other CNS depressant drug: enhanced depressant effects

Organophosphorus compounds

Combinations of 2 or more organophosphorus compounds or compounds with anticholinesterase activity: enhanced toxicity

Muscle relaxants: enhanced neuromuscular blockade with depolarising muscle relaxants

See also under individual drugs

Oxymetholone *see* Anabolic steroids

Paracetamol

Metoclopramide: increased paracetamol absorption

Warfarin: enhanced anticoagulant effect with regular high doses of paracetamol

Penicillamine
Antacids, iron salts, zinc salts: reduced penicillamine absorption

Pentazocine *see* Opioid analgesics

Pethidine
Cimetidine: increased plasma-pethidine concentration
See also under Opioid analgesics

Phenobarbitone, primidone
Cardiac glycosides: reduced effect of digitoxin
Chloramphenicol, metronidazole, progestogens: phenobarbitone (or primidone) causes reduced plasma concentration of interacting drug
Griseofulvin: increased griseofulvin metabolism
Phenytoin, sodium valproate: increased sedation
Warfarin: reduced anticoagulant effect

Phenothiazine derivatives
Antiepileptic drugs: antagonism of anticonvulsant effect
Antimuscarinic drugs: reduced plasma-phenothiazine concentration
Metoclopramide: increased risk of extrapyramidal effects
Combination with any other CNS depressant drug: enhanced depressant effects

Phenoxymethylpenicillin
Neomycin: reduced penicillin absorption

Phenylbutazone
Methotrexate: reduced methotrexate excretion
Phenytoin: reduced phenytoin metabolism
Sulphonylureas: enhanced hypoglycaemic effect
Thyroxine: falsely low total plasma-thyroxine concentration
Warfarin: enhanced anticoagulant effect

Phenylephrine *see* Sympathomimetics

Phenytoin
Aspirin, sodium valproate: transient potentiation
Cardiac glycosides: reduced effect of digitoxin
Chloramphenicol, cimetidine, diazepam, ketoconazole, metronidazole, miconazole, phenylbutazone: reduced phenytoin metabolism
Corticosteroids, corticotrophin: increased potassium loss; increased corticosteroid metabolism

Ketoconazole: increased plasma-phenytoin concentration; reduced plasma-ketoconazole concentration
Methotrexate: increased anti-folate effect
Phenobarbitone, primidone, sodium valproate: increased sedation
Progestogens, theophylline: phenytoin causes reduced plasma concentration of interacting drug
Thyroxine: increased thyroxine metabolism
Warfarin: both enhanced and reduced anticoagulant effects have been reported
See also under Antiepileptic drugs

Phosmet *see* Organophosphorus compounds

Pindolol *see* Beta blockers

Polymyxin B sulphate
Muscle relaxants: enhanced neuromuscular blockade with non-depolarising muscle relaxants

Potassium
Diuretics: increased risk of hyperkalaemia with potassium-sparing diuretics

Potentiated sulphonamides *see* Sulphonamides, potentiated

Prednisolone *see* Corticosteroids

Primidone *see* Phenobarbitone

Prochlorperazine *see* Phenothiazine derivatives

Progesterone *see* Progestogens

Progestogens
Antidiabetic drugs: antagonism of hypoglycaemic effect
Barbiturates, griseofulvin, phenytoin: reduced plasma-progestogen concentration
Theophylline: increased plasma-theophylline concentration
Warfarin: reduced anticoagulant effect

Proligestone *see* Progestogens

Propantheline *see* Antimuscarinic drugs

Propoxur
Combinations of 2 or more compounds with anticholinesterase activity such as organophosphorus compounds: enhanced toxicity

Propranolol
Cimetidine: increased plasma-propranolol concentration

Quinidine
Acetazolamide, antacids: increased plasma-quinidine concentration reported rarely
Cardiac glycosides: enhanced effect of digoxin
Cimetidine: increased plasma-quinidine concentrations

Diuretics: toxicity increased by hypokalaemia with loop and thiazide diuretics

Muscle relaxants: enhanced neuromuscular blockade

Neostigmine: antagonism of neostigmine

Warfarin: enhanced anticoagulant effect

Ranitidine

Ketoconazole: reduced ketoconazole absorption

Salinomycin

Tiamulin: severe growth retardation

Sodium valproate

Phenobarbitone, phenytoin, primidone: increased sedation

See also under Antiepileptic drugs

Spectinomycin *see* Aminoglycosides

Spironolactone *see* Diuretics

Stilboestrol *see* Oestrogens

Streptomycin *see* Aminoglycosides

Sulphonamides

Thiopentone sodium: enhanced effect of thiopentone

Warfarin: enhanced anticoagulant effect

Sulphonamides, potentiated

Detomidine: increased risk of cardiac arrhythmias

Sulphonylureas

Chloramphenicol, miconazole, phenylbutazone: enhanced hypoglycaemic effect

See also under Antidiabetic drugs

Suxamethonium *see* Muscle relaxants

Sympathomimetics

Beta blockers: enhanced hypertensive effect, especially with non-selective beta blockers

Cyclopropane, enflurane, halothane, isoflurane, methoxyflurane: arrhythmias with adrenaline or isoprenaline

Tetracyclines

Antacids, dairy products: reduced tetracycline absorption (doxycycline is not affected by dairy products)

Calcium salts, iron salts, magnesium salts, zinc salts: reduced absorption of interacting drugs

Warfarin: enhanced anticoagulant effect

Theophylline

Barbiturates, phenytoin: reduced plasma-theophylline concentration

Cimetidine, erythromycin, progestogens: increased plasma-theophylline concentration

Thiopentone

Sulphonamides: enhanced effect of thiopentone

See also under Barbiturates

Thyroxine

Phenylbutazone: falsely low total plasma-thyroxine concentration

Phenytoin: increased thyroxine metabolism

Warfarin: enhanced anticoagulant effect

Tiamulin

Maduramicin, narasin, salinomycin: severe growth retardation

Monensin: reduced monensin metabolism; severe growth retardation

Timolol *see* Beta blockers

Tolbutamide *see* Sulphonylureas *and* Antidiabetic drugs

Trenbolone *see* Anabolic steroids

Triamcinolone *see* Corticosteroids

Triamterene *see* Diuretics

Trimeprazine *see* Phenothiazine derivatives

Trimethoprim *see* Sulphonamides, potentiated

Tubocurarine *see* Muscle relaxants

Verapamil

Beta blockers: atrioventricular block

Vitamin K

Warfarin: reduced anticoagulant effect

Warfarin

Aspirin: increased risk of bleeding due to antiplatelet effect

Barbiturates, griseofulvin, progestogens, phenobarbitone, vitamin K: reduced anticoagulant effect

Anabolic steroids, chloramphenicol, cimetidine, erythromycin, ketoconazole, metronidazole, miconazole, nalidixic acid, neomycin, paracetamol (regular treatment with high doses), quinidine, sulphonamides, tetracyclines, thyroxine, aspirin, phenylbutazone, and possibly other NSAIDs: enhanced anticoagulant effect

Phenytoin: both enhanced and reduced anticoagulant effects reported

Zinc salts

Iron salts, tetracyclines: reduced absorption of interacting drugs

Penicillamine: reduced penicillamine absorption

Appendix 2: Drug Incompatibilities

Drugs intended for parenteral administration may interact *in vitro* due to physical or chemical incompatibility. This may result in loss of potency, increase in toxicity, or other adverse effects. The solution may become opalescent or precipitation may occur, but in many instances there may be no visual indication of incompatibility. Precipitation reactions are numerous and varied and may occur as a result of pH changes, concentration changes, 'salting-out' of insoluble anion-cation salts, complexation, or other chemical changes.

In general, drugs should only be added to infusion containers when constant plasma concentrations are needed or when the administration of a more concentrated drug solution would be harmful.

Drugs should not be mixed in infusion containers or syringes unless the components are of known compatibility. In general, drugs should not be added to blood, mannitol, or sodium bicarbonate solutions. Information on drug incompatibilities is given below. The suitability of additions may also be checked by reference to manufacturer's literature. Where drug solutions are added together they should be thoroughly mixed by shaking and checked for absence of particulate matter before use. A strict aseptic procedure should be adopted in order to prevent accidental entry and subsequent growth of micro-organisms in the infusion container or syringe. Ready prepared solutions should be used whenever possible.

List of drug incompatibilities

The following is an alphabetical list of drugs and their incompatibilities with other drugs and common intravenous infusion fluids. To avoid excessive cross-referencing, those drugs that should not be mixed with any other drugs are only listed once. Therefore, when checking a potential incompatibility, it may be necessary to refer to the entries for each of the drugs involved.

Acepromazine maleate Atropine sulphate, phenylbutazone sodium

Adrenaline Potassium chloride, sodium bicarbonate intravenous infusion, and other solutions with pH > 5.5

Aminoglycosides Heparin sodium, hydrocortisone sodium succinate, noradrenaline acid tartrate

Ampicillin (and other semi-synthetic penicillins) Dextran solutions, glucose intravenous infusion
Should not be mixed with other drugs

Atropine sulphate Acepromazine maleate, chlorpromazine hydrochloride, heparin sodium

Barbiturates Should not be mixed with other drugs

Benzylpenicillin sodium Glucose intravenous solutions†
Should not be mixed with other drugs

Calcium gluconate (and possibly other calcium-containing solutions) Menbutone, methylprednisolone sodium succinate, prednisolone sodium phosphate, promethazine hydrochloride, sodium bicarbonate intravenous infusion, streptomycin sulphate, tetracyclines
Drugs in the form of carbonate, phosphate, or sulphate salts

Carbenicillin   Gentamicin sulphate

Cephalosporins   Gentamicin sulphate, tetracyclines

Chloramphenicol sodium succinate   Chlorpromazine hydrochloride, erythromycin, gentamicin sulphate, heparin sodium, hydrocortisone sodium succinate, penicillins, tetracyclines, vitamins B & C

Chlorpromazine hydrochloride   Atropine sulphate, chloramphenicol sodium succinate, hydrocortisone sodium succinate, phenylbutazone sodium, tetracyclines, vitamins B & C

Cloxacillin sodium   Glucose intravenous solutions > 5%

Compound sodium lactate intravenous infusion   Methylprednisolone sodium succinate, sodium bicarbonate intravenous infusion

Dextran solutions   Ampicillin, oxytocin

Diazepam   Should not be mixed with other intravenous fluids or drugs

Electrolyte solutions   Sulphadiazine sodium, sulphisoxazole diolamine

Erythromycin   Chloramphenicol sodium succinate

Gentamicin sulphate   Carbenicillin and other penicillins, cephalosporins, chloramphenicol sodium succinate, heparin sodium, any solution in which the concentration of gentamicin exceeds 1 g/litre

Glucose intravenous infusion   Ampicillin, benzylpenicillin sodium, cloxacillin sodium, heparin sodium, sulphadiazine sodium, tetracyclines

Heparin sodium   Aminoglycosides, atropine sulphate, benzylpenicillin sodium, chloramphenicol sodium succinate, gentamicin sulphate, glucose intravenous infusions†, hydrocortisone sodium succinate, pethidine hydrochloride, promethazine hydrochloride, streptomycin sulphate, tetracyclines, tylosin

Hydrocortisone sodium succinate   Aminoglycosides, chloramphenicol sodium succinate, chlorpromazine hydrochloride, heparin sodium, noradrenaline acid tartrate, promethazine hydrochloride, tetracyclines, tylosin

Lincomycin   Penicillins

Magnesium sulphate   Sodium bicarbonate intravenous infusion, tetracyclines

Menbutone   Calcium salts, procaine penicillin, vitamin B complex

Methylprednisolone sodium succinate   Benzylpenicillin sodium, calcium gluconate, compound sodium lactate intravenous infusion, pethidine hydrochloride, tetracyclines, thiopentone sodium, vitamins B & C

Noradrenaline acid tartrate   Aminoglycosides, hydrocortisone sodium succinate, sodium bicarbonate intravenous infusion, sodium chloride intravenous infusion 0.9%

Oxytocin   Dextran solutions

Penicillins   Chloramphenicol sodium succinate, gentamicin sulphate, lincomycin, tetracyclines

Pethidine hydrochloride   Heparin sodium, methylprednisolone sodium succinate, sodium bicarbonate intravenous infusion

Phenylbutazone sodium   Acepromazine maleate, chlorpromazine hydrochloride

Polysulphated glycosaminoglycan   Should not be mixed with other drugs

Potassium chloride   Adrenaline, sulphadiazine sodium

Prednisolone sodium phosphate   Calcium gluconate, promethazine hydrochloride

Procaine penicillin   Menbutone

Promethazine hydrochloride   Should not be mixed with other drugs

Ringer's solution   Sodium bicarbonate intravenous infusion

Sodium bicarbonate intravenous infusion   Adrenaline, compound sodium lactate intravenous infusion, magnesium sulphate, noradrenaline acid tartrate, pethidine hydrochloride, Ringer's Solution, streptomycin sulphate, tetracyclines, vitamins B & C, calcium-containing solutions

Sodium chloride intravenous infusion 0.9%   Noradrenaline acid tartrate

Streptomycin sulphate   Calcium gluconate, heparin sodium, sodium bicarbonate intravenous infusion, tylosin

Sulphadiazine sodium   Electrolyte solutions, glucose 10% intravenous infusion, potassium chloride

Sulphisoxazole diolamine   Electrolyte solutions

Sulphonamides   Should not be mixed with other drugs

Suxamethonium chloride Thiopentone or other alkaline solutions

Tetracyclines Calcium gluconate, cephalosporins, chloramphenicol sodium succinate, chlorpromazine hydrochloride, glucose intravenous infusion†, heparin sodium, hydrocortisone sodium succinate, magnesium sulphate, methylprednisolone sodium succinate, penicillins, sodium bicarbonate intravenous infusion, tylosin, any solution with high sodium, calcium, or magnesium content

Thiopentone sodium Methylprednisolone sodium succinate, suxamethonium chloride

Tylosin Heparin sodium, hydrocortisone sodium succinate, streptomycin sulphate, tetracyclines

Vitamin B complex Should not be mixed with other drugs

Vitamins B & C Chloramphenicol sodium succinate, chlorpromazine hydrochloride, methylprednisolone sodium succinate, sodium bicarbonate intravenous infusion

† **Caution**: conflicting literature

Appendix 3: Conversions and Units

Mass

kg	lb
1.0	2.2
2.0	4.4
3.0	6.6
4.0	8.8
5.0	11.0
6.0	13.2
6.35	14.0 (1 stone)
10.0	22.05
20.0	44.1
50.0	110.23
50.8	112.0 (1 hundredweight, 1 cwt)
100.0	220.46
200.0	440.9
500.0	1102.3
1000.0	2204.6
1016.0	2240.0 (1 ton)

1 tonne	= 1000 kilograms (kg)
1 kilogram (kg)	= 1000 grams (g)
1 gram (g)	= 1000 milligrams (mg)
1 milligram (mg)	= 1000 micrograms (μg)
1 microgram (μg)	= 1000 nanograms (ng)
1 nanogram (ng)	= 1000 picograms (pg)

Volume

mL	fl oz
50	1.8
100	3.5
150	5.3
200	7.0
500	17.6
568	20.0 (1 pint)
1000	35.2

litres	gallons
1.0	0.22
4.55	1.0
10.0	2.2
100.0	22.0
1000.0	220.0

1 litre	= 1000 millilitres (mL)
1 millilitre (mL)	= 1000 microlitres (μL)

Temperature

°C	°F
0	32
10	50
25	77
35	95
36	96.8
37	98.6
38	100.4
39	102.2
40	104.0
41	105.8
42	107.6
43	109.4
44	111.2
45	113.0

Other conversions and units

1 kilocalorie (kcal)	=	4186.8 joules (J)
1 gallon of water	=	10 pounds
	=	4.55 kg
1 gallon	=	0.16 cu. feet
1 inch (in)	=	25.4 mm
1 foot (ft)	=	0.305 metre (305 mm)
1 yard (yd)	=	0.914 metre (914 mm)
1 metre (m)	=	39.37 in
	=	3.28 ft
	=	1.09 yd

Moles, millimoles, and milliequivalents

A **mole** (mol) is the amount of substance that contains as many entities (atoms, molecules, ions, electrons, or other particles or specified groups of particles) as there are atoms in 0.012 kg of carbon-12. A **millimole** (mmol) is one thousandth of this amount and for ions is the ionic mass (the sum of the relative atomic masses of the elements of an ion) expressed in milligrams. A **milliequivalent** is this quantity divided by the valency of the ion. Non-ionic compounds such as dextrose cannot be expressed in terms of milliequivalents.

Thus one mole of NaCl (molecular weight 58.45) weighs 58.45 g, and 58.45 mg of NaCl contains one millimole. This amount of NaCl contains 23.0 mg of Na^+ (1 mmol of Na^+) and 35.45 mg of Cl^- (1 mmol of Cl^-).

Tonicity

When two solutions, each containing the same number of solute particles are separated by a *perfect* semipermeable membrane, they are stated to be **iso-osmotic**, that is they are in osmotic equilibrium. There is no net movement across the membrane. However, in biological systems semipermeable membranes permit the passage of some solute particles. When two solutions, separated by such a membrane, are in osmotic equilibrium they are said to be **isotonic** with respect to that membrane. Solutions administered parenterally or applied to mucous surfaces should be isotonic if used in large volume. For small volumes, such as eye drops, nasal drops, or subcutaneous injections, isotonicity is desirable but not essential.

Index of Manufacturers and Organisations

This index comprises a list of manufacturers of preparations included in the veterinary formulary and organisations associated with veterinary practice.

A B Pharmaceuticals
A B Pharmaceuticals Ltd,
The Red House, Ashendon,
Aylesbury, Bucks HP18 0HE.
Aylesbury (0296) 658833

A&H
Allen & Hanburys Ltd,
Horsenden House, Oldfield Lane
North, Greenford, Middx UB6 0HB.
081-422 4225

Abbott
Abbott Laboratories Ltd,
Abbott House, Moorbridge Rd,
Maidenhead, Berks SL6 8JG.
Maidenhead (0628) 773355

Agricultural and Veterinary
Pharmacists Group
Royal Pharmaceutical Society of Great
Britain,
1 Lambeth High St, London SE1 7JN.
071-735 9141

Agrimin
Agrimin Ltd,
379 Victoria St, Grimsby, South
Humberside DN31 1PX.
Grimsby (0472) 44766

Alcon
Alcon Laboratories (UK) Ltd,
Imperial Way, Watford, Herts
WD2 4YR.
Watford (0923) 246133

Aldrich
Aldrich Chemical Co Ltd,
The Old Brickyard, New Rd,
Gillingham, Dorset SP8 4JL.
Gillingham (0747) 822211

Alfa Laval
Alfa Laval Agri Ltd,
Cwmbran, Gwent NP44 7XE.
Cwmbran (0633) 838071

Allergan
Allergan Ltd,
Coronation Rd, High Wycombe,
Bucks HP12 3SH.
High Wycombe (0494) 444722

Animal Health Trust
Animal Health Trust,
PO Box 5, Newmarket, Suffolk
CB8 7DW.
Newmarket (0638) 661111

Animalcare
Animalcare Ltd,
Common Rd, Dunnington, York
YO1 5RU.
York (0904) 488661

Animax
Contact **Bayer** (Agrochem)

Antec
Antec International Ltd,
Chilton Industrial Estate, Sudbury,
Suffolk CO10 6XD.
Sudbury (0787) 77305

Aqua Health
Contact **Vetrepharm**

Aqua Med
Aqua Med Ltd,
14 Boxhill Way, Strood Green,
Betchworth, Surrey RH3 7HY.
Betchworth (073 784) 2921

Arnolds
Arnolds Veterinary Products Ltd,
Cartmel Drive, Harlescott,
Shrewsbury SY1 3TB.
Shrewsbury (0743) 231632

Astra
Astra Pharmaceuticals Ltd,
Home Park Estate, Kings Langley,
Herts WD4 8DH.
Watford (0923) 266191

AVL
Aquaculture Vaccines Ltd,
24-26 Gold St, Saffron Walden, Essex
CB10 1EJ.
Saffron Walden (0799) 28167

Babson
Babson Bros Co. (UK),
5 Aragon Court, Tudor Rd, Manor
Park, Runcorn, Cheshire WA7 1SR.
Runcorn (0928) 719971

BASF
BASF plc,
PO Box 4, Earl Road, Cheadle
Hulme, Cheadle, Cheshire SK8 6QG.
061-488 5314

Battle Hayward & Bower
Battle Hayward and Bower Ltd,
Crofton Drive, Allenby Rd Industrial
Estate, Lincoln, Lincs LN3 4NP.
Lincoln (0522) 529206

Bayer
Bayer UK Ltd,
Agrochem Business Group, Eastern
Way, Bury St Edmunds, Suffolk
IP32 7AH.
Bury St Edmunds (0284) 763200
For information on human medicines
contact
Pharmaceutical Business Group,
Bayer House, Strawberry Hill,
Newbury, Berks RG13 1JA.
Newbury (0635) 39000

BDH
BDH Ltd,
Broom Rd, Poole,
Dorset BH12 4NN.
Poole (0202) 745520

BCL
British Cod Liver Oils Ltd,
Contact **Seven Seas**

Beecham
Contact **SmithKline Beecham**
For information on human medicines,
same address

Bimeda
Bimeda UK Ltd,
Unit F, Gores Rd, Knowsley
Industrial Park, Liverpool L33 7XS.
051-547 3711

Bioglan
Bioglan Laboratories Ltd,
1 The Cam Centre, Wilbury Way,
Hitchin, Herts SG4 0TW.
Hitchin (0462) 38444
For information on human medicines,
same address

BK
BK Veterinary Products Ltd,
Minster House, Western Way, Bury St
Edmunds, Suffolk IP33 3SU.
Bury St Edmunds (0284) 761131

Boehringer Ingelheim
Boehringer Ingelheim Vetmedica Ltd,
Ellesfield Avenue, Bracknell, Berks
RG12 4YS.
Bracknell (0344) 424600
For information on human medicines,
same address

Boots
The Boots Co. plc,
1 Thane Rd West, Nottingham
NG2 3AA.
Nottingham (0602) 506255

BP(Vet)
Contact British Pharmacopoeia
Commission, Market Towers, 1 Nine
Elms Lane, London SW8 5NQ.
071-720 9844

Bridge
Contact **SmithKline Beecham**

Bristol-Myers
Bristol-Myers Pharmaceuticals,
Swakeleys House, Milton Rd,
Ickenham, Uxbridge, Middx
UB10 8NS.
081-572 7422

British Equine Veterinary Association
Hartham Park, Corsham, Wilts
SN13 0QB.
Corsham (0249) 715723

British Horse Society
British Equestrian Centre, Stoneleigh,
Kenilworth, Warwick CV8 2LR.
Coventry (0203) 696697

**British Small Animal Veterinary
Association**
Kingsley House, Church Lane,
Shurdington, Cheltenham, Glos
GL51 5TQ.
Cheltenham (0242) 862994

British Veterinary Association
7 Mansfield St, London W1M 0AT.
071-636 6541

Calmic
Contact **Wellcome**

Cambridge VS
Cambridge Veterinary Services Ltd,
Henry Crabb Rd, Littleport, Ely,
Cambs CB6 1SE.
Ely (0353) 861911

Charwell
Charwell Pharmaceuticals Ltd,
Charwell House, Wilsom Rd, Alton,
Hants GU34 2TJ.
Alton (0420) 84801

Cheminex
Cheminex Laboratories Ltd,
7 Godwin Rd, Earlstrees Industrial
Estate, Corby, Northants NN17 2DS.
Corby (0536) 65444

Ciba
Contact **Ciba-Geigy**

Ciba-Geigy
Ciba-Geigy Agrochemicals,
Whittlesford, Cambridge CB2 4QT.
Cambridge (0223) 833621
For information on human medicines
contact Ciba Laboratories,
Wimblehurst Rd, Horsham, West
Sussex RH12 4AB.
Horsham (0403) 50101

Colborn-Dawes
Colborn-Dawes Nutrition Ltd,
Heanor Gate, Heanor, Derbyshire
DE7 7SG.
Langley Mill (0773) 530300

Connan & Wise
Connan & Wise,
Monkfield Game Farm, Bourn,
Cambs, CB3 7TD.
Caxton (09544) 298

Coopers Pitman-Moore
Coopers Pitman-Moore,
Crewe Hall, Crewe, Cheshire
CW1 1UB.
Crewe (0270) 580131

CooperVision
CooperVision Optics Ltd,
Permalens House, 1 Botley Rd, Hedge
End, Southampton SO3 3HB.
Botley (04892) 5155

Cowie
W H Cowie Ltd,
26A Dene St, Dorking, Surrey
RH4 2BZ.
Dorking (0306) 887074

Cox-Surgical
Alfred Cox (Surgical) Ltd,
Edward Rd, Coulsdon, Surrey
CR5 2XA.
081-668 2131

Creg
Creg Petfoods,
3 Bromwich Avenue, Highgate,
London N6 6QH.
081-340 2926

Crown
Crown Veterinary Pharmaceuticals
Ltd,
Minster House, Western Way, Bury St
Edmunds, Suffolk IP33 3SU.
Bury St Edmunds (0284) 61131

CP
CP Pharmaceuticals Ltd,
Red Willow Rd, Wrexham Industrial
Estate, Wrexham, Clwyd LL13 9PX.
Wrexham (0978) 661261
Also Medical Dept,
Loughborough (0509) 611001

C-Vet
C-Vet Ltd,
Minster House, Western Way, Bury St
Edmunds, Suffolk IP33 3SU.
Bury St Edmunds (0284) 761131

Cyanamid
Cyanamid UK, Animal Health
Division,
Cyanamid House, Fareham Rd,
Gosport, Hants PO13 0AS.
Fareham (0329) 224000
For information on human medicines
contact **Lederle** (same telephone
number)

Dalgety
Dalgety Agriculture Ltd,
180 Aztec West, Almondsbury, Bristol
BS12 4TH.
Bristol (0454) 201511

Dallas Keith
Dallas Keith Ltd,
Bromag Industrial Estate, Burford Rd,
Witney, Oxon OX8 5SR.
Witney (0993) 773061

Day Son & Hewitt
Day Son & Hewitt Ltd,
St George's Quay, Lancaster
LA1 5QJ.
Lancaster (0524) 381821

Degussa
Degussa Pharmaceuticals Ltd,
168 Cowley Rd, Cambridge CB4 4DL.
Cambridge (0223) 423434

Deosan
Deosan Ltd,
Weston Favell Centre, Northampton
NN3 4PD.
Northampton (0604) 414000

**Department of Agriculture for
Northern Ireland**
Dundonald House, Belfast BT4 3SF.
Belfast (0232) 650111

DF
Duncan, Flockhart & Co. Ltd,
700 Oldfield Lane North, Greenford,
Middx UB6 0HE.
081-422 2331

Dispersa
Dispersa (United Kingdom) Ltd,
Lockwood Fold, Buxton Rd,
Heaviley, Stockport, Cheshire
SK2 6LS.
061-474 1526

Dista
Dista Products Ltd,
Kingsclere Rd, Basingstoke, Hants
RG21 2XA.
Basingstoke (0256) 52011

Duck Producers Association
High Holborn House, 52-54 High
Holborn, London WC1 6SX.
071-242 4683

Dumex
Dumex Ltd,
Longwick Rd, Princes Risborough,
Aylesbury, Bucks HP17 9UZ.
Princes Risborough (0844) 274414

Du Pont
Du Pont (UK) Ltd,
Wedgwood Way, Stevenage, Herts
SG1 4QN.
Stevenage (0438) 734549

Duphar
Duphar Veterinary Ltd,
Solvay House, Flanders Rd, Hedge
End, Southampton SO3 4QH.
Botley (0489) 781711
For information on human medicine
contact
Duphar Laboratories Ltd, Gaters Hill,
West End, Southampton SO3 3JD
Southampton (0703) 472281

Ecolab
Ecolab Ltd,
799 Western Rd, Slough, Berks
SL1 4HR
Slough (0753) 22599

Efamol
Efamol Vet,
Woodbridge Meadows, Guildford,
Surrey GU1 1BA.
Guildford (0483) 578060

Elanco
Elanco Products Ltd,
Dextra Court, Chapel Hill,
Basingstoke, Hants RG21 2SY.
Basingstoke (0256) 53131

Equine Products
Equine Products (UK) Ltd,
22-23 Riversdale Court,
Newburnhaugh Industrial Estate,
Newcastle-upon-Tyne NE15 8SG.
091-264 5536

Evans
Evans Medical Ltd,
Longhurst, Horsham,
Sussex RH12 4QD.
Horsham (0403) 41400

Evans Vanodine
Evans Vanodine International Ltd,
Brierley Rd, Walton Summit Centre,
Bamber Bridge, Preston, Lancs
PR5 8AH.
Preston (0772) 322200

Farillon
Farillon Ltd,
Ashton Rd, Romford, Essex
RM3 8UE.
Ingrebourne (04023) 71136

Farmitalia Carlo Erba
Farmitalia Carlo Erba Ltd,
Italia House, 23 Grosvenor Rd, St
Albans, Herts AL1 3AW.
St Albans (0727) 40041

FEI
Fédération Equestre Internationale,
Bolligenstrasse 54, Boîte Postale CH-
3000, Berne 32, Switzerland

Ferring
Ferring Pharmaceuticals Ltd,
11 Mount Rd, Feltham, Middx
TW13 6JG.
081-898 8396

Fisons
Fisons Animal Health, Fisons plc,
Pharmaceutical Division,
12 Derby Rd, Loughborough, Leics
LE11 0BB.
Loughborough (0509) 611001
For information on human medicines,
same address

Geigy Contact **Ciba-Geigy**

Glaxo
Glaxo Laboratories Ltd,
Greenford Rd, Greenford, Middx
UB6 0HE.
081-422 3434

Glenwood
Glenwood Laboratories Ltd,
Jenkins Dale, Chatham, Kent
ME4 5RD.
Chatham (0634) 830535

Goat Nutrition
Goat Nutrition Ltd,
Tenterden Rd, Biddenden, Ashford,
Kent TN27 8BL.
Biddenden (0580) 291545

Gold Cross
Gold Cross Pharmaceuticals,
PO Box 53, Lane End Rd, High
Wycombe, Bucks HP12 4HL.
High Wycombe (0494) 21124

Hand/PH
Peter Hand Animal Health Ltd,
15-19 Church Rd, Stanmore, Middx
HA7 4AR.
081-954 7422

Harkers
Harkers Ltd,
Minster House, Western Way, Bury St
Edmunds, Suffolk IP33 3SU.
Bury St Edmunds (0284) 761131

Hill's
Hill's Pet Products Ltd,
Sherwood House, 33-35 Wellfield Rd,
Hatfield, Herts AL10 0BS.
Hatfield (07072) 76660

Hoechst
Hoechst Animal Health, Division of
Hoechst UK Ltd,
Walton Manor, Walton, Milton
Keynes, Bucks MK7 7AJ.
Milton Keynes (0908) 665050
For information on human medicines
contact
Pharmaceutical Division, Hoechst
House, Salisbury Rd, Hounslow,
Middx TW4 6JH.
081-570 7712

Hurlingham Polo Association, The
Winterlake, Kirtlington, Oxon
OX5 3HG.
Kirtlington (0869) 50044

IDIS
IDIS Ltd,
51 High St, Kingston-upon-Thames,
Surrey KT1 1LQ.
081-549 1355

IMS
International Medication Systems
(UK) Ltd,
11 Royal Oak Way South, Daventry,
Northants NN11 5PJ.
Daventry (0327) 703231

IndChemNI
Industrial Chemical NI Ltd,
42 John St Lane, Newtownards,
County Down, Northern Ireland
BT23 4LY.
Newtownards (0247) 812727

Intervet
Intervet UK Ltd,
Science Park, Milton Rd, Cambridge
CB4 4FP.
Cambridge (0223) 420221

Invicta
Contact **Pfizer**

Ivex
Ivex Pharmaceuticals,
Old Belfast Rd, Millbrook, Larne, N.
Ireland BT40 2SH.
Larne (0574) 73631

Janssen
Janssen Animal Health, Janssen
Pharmaceutical Ltd,
Grove, Wantage, Oxon OX12 0DQ.
Wantage (0235) 772966
For information on human medicines,
same address

Jockey Club, The
42 Portman Square, London
W1H 0EN.
071-486 4921

Kalium
Kalium Products Ltd,
West Court, Morton Bagot, Studley,
Warwick B80 7EL.
Studley (0527) 857870

Kennel Club, The
1-5 Clarges St, Piccadilly, London
W1Y 8AB.
071-493 6651

Kilco
Kilco Dairyfarm Chemicals Ltd,
33 Breck Road, Wallasey, Merseyside
L44 3BB.
051-638 0076

Kirby-Warrick
Contact **Schering-Plough**

Knoll
Knoll Ltd,
Fleming House, 71 King St,
Maidenhead, Berks SL6 1DU.
Maidenhead (0628) 776360

LAB
Laboratories for Applied Biology Ltd,
91 Amhurst Park, London N16 5DR.
081-800 2252
For information on human medicines,
same address

Lagap
Lagap Pharmaceuticals Ltd,
37 Woolmer Way, Bordon, Hants
GU35 9QE.
Bordon (0420) 478301

Lakenlabs
Lakenlabs Ltd,
67 Lakenheath, London N14 4RR.
081-886 1371

Lederle
Lederle Laboratories,
Fareham Rd, Gosport, Hants
PO13 0AS.
Fareham (0329) 224000
For information on veterinary
medicines contact **Cyanamid** (same
telephone number)

Leo
Leo Laboratories Ltd,
Longwick Rd, Princes Risborough,
Aylesbury, Bucks HP17 9RR.
Princes Risborough (08444) 7333
For information on human medicines,
same address

Lever
Lever Industrial Ltd,
PO Box 100, Runcorn, Cheshire
WA7 3JZ.
Runcorn (0928) 719000

Lilly
Eli Lilly & Co Ltd,
Kingsclere Rd, Basingstoke, Hants
RG21 2SY.
Basingstoke (0256) 473241
For information on veterinary
medicines contact **Elanco**

Loveridge
J M Loveridge plc,
Southbrook Rd, Southampton
SO9 3LT.
Southampton (0703) 228411
For information on human medicines,
same address

Lundbeck
Lundbeck Ltd,
Lundbeck House, Hastings St, Luton
LU1 5BE.
Luton (0582) 416565

M&B
(May and Baker)
Contact **Rhône Poulenc** for
information on human medicines,
contact **RMB** for information on
veterinary medicines

MAFF
Ministry of Agriculture, Fisheries and
Food,
Whitehall Place, London SW1 2HH.
071-270 8080

Mansi
Mansi Laboratories Ltd,
Herons Way, Wey Rd, Weybridge,
Surrey KT13 8HS.
Weybridge (0932) 845354

Martindale
Martindale Pharmaceuticals Ltd,
Chesham House, Chesham Close,
Romford, Essex RM1 4JX.
Romford (0708) 746033

Meat and Livestock Commission
PO Box 44, Winterhill House,
Snowdon Drive, Milton Keynes
MK6 1AX.
Milton Keynes (0908) 677577

Micro-Biologicals
Micro-Biologicals Ltd,
Salisbury St, Fordingbridge, Hants
SP6 1AE.
Fordingbridge (0425) 652205

Milk Marketing Board
Head office, Thames Ditton.
081-398 4101

Mill Feed
The Mill Feed Company Ltd,
Stow Park, Lincoln LN1 2AN.
Lincoln (0427) 788554

Millpledge
Millpledge Ltd,
Whinleys Estate, Church Lane,
Clarborough, Retford, Notts
DN22 9NA.
Retford (0777) 708440

**Ministry of Agriculture Fisheries and
Food**
See **MAFF**

MMB
See **Milk Marketing Board**

MSD
Merck Sharp & Dohme Ltd
Address and telephone no. as for
MSD Agvet

MSD Agvet
MSD Agvet, Division of Merck Sharp
& Dohme Ltd,
Hertford Rd, Hoddesdon, Herts
EN11 9BU.
Hoddesdon (0992) 467272

Mycofarm
Mycofarm UK Ltd,
Science Park, Milton Rd, Cambridge
CB4 4FP.
Cambridge (0223) 423971

National Greyhound Racing Club
24-28 Oval Rd, London NW1 7DA.
071-267 9256

Nicholas
Nicholas Laboratories Ltd,
225 Bath Rd, Slough SL1 4AU.
Slough (0753) 23971

NOAH
National Office of Animal Health Ltd,
3 Crossfield Chambers, Gladbeck
Way, Enfield, Middx EN2 7HF.
081-357 3131

Norbrook
Norbrook Laboratories (GB) Ltd,
Bridge House, Severn Bridge,
Bewdley, Worcs DY12 1AB.
Bewdley (0299) 400939

Nordisk
Contact **Novo Nordisk**

Norton
H N Norton & Co. Ltd,
Gentec House, Gothic Centre, Angel
Rd, Edmonton, London N18 3AH.
081-807 9999

Novo Nordisk
Novo Nordisk Pharmaceutical Ltd,
Novo Nordisk House, Broadfield
Park, Brighton Rd, Pease Pottage,
Crawley, West Sussex RH11 9RT.
Crawley (0293) 613555

Organon
Organon Laboratories Ltd,
Cambridge Science Park, Milton Rd,
Cambridge CB4 4FL.
Cambridge (0223) 423445

Organon-Teknika
Address as for **Organon**
Cambridge (0223) 423650

Paines & Byrne
Paines & Byrne Ltd,
Pabyrn Laboratories, 177 Bilton Rd,
Perivale, Greenford, Middx
UB6 7HG.
081-997 1143
For information on human medicines,
same address

Pan Britannica
Pan Britannica Industries Ltd,
Britannica House, High St, Waltham
Cross, Herts EN8 7DY.
Waltham Cross (0992) 23691

Panpharma
Panpharma Ltd,
Hayes Gate House, 27 Uxbridge Rd,
Hayes, Middx UB4 0JN.
081-561 8774

Parke-Davis
Parke-Davis Veterinary, Usk Rd,
Pontypool, Gwent NP4 0YH.
Pontypool (0495) 762468
For information on human medicines
contact
Parke-Davis Medical,
Lambert Court, Chestnut Ave,
Eastleigh, Hants SO5 3ZQ.
Eastleigh (0703) 620500

PDSA
See **People's Dispensary for Sick
Animals**

Pedigree
Pedigree Petfoods,
Breeder and Veterinary Services,
Waltham-on-the-Wolds, Melton
Mowbray, Leics LE14 4RS.
Melton Mowbray (0664) 410000

Penn
Penn Pharmaceuticals Ltd,
Buckingham House, Church Rd,
Penn, High Wycombe, Bucks
HP10 8LN.
Penn (049481) 3340

People's Dispensary for Sick Animals
PDSA House, South St, Dorking,
Surrey RH4 2LB.
Dorking (0306) 888291

Pet Health Council
4 Bedford Square, London
WC1B 3RA.
071-255 2424

Pettifer
Thomas Pettifer & Co. Ltd,
72-76 River Rd, Barking, Essex
IG11 0DY.
081-594 4074

Pfizer
Pfizer Ltd,
Ramsgate Rd, Sandwich, Kent
CT13 9NJ.
Sandwich (0304) 616161
For information on human medicines,
same address

Pharmax
Pharmax Ltd,
Bourne Rd, Bexley, Kent DA5 1NX.
Dartford (0322) 91321

Porton
Porton Products Ltd,
Porton House, Vanwall Rd,
Maidenhead, Berks SL6 4UB.
Maidenhead (0628) 771417

Radiol
Contact **Fisons**

Reckitt & Colman
Reckitt & Colman, Pharmaceutical
Division,
Dansom Lane, Hull HU8 7DS.
Hull (0482) 26151

Rhône-Poulenc
Rhône-Poulenc Pharmaceuticals,
Rhône-Poulenc Ltd,
Rainham Rd South, Dagenham, Essex
RM10 7XS.
081-592 3060
For information on veterinary
medicines contact **RMB** (same
address)

Rhône-Poulenc AN
Rhône-Poulenc Chemicals Ltd,
271 High St, Uxbridge, Middx
UB8 1LQ.
Uxbridge (0895) 74080

Ritchey Tagg
Ritchey Tagg Ltd,
Masham, Nr. Ripon, North Yorkshire
HG4 4ES.
Ripon (0765) 89541

RMB
RMB Animal Health Ltd,
Rainham Rd South, Dagenham, Essex
RM10 7XS.
081-593 7634
For information on human medicines
contact **Rhône-Poulenc**, same address

Roche
Roche Products Ltd,
PO Box 8, Welwyn Garden City,
Herts AL7 3AY.
Welwyn Garden (0707) 328128
For information on human medicines,
same address

Rorer
Rorer Pharmaceuticals,
St Leonards House, St Leonards Rd,
Eastbourne, East Sussex BN21 3YG.
Eastbourne (0323) 21422

Rosen
66 Bathgate Rd, Wimbledon, London
SW19 5PH.
081-946 9575

Roussel
Roussel Laboratories Ltd,
Broadwater Park, North Orbital Rd,
Uxbridge, Middx UB9 5HP.
Uxbridge (0895) 834343

**Royal College of Veterinary Surgeons,
The**
32 Belgrave Square, London
SW1X 8QP.
071-235 4971

**Royal Society for the Prevention of
Cruelty to Animals**
Causeway, Horsham, West Sussex
RH12 1HG.
Horsham (0403) 64181

Rumenco
Rumenco Ltd,
Stretton House, Derby Rd, Stretton,
Burton-on-Trent, Staffs DE13 0DW.
Burton-on-Trent (0283) 511211

Rybar
Rybar Laboratories Ltd,
30 Sycamore Rd, Amersham, Bucks
HP6 5DR.
Amersham (0494) 722741

Salsbury
Salsbury Laboratories Ltd,
Solvay House, Flanders Rd, Hedge
End, Southampton SO3 4QH.
Botley (0489) 781711

S&N Pharm.
Smith & Nephew Pharmaceuticals Ltd,
Bampton Rd, Harold Hill, Romford,
Essex RM3 8SL.
Ingrebourne (04023) 49333

Sandoz
Sandoz Pharmaceuticals,
Frimley Business Park, Frimley,
Camberley, Surrey GU16 5SG.
Camberley (0276) 692255

Sanofi
Sanofi Animal Health Ltd,
PO Box 209, Rhodes Way, Watford,
Herts WD2 4QE.
Watford (0923) 35022
For information on human medicines
contact
Sanofi Pharma,
Floats Rd, Wythenshawe, Manchester
M23 9NF.
061-945 4161

ScanVet
ScanVet UK Ltd,
Stanstead House, The Avenue,
Newmarket, Suffolk CB8 9AA.
Newmarket (0638) 67751

Schering-Plough
Schering-Plough Animal Health,
Mildenhall, Bury St. Edmunds,
Suffolk IP28 7AX.
Mildenhall (0638) 716321
For information on human medicines,
same address

Seven Seas
Seven Seas Ltd, Veterinary Division,
Hedon Rd, Marfleet, Hull HU9 5NJ.
Hull (0482) 75234

Shep-Fair
Shep-Fair Products Ltd,
Trefecca Fawr, Trefecca, Brecon,
Powys LD3 0PW.
Brecon (0874) 711673

Sinclair
Sinclair Pharmaceuticals Ltd,
Borough Rd, Godalming, Surrey
GU7 2AB.
Guildford (0483) 426644

SK&F
Contact **SmithKline Beecham**

Smith & Nephew
See **S&N Pharm.**

SmithKline Beecham
SmithKline Beecham Animal Health
Ltd,
Hunters Chase, Walton Oaks,
Dorking Rd, Tadworth, Surrey
KT20 7NT.
Tadworth (0737) 364700
For information on human medicine
contact
SmithKline Beecham plc,
Mundells, Welwyn Garden City, Herts
AL7 1EY.
Welwyn Garden (0707) 325111

Sorex
Sorex Ltd,
St Michaels Industrial Estate, Widnes,
Cheshire WA8 8TJ.
051-420 7151

Spencer
Brian G Spencer Ltd,
Common Lane, Fradley, Lichfield,
Staffs WS13 8LA.
Lichfield (0543) 262882

Spodefell
Spodefell Ltd,
5 Inverness Mews, London W2 3QJ.
071-229 9125

Squibb
E R Squibb & Sons Ltd,
Squibb House, 141 Staines Rd,
Hounslow, Middx TW3 3JA.
081-572 7422

Stafford-Miller
Stafford-Miller Ltd,
Broadwater Rd, Welwyn Garden City,
Herts AL7 3SP.
Welwyn Garden (0707) 331001
For information on human medicines,
same address

Sterling Research
Contact **Sterling-Winthrop**

Sterling-Winthrop
Sterling-Winthrop Group Ltd,
Sterling-Winthrop House, Onslow St,
Guildford, Surrey GU1 4YS.
Guildford (0483) 505515

Syntex
Syntex Animal Health, Syntex
Pharmaceuticals Ltd,
Syntex House, St Ives Rd,
Maidenhead, Berks SL6 1RD.
Maidenhead (0628) 33191
For information on human medicine,
same address

Synthite
Synthite Ltd,
Ryders Green Rd, West Bromwich,
West Midlands B70 0AX.
021-557 2245

Thomson and Joseph
Thomson and Joseph Ltd,
Thomson and Joseph House, 119
Plumstead Rd, Norwich NR1 4JT.
Norwich (0603) 39511

Thornton & Ross
Thornton & Ross Ltd,
Linthwaite Laboratories, Huddersfield
HD7 5QH.
Huddersfield (0484) 842217

Torbet
Torbet Laboratories,
Boughton Lane, Maidstone, Kent
ME25 9QQ.
Maidstone (0860) 319350

Trident
Trident Pharmaceuticals Ltd,
137 Malling St, Lewes, Sussex
BN7 2RB.
Lewes (0273) 480665

Trilanco
Trilanco,
Bracewell Ave Industrial Estate,
Poulton-le-Fylde, Nr Blackpool, Lancs
FY6 8JF.
Blackpool (0253) 891697

UFAW
Universities Federation for Animal
Welfare,
8 Hamilton Close, South Mimms,
Potters Bar, Herts EN6 3QD.
Potters Bar (0707) 58202

UKASTA
United Kingdom Agricultural Supply
Trade Association Ltd,
3 Whitehall Court, London
SW1A 2EQ.
071-930 3611

Unifeeds
Unifeeds International Ltd,
BOCM Silcock House, Basing View,
Basingstoke, Hants RG21 2EQ.
Basingstoke (0256) 29211

Univet
Univet Ltd,
Wedgwood Rd, Bicester, Oxon
OX6 7UL.
Bicester (0869) 241287

Upjohn
Upjohn Ltd, Animal Health Division,
Fleming Way, Crawley, West Sussex
RH10 2NJ.
Crawley (0293) 31133
For information on human medicine,
same address

Vetbed
Vetbed (Animal Care) Ltd,
Lotherton Way, Garforth, Leeds
LS25 2JY.
Leeds (0532) 870723

Vetchem
Contact **Spencer**

Veterinary Medicines Directorate
Woodham Lane, New Haw,
Weybridge, Surrey KT15 3NB.
Weybridge (0932) 336911

Vetrepharm
Vetrepharm Ltd,
Unit 15, Sandleheath Industrial
Estate, Fordingbridge, Hants
SP6 1PA.
Fordingbridge (0425) 656081

Vetsearch
Vetsearch International Pty Ltd,
PO Box 2405, North Parramatta,
NSW 2151, Australia.
Products distributed in UK by
Millpledge

Virbac
Virbac Ltd,
Cape House, 60a Priory Rd,
Tonbridge, Kent TN9 2BL.
Tonbridge (0732) 360055

VMD
See **Veterinary Medicines Directorate**

Volac
Volac Ltd,
Fishers Lane, Orwell, Royston, Herts
SG8 5QX.
Cambridge (0223) 208201

Wafcol
Wafcol Ltd,
The Nutrition Bakery, Haigh Ave,
Stockport, Cheshire SK4 1NU.
061-480 2781

Webster
Webster Animal Health (UK),
Jaykay House, 39-43 High Rd,
Ickenham, Middx UK10 8LF.
Ickenham (0895) 622322

Wellcome
Wellcome Medical Division, The
Wellcome Foundation Ltd,
Crewe Hall, Crewe, Cheshire
CW1 1UB.
Crewe (0270) 583151

Willows Francis
Willows Francis Ltd, 3 Charlwood
Court, County Oak Way, Crawley,
West Sussex RH11 7XA.
Crawley (0293) 614141

Winthrop
Contact **Sterling-Winthrop**

Wyeth
Wyeth Laboratories,
Huntercombe Lane South, Taplow,
Maidenhead, Berks SL6 0PH.
Burnham (06286) 4377

Young's
Young's Animal Health Ltd,
Elliot St, Glasgow G3 8JT.
041-204 1301

Index

Where an entry is followed by more than one page reference, the principal reference is printed in **bold** type. Proprietary (trade) names are printed in *italic* type.